Fundamentals of

COMPLEMENTARY AND ALTERNATIVE MEDICINE

Fundamentals of

COMPLEMENTARY AND ALTERNATIVE MEDICINE

Edited by

MARC S. MICOZZI, MD, PhD

Executive Director
The College of Physicians of Philadelphia
Adjunct Professor of Medicine and of Rehabilitation Medicine
University of Pennsylvania
Philadelphia, Pennsylvania

with foreword by C. EVERETT KOOP, MD, ScD

SECOND EDITION
with 26 black-and-white and 22 color illustrations

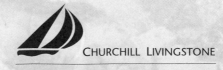

CHURCHILL LIVINGSTONE

A Harcourt Health Sciences Company
New York Edinburgh London Philadelphia

CHURCHILL LIVINGSTONE
A Harcourt Health Sciences Company

The Curtis Center
Independence Square West
Philadelphia, Pennsylvania 19106

Editor in Chief: John A. Schrefer
Editor: Kellie F. White
Associate Developmental Editor: Jennifer L. Watrous
Project Manager: John Rogers
Senior Production Editor: Mary Turner
Design: Renée Duenow

FUNDAMENTALS OF COMPLEMENTARY AND ALTERNATIVE MEDICINE   ISBN 0-443-06576-4

Printed in the United States of America.

Last digit is the print number: 9   8   7   6   5   4   3   2   1   GW/MVY

Contributors

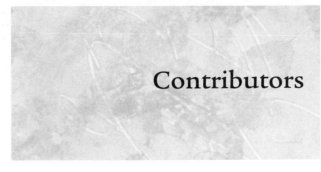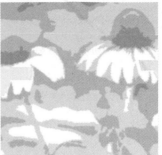

PATCH ADAMS, MD
Gesundheit Institute
Arlington, Virginia

GERARD C. BODEKER, EdD
Chair, GIFTS of Health
Green College
University of Oxford
Oxford, United Kingdom

CLAIRE MONOD CASSIDY, PhD
President, Paradigms Found Consulting
Bethesda, Maryland

PATRICK COUGHLIN, PhD
Department of Anatomy
Philadelphia College of Osteopathic Medicine
Philadelphia, Pennsylvania

ELLIOTT DACHER
Institute of Noetic Sciences
Sausalito, California

VICTOR DOUVILLE (Sicangu-Lakota)
Recognized Expert in Lakota Studies
Sinte Gleska University
Lakota Studies Department
Mission, South Dakota

KEVIN V. ERGIL, MA, MS, LAc
Director, School of Oriental Medicine
Associate Professor, Division of Health Sciences
Touro College
New York, New York

HOWARD HALL, PhD
Rainbow Babies and Childrens Hospital
Cleveland, Ohio

MARIANA HEWSON, PhD
Division of Education
The Cleveland Clinic Foundation
Cleveland, Ohio

WENDY L. HURWITZ, MD
Private Practice
Orange, Connecticut
Member, Medical, Scientific, and Academic Council
International Society for the Study of Subtle Energies
    and Energy Medicine

JENNIFER JACOBS, MD, MPH
Clinical Assistant Professor
Department of Epidemiology
University of Washington School of Public Health and
    Community Medicine
Seattle, Washington

TED J. KAPTCHUK, OMD
Associate Director, Center for Alternative Medicine
    Research
Beth Israel Hospital
Boston, Massachusetts

RICHARD A. LIPPIN, MD
President, The Lippin Group
Founder, International Arts-Medicine Association
Philadelphia, Pennsylvania

LISA MESEROLE, MS, RD, ND
Naturopathic Physician
One Sky Medicine
Seattle, Washington

MARC S. MICOZZI, MD, PhD
Executive Director
The College of Physicians of Philadelphia
Adjunct Professor of Medicine and of Rehabilitation
    Medicine
University of Pennsylvania
Philadelphia, Pennsylvania

DANIEL E. MOERMAN, PhD
Professor, Behavioral Sciences Department
University of Michigan
Dearborn, Michigan

RICHARD MOSKOWITZ, MD
Instructor, Homeopathy
National Center for Homeopathy
Alexandria, Virginia

JOSEPH E. PIZZORNO, Jr., ND
President Emeritus
Bastyr University of Natural Health Sciences
Kenmore, Washington

DENISE RODGERS
Association for the Development of Mind Body
    Potential
Tulsa, Oklahoma

HARI M. SHARMA, MD
Professor Emeritus
Former Director, Division of Cancer Prevention and
    Natural Products Research
Department of Pathology
The Ohio State University College of Medicine
Columbus, Ohio

VICTOR S. SIERPINA, MD
Assistant Professor, Clinic Medical Director
Department of Family Medicine
University of Texas Medical Branch
Galveston, Texas

PAMELA SNIDER, ND
Associate Dean, Naturopathic Medicine
Bastyr University of Natural Health Sciences
Kenmore, Washington

CAROLINE J. STEVENSEN, PhD
Macmillan Specialist and Lecturer in Complementary
    Therapies
Academic Unit
Royal London Homeopathic Hospital
London, England

GEORGIA TETLOW
University of North Carolina at Chapel Hill
Department of Medicine
Chapel Hill, North Carolina

ROBERT T. TROTTER II, PhD
Department of Anthropology
Northern Arizona University
Flagstaff, Arizona

GAYLA TWISS, MPH (Sicangu-Lakota)
Health Systems Administrator, Rosebud PHS
    Indian Hospital
Rosebud, South Dakota

CHRISTINE VLAHOS, MSPT
Englewood Hospital Medical Center
Englewood, New Jersey

RICHARD W. VOSS, DPC, MSW
Assistant Professor
Department of Social Work
West Chester University
West Chester, Pennsylvania

ALAN D. WATKINS, MD
University Medicine
Southampton General Hospital
Southampton, United Kingdom

KENNETH G. ZYSK, PhD
University of Copenhagen
Department of Asian Studies
Copenhagen, Denmark

To my teachers at the University of Pennsylvania
who instructed me in both the art and science of medicine,
and who maintain the traditions on which American medicine was founded
and upon which the future of American medicine will be built.

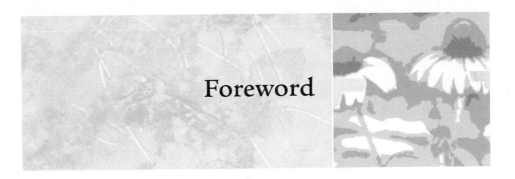

Foreword

THE ART AND SCIENCE OF MEDICINE

For more than 40 years I have tried to identify the mix of personal attributes and technical skills that make one an outstanding doctor. I am sure that most physicians in the United States have pondered the same question. Now, through the work of the C. Everett Koop Institute at Dartmouth I have an opportunity to influence the way medical students are trained. The Institute, working in partnership with the Dartmouth Medical School and the Dartmouth-Hitchcock Medical Center, is actively engaged in training physicians for the next century.

Because doctors must remain abreast of a growing volume of new information, our medical schools help both their graduates and society by producing physicians who are computer literate and comfortable with telemedicine. As a scientific pursuit, medicine should take advantage of the technologic innovations that allow us to better serve the lifetime learning needs of physicians as well as the health education needs of patients. Nonetheless, because medicine is also an art, doctors still need to listen to their patients. This aspect of medical practice has not changed.

As I travel across the country many of the people I meet are eager to share their ideas for improving the nation's health care system. The most common complaint I hear focusses on poor communication in the doctor-patient relationship. Too many patients feel that their physician does not really listen to them.

When the patient attempts to explain his or her problem, the doctor interrupts. Subsequently, when the doctor tries to explain what conditions the patient has and attempts to outline a treatment regimen, the patient is confused because the physician does not communicate to the level of the patient's understanding.

From my perspective, medical students need to master the art of listening to and communicating with their patients just as much as they need to learn the fundamentals of human biology. We have found at the Koop Institute that a student's communication skills are greatly improved by having to explain the first principles of health promotion and disease prevention to second graders. Medical students who choose to participate in programs sponsored by the Koop Institute work in and with local communities from their very first year. Some choose to advise junior high and high school students on the risks associated with alcohol, tobacco, and sexually transmitted diseases; others help rural physicians take better advantage of the computer revolution.

Just as a physician should be sensitive to the feelings of a patient and the needs of the community, he or she must be conversant with major trends and developments in society. I would like to tell you about one current trend that is of interest to me. Studies conducted at Harvard Medical School and reported in the *New England Journal of Medicine* focussed on attitudes toward complementary and alternative medicine in the United States. They indicate that one third of adult Americans regularly use some kind of complementary or alternative treatment even though it was not covered by insurance and they had to pay for it themselves. This is an opportune time for us to take a second look at such alternative treatment approaches as acupuncture, botanical medicine, homeopathy, and others; not to offer these treatment modalities blindly but to expose them to the scientific method. Physicians have to depend on facts—on empirical data—when they determine treatment strategy for a particular patient. Today we do not have enough data on the potential of alternative approaches to help or harm human health. It is time to discover the value of these treatment regimens. We can conduct the necessary studies and assemble the data that doctors and health policy makers need; a type of biomedical research that would be a prudent long-term investment.

In my lifetime we have achieved great successes in the fight against infectious diseases. We have more work to do in our effort to improve the quality of life and make people more comfortable as they endure chronic health problems such as cancer, heart disease, and arthritis. Drugs and surgery can be useful tools in the effort to treat these diseases, but when possible I would like to see us increase the range of approaches that can be used. My experience as a doctor has taught me that often a mix of different approaches is necessary to achieve success. We need to be flexible and adaptable because the diseases that challenge us certainly are not static.

A recent trend that concerns me is the growth of drug resistant bacteria. Today it is easy to forget that prior to the development of antibiotics in the 1940s a child's ear infection could be a frightening and fatal experience. I well remember patients with serious complications and death caused by the lack of antibiotics. If drugs we have depended on for decades are compromised, we may return to a time when even routine infections could be dangerous. As both a grandfather and a physician, I would hate to see that happen.

There is an element of good news in this picture. If some of the synthetic drugs we have developed are no longer as dependable as they once were, studies have shown that the botanical substances these drugs are based on are still effective in treating disease. I have never claimed to be an expert on botany or ecol-

ogy, but current trends suggest that we need to do more. We need to conserve the plants that may contain the medicines of the future and more importantly we need to learn what local experts seem to understand about the pharmacologic properties and uses of these medicines.

Reduced health care costs is an important by-product of the work we are doing at the Koop Institute. Our students know that the physician of the future must be a health educator first and foremost. Today, the challenge is to treat the patient once he or she has gone to the hospital. Tomorrow, the challenge will be to keep the patient out of the hospital in the beginning.

Preventive medicine means education, empowerment, and personal responsibility. Many patients want alternatives to invasive medical procedures and long stays in the hospital. Physicians can conserve time and resources by teaching patients how to reduce their risk of cancer, heart disease, and other life-threatening diseases. As our students know, the most inexpensive treatment is to keep the patient from becoming sick in the first place. Demand reduction in the health care system is the most immediate cost saving effort.

I think that alternative/complementary therapies may potentially be an important part of this overall educational process. One must have an open mind about complementary therapies and understand belief systems that emphasize the mind-body connection. At a time when many Americans complain of stress, make poor nutritional choices, and are increasingly concerned about environmentally induced illnesses these messages could hardly be more timely.

Many people are confused about alternative medicine, and I do not blame them. For many Americans alternative therapies represent a *new* discovery, but in truth, many of these traditions are hundreds or thousands of years old and have been used by millions of people worldwide. To ease the uncomfortableness of the word *alternative* one must realize that while treatments may look like alternatives to us, they have long been part of the medical mainstream in their cultures of origin.

When I worked in Washington as Surgeon General for eight years, President Reagan had an important credo in his approach to foreign policy: "Trust but verify!" So it is with complementary and alternative medicine. So many people have relied on these approaches for so long that they may have something of value to offer. Let us begin the necessary research so that we could have substantive answers in the near future.

One reason such research is worth doing is that eighty percent of the world's people depend on these alternative approaches as their primary medical care. For years, we have attempted to export Western medicine to the developing world. The sad truth is that the people we are attempting to help simply cannot afford it. I have doubts about how much longer we can afford some of it ourselves. It is possible that in this new millenium, we may be more ready to ask the peoples of the developing world to share their wisdom with us.

During the nineteenth century, American medicine was an eclectic pursuit where a number of competing ideas and approaches thrived. Doctors were able to draw on elements from different traditions in attempting to make people well. Perhaps there is more to this older model of American medicine than we in the twentieth century had been willing to examine. My experience with physicians has convinced me that they are healers first. As such, they are willing to use any ethical approach or treatment that has been proven to work. However, in the opinion of many doctors, there is not yet a definitive answer on the value of complementary and alternative medicine. I would like us to undertake the study and research that will provide definitive answers to prudent questions about the usefulness of complementary and alternative medicine for society at large.

C. EVERETT KOOP, MD, ScD
Former Surgeon General of the United States
Senior Scholar, The Koop Institute at Dartmouth,
Hanover, New Hampshire

Preface to Second Edition

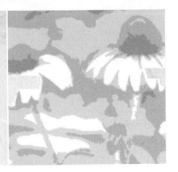

A NEW ECOLOGY OF HEALTH: A COMMON SENSE GUIDE TO COMPLEMENTARY AND ALTERNATIVE MEDICINE

The history of both medicine and physical science over the last 100 years has been the history of relentlessly breaking material reality into smaller and smaller parts.

In the effort to reduce reality to the smallest components physics encountered a point at which it is impossible to observe matter without influencing the reality of what one is trying to observe. It also became clear that all matter also has an energetic nature—and that the further one looks the more the matter-energy duality becomes impossible to separate.

We have also begun to perceive that not all physical phenomena may be explained by reducing matter to its smallest constituent parts and explanations at this end point become increasingly elusive.

THE NATURE OF MEDICINE

The central idea in medicine over the past 100 years, propagated as part of general science, is that health can also be broken down into its smallest component parts and studying the parts can be made relevant to the experience of the health of the whole. In its "reduced" state modern medicine has focused on cells, genes, and molecules—an understanding of which is central to the modern practice of biomedical science. While much of science is necessarily beginning to move beyond basing all understanding of reality on reductionist studies, modern Western medicine remains rooted in this central idea.

In the meantime contemporary studies in biology and ecology increasingly demonstrate that the behavior of biological systems, whether at the level of the whole organism, the whole community or population, or the whole planet, is not predicated, predicted, or perceivable on the basis of the isolated parts—but can be observed and understood only as phenomena at the level of the whole. Likewise, "health" is not a property that can be ascribed to or experienced by cells or molecules but only at the level of the whole person in the context of his or her physical and social environment.

Science has also attempted to produce laws to explain and predict observable behavior. The most obvious and successful examples have been in the physical sciences. In the biological sciences we have found scientific laws alone to be often insufficient in the interpretation of the natural reality that surrounds us. For in nature it has become clear that what we observe is based not only on scientific law but also on the history of everything that has ever happened before in nature. As stated by the natural scientist Stephen Jay Gould, "biology is a science with a history," and in this way biological phenomena can be made sense of only by a reading of the history of nature—a truly natural history. If one thinks of life on earth as part of a continuum connected to all other forms of life at every point in time and through time, it is not possible to think of human life or health as separate from nature. Certainly, the celebrated gene provides the mechanism by which life is linked to nature through individuals and communities through time, but it does not provide a new central idea in biomedical science.

Similarly, modern biomedicine is a science with a history and the modern practice of medicine and medical science is as influenced by social history as it is by scientific laws. The central idea of modern medicine has been to master the minutiae while missing the whole—and it is the whole that people are missing most in modern medicine. In the laudable effort to make medicine scientific, we have emphasized that knowledge about the world, including nature and human nature, must be pursued by the following criteria: (1) *objectivism*—the observer is separate from the observed, (2) *reductionism*—complex phenomena are explainable in terms of simpler, component phenomena, (3) *positivism*—all that can be known is derivable from physically measurable data, (4) *determinism*—phenomena can be predicted from a knowledge of scientific law and initial conditions. This is not the only way of knowing things, but it has become the modern test to determine whether such knowledge is "scientific" (see Chapter 1).

In fact, science requires only empiricism—making and testing models of reality by what can be observed, guided by certain values and based on certain metaphysical assumptions. Science itself is not reality but a system of human knowledge like any other human knowledge system. Often we cannot tell the difference between metaphysical reality and the scientific model that has been constructed through human intellectual activity to describe it. In this way new thoughts about the nature of medicine do not represent a "new science" so much as a new philosophy.

In the fundamental science of physics we already know that objectivism is ultimately not possible at the fundamental level because of the Heisenberg uncertainty principle—the act of observing phenomena necessarily influences the behavior of the observed. Modern biological and ecological science has produced a wealth of observations about how living organisms and communities interact with each other and their environment in transactional, multidirectional, and synergic ways that are ultimately not subject to reductionist explanations. For positivism and determinism to provide a complete explanation we must assume that science has all the physical and intellectual tools to ask the right questions, and knows the right questions to ask. However, the tools we have and the questions we ask are based on the history of science itself as part of the history of human intellectual enquiry.

Nature and Human Nature

The self-conscious experience of humans in their natural and social environments is a common and ancient topic of human enquiry. Virtually every human society around the world through time has had ways of describing and understanding the experience of the human condition—a broad and general way of describing "health." Without modern biomedical science, the ancients and the elders of human society came to understand the experience of the human condition at the level of the experience itself. And all human experience has a material nature and an energetic nature. The ancients and elders did not know that mind is separate from the body and did not know that experience could be reduced to cells and molecules, so their explanations were based on whole phenomena. The ancients and elders also did not know about the new physics, but they knew that the human body and living things have energy, as well as matter, whereas we now know that fundamental particles have a material nature and a wave (energy) nature. And despite the fact that the ancients and elders of human society did not always have sophisticated technology (although the appropriateness of many of their technologies is amazingly sophisticated) their central idea of medicine, their philosophy of health, was perhaps more sophisticated than ours has become.

Ancient and indigenous medical systems think of the human body as having energy, the balance of which is critical for health and the flow of which can be manipulated to maintain and restore health. In this way medicine is not about the putting of things into the body but using outer resources to help mobilize the inner resources of the body. The body heals itself and maintains its own health.

Modern Western medicine works on the material aspects of the body: sending in drug molecules to affect cell receptors, cutting out parts that do not work, replacing parts that fail. But the body is not a machine. Although these mechanistic approaches have clearly had great success in fixing problems, they do not always provide the best approaches to maintaining health.

Modern Western medicine knows that body has its own energy. We know the body can heal itself. Practitioners know that the "placebo" effect is real. They know that the "laying on of hands" can heal. But these things have not been in the realm of science for modern biomedicine, and even though we know they exist, they have not been studied until now. And although we know the body has energy, we have not until now used energy to heal. We measure the energy of the heart (ECG), and muscle (EMG) to help address the material aspects of the body. We know now that bones can heal by using energy. However, this has not changed the central idea of modern medicine.

Alternative Medicine Means Medical Choices

What today is called *complementary* and *alternative medicine* in the United States and Europe covers a broad range of health and medical systems often derived from ancient and indigenous societies and variously called in recent years unconventional, nontraditional, integral, holistic, and wholistic. Most have in common the idea that the body has energy, as well as material, reality. So what is really an old idea has become a new idea consistent with the frontiers of physics but not yet the frontier of modern medicine, which still operates with 100-year-old central ideas. Although alternatives are very diverse in terms of cosmology in the *causes* of disease, they generally share an idea about the cures of disease—that the body can heal itself (as modern medicine knows) and that healing comes only from the inner resources of the body, which can be mobilized by external manipulation.

When focusing on the energetic aspects of the body, the emphasis is on the flow of energy and the balance of energy, implying a dynamic interaction that is different from the static grasp of matter. Much of our modern knowledge of medicine comes from the historically important idea more than 100 years ago that diseases of the whole organism can be understood at the cell level and that observations at the cell level are directly related to diagnosis, prognosis, and therapy of the patient. Great advances have come from this approach to the material aspects of disease. When studying the dynamic energy of life processes, however, we may have reached our limits in what can be understood through the study of dead tissue cells. Many neuroscientists now believe that we will further advance our fundamental understanding of the brain only when we "remap" what we know about the brain from studying dead brain cells to studying living brain tissue.

Many believe that a new central idea, a new philosophy, is needed for medicine to maintain its relevance to a broadened definition of health. Today there are many approaches through different models and medical philosophies. It is not so much that there are many alternatives to modern Western (allopathic) medicine, but that allopathic medicine is one of many alternatives. How can we make sense of so many different modalities of health and healing? It makes sense only if we realize that the final common pathway for the way that all medical systems work is by their ability to influence the body to heal itself, to mobilize inner resources, and to address the energetic, as well as material, aspects of a living human organism.

Alternative medicine means having choices that people want and are willing to pay for. Americans are not primarily interested in propagating any particular model of medical practice or science. People want what works. Increasingly, medical practitioners who know and respect the power of the placebo effect, the laying on of hands, and other "nonscientific" medicine also are on a search for what works for their patients and what works for their own personal perceptions as healers.

Healing is not solely about a given medical system or tradition. It is about the human body, human biology, and human physiology—how the body works and how it heals. Formulary approaches to alternative medicine (e.g., acupuncture, herbalism, homeopathy) taken out of the complete context of their traditional practices still are observed to work because they draw on the body's biology in the same ways. These formulary approaches provide evidence that empirical traditions of alternative medicine have discovered certain truths about human physiology and encoded them into their medical practice and/or cultural knowledge systems.

Nonetheless, no medicine works as well if the patient (and practitioner) does not believe it. And any medicine works better if patient and practitioners share a belief in its efficacy. As stated in the foreword by Dr. C. Everett Koop, the health care practitioner operates within and between the realms of the art and the science of medicine. Integration of complementary and alternative therapies into medical practice affords the opportunity to expand our knowledge and utilization of both.

MARC S. MICOZZI, MD, PhD

Preface to First Edition

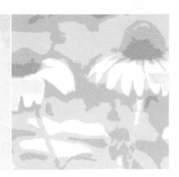

*F*undamentals of Complementary and Alternative Medicine provides the reader with a basis of knowledge about systems of medical thought and practice referred to today in the United States as complementary and alternative medicine. The book's approach is to present medical, health, and science students and practitioners, as well as other interested individuals, with the intellectual foundations and tools to understand and make sense of these various fields that demonstrate great diversity and yet can be unified around certain themes. To provide a useful introduction to these topics, the book is carefully organized with subjects presented in the order in which they should be read for a progressive, comprehensive overview and understanding of the material.

Alternative and complementary medicine, natural medicine, and the use of natural products represent a classic consumer movement and a current social phenomenon of significant dimensions. Students, practitioners, patients, and consumers need a common language for understanding this movement. Physicians and patients are becoming increasingly involved in *alternatives* driven by the perceived need for health care reform, the desire to move toward a wellness orientation in medical practice, and an intellectual interest and curiosity about the ability of what well-established ancient and historic medical systems continue to offer us today.

In sum, this book presents the contemporary complementary and alternative medical approaches that come from observations within, around, and beyond the current Western, biomedical paradigm. The approaches discussed expand our view of the possibilities for light, time, touch, sensation, energy, and mind to enter into health and medicine. The ultimate goal is a synthesis of mind-body medicine, its relation to the emerging field of psychoneuroimmunology, and a possible model for a final common pathway among complementary and alternative medical systems.

MARC S. MICOZZI, MD, PhD

And new philosophy calls all in doubt
The element of fire is quite put out
The sun is lost, and the earth, and no man's wit
Can well direct him where to look for it

And freely men confess that this world's spent
When in the planets, and the firmament
They seek so many new; then see that this
Is crumbled out againe to his atomies

'Tis all in pieces, all cohaerence gone;
All just supply, and all relation . . .

John Donne (1572-1631)

About the Author

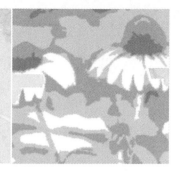

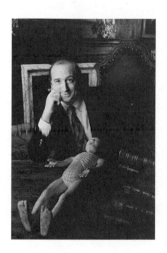

MARC S. MICOZZI, MD, PhD, is the Executive Director of The College of Physicians of Philadelphia (the nation's first medical society, founded 1787) and Adjunct Professor of Medicine and of Rehabilitation Medicine at the University of Pennsylvania (the nation's first medical school, founded 1765). He was previously the Founding Director of the National Museum of Health and Medicine in Washington, DC, and a Senior Investigator at the National Cancer Institute, National Institutes of Health (NIH). He has published six books and over 200 articles in medical and health topics. He was the founding editor-in-chief of the first medical journal on complementary and alternative medicine and is editor of the first textbook, *Fundamentals of Complementary and Alternative Medicine,* now in its second edition. He serves as consultant to the U.S. Federal Trade Commission and the Commonwealth of Pennsylvania Bureau of Professional and Occupational Affairs on complementary and alternative medicine and is Principle Investigator on a grant from the NIH for developing a professional reference resource on alternative therapies in cancer. He has been a frequent speaker to medical and consumer audiences worldwide on complementary medicine.

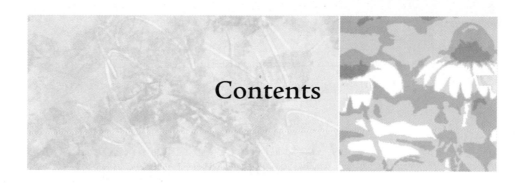

Contents

IV TRADITIONAL MEDICAL SYSTEMS, 301

Fundamentals of
COMPLEMENTARY AND ALTERNATIVE MEDICINE

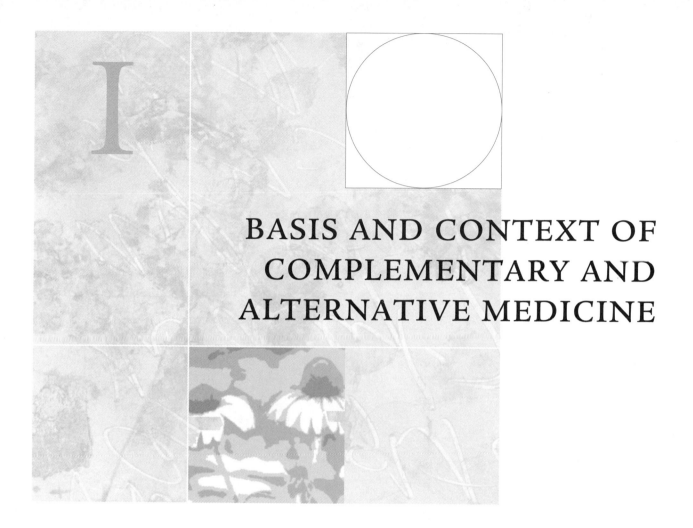

I

BASIS AND CONTEXT OF COMPLEMENTARY AND ALTERNATIVE MEDICINE

This section provides an introduction to the whole topic of complementary and alternative medicine, its themes and terminology, and the various contexts relative to its proper interpretation. The chapters provide a social and cultural recontextualization of complementary and alternative medicine. The ubiquitous use of plants and natural products among alternatives is reviewed through underlying themes from both the social and biological sciences. The social history of the use of complementary and alternative medicine is provided through a review of the concept of "vitalism" in intellectual and medical discourse, which is important to understanding the common themes of bioenergy and self-healing among complementary and alternative medical systems. ∾

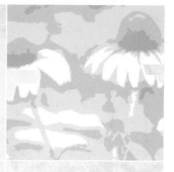

CHAPTER

1

Characteristics of Complementary Medicine

MARC S. MICOZZI

The different medical systems subsumed under the category *complementary and alternative* are large and diverse, but these systems have some common ground in their views of health and healing. I call this overall philosophy *a new ecology of health,* sustainable medicine, or *medicine for a small planet.*

ROLE OF SCIENCE

Allopathic medicine is considered the "scientific" healing art, whereas the alternatives are considered "nonscientific." However, perhaps what is needed is not *less*

science but *more sciences* in the study of complementary and alternative medicine. Some of the central ideas of biomedicine are very powerful but are becoming intellectually stale. The study of dead tissue cells, components, and chemicals to understand life processes and the quest for "magic bullets" to combat disease are based on a reductionist, materialist view of health and healing. We have made tremendous advances over the past 100 years by applying these concepts to medicine. However, the resulting biomedical system is not always able to account for and use many observations in the realms of clinical and personal experience, natural law, and human spirituality.

3

Contemporary biomedicine is a scientific paradigm with a particular history, as much influenced by social history as it is by scientific laws. In the laudable effort to make medicine scientific, we have emphasized that knowledge about the world—including nature and human nature—must be pursued by the following criteria: (1) objectivism—the observer is separate from the observed, (2) reductionism—complex phenomena are explainable in terms of simpler, component phenomena, (3) positivism—all information can be derived from physically measurable data, and (4) determinism—phenomena can be predicted from a knowledge of scientific law and initial conditions. We all know that this is not the only way of "knowing" things but it has become the twentieth century test to determine whether such knowledge is "scientific."

In fact, science simply requires empiricism—making and testing models of reality by what can be observed, guided by certain values, and based on certain metaphysical assumptions. Science itself is not reality but a system of human knowledge. Scientists often detect differences between metaphysical reality and the scientific models constructed through human intellectual activity. These new thoughts about the nature of medicine do not represent a new science so much as they represent a new philosophy.

Therefore the aforementioned criteria are not always applicable. In the science of physics, objectivism is ultimately not possible at the fundamental level because of the Heisenberg uncertainty principle, which states that the act of observing phenomena necessarily influences the behavior of the phenomena being observed. Contemporary biological and ecological science has produced a wealth of observations about interactions between living organisms and their environments in transactional, multidirectional, and synergic ways that are not ultimately subject to reductionist explanations. For positivism and determinism to provide a complete explanation, we must assume that science has all the physical and intellectual tools to ask the right questions. However, the questions we ask are based on the history of science itself as part of the history of human intellectual inquiry.

Contemporary biomedicine conceptually uses Newtonian physics and pre-Darwinian biology. Newtonian physics explains and can reproduce many observations on the mechanics of everyday experience. Contemporary quantum physics (quantum mechanics) recognizes aspects of reality beyond Newtonian mechanics, such as matter-energy duality, "unified fields" of energy and matter, and wave functions (see Chapter 15). Quantum physics and contemporary biology-ecology may be needed to understand alternatives. Nuclear medicine uses the technology of contemporary physics but does not yet incorporate the concepts of quantum physics in its fundamental approach to patient health. Contemporary medicine does measure the body's energy using electrocardiography, electroencephalography, and electromyography for diagnostic purposes, but it does not enlist the body's energy for the purpose of healing.

The biomedical model relies on a projection of Newtonian mechanics into the microscopic and molecular realms.

As a model for everything, Newtonian mechanics has limitations. It works within the narrow limits of everyday experience. It does not always work at a macro (cosmic) level as shown by Einstein's theory of relativity or at a micro (fundamental) level as illustrated by quantum physics. However useful Newton's physics has been in solving mechanical problems, it cannot explain the vast preponderance of nature: the motion of currents; the growth of plants and animals; or the rise, functioning, and fall of civilizations. Per Bak once stated that mechanics could explain why the apple fell but not why the apple existed or why Newton was thinking about it in the first place.

Mechanics works in explaining machines. But no matter how popular this metaphor has become (with apologies to *National Geographic's* "incredible machine" imagery), the body is not a machine and it cannot be entirely explained by mechanics. It is becoming increasingly clear that an understanding of energetics is required. This duality between the mechanical and the energetic has been accepted in physics for most of the past century. This duality is famously illustrated by the fact that J.J. Thomson won the Nobel Prize for demonstrating that the electron is a particle. His son, George P. Thomson, won the Nobel Prize a generation later for demonstrating that the electron is a wave.

"Hard scientists" such as physicists and molecular biologists accept the duality of the electron but have a hard time accepting the duality of the human body. The "soft sciences," which attempt to be inclusive in their study of the phenomena of life and nature, are often looked on with disdain according to the folklore of the self-styled real scientists. However, real science must account for all of what is observed in nature, not just the conveniently reductionistic part.

The biological science of contemporary medicine is essentially pre-Darwinian in that it emphasizes typology rather than individuality and variation. Each patient is defined as a clinical entity by a diagnosis, with treatment prescribed accordingly. The modern understanding of the human genome does not make this approach to biomedical science less pre-Darwinian. Both the fundamentals of inheritance (Mendel) and natural selection (Darwin and Alfred Russel Wallace) were explained long before the discovery of the structure of the gene itself. Although modern biology-ecology continues to explore the phenomena of how living systems interact at the level of the whole—which cannot be seen under a microscope or in a test tube—molecular genetics continues to dissect the human genome.

It may seem outrageously complex to construct a medical system based on the concepts of modern physics and biology-ecology while maintaining a unique diagnostic and therapeutic approach to each individual. This would indeed be complex if not for the fact that the body is its own entity, a part of nature, and each body has an innate ability to heal itself.

If biomedicine cannot explain scientific observations of alternatives, the biomedical paradigm will be revised. ∾

One way of studying and understanding alternative medicine is to view it in light of contemporary physics and biology-ecology and to focus not just on the subtle manipulations of the alternative practitioners but on the physiological response of the body. When homeopathy or acupuncture is observed to result in a physiological or clinical response that cannot be explained by the biomedical model, it is not the role of the scientist to deny this reality but rather to modify our explanatory models to account for it. In this way science itself progresses. In the end there is

only one reality. Alternative medical systems, which are relatively old in terms of human intellectual history, always have been trying to describe, understand, and work with the same reality of health and healing as biomedicine. Furthermore, whereas contemporary biomedicine uses new technologies in the service of relatively old ideas about health and healing, alternative methods use old technologies whose fundamental character may reflect new scientific ideas on physical and biological nature (Box 1-1).

Science must account for all of what is observed, not just part of it. That is why physics has moved be-

BOX 1-1

A Note About Nomenclature

The word *alternative,* or the term *complementary and alternative medicine,* now seems to be culturally encoded in the English language. Workers at Harvard Medical School have provided a basis for a functional definition of the term:

Alternative medicine refers to those practices explicitly used for the purpose of medical intervention, health promotion or disease prevention which are not routinely taught at U.S. medical schools nor routinely underwritten by third-party payers within the existing U.S. health care system.

The Harvard definition seems to be a diagnosis of exclusion, meaning that alternative medicine is everything not being presently promoted in mainstream medicine. This definition may remind us of a popular song from the 1960s called, "The Element Song," which offers a complete listing of all the different elements of the periodic table (set to the tune of "I Am the Very Model of a Modern Major General" from Gilbert and Sullivan's *The Pirates of Penzance*). It ends with words to this effect: "These are the many elements we've heard about at Harvard. And if we haven't heard of them, they haven't been disco-vard." I have likened the recent "discovery" of alternative medicine to Columbus's discovery of the Americas. Although his voyage was a great feat that expanded the intellectual frontiers of Europe, Columbus could not really discover a world already known to millions of indigenous peoples who used complex systems of social organization and subsistence activities. Likewise, the definitional statement that alternatives are not "within the existing U.S. health care system" is a curious observation for the millions of Americans who routinely use them today.

yond Newtonian mechanics—biology beyond typology. Is it possible for a biomedical model to be constructed for which its validity includes observations from alternative medicine? Although it may be necessary to wait for new insights from physics and biology to understand alternatives in terms of biomedicine, clinical pragmatism dictates that successful therapeutic methods should not be withheld while mechanisms are being explained—or debated. We live in a world filled with opportunities to observe the practice of alternatives. It only remains to apply scientific standards to their study. In the meantime, patients are now waiting for mainstream physicians to understand the mechanisms of alternatives. Also in the meantime we can come to understand the underlying intellectual content and history of alternatives as complete systems of thought and practice.

WELLNESS

The complementary and alternative systems generally emphasize what might be called wellness by the mainstream medical system. The goal of preventing disease is shared by alternative and mainstream medicine alike. In the mainstream medical model this involves using drugs and surgery to prevent disease in those who are only at risk rather than reserving these powerful methods for the treatment of disease. I have called this trend the medicalization of prevention. One can continue to engage in risky lifestyle behaviors while medicine provides "magic bullets" to prevent diseases that it cannot treat. Wellness in the context of complementary medicine is more than the prevention of disease. It is a focus on engaging the inner resources of each individual as an active and conscious participant in the maintenance of his or her own health. By the same token, the property of being healthy is not conferred on an individual solely by an outside agency or entity but results from the balance of internal resources with the external natural and social environment. This latter point relates to the alternative approach that relies on the abilities of the individual to get well and stay healthy.

SELF-HEALING

The body heals itself. This might seem to be an obvious statement because we are well aware that wounds heal and cells routinely replace themselves. Nonetheless, this is a profound concept among alternatives because self-healing is the basis of *all* healing. External manipulations simply mobilize the body's inner healing resources. Instead of wondering why the body's cells are sick, we ask why the body is not replacing its sick cells with healthy ones. The ability to be well or to be sick is largely tied to inner resources, and the external environment—social and physical—has an impact on the body's ability.

What is the evidence for self-healing? The long and common history of clinical observations of the "placebo" effect or the "laying on of hands." To paraphrase Jung: Summoned or unsummoned, self-healing will be there. It is so powerful that biomedical methodology mainly designs double-blind, controlled clinical trials to see what percentage of benefit can be added by powerful drugs to the healing encounter.

BIOENERGY

A related concept is that the body has energy (see Chapter 15). Accordingly, as a living entity, the body is an energetic system. Disruptions in the balance and flow of energy cause illness, and the body's response to energetic imbalance leads to perceptible disease. Because the body heals itself, the body can also make itself sick. Restoring or facilitating the body to restore its own balance restores health. The symptoms of a cold, flu, or allergy are caused by the body's efforts to rid itself of the offending agent. For example, by raising the body's temperature, a fever reduces bacterial reproduction, and sneezing physically expels offending agents (see Chapter 7).

Pathologists know that there are only so many ways that cells can look sick because cellular reactions have a defined repertoire for manifesting the body's disease. We have also learned a great deal over the past 100 years by correlating the appearance of dead tissue cells under the microscope with clinical diagnosis and prognosis. However, studying dead tissue cells for clinical significance does not allow direct observation of the dynamic energy of living cells, systems, organisms, and communities. Although correlation of the appearance of stained tissue cells under a microscope to clinical conditions is a very powerful concept in medicine, alternatives appear to provide a path to study the energy of living systems for health and healing (see Chapter 4).

NUTRITION AND NATURAL PRODUCTS

The reliance on nutrition and natural products is fundamental to alternatives and does not play merely a supportive or adjunctive role. Nutrients and natural products are taken into the body and incorporated in the most literal sense. They provide the body with energy in the form of calories and with the material resources to stay healthy and get well.

Because the basic plan of the body, as a physical entity and as an energy system, evolves and exists in an ecological context, what the body needs it gets from the environment in which it grew. Lao Tzu states that "what is deeply rooted in nature cannot be uprooted." The human organism is designed to obtain nutrients from natural food sources present in the natural environment, and the body is best suited to obtain nutrients in their natural forms (see Chapter 9).

PLANTS

Plants are an important part of nature relative to health and a dominant part of the nature in which humans evolved. In addition to producing the oxygen that we breathe, they are seen as sources of nutrients, medicines (such as phytochemicals), essential oils (volatiles for inhalation and/or transdermal absorption), and, by some systems, as sources of vibrational energy. Many systems see the use of plants as source of nutrients in continuity with their use as sources of medicine, paralleling contemporary biomedical guidelines for nutrition as disease prevention.

INDIVIDUALITY

The emphasis of alternatives is on the whole person as a unique individual with his or her own inner resources. Therefore the concepts of normalization, standardization, and generalization are more difficult to apply to research and clinical practice compared with the allopathic method. Some believe that alternatives restore the role of the individual patient and practitioner to the practice of medicine; the biomedical emphasis on standardization of training and practice to ensure quality may leave something lost in the translation back to restoring the health of the individual (see Chapter 7).

The focus on the whole person as a unique individual provides new challenges to the scientific measurement of the healing encounter. Mobilizing the resources of each individual to stay healthy and get well also provides new opportunities to move health care toward a model of wellness and toward new models for helping solve our current health care crisis, which is largely driven by costs.

If the body heals itself, has its own energy, and is uniquely individual, then the focus is not on the healer but on the healed. Although this concept may be humbling to the practitioner as heroic healer, it is liberating to realize that in the end each person heals himself or herself. If the healer is not the sole source of health and healing, there is room for humility and room for both patient and practitioner to participate in the interaction.

For the purposes of this book I offer my own functional definition of alternative medicine, which (to further these purposes) here is called complementary medical systems. Complementary medical systems are characterized by a developed body of intellectual work that underlies the conceptualization of health and its precepts; that has been sustained over many generations by many practitioners in many communities; that represents an orderly, rational, conscious system of knowledge and thought about health and medicine; that relates more broadly to a way of life (or lifestyle); and that has been widely observed to have definable results as practiced.

Although the term *holistic* has been applied to the approach to the "body as person" among alternative medical systems, I apply holism to the medical system itself as a complete system of thought and practice (what I have elsewhere called health beliefs and behaviors). This system of knowledge is therefore shared by patients and practitioners—the active, conscious engagement of "patients" is relative to the focus on *self-healing* and *individuality* that are among the common characteristics of these systems.

In this regard it might be considered that we are trying to document here the classic practice of complementary and alternative medical systems. In trying to build a bridge between a well-developed system of allopathic medicine and complementary medical systems, it is necessary to have strong foundations on both sides of this bridge. It is, of course, not possible to apply these criteria to the work of individual alternative practitioners who have unilaterally developed their own unique techniques over one or two generations (what might be called unusual) just as it is not possible to build a bridge to nowhere. My definition is meant to apply to systems of thought and not just techniques of practice. Often there is an underlying philosophy of individual practitioners surrounding new techniques they have developed. Or new techniques may be subsumed under existing systems of practice.

Eclecticism itself is a historical form of alternative medicine that drew from among different traditions and was popular in the United States in the last century. In such a system treatment is determined by the needs of each individual patient, not just by what one given system has to offer. Today a chiropractor might practice in an Ayurveda clinic, osteopaths might practice in allopathic clinics, and chiropractors or allopaths might use acupuncture. *Naturopathy,* in some ways the most recent of homegrown alternatives from the Euro-American tradition, consciously uses a variety of traditions ranging from acupuncture to herbal medicine. I have termed naturopathy as *neoeclecticism* with the underlying philosophy that the body heals itself using resources found in nature (see Chapter 11).

In the end a given system develops in answer to human needs. Alternatives vary widely, but their characteristics cluster around the self-healing capabilities of the human organism and the ability (and reliance) of the human organisms to use resources present in nature. What is constant and at the center of such alternative systems is the individual human being. Therefore if the focus is not on the medical system itself but on the human being at the center, there is really only one system.

A final point about alternatives: In a way, perhaps particular to the United States, they imply the importance of individuality and choice. In an era when the active engagement of the individual in his or her own health is a paramount goal, the importance of individuality and of choice could not be more salient. ∽

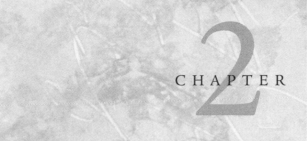
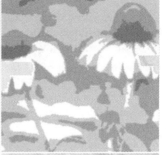

CHAPTER 2

Translational Issues in Conventional and Complementary Medicine

MARC S. MICOZZI

What has been labeled alternative medicine in the United States is, first of all, a social phenomenon and consumer movement of significant dimensions. The term *complementary medicine* has been used interchangeably and is a more accurate functional description of this social phenomenon because patients in the United States generally use "alternative medicine" as an adjunct to (not a replacement for) conventional medical care. Much of what we call complementary and alternative medicine in the United States, in fact, represents time-honored traditions of medical practice originating from other countries and other cultures or from the history of European and American society.

One of the most important distinctions we can make in studying and understanding alternatives is to note the differences between two types of practices: (1) practices that are many years or centuries old and have a large body of practitioners and patients and a well-developed fund of clinical "wisdom" that is encoded into the belief system of a particular society or subgroup of people and (2) practices that have been developed recently by one or few practitioners in isolation from peers and without benefit of scientific testing and clinical studies (what may be called unusual therapy). Practices in this second category often fit conceptually within the biomedical model but simply have not been tested by use of the standards of biomedical research and practice.

For example, for the topics in this volume, alternatives in the first category of time-tested traditions include the traditional medicine of China (with heterogeneous practice styles), manual therapies (osteopathy, chiropractic, massage), and homeopathy.

Many time-tested traditions have in common, to a greater or lesser extent, aspects of mind-body medicine, a focus on nutrition and natural products, hands-on interaction between practitioner and patient, and an emphasis on listening to the patient. The five common characteristics of complementary and alternative medicine (CAM) described in this book are (1) a wellness orientation, (2) a reliance on self-healing, (3) an interference that bioenergetic mechanisms play a role, (4) the use of nutrition and natural products in a fundamental role, and (5) an emphasis on individuality.

Because homeopathy, for example, stresses the importance of eliciting detailed symptoms and symptom complexes from the patient (and is not a system for placing patients into disease-based diagnostic categories), the practitioner must spend a great deal of time listening to the patient. The therapeutic benefits (and diagnostic value) of listening to the patient continue to be actively used among the "talk therapies" of contemporary mainstream medical practice in psychiatry and psychology, as well as general clinical practice (Adler, 1997).

Because complementary and alternative therapies do not necessarily stress the assignment of patients to disease-based diagnostic categories, they are routinely prepared to deal with "functional" disorders and complaints (such as pain, gastrointestinal dysfunction, menstrual dysfunction, and other "subjective" symptoms) that do not carry a pathological diagnosis. Many complementary medical systems see these functional disorders as precursors of disease (rather than, for example, results of disease) and approach the clinical intervention on that basis.

VITALISM AND HOLISM

Various complementary medical systems also make reference to the importance of "energy" in the development of disorders and diseases and in their treatment and cure. Energy has a dynamic quality and is not measured in the usual ways that conventional medicine is accustomed to describing on the basis of materialist, reductionist biomedical mechanisms. The idea that whole living systems and organisms have a "vital energy" that may not be present in nonliving entities or in parts or portions of an organism is an ancient one among human cultures that is also

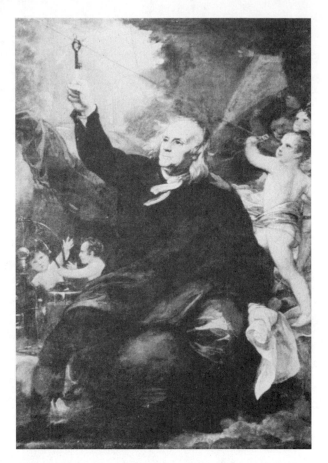

Figure 2-1 Poets, philosophers, and scientists of the late eighteenth and early nineteenth centuries were all interested in vitalism—the energy that animated life and the universe. Here Benjamin Franklin is shown in this heroic pose by Benjamin West figuratively "taming lightning." In fact, Franklin like his contemporaries was searching for insights into nature and human nature, not just exploring electricity in a contemporary utilitarian sense. Later, scientists felt that reductionist, materialist explanations substituted for the need for vitalist interpretations.

reflected in European and U.S. intellectual traditions (Figure 2-1).

Complementary and alternative medical systems are sometimes considered vitalistic and holistic compared with allopathic medicine, which is considered materialistic and reductionistic (Table 2-1). Vitalism contends that there is an "energy" to living organisms that is nonmaterial. Vitalism is a nonecological concept historically and posits nonnaturalistic explana-

TABLE 2-1

Vitalism and Holism in Complementary Medicine

Biomedicine	Complementary medicine
Reductionist Materialist	Holistic Vitalist

tions for life. Holism is an ecological concept that the totality of biological phenomena in a living organism or system cannot be reduced, observed, or measured at a level below that of the whole organism or system (Smuts, 1926). Holism as an ecological concept is not consistent with the vitalist idea that living systems are independent of nature. Holism was meant to be both antimechanistic and antivitalist. However, it is generally interpreted that vitalism and holism go together in studying the characteristics of CAM. However, some interpretations of homeopathy, for example, rely on a vitalist mechanism while basing therapy on an essentially reductionist approach (meaning that a whole organism's energetic mechanism is postulated for the effect that is elicited by minute doses of specific materia medica in pills). Likewise, in Chinese medicine the post-1949 Traditional Chinese Medicine (TCM) "style" of practice veers toward a reductionist model while maintaining an essentially vitalist mechanism. Since 1978 the World Health Organization (WHO) has referred to traditional (cultural) medical systems as holistic, meaning "viewing humans in totality within a wide ecological spectrum, and emphasizing the view that ill health or disease is brought about by imbalance or disequilibrium of humans in the total ecological system and not only by the causative agent and pathogenic mechanism" (World Health Organization, 1998).

Historically, we might say that premodern medical systems could understand medicine only on the basis of observations of the whole organism, whose components were not well known or understood. Modern reductionist biomedical science has allowed knowledge to be built on the basis of studying dead parts and pieces of the whole organism, such as tissue cells and DNA. A postmodern medicine might permit translation of the biomedical model back to the realm of the whole, vital organism. New imaging technologies that permit observation of living cells for diagnostic and therapeutic purposes may provide one mechanism, for example.

In this view it might be considered that biomedicine has new technologies that are generally in the service of old ideas about health and healing, whereas complementary medical systems represent old technologies that may be interpreted in light of new ideas about health and healing.

Outcomes-based research has begun to be helpful in demonstrating the therapeutic benefit (or lack thereof) of alternative practices that are unexplainable on the basis of postulated mechanisms of action foreign to the biomedical model. In this way, it is regarded by some that such ideas are nonsense or perhaps more accurately, "unsense." However, some sense may be made of these ideas by considering a medical ecological or adaptational model.

The medical ecological or adaptational conceptual models around the ideas of vitalism and holism in translation from complementary to conventional medicine will be described further.

MEDICAL ECOLOGICAL AND ADAPTATIONAL MODEL

With medical traditions that have been encoded and carried as knowledge in different cultures for many years, it is possible to study the adaptiveness and adaptive value of such practices. What benefits do they confer on members of a society who follow certain health-related beliefs and practices?

Human physiology allows adaptation to occur in response to environmental pressures in the short term in the individual. Evolution allows adaptation to occur over the long term in the population. Human culture is learned behavior that also has adaptive value.

At the end of the nineteenth century, European interpretations regarded traditional medical practices as myth, superstition, or magic (and sometimes madness), as illustrated in Sir James Frazer's *The Golden Bough* (Frazer, 1890, 1959). During the twentieth century, social scientists searched for the functional meanings and purposes of medically related traditions. European and North American social scientists began describing the meanings of traditional medical practices in the 1920s. For example, if traditional societies through plant domestication and agriculture learn to obtain nutrients (foods) from the environment in which they live, they may also learn to obtain medicines from their environments and to develop therapeutic techniques to provide medical care.

As previously stated, many contemporary complementary and alternative medical paradigms and practices derive from complex and sophisticated ancient health systems and/or from indigenous cultures closely in touch with their natural and social environments. These health systems form part of the adaptation of these societies and cultures to their respective environments, representing integral components of traditional societies (Micozzi, 1983). Beliefs and behaviors relating to health that are widespread and persistent merit study to determine their adaptive value (Table 2-2).

To accept the validity of the premise for scientific investigation of alternative medical systems, one need only accept the possibility (or probability) of the adaptiveness of human belief and behavior systems that are persistent and widespread. The adaptiveness of human behavior is an important concept to both social and biological scientists. Whether human behavior is adaptive represents a persistent question in intellectual discourse. Cultural practices that are widespread and persist over generations have been taken by some as evidence of the adaptiveness of such practices.

Although many hold out the symbolic power of beliefs and the transcendental value of ideas regardless of "adaptive" value, belief and behavior systems can often be demonstrated in a scientific sense to have associated outcomes relative to human health and disease. The British anthropologist-physician W.H.R. Rivers demonstrated that traditional health systems are not magic or superstition but represent rational, ordered systems of knowledge and useful ways of understanding and interacting with the environment (Rivers, 1924).

Bringing together social science and biomedical science in a more effective and integrated way must be rigorous in the application of the social sciences to the study of health and medicine. Social scientists often study health belief systems without adequately measuring health outcomes in a scientific sense, whereas biomedicine measures outcomes scientifically without being able to study the underlying belief systems. Social and cultural factors are amenable to study by techniques extrinsic to biomedical science. A conceptual paradigm may be considered to have reached the limits of explanation or inquiry when dependent variables can be measured, but independent variables are unknown or immeasurable in the system of study (Kuhn, 1973). If health outcomes are considered dependent variables, the explanatory limits of biomedical science are exceeded because relevant independent variables are not made an explicit component of the explanatory model.

There are different ways of explaining how manual therapies work, for example. Although their clinical applications and associated health outcomes have been accepted on the basis of biomechanical mechanisms, many manual therapy traditions invoke the manipulation of bioenergy as the mechanism.

TABLE 2-2

Representation of Traditional Health Systems

Conceptual paradigm	Health system component	Methodology	Representation

"Social reality"	Health beliefs
	Health behaviors
	  Health practices, *wellness*
	    maintenance
	  Care seeking, *illness* perceived
	    Structural-functional access
	    Cultural access
		Informant interview/survey
		Participant-observation
			Cognitive
			Observational

"Scientific reality"	Health outcomes, *disease* defined	Technical evaluation: health and nutrition status indicators	Analytical

BIOENERGETIC EXPLANATIONS FOR MANUAL THERAPIES

First, all manual therapies imply that touching the patient in a particular manner is a primary means of therapy. The traditional view of the "laying on of hands" is to focus the attention of both practitioner and patient on the intention to heal and undertaking to treat the patient by the practitioner.

Manual therapies as complementary medicine combine several approaches to healing traditions. Manual therapies can be seen to include North American historic traditions such as osteopathy and chiropractic and more recently "body work" (for example, massage therapy, rolfing, the Trager method, applied kinesiology, and the Feldenkrais method). Asian manual systems include Chinese tui na and Japanese shiatsu. Techniques that are often seen as manual therapy but more explicitly relate to manipulation of bioenergy are the Asian systems of qi gong and reiki and the North American technique of therapeutic touch.

The founder of chiropractic, Daniel David Palmer, was originally an "energy healer" or "magnetic healer," as was the founder of traditional osteopathy, Andrew Taylor Still (Palmer, 1910; Still, 1902). Both traditions were established within a few years and a few hundred miles of each other in the American Midwest of the 1890s. In addition to embracing the concept of "vital energy," both Palmer and Still also rejected the use of drugs, which were especially toxic during that period of history. In this regard, Still and Palmer were joined by such mainstream medical figures as Sir William Osler and Oliver Wendell Holmes. In a famous statement Holmes opined that if the entire materia medica of contemporary medicine were thrown to the bottom of the sea, it would be better for mankind and worse for the fishes. However, chiropractic and traditional osteopathy went further by specifically identifying themselves as "drugless healing," which found many adherents in reaction to the therapeutic excesses of the day in mainstream medicine. After World War II, osteopathy was largely mainstreamed into modern medicine, partially driven by the chronic shortage of medical manpower in the U.S. military (who recruited DOs to supplement MDs), as well as the desire of osteopaths to participate in the full benefits of medical mainstream training and practice.

Therapeutic touch and healing touch are more recent developments initially largely promulgated by two nurses in the United States, Dolores Krieger (Krieger, 1979) and Dora Kunz (Kunz, 1991). Healing "touch" is notable in that the patient is not actually physically touched. The technique therefore may be explained as a form of energy healing (perhaps the form most in practice in clinical settings in the United States) rather than manual therapy. The flow of energy is thought to be manipulated around the body of the patient by the hands of the practitioner.

Other forms of hand-mediated healing modalities include polarity therapy, Tibetan-Japanese reiki, Japanese jin shin jyutsu, external qi gong, touch for health, reflexology, acupressure, and shiatsu massage.

Bioenergetic mechanisms are invoked to explain clinical observations of the efficacy of therapeutic touch. These concepts are difficult to translate in clinical medicine, which at the same time recognizes that there is experimental reality beyond the realm of the contemporary biomedical paradigm.

AYURVEDA

Bioenergetic mechanisms have also been invoked in attempting to understand some aspects of Ayurveda, or the traditional medicine of India (see also Chapters 19 and 20). Traditionally, Ayurveda is not just a medical system per se but is described as the science of longevity and relates more to what we would think of as a way of life or "lifestyle." A contemporary view of Ayurveda is provided by Maharishi Ayurveda, which represents a revival of Ayurvedic traditions lost through centuries of foreign rule (Moslem/Mogul and European/British) in India, blended with "bioenergetic" interpretations of mechanism.

Empirically, Ayurveda makes use of correspondences among five cosmic elements of earth, air, fire, water, and space (similar to ancient Greek concepts and "humoral" Western medical systems extending into the nineteenth century). There are three constitutional body types based on the balance of three *doshas*, which represent these five elements as they occur in the human body (Table 2-3). The three primary body types (*prakriti*) represent an empirical system for describing predisposition to illness, proscribing against unhealthy behavior, and prescribing for treatment of disease. The three primary body types of vata, pitta, and kapha may be roughly translated to the

TABLE 2-3

Characteristics of Three Constitutional Types in Ayurveda

	Dosha		
	Vata	Pitta	Kapha
Somatotype (Sheldon)	Ectomorph	Mesomorph	Endomorph
Body type	Light, thin	Moderate	Solid, heavy
Skin type	Dry	Reddish	Oily, smooth
Personality	Anxious	Irritable	Tranquil, steady
Digestion	Irregular, constipation	Sharp	Slow
Activity	Quick	Medium	Slow, methodical
Season	Winter	Fall	Spring
Diseases	Hypertension	Inflammation	Sinusitis
	Arthritis	Inflammatory bowel disease	Respiratory diseases
	Rheumatism	Skin diseases	Asthma
	Cardiac arrhythmia	Heartburn	Obesity
	Insomnia	Peptic ulcer	Depression

Sheldon somatotypes of twentieth century Western science describing body constitution as ectomorph, mesomorph, and endomorph. Ayurveda also demonstrates systematic correspondences among a number of cosmic elements, seasons, constitutions, personalities, diseases, and treatments.

The idea that body constitution predisposes to certain diseases is an old one, and in biomedicine it now finds expression in the association of genetic factors with disease, a current preoccupation of contemporary biomedical science.

CHINESE MEDICINE

We can also think of Chinese medicine as an empirical tradition of systematic correspondences making reference to five cosmic elements extending back to roughly 3000 BC (Table 2-4). Although for comparative purposes Chinese medicine is often treated as a homogeneous monolithic structure, this view neglects the changing interpretations of basic paradigms offered by Chinese medicine through the ages and the synchronic plurality of differing opinions and ideas over thousands of years (Unschuld, 1985).

Likewise, I prefer to use the term *China's Traditional Medicine* or *Traditional Medicine of China*. The popular term *Traditional Chinese Medicine* is a twentieth century invention, concoction, or perhaps convention that blends certain aspects of Chinese medicine with a scientific underpinning put into place by the Communist government of Mao Tse-Tung to provide basic health care to the Chinese population.

Much of what the Chinese medical practitioner does is thought to influence the flow or balance of the body's energy called "qi." In my view, the Chinese concept of qi, which is translated as energy, bioenergy, or vital energy, has a metabolic quality because the Chinese character for qi (Figure 2-2) may be described as vapor or steam rising over rice. The term *rice* has a specific quality that we associate with a specific food, but it also has a generic meaning, "food" or "foodstuff." For example, the character "rice hall" is used to describe a restaurant in Chinese. The elusive meaning of qi may therefore be likened more to living metabolism than to the energy that we associate with electromagnetic radiation.

Energy or qi also has the dynamic qualities of "flow" and "balance." Because flow and balance are dynamic, they may be described in changing terms from one patient to the next or in the same patient from one day to the next (again, not using static, fixed pathological diagnostic categories). Such concepts present great challenges in translation to the biomedical model. Acupuncture is a major modality for the manipulation of qi. Clinical observations of efficacy are increasing, and some biomedical explanations focus on the physiological effects of skin puncture

TABLE 2-4

Five Phase Correspondences in Chinese Medicine

	Category				
	Wood	Fire	Earth	Metal	Water
Organ	Liver	Heart	Spleen	Lungs	Kidney
Bowel	Gallbladder	Small intestine	Stomach	Large intestine	Urinary bladder
Season	Spring	Summer	Late summer	Autumn	Winter
Time of day	Before sunrise	Forenoon	Afternoon	Late afternoon	Midnight
Climate	Wind	Heat	Damp	Dryness	Cold
Direction	East	South	Center	West	North
Development	Birth	Growth	Maturity	Withdrawal	Dormancy
Color	Cyan	Red	Yellow	White	Black
Taste	Sour	Bitter	Sweet	Pungent	Salty
Sense organ	Eyes	Tongue	Mouth	Nose	Ears
Odor	Goatish	Scorched	Fragrant	Raw fish	Putrid
Vocalization	Shouting	Laughing	Singing	Weeping	Sighing
Tissue	Sinews	Vessels	Flesh	Body hair	Bones

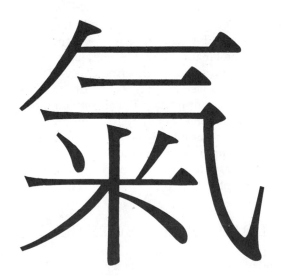

Figure 2-2 The Chinese character qi, described as vapor or steam rising over rice.

and/or modulation of neurotransmitter substances. Some experiments indicate that the acupuncture needle has the same effect when it is merely held in place over the appropriate point (without puncturing the skin). If acupuncture needles operate by influencing the flow of energy, which is not limited by internal-external barriers, then puncturing the skin is not a necessary part of the mechanism of action. It strikes one that perhaps practical Chinese acupuncturists simply found a way to hold the needles in place by puncturing the skin when they were trying to influence more than two acupuncture points simultaneously (and of course, had only two hands to hold the needles in place).

HOMEOPATHY

Homeopathy challenges certain assumptions of allopathic medicine with the concept that "like cures like." A symptom may be seen as an attempt on the part of the body to correct itself, to fight disease, and/or to restore balance (homeostasis). For example, in the case of fever this may be seen as an adaptation to bacterial infection. (Increased temperatures [above normal body temperature] are seen to significantly slow the rate of bacterial reproduction.) In this way, raising body temperature above normal is bacteriostatic and, like many antibiotics, may slow bacterial growth, giving the immune system a chance to clear the infection.

Homeopathy originally gave the name "allopathic" medicine to the "regular" medical mainstream approaches of the time (early nineteenth century) because the medical focus is on the elimination or control of symptoms. In homeopathy, symptoms are everything, and describing them is the primary goal and guide to therapy. In classical homeopathy an empirical approach is taken by administering "provings"of substances (largely materia medica) in minute doses and observing whether there is clinical improvement. This practice may also be considered reductionistic. Because there is a tendency of many symptoms to improve over time, these "provings" cannot be considered controlled experiments, but the same observation may be applied to the administration of "cures" in other traditions as well.

NATUROPATHIC MEDICINE AND HERBALISM

Naturopathy is the most recent of alternative approaches to have developed as a complete system in North America (see Chapter 11). It emphasizes the healing power of nature and can also be understood in terms of the adaptational model. In practice, contemporary naturopathy is eclectic, consciously drawing on a number of models and systems (for example, Chinese, Ayurveda, homeopathy, manual therapies, Islamic healing) in an effort to fit the patient profile and the clinical problem with appropriate medical systems and techniques. Naturopathy is well organized in a few western states (notably Oregon, Washington, and Montana) and in Connecticut and northern New England but may be practiced in a less formal fashion in other parts of the country.

The use of nutrition, herbs, natural remedies, and other natural products is an important component of naturopathic medicine. Medical traditions around the world, from the most basic shamanistic approaches to healing to the highly complex and sophisticated systems of Chinese and Ayurvedic medicine, make use of medicinal plants in light of their biological activity. Homeopathy (often included in the range of practice of naturopathic medicine) is also based largely on minute doses of materia medica.

From the standpoint of evolutionary biology, it is not surprising that plants develop biologically active constituents as an adaptation to compete in nature with each other and with animal species. Because plants form a primary feature of the terrestrial environment in which humans evolved, it is also not surprising that human physiology and metabolism are adapted to obtaining nutrients and medicines from plants in their environments. Societies learn over time which plants have value, and how to obtain, harvest, and prepare them and encode this knowledge

TABLE 2-5

Medicinal Plant Constituent Actions

Respiratory	Gastrointestinal	Neural
Expectorant	Emetic	Sedative
Antitussive	Antiemetic	Stimulant
Immuno-	Laxative	Cardiotonic
modulative	Spasmolytic	Antidepressant

and behavior into their cultures. In addition to the traditional medical settings for the use of medicinal plants, an eclectic system of herbal medicine has historically developed in the West, which can be referred to as Western herbalism. Biologically active constituents of plants include carbohydrates, glycosides, tannins, lipids, volatile oils, resins, steroids, alkaloids, peptides, and enzymes.

Volatile oils form the primary basis of the practice of aromatherapy. The active constituents have various physiological effects throughout the body (Table 2-5). Because biologically active constituents are present in combination in medicinal plants, they are often observed to have synergistic effects. These synergistic effects have been useful in the application of crude extracts of medicinal plants to antibiotic-resistant bacterial infections and to chloroquine-resistant malaria, for example. However, it is difficult to translate this approach to the active ingredient model of reductionist biomedical research, as described in the next section.

GLOBAL PERSPECTIVES

Understanding complementary medical systems described here as traditional or cultural medicine in an ecological model, we can compare and contrast how they "fit" in their indigenous settings with the interpretations made in the contemporary United States. In the U.S. health care system, we assume traditional herbal medicines are of value only when their active principal or ingredient is known and can be purified for mass production. However, this "active ingredient" approach to medicinal plants and traditional medicine reflects a particular conceptual paradigm rather than a particular truth about how natural medicines may work. On the basis of findings from U.S. biomedical plant screening programs, therapeu-

TABLE 2-6

Old Assumptions and New Perspectives on Complementary Medical Systems

Old assumptions	New perspectives
"Primitive"	Holistic
Ineffective	Cost-effective
Marginalized	Locally available
Extinct	Renewed
Should be regulated	Should be studied
Prospects for biomedicine	Valid in own right
Active ingredient model	Synergistic activity

tic benefits are often observed to be limited. However, methodologies used in biomedicine often overlook the effects by which traditional medicines produce results because of a fixed and defined view of what constitutes therapeutic action. Although traditional health systems have acknowledged use in chronic, low-level conditions, they are assumed to be of no value in providing acute or emergency care. However, in some countries (China, Vietnam, Nicaragua) traditional medicine is mandated and used effectively for trauma and major acute diseases; historically this was caused by political and/or economic exclusion from other health care technologies. Much research already exists in other countries (often in other languages besides English).

Traditional medicines are now seen as valuable because they serve as sources of leads for new pharmaceuticals (so-called biodiversity prospecting), and the potential medical value of tropical rainforest species provides a basis for support to preserve and conserve regional biodiversity. However, this "biodiversity prospecting" assumption overlooks the role of traditional medical systems in addressing the needs of the people from whence come the medicinal plants and the knowledge about their appropriate use. Whereas old views assume the marginalization of traditional medical systems, a new perspective looks to them to provide complementary therapies and, in

some cases, new solutions to our contemporary "health care crisis" (Table 2-6).

Much of what is called complementary medicine in the United States represents primary care for 80 percent of the world's people (World Health Organization, 1998). In this way it may be considered to represent appropriate technology and affordable, sustainable medicine both for indigenous people traditionally and now for industrialized societies as well on a global basis.

References

Adler, H.M. 1997. The history of the present illness as treatment: who's listening, and why does it matter? Journal of American Board of Family Medicine 10:28-34.

Frazer, J.G. 1890, 1959. The Golden Bough, new ed. Gaster, T.H., trans., New American Library, New York.

Hahnemann, S. 1933, 1980. Organon of Medicine, 6th ed. Boericke, W, trans., B. Jain Publishers, New Delhi.

Krieger, D. 1979. The Therapeutic Touch. How to Use Your Hands to Help or to Heal. Prentice-Hall, New York.

Kuhn, T. 1973. The Structure of Scientific Revolutions. Yale University Press, New Haven, Connecticut.

Kunz, D. 1991. The Personal Aura. Quest, Wheaton, Illinois.

Lust, B. 1918. Universal Directory of Naturopathy. Lust Publisher, Butler, New Jersey.

Micozzi, M.S. 1983. Anthropological Study of Health Beliefs, Behaviors and Outcomes. Human Organization 42:351-353.

Palmer, D.D. 1910. Textbook of the Science, Art and Philosophy of Chiropractic. Portland Printing House, Portland, Oregon.

Rivers, W.H.R. 1924. Medicine, Magic and Religion. Harcourt and Brace, New York.

Smuts, J.C. 1926. Holism and Evolution. Macmillan, New York.

Still, A.T. 1902. Philosophy and mechanical principles of osteopathy. Hudson-Kimberly Publishing, Kansas City, Missouri.

Unschuld, P. 1985. Medicine in China: A History of Ideas. University of California, Berkeley.

World Health Organization. 1998. Traditional Medicine. Geneva, Switzerland, WHO Publications.

CHAPTER 3

Social and Cultural Context of Complementary and Alternative Medicine Systems

CLAIRE MONOD CASSIDY

There are a great many health care systems in the world. All share the goals of alleviating the suffering of the sick, promoting health, and protecting the wider society from illness.

Despite this underlying universality, systems differ profoundly. They differ in degree of expansion into the world, so that some systems are practiced only locally, as among a single rainforest tribe, whereas others have spread to every corner of the globe. They differ in degree of technology, from systems that require none at all, to others that can barely function in the absence of electricity and perfect sanitation. Most importantly, they differ in their perceptions of the sick and well human body and in how they deliver health care.

These similarities and differences among health care systems have been systematically studied for more than 100 years. As a result, we can now discuss both why so many systems exist and how differences among them matter. Basically, systems arise and persist because each one serves a need. Moreover, patients report satisfaction with care—no matter what kind—if that care is delivered in a manner that meshes with their cultural expectations. The form health care takes is first and fundamentally a matter of sociocultural interpretation. In other words, the "truth" that guides any health care system is relative and is learned.

This point, although implied by the very existence of numerous health care systems, surprises us—particularly in North America, where we have hoped and assumed that we have had only one real health care system since early in this century. This hope has been couched in language that still argues for the primacy of scientific medicine, including the claim that "biomedicine" is scientific. But as the voices of other types of practitioners gain strength, and as the world's cultural diversity increasingly bears in on American culture, it becomes clear that most of what we know, even scientific fact, is culturally modeled. We remain unaware of this situation most of the time because our cultural assumptions are learned at an early age and are embedded within us to the point that we take them for granted. Only when they are challenged—as they will be by the material in this text—do we become aware of them. Once aware, we can choose either to expand our thinking or to defend the status quo.

Biomedicine is the formal name for the health care system in which the primary practitioners earn the degree of MD; it also is called allopathy. These names emphasize aspects of this system's explanatory model. Other names are flavored by cultural politics and emphasize biomedicine's expanded or dominant position. Examples include Western, cosmopolitan, modern, orthodox, and conventional. In this chapter all health care practices, including biomedicine, are treated as alternatives, meaning that all are options available to users. They are complementary to the extent that they can be and are used together. ೋ

This chapter offers an opportunity to expand thinking through a series of conceptual models that contextualize the variety of health care systems. It considers three questions:

1. What are the many health care realities?
2. How do they resemble each other?
3. What are the implications of the differences?

REALITY, INTERPRETATION, AND RELATIVITY

A psychiatrist once told me about a Mormon woman who came to him deeply distressed because 20 years and four children into her second marriage she realized that she would be spending eternity with her first husband, a man who had died 6 months after their wedding. Mormon couples can be married both for this life and for "eternity," and she and her first husband had chosen to be linked in both ways. Now her first husband was a stranger to her, and she desperately wanted to spend the afterlife with her present husband and children. To his credit the psychiatrist realized that he could not help this patient. He called a Mormon colleague who quickly linked the patient with a bishop of the Mormon church. In a single visit the bishop helped the woman straighten out her fears about the afterlife.

Why could the first psychiatrist not help the patient himself? He did not share her reality model. Instead of telling her not to be so silly, he took a logical and compassionate step and linked the sick woman with health care workers who did share her reality model.

Another example: On a chilly wet day, a young woman laughingly pointed out her red tights and red boots to me, saying, "I always wear red on my feet on days like this, to keep me cooking from below up." Was this an amusing poesy shared on an elevator? A sign of psychosis? Certainly, this remark did not make sense from within the biomedical model. But an acupuncturist would understand that the cold element, water, is chased by the hot element, fire, and the symbolic color of fire is red. A similar behavior pattern would be recognized by practitioners of Ayurveda, the traditional medicine of India, or Curanderismo, the folk medicine tradition of Mexico, Central America, and many Hispanic people in the United States. It also survives in mainstream America when a mother boots up her kids on rainy days to keep them warm and prevent colds.*

These stories provide small illustrations of the statement that the form health care takes is first and fundamentally a matter of interpretation. The wide variety of lifeways shows that humans have found many different ways to answer the same life questions. We can enjoy these differences much as we enjoy a good conversation, or we can grapple with their meanings and implications. Those involved in delivering health care must grapple with them.

---

*That the remark makes sense within the logic of humoral models does not mean that practitioners would say that red boots work, that is, that they themselves, or their color specifically, prevented the young woman from being invaded by cold damp. To determine whether an action is instrumental requires an entirely different level of analysis.

Unfortunately, the same derisive tone that labels the interpretation of personal experience as merely superstition is also found in comparisons of medical belief systems. If one is modern then others are, by inference, outmoded; if one is based on fact then others must be laced with superstition. In this way, biomedicine is seen as somehow more true than any alternative system could possibly be. . . . Such a view . . . fails to consider the internal logic of other explanatory models. But most health systems are logical and rational systems of thought if the underlying assumptions are known; this does not necessarily mean that these assumptions are correct, only that they can be viewed as having been reached by the coherent use of reason (Snow, 1993).

This can be difficult if we do not even know why we are reacting with laughter, anger, or defensiveness. The process of socialization—into our culture as children and into our profession as adults—provides us with truths and logical structures that hang together and answer life's questions well. We even learn to deal with the ambiguities and inconsistencies of what we have learned: We may not notice that we believe two mutually incompatible things before breakfast until someone who has a different perspective points it out to us. Even then, why should we question our own truths or pay other truths heed? Strange answers make no sense and provide no guidance or comfort. It is tempting to think that others are irrational or ignorant:

Mothers may not believe this, but colds are *not* caused by standing in drafts, going without a hat, or getting feet wet. They occur when one sneezing, coughing child shares germs with another (Sears, 1991).

The fact that there are numerous cogent *models* of reality is not trivial to Western thinkers. In this cultural region, battles have been fought and lives lost in defense of the ideal of a singular reality (Ames, 1993). Earlier in our history the search for this reality was mainly expressed in religious terms, but for the last 150 years or more many have believed that science holds the key. By this logic, health care practices that are not considered scientific are not as trustworthy because they are not seeking the singular reality.

This situation helps explain why the preceding psychiatric example might be shrugged off. Laypeople are known to have beliefs, and clinicians must deal with them. The point of this discussion is that *everyone* has beliefs, and *all* realities are constructed; the facts of science are as culturally contextualized as those of law, theology, or social manners. Scientific fact is only as stable as the logic that produced it and the systems that apply it. Thus, science itself is rapidly experiencing a paradigm shift. Plasma physics operates by a different logic and perceives reality differently from how Newtonian physics does; population biology is quite a different kettle of fish from Linnaean systematics (see Chapters 1, 2, and 15).

The curious thing about modular reality is that you are likely to find exactly what you expect. The observer is not separate from the observed (see Heisenberg Principle, Chapter 1). Expectations are based on assumptions and the application of logic. When the assumptive base changes, so does the logic and as a result the appropriate response. Consider, for example, streptococcal pharyngitis. According to biomedicine the *streptococcal bacterium* causes the sore throat. Logically, one could treat with antibiotics to destroy that bacterium. However, approximately 20 percent of the population carries this germ in their throat without developing an illness (Greenwood & Nunn, 1994). Indeed only a minority of people who are exposed to the sore throat contract it. Thus other factors must be involved; the presence of bacterium, although necessary, is not sufficient. Health care systems such as homeopathy understand this concept and focus more attention on the other factors—the reacting body, the person—than on infectious microorganisms. Care is aimed at strengthening the person, rather than at destroying bacteria.

But surely, people use universal definitions for such material body parts as the heart or blood? No, not quite. Although everyone might agree that the heart is a pulsating organ located in the center of the chest, its energetic and spiritual capabilities are debated. Biomedical thinkers describe the heart as a pump, using a material and mechanical metaphor. Once even doctors thought of it as the seat of the soul, a memory our society revisits in many romantic songs. This idea still is active in Chinese medical thought, in which the physical heart beats while the energetic heart fills the role of sovereign ruler from whom directing influence and clear insight emanate (Porkert, 1974) for all other organs. In Chinese anatomy the heart even has a special protector, an organ unknown in biomedical anatomy.

In biomedicine, blood is a living red substance that contains red and white cells and carries food, enzymes, hormones, and oxygen; it is complex and constantly renews itself. In popular Jamaican thought, however, blood does not renew itself. Its purity (a social rather than medical concept) determines one's success in life (Sobo, 1993). Following this logic, many Jamaicans are loath to give or receive blood for transfusions.

Cultural Relativity

In each of the preceding examples a reader might ask, who's right? But that is not the most useful question because all answers are right from within the logic of the model in use. Rightness also is modular or relative.

A much more useful question is, How does this model serve its users? To be able to ask this question demands that one stand back dispassionately from one's own beliefs and models and recognize them as constructed and not exclusively correct. To ask this question is to practice *cultural relativity*.

Cultural relativity is a technique for dealing with the many ways in which people explain themselves. It tells practitioners and researchers to remain in a fairly neutral, nonjudgmental stance, *knowing the values of people without adopting or rejecting them* (Kaplan, 1984). From this position, clinicians, researchers, or students can observe their own perceptions and those of others and understand how these interpretations serve users' lives. They can avoid becoming mired in determining which method is true because nothing is really true when all realities are constructed.

On the other hand, ideas can be true in certain contexts or situations; that is, they make sense to their users. Therefore the observer must learn to synthesize his or her position with those of others, so as to design an effective response strategy. For example, if people think of penicillin as a cooling drug and therefore hesitate to use it to treat a "cold" illness such as pneumonia, the practitioner neutralizes the cold of penicillin by suggesting that the patient take the medicine along with a food perceived as "hot" (Harwood, 1977). Or, as in the first example cited previously, the clinician can refer a patient to a practitioner whose reality model more closely resembles that of the patient.

The practice of cultural relativity is pivotal to the study of alternative medicine because each alternative system of medicine provides a different set of ideas about the body, disease, and medical reality. Readers will find it much easier to absorb and use this material if they can willingly—even playfully—step aside

from their current beliefs and appreciations to let in new ones.

THE BEHAVIORAL FIELD OF HEALTH CARE

What belongs under the rubric of health care? Once we know, we can examine which components are addressed by which particular health care system because no single system addresses the whole.

The Field of Health Care From Ego's Point of View

Imagine that each person is immersed in a potential field of health care that instructs how to prevent illness, treat illness, and, more positively, enhance wellness. Figure 3-1 depicts this idea as three triangles (shown as nonoverlapping, although in reality they do overlap, at least partially). The three triangles are embedded in a semicircle labeled historical, cultural, and social environment, which reminds us that all health care is delivered within a context of experience, belief, and expectation that is not always obvious to us.

The central triangle deals with health care as it is delivered to groups of people, and the right and left triangles deal with health care that is received primarily by individuals or families. The small circle in the center represents a person, Ego,* to whom all the contents of the field are available. Lines at the bottom of the drawing mark the health condition, from increasing health (left) to decreasing health (right). The central triangle covers prevention, that is, the avoidance of sickness without seeking high-level wellness.

Each triangle is divided into three sections. Section 1 represents the forms of health care that Ego can seek and deliver without the intervention of a specialist. Some examples include praying, exercising, brushing teeth, bathing, drinking fruit juice, cleaning house, paying utility bills for receipt of electricity and pure water, taking dietary supplements, washing and bandaging minor wounds, and taking an analgesic or sleeping to treat a headache.

---

*Ego is used in the anthropological or geneological sense, that is, the person from whose point of view the figure is to be understood. It is not used in the common psychiatric sense, that is, the "I" that deals with reality.

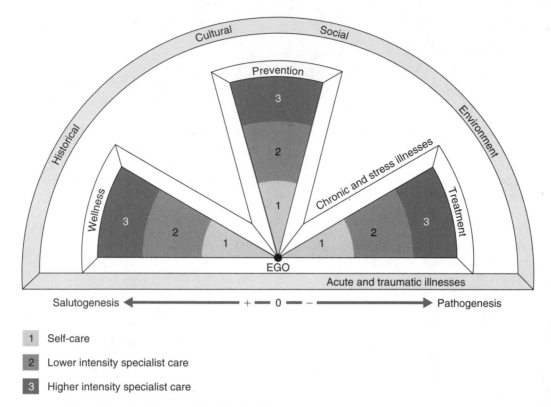

Figure 3-1 The behavioral field of health care from the perspective of an individual.

Section 2 represents a degree of complexity or severity that requires specialist intervention. Most health care needs fall at this level, and most health care systems deliver most care at this level. At this level of wellness we might find Ego seeking help with finding appropriate work, consulting a dietary specialist, taking a parenting class, or learning meditation techniques. Under treatment, we would find Ego seeking help for traumas, discomforts, or malfunctions that have not responded to home remedies or that Ego recognizes as requiring the attention of a specialist. This section also includes ongoing care and control of chronic conditions and handicaps. Prevention at this level involves preventive dental care, screening tests, vaccinations, and community prevention activities such as pure food and drug controls and pollution prevention—activities of which Ego is generally unaware and over which he or she has little control.

Section 3 represents a high degree of complexity and intensity that few specialists emphasize and that Ego calls on rarely. This level of treatment deals with extreme illnesses, malformations, and trauma, includ-

ing care that is delivered in emergency departments, operating rooms, and intensive care units. This level in the prevention triangle deals with responses to major catastrophes such as epidemics and earthquakes. In the wellness triangle it deals with an issue that is not easily expressed in English and is generally described in terms with psychological and spiritual overtones such as *self-actualization, enlightenment,* or *awakening.*

Note that the cost of health care rises from level 1 to 3, attaining the highest cost in the prevention and treatment triangles at level 3 but paradoxically potentially the lowest cost at wellness level 3.

Now having drawn and laid out this concept in a linear form, I must critique it. The alert reader already will be asking such questions as, What if Ego has diabetes and is taking all kinds of proactive steps to increase wellness despite his or her condition? What about healing communities that increase wellness for terminally ill patients? Where do healthy, pregnant women belong on this figure? These are appropriate criticisms: distinctions between the sections are not as precise in real life. A healthy woman who seeks a midwife's care during

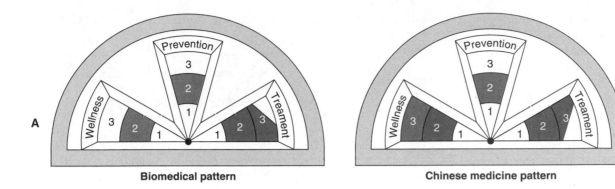

■ Strong emphasis
■ Moderate emphasis

Figure 3-2 The behavioral field of health care, highlighting the components addressed by two particular health care systems. **A,** Biomedical. **B,** Chinese medicine.

delivery might belong in wellness section 2, whereas one who delivers in a hospital with medical intervention belongs in treatment section 2—not because she is sick but because her pregnancy is being treated as if it were an illness, as it has been for most North American women in the latter half of the twentieth century. Only in the last few years has the situation been recognized and some effort toward demedicalizing it been made.

The Field of Health Care From the Point of View of the Variant Practices or Systems

Activities included in the wellness triangle in Figure 3-1 range from those that are widely accepted in our society such as diet and exercise to behaviors such as praying that many do not classify as health related. Why include them here?

The dominant biomedical system's materialist effort to segregate medicine from religion grew out of the secularist urge to embrace science at the turn of the century; this concept is artificial and is not shared by most of the world's health care systems. Indeed most systems accept the reality of the nonmaterial aspects of the body-person.

Sister Erma Allen once told me of having healed a small boy who had cut his head; she had silently said the [bloodstopping] verse over and over while at the same time applying ice to the wound. I asked how she knew

that it was not the *ice* that had stopped the bleeding. After a pause she reprimanded me gently, "God sewed it with *His* needle, darlin'" (Snow, 1993).

The fact that biomedicine prefers materialist explanations also implies that it does not deliver care in all parts of the triangles. Indeed this also is true for all other systems. Each emphasizes a distinctive viewpoint (explanatory model) and develops expertise in just some of the potential areas of health care. For example, biomedicine has had great success in treating acute illness and trauma. Its control of technology also allows for remarkable success in extending life and in producing pharmaceuticals and technology to address the physical and physiological components of chronic conditions. Simultaneously, however, biomedicine has been criticized for its relatively ineffective care of many chronic conditions and for repeated inefficiencies in human kindness and humane development, areas that tend to escape its materialist model.

Other systems, notably the so-called holistic systems, integrate human development into their usual care patterns. These systems also control technologies and techniques that address physical and physiological functioning. Patients praise these systems for their care of chronic conditions and for their efforts to enhance wellness, which include weaning patients from excessive dependence on health care specialists.

Figure 3-2 portrays these different approaches. Note that neither the biomedical system nor the

Chinese medical system deals much with prevention on a mass scale. That is the prerogative of different specialists, especially of public health specialists.

Two vital points emerge from the field discussion and will recur throughout this chapter:

1. No one health care system addresses the whole field.
2. All health care systems address a considerable part of it.

No one system is best for everything, and existing systems overlap considerably in what they offer. There is a temptation to argue that societies ought to achieve economies of scale by making sure only the best survive. However, considering our discussion of cultural relativity, it is impossible to define the "best" in a manner that satisfies everyone. Logic demands that we determine who will be served well by which system and why. We will return to this issue after discussing some of the important ways in which health care systems differ.

THE CULTURAL CONCEPT OF THE HEALTH CARE SYSTEM

A cultural medical system is a complex of beliefs, models, and linked activities that providers and users consider useful in bettering health or well-being and in relieving stress and disease (Box 3-1).

This definition makes it clear that a health care system is complex and multilayered. Even simple systems, such as those limited in scope to one self-defined ethnic group, are difficult for one person to master or describe. Larger systems are correspondingly more complex, encompassing a wide range of viewpoints, numerous subspecialties, and distinctive styles of practice. Biomedicine includes specialties ranging from the intensely material practice of surgery to the far more relational specialties of family medicine and psychiatry. Biomedical complexity is compounded by the fact that it is practiced rather differently in different countries.

Even the best simultaneous translator is going to have trouble dealing with the fact that *peptic ulcer* and *bronchitis* do not mean the same things in Britain that they do in the United States; that the U.S. *appendectomy* becomes the British *appendicectomy;* that the French tendency to exaggerate means there are never headaches in France, only

BOX 3-1

Components of a Health Care System

A developed theory of the body-person, known as the explanatory model (Kleinman, 1980). This theory includes the causes of malfunction, as well as appropriate ways to address this malfunction

Plans to educate and train new practitioners through apprenticeship, schooling, or both

A health care subsystem that delivers care to the needy

Associated means of producing substances or technologies necessary to delivery and educational subsystems

Professional organizations of practitioners who monitor each other's practices and promote the system to potential users

A legal mandate that provides for the official recognition of practitioners and maintains a minimum standard of quality

A social mandate that informally reveals levels of community acceptance, as by frequency of use, willingness to pay, and stereotypes about practitioners, among other markers

migraines, and that the French often refer to real migraines as 'liver crises'; that the German language has no word for chest pain, forcing the German patient to talk of heart pain, and that when a German doctor says 'cardiac insufficiency' he may simply mean that the patient is tired. . . . How can [bio]medicine, which is commonly supposed to be a science, . . . be so different in four countries whose peoples are so similar genetically? The answer is that while [bio]medicine benefits from a certain amount of scientific input, culture intervenes at every step of the way (Payer, 1988).

This complexity is equally true of Chinese medicine, which embraces many styles, including traditional Chinese medicine, Five Element style, and Japanese, Korean, and French styles. Even community-based or folk systems may have different specialties. Lakota (Sioux) people distinguish medicine men and women who emphasize herbal treatment from holy men and women who practice shamanically (Hultkrantz, 1985). The Dineh (Navajo) recognize three types of diagnosticians and singers who work with ritual, herbs, and the psychosocial body to deliver health care (Morgan, 1977).

On a much smaller scale than the system or the style is the technique of health care (Figure 3-3). A technique is comparatively simple; it might be single therapy and often can be practiced without being linked to an explanatory model, detailed training, or professional oversight. Some practitioners specialize in offering single therapies, such as bee-sting injections, colonic irrigations, biofeedback, specific dietary supplements, or Swedish massage.

Single-therapy practitioners can provide *symptomatic relief* to their patients, but they cannot provide *systematic care,* that is, care guided by a well-developed model of how the body-person works, how the malfunction arose, and how the technique can help. Indeed the expansive power and persistence of health care systems correlate with the effectiveness of their explanatory models and linked therapeutic modalities.

Systems Embedded in Larger Constructs

But where do explanatory models come from? As noted earlier, health care systems are embedded in the sociocultural system surrounding them. This provides not only access to natural resources but also ideas, assumptions, and patterns of logic. All these are reflected in explanatory models and health care delivery formats. In formal terms, health care systems are guided by the worldview principles of their society. The larger and more heterogeneous the surrounding society, the wider the range of health care ideas that society can encompass.

Nevertheless certain worldviews tend to predominate. In the United States and Europe the hierarchical or reductionistic worldview dominates. This worldview model emphasizes hierarchies of value (judgmentalism), a tendency to be judgmental, competition, forcefulness, and materialism (Cassidy, 1994). Biomedicine reflects these patterns in its concern for the expertise of the practitioner over that of the layperson or patient; its tendency to magnify the importance of some specialties or diseases over others (cardiology over pediatrics, cancer over asthma); its preference for treatment modalities that cause obvious reactions in the physical body; and its focus on end-stage physical malfunction while generally ignoring less-developed conditions and rejecting nonmaterial explanations of cause.

[Cartesian] assumptions permeate Western society and form the modus operandi of conventional medicine. They have led to our belief in rationalism, causality, objectivity, and the separation of [bio]medicine and psychiatry. The assumptions work very well in acute emergency situations, but are limited when illness becomes chronic. . . . Cartesian thinking can be classified broadly as yang, and its inferred opposite as yin. Chinese philosophic thought can therefore be seen to be inclusive of Western thought, while Western thought has no way of incorporating Chinese holistic thinking (Greenwood & Nunn, 1994).

Other Western health care systems literally originated in reaction to biomedicine (allopathy), including homeopathy, osteopathy, naturopathy, chiropractic, and Christian Science. Others have been imported from the East, like Chinese medicine and Ayurveda. All argue (not always convincingly) that their approaches to care are more egalitarian, less judgmental, and gentler than biomedicine. Several offer nonmaterialist explanations of cause and care. In making such arguments, these systems are calling on another worldview currently held in the United States, namely, the relational (ecological or holistic) worldview. This worldview sees all things as connected in a network of relationships and deals with how people, things, and energy interact and how these interactions can better the whole. Reflected into health care this idea means that practitioners model health in terms of achieving bal-

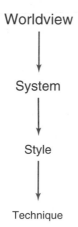

Worldview

System

Style

Technique

Figure 3-3 Scale of complexity in understanding health care.

ance, and patients are seen to have expertise different from that of the practitioner but expertise nonetheless. Thus practitioner and patient form a partnership, and patients take some responsibility for their own care and development.

Professionalized and Community-Based Systems

The terms *professionalized* and *community-based systems* distinguish between systems that serve large, heterogeneous patient populations and those smaller, more localized systems that serve culturally homogeneous populations.

A professionalized system tends to be found in an urban setting, is taught in schools with the aid of written texts, and demands formal, usually legal, criteria for practice (Foster & Anderson, 1978). Students enter the system by choice and are approved by entrance examinations. They become practitioners on completing a designated plan of study, passing more examinations, and, often, being licensed by the state or nation. Health care typically is delivered on a one practitioner–to–one patient basis in locales that have been set aside for this purpose, such as offices, clinics, and hospitals. Practitioners form membership organizations dedicated to policing their respective specialties and presenting them in a positive light to outsiders. The dominant health care systems of modern nations always are professionalized systems. Examples include Ayurveda, biomedicine, Chinese medicine, chiropractic, homeopathy, osteopathy, and Unani (the traditional system of Pakistan and neighboring Muslim nations).

Community-based systems, also known as folk or tribal systems, are less expanded than professionalized systems, although they may have equally complex explanatory models and equally lengthy histories. These systems are found in both urban and rural settings, and training is often by apprenticeship. People enter training sometimes by inheritance but most often by receiving a call from the unseen world, indicating that he or she has the special capacity necessary to become a healer. Training ends when the teacher considers the student ready to practice. Rather than written examinations, students are tested by practicing medicine under guidance; essentially the community itself determines

BOX 3-2

Community-Based Systems in North America

American Folk Medicine (Hand, 1976)
Black Elk, The Sacred Ways of a Lakota (Black Elk & Lyon, 1990)
Cry of the Eagle, Encounters with a Cree Healer (Young et al., 1989)
Ethnic Medicine in the Southwest (Spicer, 1979)
Healing Traditions, Alternative Medicine and the Health Professions (O'Conner, 1995)
Herbal and Magical Medicine (Kirkland et al., 1992)
Masters of the Ordinary (Scott, 1993)
Powwowing in Union Country, A Study of Pennsylvania German Folk Medicine in Context (Reimansnyder, 1989)
Ritual Healing in Suburban America (McGuire, 1994)
Susto (Rubel et al., 1984)
This Other Kind of Doctors (Terrell, 1990)
Walkin' Over Medicine (Snow, 1993)

whether a student is "good enough." Care is often offered in people's homes, and community-based healers often practice on a part-time basis. Some folk healers form professional associations, with the same goals as professionalized doctors. Examples of community-based systems include Alcoholics Anonymous and similar urban self-help groups, Curanderismo (among the most expanded of folk systems), rootwork (an African-derived system used by some African-Americans), and traditional health care in Native American and Euro-American rural groups.

Box 3-2 provides sources for details about community-based systems in North America.

A third type is often called popular health care. Popular health care is not organized systematically; rather, it consists of simple techniques associated with the care of particular conditions. Examples include using cranberry juice for bladder infections, chicken soup for colds, and hot toddies for sore throats. Much of what is published in general-reader magazines or discussed on talk shows is popular medicine. It is typically presented using biomedical terminology and is often simplified biomedicine.

Distinctions of complexity among health care systems are not absolute. For example, most professionalized systems continue to insist on considerable hands-on training, similar to apprenticeships. Some folk systems, especially urbanized ones, train practitioners in schools and do not expect students to have received a call to practice; these practitioners often earn their living through full-time health care work.

Language Issues

Distinctions made in this section deal with differences of scale. A system is remarkably more complex than a technique or a single therapy; a professionalized system is expanded further than a community-based system. Failing to understand this point can lead to confusion. For example, one writer claims that "Subjects were presented with a list of 32 alternative therapies" (Furnham, 1992). The list includes practices of completely different scale, from systems that take years to learn (acupuncture, homeopathy, and anthroposophical medicine) to techniques that one receives as a gift (dowsing) or can learn in a few weeks (reflexology, iridology). The worst form of confusing scalars occurs when someone directly compares a technique and a system, does not account for differences of complexity, and concludes that the system failed.

One must be aware of terms that lend themselves to scalar confusion. The single term *acupuncture* can refer to a system, an approach, or simply a needling technique. Which does a given writer or speaker mean? Massage can mean a single technique, or it can refer to a rapidly professionalizing and systematizing practice. Some people use the term *medicine* to refer exclusively to biomedicine; for most, however, medicine is a term that encompasses all the ways in which people deliver health care.

Another confusing term is *traditional*. Biomedical publications often refer to their own practice as traditional medicine, categorizing all other practices by a term such as *alternative*. However, when biomedicine is referred to as modern medicine, its worldwide nature is being contrasted with the indigenous systems of non-Western societies, which are then called traditional. Of course, systems other than biomedicine are used worldwide, so all major

systems are sometimes classified as the "Great Tradition" systems and other systems, in contrast, as little tradition or folk systems.

In summary, it is most effective to refer to health care systems by their specific names and to clearly distinguish the scale of which one wishes to speak or write.

MODALITIES OF HEALTH CARE

Whatever the other aspects of their character, all health care systems and techniques care for people by trying to change some aspect of their functioning. Common interventions include surgery, pharmaceutical injection or ingestion, biologicals or botanicals, needling, dietary management, manipulation, massage, meditative exercises, dancing, music therapy, art therapy, water and heat treatments, bioenergetic manipulation (touch therapy), talk therapy, shamanic journeying, sitting meditation, and prayer.

Most health care systems use several of these modalities. A community-based system like Curanderismo uses dietary manipulation, herbs, first aid techniques, and shamanic techniques to treat a wide range of physical, psychosocial, and spiritual malfunctions. Ayurveda offers surgery, a variety of water treatments from purges to baths, numerous biological and herbal remedies, dietary management, and both sitting and moving forms of meditation.

Some modalities are more invasive than others. Some enter the physical body by cutting, pricking, or ingesting, and others do not break even this barrier. The second break is between those that touch the surface of the body and others that work with energetic or spiritual levels of the body that can be accessed without touching the skin. Even among those that break into the body there are differing degrees of intensity: Replacing a hip is more intrusive than removing a cataract. Pharmaceutical drugs generally are more toxic than phytomedicines (semipurified plant medicines), which are in turn more forceful than herbs. Forcefulness does not connote effectiveness: Mild and gentle modalities can be as effective as intrusive ones if properly administered.

Figure 3-4 sorts the modalities along a line indicating the level of invasiveness into the physical body. Sorting from intensely to lightly invasive procedures

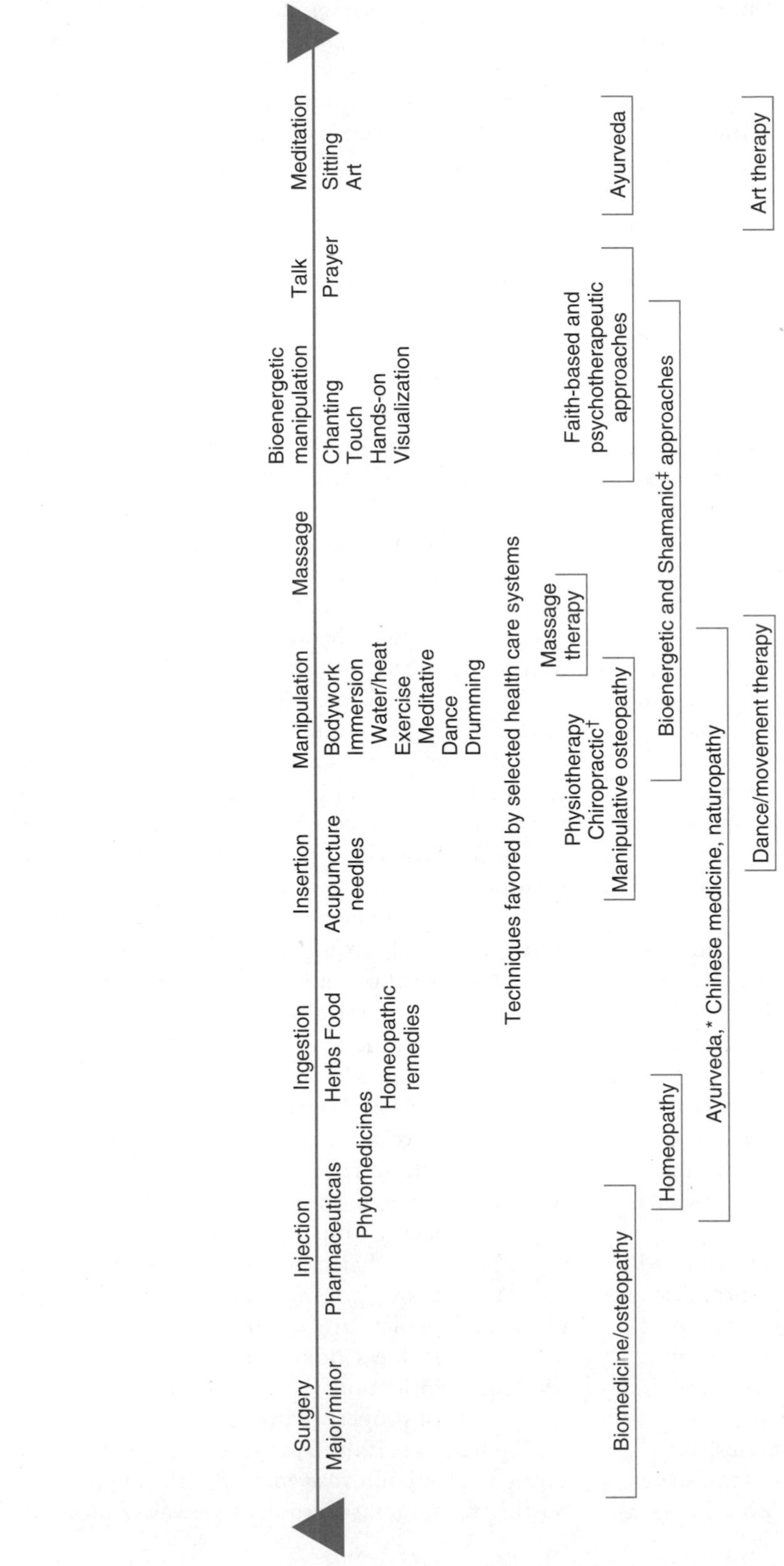

Surgery	Injection	Ingestion	Insertion	Manipulation	Massage	Bioenergetic manipulation	Talk	Meditation
Major/minor	Pharmaceuticals Phytomedicines	Herbs Food Homeopathic remedies	Acupuncture needles	Bodywork Immersion Water/heat Exercise Meditative Dance Drumming		Chanting Touch Hands-on Visualization	Prayer	Sitting Art

Techniques favored by selected health care systems

Biomedicine/osteopathy

Homeopathy

Ayurveda,* Chinese medicine, naturopathy

Physiotherapy
Chiropractic†
Manipulative osteopathy

Massage therapy

Bioenergetic and Shamanic‡ approaches

Dance/movement therapy

Faith-based and
psychotherapeutic
approaches

Ayurveda

Art therapy

* Ayurveda also provides minor surgery.
† Some chiropractors offer dietary management, acupuncture needling, etc.
‡ Many Shamanic practitioners also provide herbs.

Figure 3-4 Relative physical invasiveness of selected therapeutic techniques.

correlates with a movement from materialist to non-materialist views of the body-person. Also, actual health care systems roughly correlate with certain areas of the line, further evidence that each system emphasizes certain parts of, but not the entire spectrum of, health care options.

EXPLANATORY MODELS

We have discussed how health care systems intervene, but we have yet to understand the "madness" behind each method. Each system has its own explanatory model that summarizes the perceptions, assumptions, beliefs, theories, and facts that guide the logic of health care delivery. To develop the idea of the explanatory model, we will explore how different systems perceive the body-person and sickness and disease, their preferred causal explanations, and the preferred relationship between patients and practitioner.

Concepts of the Body-Person

There is not one human body, not one anatomy, not one physiology, but many. To understand any system, we must understand its concept of the body. Figure 3-5 depicts the body-person as four intersecting circles. The figure is simplified, for even within each of the circles there are many ways in which systems can phrase their material, energetic, spiritual, or social perceptions of the body.

The biomedical model of the body-person focuses on the physical body, concerning itself with the structure of its tissues and the movement and transformation of chemicals within cells. Classic chiropractic and osteopathic* models of the body are equally materialistic, emphasizing connections and communications between bones, nerves, and muscles and the rest of the physical body.

Homeopathy views the physical body as having three significant layers and the body-person as having three distinct aspects (Vithoulkas, 1980). Each of these layers and aspects is imbued with *vital spirit* or *vital energy,* and this energy is the ultimate focus of health care delivery. Acupuncture analyzes the physical body in terms of the flow of energy through pathways, or *meridians,* that have not yet been shown to have material counterparts. The energy that flows through and animates the material body is called *qi (ch'i, ki)* and closely resembles the homeopathic concept of vital spirit or the Ayurvedic concept of *prana.*

Biofield or bioenergetic therapies intervene in bodies outside the physical body that are sometimes spoken of as emanations and that can be perceived as *auras.* Different specialists perceive and name auras somewhat differently. Wirkus, using bioscience terminology, writes of the thermal, electromagnetic, and acoustic fields (Wirkus, 1993), whereas Brennan, using esoteric science terminology, labels the same three

---

*Osteopathy originated as a manipulative system. Today only a minority of practitioners maintain this tradition; the remainder practice biomedicine (allopathy) or a combination.

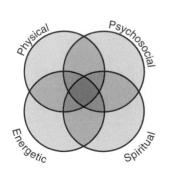

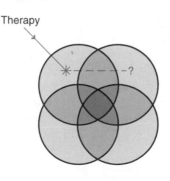

**Therapeutic goal assumption
of materialist systems**

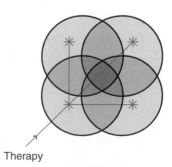

**Therapeutic goal assumption
of nonmaterialist systems**

Figure 3-5 The four bodies addressed by health care.

auras the etheric, astral, and mental bodies (Brennan, 1988).

Spiritual and shamanic healers also work with nonmaterial and normally invisible bodies. Most of these healers believe that these spiritual forces imbue the physical body, although some say they extend beyond it, and some say that parts can travel (as during sleep), be removed (exorcism), or lost (Eliade, 1964; Ingerman, 1991).

Psychotherapists and shamanic healers typically work with the psychosocial body, that is, the "person" who lives within the other bodies and interacts with the world outside. Terms for this being include *mind* and *emotions,* as well as technical terms that each subspecialty uses to showcase its particular explanatory model.

The several bodies are not, of course, separate: only one body-person stands before the practitioner seeking help. But who can say where the physical body, with its ongoing chemical and electrical changes, merges into the energetic body and where the latter extends into the spiritual body? All are immersed in the psychosocial body; what a person believes markedly affects how he or she will respond to illness and to treatment or what he or she will deliver in the way of health care.

With the exception of heavily materialist models that perceive themselves as treating the physical body and only reluctantly acknowledge the psychosocial body, all health care systems argue that there are both material and nonmaterial aspects to the body (see Figure 3-5). Intervention in one area will affect all others. When a Five Element acupuncturist needles a patient who is having an asthma attack, he or she enters the energetic body and moves energy. In addition, he or she expects the physical, psychosocial, and spiritual bodies to respond: the bronchial tubes will dilate, and pain, anxiety, and fear will dissipate. These changes do not occur coincidentally; according to this system's explanatory model, all the aspects of the body can work at ease when energy flows smoothly.

CONCEPTS OF SICKNESS, DISEASE, AND IMBALANCE

Although often used generically, the term *sickness* formally refers to an experience of discomfort or malfunction. Disease and imbalance, however, are abstracted concepts. Thus a person has an illness or sickness, and a practitioner assigns meaning to this experience by diagnosing and explaining what has happened. The answers provided by the practitioner are guided by the explanatory model of his or her health care system. Cultural learning also guides the expression of the patient's illness and the practitioner's diagnostic values, so much so that even the pain people feel and report is related to such learned aspects of being as gender and ethnicity (Bates et al., 1995).

A system's preferred malfunction concept is closely linked to its perception of the body-person, particularly whether a system tends to perceive cause as primarily external or internal (Cassidy, 1982, 1995; Fabrega, 1974; Foster & Anderson, 1978; Murdock, 1980). Most health care systems accept that both occur, although most also prefer to emphasize either the invader or the responding organism. External models argue that malfunctions attack from outside the body-person, invading and destroying. Internal models argue that something must first go wrong internally, thereby allowing outer influences to penetrate where they could not have before. These conceptual differences affect each system's views of patient and practitioner. External theorists see the patient as passive and the practitioner as authority, whereas internal ideology interprets the patient as responsible and the practitioner as partner to that responsibility.

Disease

The concept of disease is preferred by external models. The body-person is relatively passive, whereas the surrounding environment is teaming with danger. Body-persons are thought to respond similarly to invaders; that is, one person with mumps, leukemia, or pneumonia experiences it much as others do. If people are similar and the environment is dangerous, emphasis is placed on the actions of the invader, and every different type of invader creates a different disease. These assumptive patterns lead to the possible existence of many different diseases, and a major function of practitioners is to distinguish between them, or diagnose. Their second job is to remove, destroy, or immobilize invaders, thereby curing the patient.

This model has long been preferred by biomedicine and has yielded familiar metaphors. Tumor cells and microorganisms that have been awaiting their chance in reservoirs invade human victims. The body wages war, and surgeons and doctors are warriors in white, battling the invaders.* Diseases that fit this classic model have distinctive symptoms and signs, single causes, and respond to specific therapies. Treatment results in cure. To emphasize the separation between ailments and patients, the former often are called *disease entities*.

Only a minority of the disease entities defined by biomedicine fits the invasion model. Chronic, degenerative, and stress-related disorders frustrate the system because they do not have specifiable boundaries, single causes, or predictable outcomes. Indeed, they force biomedicine to consider explanations that fall outside the usual framework: that the body-person is not passive but plays some part in the genesis of disease; that many (often unspecifiable) factors must interact before disease arises; that some of these factors might be psychosocial; and that the practitioner's role is less to prescribe than to educate. The area of biomedicine that best reflects this opening state of mind is that of "lifestyle" diseases, or conditions that arise from and can be ameliorated by changes in how people behave and believe. Interestingly, even this door has not opened too widely: most lifestyle discussions still focus on ameliorative factors that address the physical body, such as diet and exercise. Biomedical practitioners who recommend visualization or meditation are likely to consider themselves avant-garde.

Chiropractic and osteopathy share biomedicine's mechanistic view of disease. In these systems, misalignment within the musculoskeletal system can cause malfunctions in other parts of the physical body. The explanatory model states that if the core misalignment can be alleviated, the distant malfunctions will resolve. The cause of misalignment is usually external (a fall, a twist, a jolt, or habitually poor posture) and sometimes internal (that poor posture is related to poor self-image). Patient instructions tend to take a physical form, such as modifications of diet and exercise.

Imbalance

A larger number of health care systems emphasize internal models of disorder and speak of imbalance

rather than disease. Their therapeutic goal is to return the person to a state of balance. These systems often name conditions according to their process within the person: For example, in Chinese medicine, *rising liver fire* describes a person's condition momentarily or repeatedly but is not a freestanding and categorical concept like the biomedical disease entity hepatitis.

Balance can be perturbed by external invaders or by interruptions in the smooth working of the internal milieu. External causes, however, cannot harm a body-person who is well. Health care therefore tends to the self-protective abilities of the body-person, maintaining and strengthening them. This is not curing but healing; the practitioner's goal is not to battle the invader or to fix the patient but rather to prune, weed, and plant within the patient, enabling him or her to grow a vibrant internal garden in which all aspects of his or her body-person coexist with the vagaries of the external environment.

Treatment within internal-cause systems is individualistic because the logic of this model is such that each person has a unique history and constitution that affects how he or she will respond to the myriad circumstances of life. The practitioner examines the current condition of the patient, relates it to his or her social and medical history, and then selects therapy on the basis of the entire assessment.

Diet, exercise, rest, and other physical interventions might be prescribed, but these recommendations usually are offered in formats that also address the spiritual and energetic bodies, such as yoga, t'ai chi, or Qigong or moving meditations might be recommended for exercise. The person might be advised to develop his or her spiritual and emotional body through creative skills such as art, dance, and chanting. Or the patient may be encouraged to minimize his or her vulnerability to psychic attack by meditation, shamanic journeying, or prayer. The patient may be counseled to modify diet not only as to nutrient content but also as to seasonal appropriateness and essential (as opposed to literal) temperature.

Constitutional Types

The disease entity and imbalance models represent ideals. Practitioners recognize that neither model works all the time. Thus biomedicine recognizes conditions such as syndromes or chronic diseases have

---

*Similar metaphors are used to describe the need for exorcism: Invasion by an evil entity demands a spiritual battle to defeat it. Faith-based systems that use exorcism therapeutically also use external models of disease causation.

multiple linked causes, not all of which can be specified. Similarly, internal-cause systems recognize that individuality is not absolute because people do present commonalities or patterned responses to similar challenges.

In fact many health care systems have developed sophisticated models to link certain constitutional types with the probability of their developing particular illnesses. In the European and Middle Eastern system that preceded biomedicine, persons were categorized as melancholic, phlegmatic, sanguine, or choleric. Although today's biomedical practitioners may view these concepts with an indulgent smile, the underlying idea is by no means absent in modern biomedicine: Earlier in this century bioscientists attempted to link physical and psychosocial diseases with the endomorphic, mesomorphic, and ectomorphic types (Sheldon et al., 1949). Today there is much interest in type A personalities, which are said to be prone to heart disease, and type C, prone to cancer. Constitutional typologies are well developed in the Ayurvedic system (the *doshas* of *pitta, vata, kapha*) and in some styles of Chinese medicine (the five central foci of Worsley-style Five Element acupuncture). The old European categories survive in the hot-cold systems of Latin America and the Philippines.

Figure 3-6 summarizes the data of this section on a linear model. The disease entities model of biomedicine forms one extreme on a continuum, with the process-related imbalance models at the other end. At the midpoint are patterned responses, including constitutional types. At the end featuring diseases the individual person essentially has been deleted from the argument "one person suffers much like others so focus on identifying the disease," whereas at the other extreme the person is the final focus and arbiter of interpretation ("in this individual these symptoms mean *x*, which I know from experience of him/her . . . they may mean *y* in another individual"). In the middle are positions that share both interpretive energies: "Certain characteristics make it more likely that he or she will experience these symptoms, so perhaps I can reduce my diagnostic chore."

Language Issues

Biomedical disease entities have become standard vocabulary, but these diseases (not the symptoms) are real only to people who use the biomedical model. Practitioners of other systems may use these terms out of familiarity to communicate with patients or granting agencies or to complete insurance claim forms, but within their own system of health care, these labels have no real cogency. Acupuncturists, for example, treat what their patients and referring physicians call "depression," but the concept does not exist in Chinese medicine. In the Five Element model there are at least five different ways people can express what biomedicine labels depression. Thus two patients with the same biomedical diagnosis of depression might receive quite different herbal or needle therapies from a Chinese medicine practitioner.

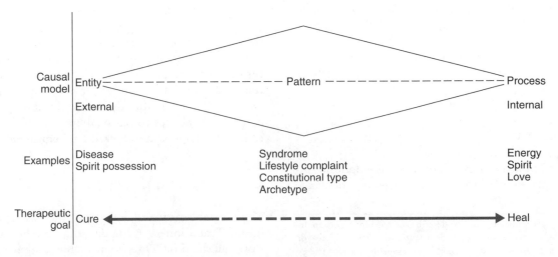

Figure 3-6 Three major approaches to interpreting symptoms.

Practitioners and scientists must be careful in their use of biomedical terminology, not assuming it is sufficient to describe what is understood by other systems. Specialists should describe the symptoms and then, if they wish, affix a biomedical label while clearly stating that the biomedical label may not reflect the way of knowing of another system. This can serve because symptoms are recognized everywhere; it is the interpretations that differ. By focusing on symptoms, the malfunction labels of the other systems would begin to take on the kind of reality that now is owned only by the biomedical labels. The medical conversation would become more accurate and broader.

Concepts of Deep Cause

External and internal causative factors mentioned so far can be understood as proximate causes of malfunction. With the issue of deep cause, we contemplate why *this* person at *this* time or in *this* place has become ill in *this* way. We want to consider sociocultural answers, not epidemiological ones. We will explore the issue first by returning to our discussion of the body-person and considering the developmental nature of sickness, and second by considering the intentional component of sickness.

The Developmental Nature of Sickness

An ancient chicken-and-egg philosophical argument questions whether the physical body comes first, giving rise to nonmaterial constructs such as emotions and mind, or whether mind (spirit, soul) comes first and animates the physical body. Materialist models prefer the first argument, whereas nonmaterialist models favor the second.

This choice affects both the theory and politics of health care. One can only deliver care in a fashion that does not conflict with one's beliefs. If one accepts as real only what one can see, hear, or measure with machines, then delivering care to the nonmaterial bodies is at the very least puzzling. Efforts to test nonmaterialist systems include designing machinery to "prove" the nonmaterial bodies exist, such as using electrical point locators to find acupuncture points and meridians, or Kirlian photography to find auras.

Materialists suspect nonmaterialist practitioners of misleading their patients or of achieving effects primarily by activating the placebo response. Cynics also argue that nonmaterialist practitioners have their greatest successes in the care of functional, or psychosomatic, diseases. Such diseases are disvalued in materialist systems precisely because they lack specific material signs such as germs, malfunctioning genes, tumor cells, abnormal metabolic values, or broken bones. Those who have functional conditions are suspected of not being really sick.

Nonmaterialist thinkers consider malfunction in the nonmaterial aspects of the body to be as real as physical malfunction. All patient complaints signal true distress; the diagnostic concern is not with triaging between the real and the imaginary but with identifying what aspect of the person will respond most efficaciously to treatment.

Many such systems use a developmental model of malfunction in which sickness starts in the nonmaterial bodies and is expressed in the physical body only later. They fault materialist systems for paying attention only to end-stage malfunction and failing to treat conditions before they become entrenched. They further argue that a focus on the material level alone provides only symptomatic relief and ignores deep cause, allowing underlying malfunctions to remain unaddressed. Nonmaterialist systems assume that care can modify all parts of the body-person. Some also claim that as the person heals, he or she cycles backward through layers of long-buried symptoms until finally they express the oldest symptoms, release them, and are well. This pattern is called the "law of cure."

From the adjoining room she heard friends, who could not see her, discussing some of the slanderous stories being circulated about her. Rachel was crushed. When she [arrived home] one of the servants thought she looked as if she had been shot through the heart. Questioned about why she looked so dejected, she started to sob and then to cry uncontrollably as she poured out her experiences of the day. . . . Several days later Rachel suffered a heart attack (Huber, 1990).

To give an example, a child might experience a spiritual trauma such as loss of intimacy. Afterward this child has eczema. Later still the child has allergies and asthma. Untreated, the original spiritual wound or deep cause has been magnified and becomes overt and disabling. Appropriate treatment of the asthma not only will relieve wheezing but also might instigate a recrudescence of eczema and grief. Depending on the system, these results may be expected to occur in sequence or simultaneously.

Thus by the logic of internal-cause systems it is advantageous to treat complaints before malfunction is manifested physically. Even nonmaterial complaints are real because any suffering affects the whole body-person.

Systems that use only nonmaterial therapies, such as bioenergetic healing, psychotherapy, and shamanism, focus care on the nonmaterial aspects of the person but expect that the physical body will respond. However, many systems use a combination of material and nonmaterial therapeutic modalities. The techniques themselves often have a layered character; needling acupuncture points have specific physical and specific spiritual and emotional effects. For example, the same is true of herbal remedies and bodywork. Patients are cared for by the material, energetic, and spiritual actions of the specific therapies, and it is assumed that their physical, mental, emotional, spiritual, and energetic bodies all will respond and change.

Nonmaterialist models also view the person as having an active role in creating and treating his or her own condition. The role of practitioner is reformulated from authority to facilitator, from the one who does the curing to the one who helps the person heal himself or herself. As treatment is administered, such practitioners encourage patients to consider what attitudes of mind or spirit may have played a part in their illness and to explore new, life-enhancing ways of believing and behaving—wellness training. The goals of nonmaterialist health care are to care for the nonsomatic aspects of the patient so completely that the somatic aspect rarely suffers.

Unfortunately, in the hands of some practitioners the focus on patient responsibility becomes excessive and patients feel guilt about their sickness. The materialist emphasis on the patient as the victim of disease can be equally harmful, resulting in patients who feel helpless to change themselves or learn health-enhancing behaviors.

The Intentional Component of Sickness

Practitioners discuss proximate and deep causes of sickness; medical social scientists recognize another cross-cutting domain of causality and contrast—naturalistic and personalistic explanatory approaches. According to the naturalistic approach, the causes of sickness are found in the natural world and lack intention; they cause malfunction by unintentionally ending up in the wrong place. Sickness is considered a normal experience of life, natural and inevitable. The personalistic approach, however, maintains that some form of intention is present, and sickness is considered to be an unnatural result of attracting the attention of the wrong energies or a response to one's own misbehavior or misperception (Foster & Anderson, 1978).

When a person says he or she has lung cancer and attributes it to 30 years of smoking, he or she speaks in a naturalistic mode. But if the person complains of having been inveigled into smoking or that this habit is an expression of weak character, he or she is moving in a personalistic direction. If people attribute their cancer to the corrective or punitive actions of a spiritual entity such as God, they speak fully in the personalistic mode.

These tendencies coexist in most health care systems, although one or the other usually is emphasized. Professionalized health care systems generally prefer such naturalistic explanations as microorganisms, malformations, toxins, age-related degeneration, winds, hot and cold, or damp and dry. But within these systems, some practitioners recognize, even specialize in, the personalistic approach. In biomedicine, psychiatry and psychology emphasize this structure, usually attributing malfunction to troubles in the psychosocial body rather than in the spiritual or energetic bodies; in other major systems, practitioners deal with expressions of self-distrust or the results of psychic attacks much as they deal with physical conditions.

Faith-based systems are primarily personalistic in approach. They ask patients to confess ways in which they have angered God, who may have retaliated by sending disease. Some also recognize invasion by evil spiritual entities and offer exorcism as a treatment. Prayer is offered to alleviate pain and prevent sickness; some faith-based systems also practice the "laying on of hands."

"But she seems to be an intelligent woman," one family practitioner kept repeating as he told me of the woman who had refused the surgical removal of uterine fibroids. What he viewed as a completely medical (and secular) situation his patient took to be a tangible sign of divine displeasure . . . God would heal her if it would be his will; no scalpels necessary (Snow, 1993).

Shamanic systems combine naturalistic and personalistic approaches. Natural events, such as experiencing a severe emotional or physical shock or fright, may cause parts of the soul to be lost. The shaman recognizes the situation from the symptoms and takes a spiritual journey to retrieve the soul parts. Again, a person with an insufficient degree of psychic protection may be psychically attacked by someone else, either purposefully, during an argument, or even by being looked at with envious eyes. The shaman's task is to heal the psychospiritual wound and then help the patient to develop stronger personal protective skills. (Shamans also serve communities by mediating arguments, changing weather, and treating physical illness with herbs and psychospiritual support.)

Notice that the naturalistic-personalistic frame cuts across the materialist-nonmaterialist frame. Naturalistic explanations often deal with causes that are nonmaterial, like temperature changes or wind invasions. Similarly, personalistic explanations can be materialist; some people see, hear, or feel entities such as ghosts or spirits, and material objects can store nonmaterial energies and can be used to heal or harm. But most importantly, even when the system and practitioner prefer naturalistic explanations, patients regularly demand to know "why me, Lord?" and offer answers couched in the personalistic framework.

CONCEPTS OF THE PRACTITIONER-PATIENT RELATIONSHIP

Systems that prefer external causative models characteristically view the body-person as passive, a victim, and, logically enough, interpret the practitioner as active, the one who cures. By contrast, systems that prefer internal causative models view the body-person as active and as already capable of healing. The job of the practitioner is to facilitate the discovery of this capacity and develop it. The patient in this model has life expertise, and the practitioner must use his or her specialized expertise in partnership with the patient.

Of course, some patients will be passive no matter what is asked of them, and equally, some always will demand a say in their care. The biomedical literature discusses this issue under the rubrics of external and internal locus of control. However, the point made in this chapter is that not just practitioners, not just patients, but entire systems are modeled to emphasize one style of caregiving. Systems that want patients to be passive find active patients frustrating, irritating, and intrusive; systems that want patients to be active find passive patients unresponsive, helpless, and in denial.

A lucid practitioner might be able to match his or her style to the patient's needs, providing either authoritarian or relational (patient-centered) care to fit the situation. But practitioners too have preferences and personal styles that cannot be modified easily. Students might even select health care practices that fit their personal styles.

MAKING SENSE OF ALL THE VARIABILITY

The chapter began with the claim that health care systems vary in many ways and that the variety can be analyzed with the help of conceptual models. How can this information be applied in a world in which patients use many health care modalities and in which practitioners are advised to understand and sympathize?

This section explores this question by discussing an example that compares biomedicine and Chinese medicine. We have developed a conceptual map that allows any system to be rapidly compared with another. We will end by summarizing what makes biomedicine unusual, yet convinced that it is normative.

A Comparison of Care in Two Medical Systems

As discussed, biomedicine prefers reductionistic, categorical explanatory models, whereas Chinese medicine prefers relational, process-related explanatory models (for more detail see Beinfield & Korngold, 1991; Kaptchuk, 1983; Lock & Gordon, 1988; Stein, 1990). Both are heterogeneous systems, so relational tendencies can be found in biomedicine, and categorical tendencies exist in Chinese medicine. How different do these preferences really make these two systems?

Similarities of Biomedicine and Chinese Medicine

Both aim to provide comprehensive health care, which includes health-enhancing, preventive, reproductive, acute and chronic illness, and trauma care.

Both prefer to deliver care in specific locales such as clinics or hospitals and in practitioner to patient dyads; group-based and home- or community-based practices are viewed as possible but non-modal.

Both prefer naturalistic explanations of malfunction, arguing that impersonal forces are the main sources of ill health. However, if sometimes reluctantly, both also recognize that personalistic explanations sometimes make sense.

Both subsume a wide range of practices or specialties. Although specialties within internal medicine represent the intensively reductionistic naturalistic components of biomedicine, psychiatry veers toward personalistic explanatory models, and immunotherapy, clinical ecology, and approaches emphasizing lifestyle intervention use a relational flavor. Again, although Five Element acupuncture aims to be primarily relational and holistic in outlook, the post-1949 traditional Chinese medicine style veers toward the reductionistic model and borrows many ideas from biomedicine.

Differences Between Biomedicine and Chinese Medicine

Biomedicine focuses on trauma, acute illness, and end-stage chronic disease intervention. Although prevention is discussed as part of biomedical care, wellness is a concept that may not always be stressed. Chinese medicine emphasizes wellness and preventive care, treats chronic and acute illness conditions, but pays little attention to trauma (see Figure 3-2).

Biomedicine emphasizes materialist explanations, whereas Chinese medicine emphasizes nonmaterialist explanations based on a distinctive concept of qi (ch'i, vital energy). Indeed, their views of anatomy and physiology and their favored bodily metaphors (machinery and warring vs gardening) are distinctly different.

Biomedicine emphasizes the physical body as the locus for intervention, recognizes but remains uncomfortable with the concept of the psychosocial body, and largely denies the existence of the energetic and spiritual bodies. By contrast, Chinese medicine uses the energetic body as the locus for intervention and assumes that interventions at that level will redound on all the other bodies.

Biomedicine sees human beings as biologically similar; therefore diseases will present similarly and can be treated similarly. Chinese medicine sees each human being as unique and assumes that even if symptoms appear to be similar, the deep cause might be dissimilar; and thus care should be delivered individualistically.

Biomedicine has defined an immense universe of distinct disease entities, assumes they will present similarly in most people, focuses much energy on diagnosis, and defines success as cure. Controlling or palliating symptoms is considered a lesser success, and death is commonly thought of as a failure. Chinese medicine focuses on the flow of energy within the body and between the patient and the cosmos. Ill health arises when this flow is disrupted or impeded or when there is insufficient energy. Because this can happen in many ways, the practitioner spends much time assessing the character of the flow, both by hearing the patient's story and by listening in to the energetic body (for example, taking the pulses). Imbalance is viewed as commonplace and natural, and there is little to cure; instead the practitioner hopes to maintain or improve the coherence of the body-person, that is, heal the person. Death is also deemed natural; the dying patient can use acupuncture to ease pain and to achieve a final energetic balance.

Conceptual Mapping of Health Care Systems

It is possible to map differences among health care systems to allow these similarities and differences to be rapidly grasped and applied. Figure 3-2 maps the systems in terms of individual needs; Figure 3-7 redraws Figure 3-2 in terms of the conceptual models explored in this chapter.

Figure 3-7 shows a matrix with the categorical (reductionistic) vs relational (process-related) worldview represented on the horizontal axis and the naturalistic to personalistic causal model on the vertical axis. A third axis (not shown) might appropriately deal with delivery issues, especially whether care is delivered to individuals or to communities.

Using this map, we can—hypothetically—locate virtually any system of health care in such a way as to rapidly compare it with another system. Knowing more about the terrain of systematic health care differences makes it easier to understand and use the insights from other systems of health care. Practitioners can use information to design research, to make themselves and their patients aware of their own prejudices, and to listen more openly to the users of different health care systems.

Figure 3-7 maps only the two systems cited in our example; readers are encouraged to map others as they learn about them in this text. Note that each of the two systems mapped, however, covers a wide area. Biomedicine, although clearly within the realm of categorical naturalistic thinking, spills over the horizontal line into personalistic models (psychology, psychiatry) and over the vertical line into relational territory (family practice, aspects of immunology, lifestyle arguments). In fact, biomedical practice overlaps the Chinese medicine outline at the center of the figure.

The map also shows that in terms of preferred worldview, Chinese medicine is opposite that of biomedicine. On the other hand, it is similar to biomedicine in its general preference for naturalistic causal explanations. These twin characteristics map it into

the upper right quadrant. Note again, however, the wide range of practice under the umbrella of Chinese medicine. The more symptomatic and categorical styles of practice map left toward the reductionistic quadrant, and the traditional shamanistic components of Chinese medicine map below the horizontal line.

We are reminded by this map that no single health care system serves the whole field, and that systems differ but also share similarities.

Biomedicine's Findings of the Other Systems to Be Unconventional

Although not drawn onto the map, the other health care systems tend to cluster more centrally or to the right of the center on both sides of the horizontal axis. Thus the mapping exercise also provides a visual clue as to why biomedicine, from its perch in the upper left quadrant, might find the other systems un-

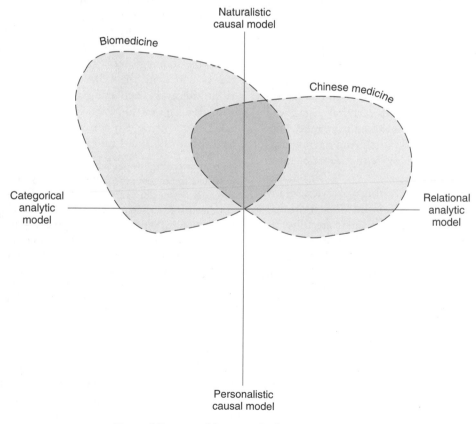

Figure 3-7 A cognitive map for health care systems.

conventional. They are nonmodal when judged from biomedicine's position. Of course, biomedicine is equally unconventional when viewed from the position of most systems. From a worldwide viewpoint biomedicine is unusual in the following ways:

1. Its intense attachment to materialist interpretive models
2. Its focus on the physical body, almost to the exclusion of other possibilities
3. Its focus on the disease, often to the virtual exclusion of the person
4. Its vast development of disease types
5. Its highly technological delivery system
6. The invasiveness of its care modalities
7. Its emphasis on acute disease, trauma, and end-stage malfunction, with relatively little focus on prevention or wellness
8. Its high cost

Despite these oddities, biomedicine considers itself conventional and other systems "alternative." How did this situation come about, and why is it not surprising to most people? Why is it difficult for people to consider biomedicine as just one more alternative?

Health care is not free of culture or politics. In the United States, we are accustomed to thinking of biomedicine as the best because it is the most expansive, being practiced in every country in the world, although acupuncture and homeopathy run close seconds. It also has the largest educational, legal, and economic mandate. Finally, its explanatory model fits the dominant European and North American worldview paradigm—categorical or reductionistic—most closely.

As part of the expression of this worldview, many say biomedicine is the most scientific. This argument is a slippery one and must be examined carefully.

Science is a particular method for gathering information and constructing knowledge. In contrast to other systems such as theology, which allows for revelation, and law, which allows for precedence, science demands that information be sought in the natural world and that interpretations be tested for accuracy. This is extremely unusual; it means that a person's opinion or mere observation and consequent certitude are not enough to make his or her position acceptable to scientists. Instead, the person must show that he or she has gathered data systematically and accounted for potential biases, and then must submit his or her interpretations to others for examination and retesting. Furthermore, the researcher is enjoined to be a relativist; that is, not to fall in love with his or her interpretations but to hold them always as models of reality, approximations. This provides remarkable training in humbleness, and to be frank, not many achieve it.

ROLE OF SCIENCE

Euro-American society in particular has developed science to be the believable knowledge method, the knowledge orthodoxy of the late nineteenth and the twentieth centuries. The determination with which Westerners cling to their cultural preference concerning the power of science approaches a religious fervor. Biomedicine gradually took on the cloak of scientism with the rise of clinical medicine in the early nineteenth century, moving toward a laboratory-based experimental model by the late nineteenth century. Although the experiment is only one way to gather valid data by use of the scientific method, this became accepted as the "scientific" approach; by the early twentieth century, American biomedicine already contrasted itself to other systems by claiming to be experimental, hence uniquely scientific. Given that the other major systems are generally not experimental—they depend on well-developed clinical observation skills and experience guided by their explanatory models—it becomes clear why a system that perceives itself as scientific can consider nonscientific systems as inferior in our cultural milieu.

The biomedical model assumes diseases to be fully accounted for by deviations from the norm of measurable biologic (somatic) variables. It leaves no room within its framework for the social, psychological, and behavioral dimensions of illness. . . . The biomedical model has thus become a cultural imperative, its limitations easily overlooked. In brief, it has now acquired the status of dogma. In science, a model is revised or abandoned when it fails to account adequately for all the data. A dogma, on the other hand, requires that discrepant data be forced to fit the model or be excluded (Engel, 1977).

But is biomedicine really scientific if judged from the perspective of science rather than cultural preference? Recent studies suggest that only 30 percent of what biomedicine achieves has been tested adequately (Altman, 1994; Andersen, 1990). A full 70 percent of practice uses the same well-developed clinical observation skills and experience guided by the explanatory model that powers the other health care systems.

Those who can stand back dispassionately—that is, those who really do think like scientists—understand that a great deal of the argument over which systems are modal or alternative is really an argument over cultural turf. As such, victory in this argument serves the usual political purpose of maintaining power by insisting on the virtue of one's own values, often by attacking the perceptions of one's rivals; these are political, not scientific, acts.

THE IMPORTANCE OF VIEWING HEALTH CARE AS A MATTER OF CULTURAL MODELING

That health care is a matter of cultural modeling rather than scientific truth matters to practitioners whose goals really are to relieve suffering. It also matters to those who wish to be scientific in their thoughts and choices. Differences must be dealt with. So, pragmatically, we end by asking, Who do the differences serve? How do the differences serve?

Users of Alternative Medicine

Demand for nonbiomedical health care in Europe and North America is at a peak that has not been met for about 150 years. Surveys of users of alternative medicine tell similar stories: People want to feel cared for, and biomedicine's emphasis on laboratory medicine, factoring the person out of the diagnostic and treatment equation, invasive treatments including high levels of painful side effects,* rushed delivery of care, and immensely high cost, all connote an uncaring system and are making biomedicine unattractive to increasing numbers of people.

Who are these people? Surveys indicate that the users of the major nonbiomedical systems are mainly urban, female, well educated, with middle to high incomes (Cassileth et al., 1984; Eisenberg et al., 1993; McGuire, 1994). These people are in excellent positions to judge the quality of the care they receive from the variety of practitioners that they consult. This point matters because mainstream practitioners and researchers often attack nonbiomedical health care by saying that the users are being misled, either purposefully by the practitioners or by their own desires, distress, and ignorance.

The defensive, politically motivated arguments of biomedical practitioners are being increasingly weakened by three facts:

1. Studies show that where health care is obviously pluralistic, laypeople are astute at matching systems with complaints (Young, 1981).
2. On the whole, patients report satisfaction with alternative health care (Emad, 1994; Hare, 1993; O'Connor, 1995; Workshop on Alternative Medicine, 1994).
3. Rapidly accumulating results of scientific research on alternative treatments show that they often are as effective or more effective than biomedical treatments of identical conditions or that they provide valuable complementary effects when biomedicine is in use (Benor, 1993; Byrd, 1988; Jacobs et al., 1994; Jobst, 1995; O'Connor, 1995; Reilly et al., 1994; Workshop on Alternative Medicine, 1994).

The Constituency for Alternative Medicine

Current biomedical discussion on the best use of nonbiomedical alternatives focuses either on annexing particular techniques (for example, jettisoning the systemic embedding of the treatments in explanatory models) or on using the alternatives adjunctively (for example, recommending acupuncture as adjunctive therapy to minimize the side effects of chemotherapy). Readers are now prepared to interpret these proposals as expressions of a biomedical perspective that claims its health care reality is superior to all others.

Of course, the situation looks a little different from the viewpoints of alternative practitioners, as well as from the perspective of potential patients, many of whom are glad that modern health care provides a menu of alternatives to choose from.

Many would benefit if the U.S. national health care system was organized such that several alternatives were widely available and people learned about them from childhood (Box 3-3).

---

*Approximately 20 percent of illnesses that lead to hospitalization are iatrogenic, that is, caused by the biomedical care itself (Greenwood and Nunn, 1994).

BOX 3-3

Beneficiaries of Widely Available Alternative Health Care Systems in the United States

Those who have a high need for affiliation and who therefore want a relational style of health care

Those who wish to alleviate symptoms gently or with fewer side effects

Those who will not take hopeless for an answer

Those who would wish to prevent disease or enhance wellness

Those who interpret the body-person as having more than a physical aspect and who want to be able to address the energetic, psychosocial, and spiritual bodies when receiving or delivering health care

Those who are concerned with the end-stage focus and invasiveness of typical biomedical care

Note that this discussion assumes that there is space for all forms of health care. This should be true in a democratic society, and it is true in the sense that all the systems already exist and serve people. The drive behind current research is to discover what services each system can provide and to compare their effectiveness in providing these services. Interestingly, this drive will fail if it is expressed soley in terms of conditions or complaints, which is only half the equation. The other half consists of the people who are to receive the care. There always will be a range of desires and needs; some patients will always prefer care that is technological and has rapid overt effects, whereas others will always prefer care that is relational, gentle, and virtually contemplative.

It is to be hoped that the world's people will become more skilled at using all our health care resources and options, to make it possible for everyone—practitioners and people—to know enough about their options to successfully triage care in a manner that maximizes patient satisfaction and health while minimizing suffering, iatrogenic disease, and cost.

It remains for you to consider your own goals for practice. Where do you fall on the various continua discussed in this chapter? Are you satisfied with the care that you deliver, or would you like to modify some rough spots? How can the alternative systems help you do so? How can they help your current or future patients?

CONCLUSION

This chapter introduces concepts that are fundamental to understanding values and issues in the practice of health care and provides a sociocultural context and models that will be useful in understanding the practices described in subsequent chapters.

We began by stating that the form health care takes is fundamentally a matter of sociocultural interpretation. As we end, it should be clear that health care systems differ in important ways and that no one system provides all the answers, or even the best answers, for all users or circumstances. Differences among systems are not random but are driven and logically organized by underlying assumptive patterns that are revealed in explanatory models, therapeutic modalities, and styles of practice.

These differences are *not* unbridgeable; the concepts developed in this chapter should allow most practitioners and researchers to approach even strange ideas with new appreciation, as well as provide them with tools that allow for better communication and understanding. After all, the deepest and most common goal of all health care systems is to relieve pain and prevent suffering.

Acknowledgments

Special thanks to Haig Ignatius, MD, MAc, and Marc Micozzi, MD, PhD, for their generous reading of this chapter in its draft stages. Continuing thanks to many colleagues whose deep thinking about medical philosophical and practice issues guides and sustains my own explorations. Thanks too, to my husband and daughter, whose love and support are most precious.

References

Altman D. 1994. The scandal of poor medical research. BMJ 308:283-284

Ames R. 1993. Sun-Tzu: The Art of Warfare. Ballantine Books, New York

Andersen B. 1990. Methodological Errors in Medical Research. Blackwell Scientific Publications, Oxford

Bates MS, Rankin-Hill L, Sanchez-Ayendez M, Mendez-Bryan R. 1995. A cross-cultural comparison of adaptation to chronic pain among Anglo-Americans and native Puerto Ricans. Med Anthropol 16(2):141-173

Beinfield H, Korngold E. 1991. Between Heaven and Earth, A Guide to Chinese Medicine. Ballantine Books, New York

Benor D. 1993. Healing Research: Holistic Energy Medicine and Spirituality. Helix Verlag GmbH, Munich

Black Elk W, Lyon WS. 1990. Black Elk, The Sacred Ways of a Lakota. Harper & Row, San Francisco

Brennan B. 1988. Hands of Light, A Guide to Healing Through the Human Energy Field. Bantam Books, Toronto

Byrd RC. 1988. Positive therapeutic effects of intercessory prayer in a coronary care unit population. South Med J 81:826-829

Cassidy CM. 1982. Protein-energy malnutrition as a culture-bound syndrome. Cult Med Psychiat 6:325-345

Cassidy CM. 1994. Unraveling the ball of string: Reality, paradigms, and the study of alternative medicine. Adv J Mind-Body Health 10:3-31

Cassidy CM. 1995. Social science theory and methods in the study of alternative and complementary medicine. J Altern Comple Med 1:19-40

Cassileth B, Lusk E, Strouse R, Bodenheimer B. 1984. Contemporary unorthodox treatments in cancer medicine, a study of patients, treatments and practitioners. Ann Intern Med 101:105-112

Eisenberg D, Kessler R, Foster C, Norlock F, Culkins D, Delbanco R. 1993. Unconventional medicine in the United States. N Engl J Med 328:246-252

Eliade M. 1964. Shamanism, Archaic Techniques of Ecstasy. Princeton University Press, Princeton, New Jersey

Emad M. 1994. 'Does acupuncture hurt?': Ethnographic evidence of shifts in psychobiological experiences of pain. Proc Soc Acupunct Res 2:129-140

Engel G. 1977. The need for a new medical model challenge for biomedicine. Science 196(4286):129-136

Fabrega H. 1974. Disease and Social Behavior: An Interdisciplinary Perspective. MIT Press, Cambridge, Massachusetts

Foster G, Anderson B. 1978. Medical Anthropology. John Wiley & Sons, New York

Furnham A. 1992. Why people choose complementary medicine, in Andritsky W (ed). Yearbook of Cross-cultural Medicine and Psychotherapy, pp 165-198

Greenwood M, Nunn P. 1994. Paradox and Healing, Medicine, Mythology and Transformation, 3rd ed. Paradox Publ, Victoria British Columbia

Hand WD (ed). 1976. American Folk Medicine: A Symposium. University of California Press, Berkeley, California

Hare M. 1993. The emergence of an urban U.S. Chinese medicine. Med Anthropol Q 7:30-49

Harwood A. 1977. The hot-cold theory of disease: Implications for treatment of Puerto Rican patients. JAMA 216:1153-1158

Huber P. 1990. Presidential candidate's wife accused of bigamy. Old News 1:5, Marietta, Pennsylvania

Hultkrantz A. 1985. The shaman and the medicine man. Soc Sci Med 20:511-515

Ingerman S. 1991. Soul Retrieval, Mending the Fragmented Self. Harper Collins, San Francisco

Jacobs J, Jimenez LM, Gloyd SS, et al. 1994. Treatment of acute childhood diarrhea with homeopathic medicine: A randomized clinical trial in Nicaragua. Pediatrics 93(5):719-725

Jobst KA. 1995. A critical analysis of acupuncture in pulmonary disease: Efficacy and safety of the acupuncture needle. J Altern Comple Med 1:57-85

Kaplan A. 1984. Philosophy of science in anthropology. Annu Rev Anthropol 13:25-39

Kaptchuk T. 1983. The Web That Has No Weaver. Understanding Chinese Medicine. Congdon & Weed, New York

Kirkland J, Mathews HF, Sullivan III CW, Baldwin K, (eds.) 1992. Herbal and Magical Medicine: Traditional Healing Today. Duke University Press, Durham, North Carolina

Kleinman A. 1980. Patients and Healers in the Context of Culture. University of California Press, Berkeley, California

Lock M, Gordon DR (eds). 1988. Biomedicine Examined. Kluwer Academic Publishers, Dordrecht, The Netherlands

McGuire MB. 1994. Ritual Healing in Suburban America. Rutgers University Press, New Brunswick, New Jersey

Morgan W. 1977 (1931). Navajo treatment of sickness; Diagnosticians, in Landy D (ed), Culture, Disease and Healing, Studies in Medical Anthropology, Macmillan Publ Co., New York, pp 163-168

Murdock GP. 1980. Theories of Illness, A World Survey. University of Pittsburg Press. Pittsburgh, Pennsylvania

O'Connor BB. 1995. Healing Traditions, Alternative Medicine and the Health Professions. University of Pennsylvania Press, Philadelphia

Payer L. 1988. Medicine and Culture, Varieties of Treatment in the United States, England, West Germany, and France. Penguin Books, New York

Porkert M. 1974. Theoretical Foundations of Chinese Medicine: Systems of Correspondence. The MIT Press, Cambridge, Massachusetts

Reilly D, Taylor MA, Bettie N, et al. 1994. Is evidence for homeopathy reproducible? Lancet 344(8937):1601-1606

Reimansnyder BL. 1989 (1982). Powwosing in Union County, A Study of Pennsylvania German Folk Medicine in Context. AMS Press Inc., New York

Rubel A, O'Nell CW, Ardon RC. 1984. Susto: A Folk Illness. University of California Press, Berkeley, California

Scott AW. 1993. Masters of the Ordinary: Integrating Personal Experience and Vernacular Knowledge in Alcoholics Anonymous. Dissertation. Michigan Microfilms, Ann Arbor, Michigan

Sheldon WH, Hartl EM, McDermott E. 1949. Varieties of Delinquent Youth, An Introduction to Constitutional Psychiatry. Harper and Brothers, New York

Snow LF. 1993. Walkin' Over Medicine. Westview Press, Boulder, Colorado

Sobo EJ. 1993. One Blood, The Jamaican Body. State University of New York Press, Albany, New York

Spicer EH (ed). 1979. Ethnic Medicine in the Southwest. University of Arizona Press, Tucson, Arizona

Stein HF. 1990. American Medicine as Culture. Westview Press, Boulder, Colorado

Terrell SJ. 1990. This Other Kind of Doctors: Traditional Medical Systems in Black Neighborhoods in Austin TX. AMS Press Inc., New York

Vithoulkas G. 1980. The Science of Homeopathy. Grove Press, New York

Wirkus M. 1993. Mietek Wirkus: School of bioenergy, the healing art. Newsletter of the International Society for the Study of Subtle Energies and Energy Balance 4(2): 8-10

Workshop on Alternative Medicine (Chantilly, VA), 1994. Alternative Medicine: Expanding Medical Horizons, Report to the National Institutes of Health on Alternative Medical Systems and Practices in the United States. NIH Publ 94-066, Government Printing Office, Washington DC

Young JC. 1981. Medical Choice in a Mexican Village. Rutgers University Press, New Brunswick, New Jersey

Young D, Ingram G, Swartz L. 1989. Cry of the Eagle, Encounters with a Cree Healer. University of Toronto Press, Toronto

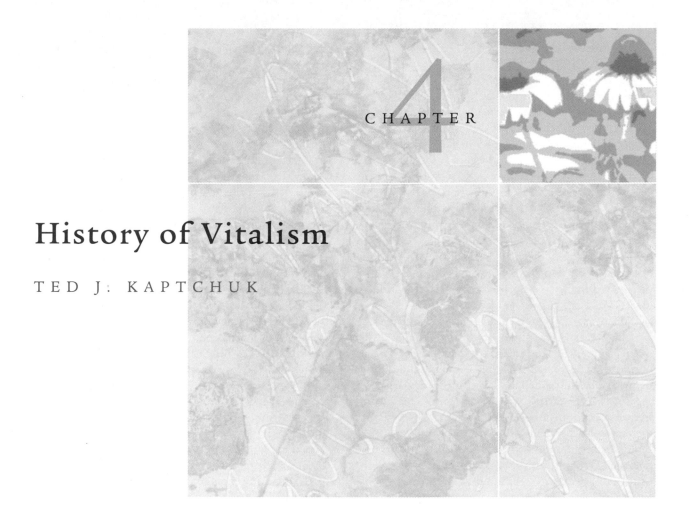

CHAPTER 4

History of Vitalism

TED J. KAPTCHUK

Practitioners of most alternative healing believe that one source of their intervention is a kind of "vital energy" their system uses that is still not appreciated by conventional biomedical science. Subtle health-promoting influences pervade the alternative healing world. Health is accessible through gentle technologies that activate, evoke, or redirect universal beneficent healing influences. The universe is thought to provide an endless influx of forces that can help to "put things right." Health is harmony in the cosmic energy; illness is cured by reordering the protective forces. A person threatened by disorder and disease is guaranteed a response from fundamentally benign, lawful, coherent, potent, and even meaningful powers. One can almost speak of a faucet that pours out healing juice. Homeopathy connects with the "spiritual vital force" (Hahnemann, 1980); chiropractic calls it "innate" or "universal intelligence" (Palmer, 1910); psychic healing manipulates "arauric," "psi," or psionic powers (Moore, 1977; Reyner, 1982); believers in New Thought are restored by correct "mind" (Braden, 1987); acupuncture uses "qi" (Eisenberg, 1987); Ayurvedic medicine and yoga teachers are in touch with "prana" (Lad, 1984); and naturopaths invoke the "vis medicatrix naturae" (Turner, 1990). Unseen powers are said to permeate the universe and have a profound effect on human beings undetectable by scientific instruments. This chapter delineates this concept of alternative medicine by tracing the historical development of the idea of vital energy. Individual alternative healing practices are described in terms of their fundamental propositions and the ontological status that they confer on the vital principle.

HISTORY: THE RISE AND FALL OF THE MAINSTREAM VITALIST PRINCIPLE

Vitalism is the proposition that more is needed to explain life than just physical or mechanical laws. It is less archaic than recent advocates or detractors of alternative medicines claim and has its origins not within alternative health care systems themselves but within the elite universities of eighteenth and nineteenth century Europe. This doctrine arose in the West as a response to the mechanistic thesis and atomistic physicochemical reductionism of the scientific revolution (Lain Entralgo, 1948).

To understand the new science and the vitalist formulation, review of the previously dominant Aristotelian worldview is helpful. In the Aristotelian universe, unlike the new scientific world, there was no such thing as totally inert matter changing because of external forces. Aristotelian physical matter had inherent tendencies, intentionality, and teleological properties. Things happened in the material universe because of latent tendencies that unfolded: fire's goal was to ascend, earth's was to descend. The future exerted a compulsion on the present. The organic universe was the model for the inorganic universe; the acorn both embodied and obeyed its future potential as an oak tree. The material realm was a continuum of the organic realm but at a reduced level of complexity.

In terms of human beings, this sense of continuation persists. Medieval biology could not conceive of an extreme dichotomy of soma (body) and psyche (mind), much less their separate existence (Gilson, 1940; cf. Hartman, 1977). This would have conflicted with theology (Kemp, 1990). Psyche had no reality apart from soma. A human being's material body overlapped and interpenetrated and was given actuality and form by a subtle substratum of souls. Each soul organized the soma into a distinct hierarchy of function and awareness. Somehow, pneuma, a mediator of the same eternal essence as the celestial bodies, allowed for both an embodied and mindful integrity of psyche and soma (Hall, 1975). Pneuma served as a common denominator of all phenomena and allowed all forms of being—from human to minerals—to maintain their cohesiveness and growth and to transform into other forms of being.

These medieval notions were replaced by the new science. Rather than conceiving nature as an organic being that matured through self-development, seventeenth-century scientists viewed nature as a machine whose parts only moved in response to other parts. Volition, intentions, cognition, and mental states were relegated to peripheral or epiphenomenal status in biology; some scientists even came to believe that all life could be explained in mechanical and physicochemical terms (Ledermann, 1989).

For some doctors and scientists, explaining life as an intricate system of levers, pulleys, or bubbling and fermenting microchemical flasks was inadequate. They criticized the new philosophy as excessively mechanical, material, and simple and argued that life was determined by more than the laws of the inanimate world. These physicians and biologists tried to animate the newly constituted passive matter of science with a vitalist hypothesis to explain the feeling and thought behind organic and human life (Roger, 1986). The most important figure in this effort was the chemist-physician George Ernest Stahl (1659-1734), whose prominent university status at Halle was enhanced by his former position as physician to Frederick Wilhelm I (Rather, 1961). He proposed the *anima,* or "sensitive soul," to fill the perceived void in the new science. Anima was the agency that made life distinct from lifeless matter. Stahlian animism was undoubtedly influenced by the earlier "archeus" of Paracelsus (1493-1541) and van Helmont (1577-1644), two pre-Cartesian chemist-physician-mystics of the Nordic renaissance who were involved in an entirely different dialogue (Lain Entralgo, 1948). Francois Boissier de Sauvages (1706-1767) introduced the anima into the teaching of Montpellier, one of Europe's oldest and most important medical schools, but he preferred using the word "soul" for this animating life force. His student, Paul Joseph Barthez (1734-1806), whose credentials included having been Napoleon's physician, believed that both words were too occult and old-fashioned and in 1778 introduced the phrase *principe vitale* or *vital principle* (Haight, 1975; Wheeler, 1939). The vitalist hypothesis could not totally obliterate the newly created Cartesian chasm of an inert matter *(res extensa)* and a mind *(res cognitans)*—it conceded too much to the new physics. But the power relationship had been reversed; in life, primary agency was no longer physicochemical or mechanical but rather a benevolent power with a self-directive healing power.

Unbound by the precise and quantifiable laws of physics and chemistry, the vitalism argument, by its very nature, quickly fractured into many interpretations. Some physicians took a phenomenal position and saw the vital principle to be a regulative principle (Lipman, 1967). Others took a realist position and postulated that a constitutive part animated matter; this approach is much more important to alternative healing (Benton, 1975). Realist theories took various forms: from various shades of incorporeal and spirit agency; to diverse mental powers; to different kinds of distinctive forces analogous and on the same plane of reality as conventional electromagnetism but still not scientifically measurable (Larson, 1979; Toulmin & Goodfield, 1962).

In the nineteenth century the mechanistic physicochemical view gained complete ascendancy in biology and medicine. From Wohler's synthesis of organic material in 1828 to Atwater and Rosa's demonstration in 1897 that the laws of thermodynamics apply to life, as well as inorganic matter, there was a gradual elimination of any need to believe in a vital principle or life force to explain perceived inadequacies of physicochemical explanations (Needham, 1955). Vitalism's main argument was the opponent's weakness; vitalism had to retreat before each new scientific discovery. This weakened vitalism migrated to the alternative medical worldview that was being created in the nineteenth century, where it was welcomed and eventually merged with other important forms of vitalism.

MESMERIC VITAL ENERGY

At the time that vitalism was being developed in elite academia and just before it received an official name, the Viennese physician Anton Mesmer (1734-1815) uncovered what he believed to be the real vital energy. In 1775 Mesmer discovered that the source of a popular religious exorcist's powers was not divine intervention but rather a vital force. The cures were due to "animal magnetism," a subtle fluid that pervades the universe and is analogous to gravitation (Ellenberger, 1970). Mesmer declared that the scientific evidence of the new vital force is the healing influx; harmony with the cosmic fluid is health. All disease was due to an unequal distribution or blockage of this fluid; healing is the restoration of equilibrium, and healers can manipulate this fluid to cure patients (Mesmer, 1980). An influx of subtle fluids from the celestial bodies is the substantive basis of all life and health, and later even mortality (Darton, 1968).

Mesmer relocated to Paris, and his popularity quickly generated controversy. In 1784 King Louis XVI, through the Royal French Academy of Science, appointed a prestigious investigatory commission including ambassador Benjamin Franklin, chemist Antoine Lavoisier, and physician-inventor J.I. Guillotin. Mesmer demanded clinical outcome comparisons. Instead the blue ribbon panel wanted to investigate mechanism. In a series of some of medicine's earliest controlled, blinded trials the panel discovered that healing occurred whenever subjects believed they were being mesmerized, and no effect occurred if subjects were ignorant of magnetic passes. The commission sentenced mesmerism to the medical fringe, where it became a critical component of alternative medical thought (Fuller, 1982)

Mesmer's followers quickly split into denominations. Mesmerists divided between those who understood the force as a physical agency and others who detected a more incorporeal power. A lower mesmeric interpretation made the force analogous to a physical electromagnetic vibration that resembled more recognized scientific energies. A higher mesmeric interpretation that quickly fused with earlier mystical and occult traditions saw the force as ethereal and reduced the physical agency to an epiphenomenon of no consequence. In addition to healing, the force had abilities for clairvoyant medical diagnosis and telepathy and became a scientific vehicle to contact spiritual forces or spiritual beings (Darton, 1968). Between the poles of lower and higher mesmerism were various intermediate versions, each spawning complex lineage; all shared the distinctive mesmeric view that life's agency and healing potential can be found in a vital energy or presence distinct from the ordinary mechanical forces. Mesmerism became the inspiration for many unconventional therapies.

Lower Mesmerism and Psychic Healing

Tracing the history of mesmerism can be difficult because many of Mesmer's descendants often changed their names, like other new arrivals on Ellis Island, to avoid the stigma associated with the term *mesmerism* since its excommunication from official science. New designations could be helpful, however. If an earlier vital energy was discredited, new forces could be discovered to take its place. For example, Robert Hare (1781-1858), a chemist at the University of Pennsylvania and the inventor of the oxyhydrogen blowpipe, was an early convert to mesmerism. In 1856 he developed a spirit-scope to measure mesmeric and spiritual presences and also coined the scientific-sounding term *psychic force* in 1856 (McClenon, 1984; Moore, 1977). In 1935 Joseph Bank Rhine (1885-1980), who spent most of his career at Duke University trying to shift psychical research from the seance room to the laboratory, adopted the more respectable "parapsychology" from German (McVaugh & Mauskupf, 1976; Moore, 1977). In 1947 Robert Thouless (1894-1984), a British psychologist and parapsychologist at Cambridge, thought psi phenomena or psionic energy was a noncommittal label for paranormal energetics (Moore, 1977). Historically, theosophists preferred the word *auric* or *astral* force (Campbell, 1980; Coddington, 1990), whereas modern researchers have recently chosen the phrase *subtle energy*. These name substitutions indicate the lower mesmeric concern for keeping vital energy on a par with other more physically established forces as the primary agency for life.

"Lower mesmeric forms of healing energy are easily recognized in the contemporary alternative therapies that speak of an electromagnetic dimension which can become depleted or unbalanced . . . [causing] the blockage of energy flow, requiring physical or spiritual cleaning in order for healing to occur" (Glick, 1988). Alternative therapies—such as therapeutic touch (Krieger et al., 1979), laying on of hands (Vlamis, 1978), polarity (Vlamis, 1978), paranormal healing (Rose, 1954), and the countless individual psychic, auric, and psionic healers—although often unaware of their heritage, all bear the characteristic mesmeric style of manipulating unseen and refined forces that evade biomedical detection. The proof of the force is healing, and secondary evidence can be sensations of heat, tingling, or vibratory motions (Fuller, 1989). Curiously, despite the suspicions—and even hostility—of colleagues, some conventional researchers hover on the edge of this type of healing and continue to scientifically investigate the phenomenon (Benor, 1990; Beutler et al., 1988).

Higher Mesmerism and Channelling

The trance states of higher mesmeric traditions were used to contact noncorporeal realities. Healing dispensations, medical diagnosis, and medical advice were common products of "tuning-in," as were clairvoyance, spirit sightings, levitations, ectoplasmic emissions, table turning, spirit tapping, and spirit photographs. This higher trance phenomenon quickly merged with earlier occult and theurgic movements (such as neo-Platonism, Renaissance occult and kabbla, pre-Christian religions, theurgic traditions, and Swedenborgianism [Galbreath, 1971]), creating a mass phenomenon in the nineteenth century (Braude, 1989; Oppenheim, 1988). This spiritualist movement was later reincarnated in various theosophical and occult movements in today's New Age scene (Beckford, 1984; Melton, 1988). Such contemporary phenomena as "experiencing the healing powers of interplanetary Brotherhoods and curing their medical ailments by soul travel to different planes of reality" (Levin & Coreil, 1988) are all direct descendants of higher mesmerism. Alternative healing methods and associations such as Spiritual Frontiers Fellowship, Edgar Cayce's Association for Research and Enlightenment (Carter, 1972), and Great White Brotherhood and modalities such as past lives therapy (Netherton & Shiffrin, 1978) are involved with a panoply of spiritual beings that are detectable by mesmeric trances, currently spoken of as altered states of consciousness, channeling, higher states of awareness, or transmissions from spiritually evolved beings. These are rarely organized as healing professions and routinely exceed the limits of healing practices, becoming instead alternative or emergent religions.

ELECTRICAL DEVICES AND CRYSTALS

Electrical devices and crystals that emit or harmonize energies for healing are important first cousins of mesmerism. Luigi Galvani's (1737-1798) experiments, which caused the severed legs of frogs to jump as if alive, coincided with Mesmer's own research. This discovery of animal electricity, or electrical body fluid, was considered to be analogous or identical with animal magnetism and all mysterious vital forces (Sutton, 1981). Electrical machines and gadgets with healing properties were ubiquitous in the nineteenth century (Marvin, 1988) and continued into the twentieth century. Contemporary radionic machines, magnetic beds, transcranial electrostimulators, neuromagnetic vibrators, and electromagnetic chairs all bear the imprint of their preceding mesmeric electrical cousins (Easthope, 1986; Schaller & Caroll, 1976). Important scientific research has been generated by scientists interested in low-frequency electromagnetic devices despite the stigma of an association with charlatanism (Macklin, 1993).

Crystal healing, a form of lithotherapeutics, has ancient roots distinct from mesmerism (Forbes, 1972). In the last 200 years, however, it has repositioned itself to become part of the vital energy family. In the 1840s and 1850s Baron Charles von Reichenbach (1788-1869), the discoverer of kerosene, also managed to detect a refined and definitive mesmeric energy in crystals. He gave it the scientifically oriented name *odic force*. Modern crystal healers continue this merged tradition and speak of crystals as "able to tap the energies of the universe" and be an especially potent "focus of healing energy" (Fuller, 1989).

MIND CURE

Mind cure, or the healing systems that consider thoughts or deep feeling to be the primary arbitrator of health, is an important offshoot of mesmerism. The discovery of the mind as the ultimate unseen force of healing is related directly to Phineas P. Quimby (1802-1866). Quimby first worked as a magnetizer or magnetic healer (reconstituted names for a mesmerist) in Portland, Maine. He decided that healing was not so much animal magnetism or an esoteric energy but rather results from changes in the mind. The force was not a physical force, but a mental state. Mesmer's fluid was really Mind, and everything was controlled by Mind, with a capital *M*. Disease is what follows the disturbance of the mind or spiritual matter (Dresser, 1969).

Quimby began the New Thought movement that believes disease is wrong thinking. Change the thought, and you have health (Judah, 1967). Divine Mind, Divine Truth, and Love are primary agency, not the physical world. Physical reality is clay in the hands of the Mind. New Thought and positive thinking all derive from Mind Cure, as do such metaphysical groups as Unity Church of Christianity, United Church of Religious Science, and International Divine Science (Braden, 1987). New and more contemporary forms of this approach to healing are constantly being offered. For example, A Course on Miracles (Perry, 1987), Prosperity Consciousness (Chopra, 1993; Cole-Whittaker, 1983), and Living Love (Cornucopia) (Keyes, 1989) are all based on the same premise. Beyond any organization, this notion of "what you think is what is real" infuses important sectors of the modern alternative health community,

resonating through history in uncanny ways. For example, the words Quimby wrote in 1859 could easily have been taken from Bernie Siegel's best-selling alternative healing book *Love, Medicine and Miracles* (Siegel, 1986): "Love is the true answer to our desire . . . it contains nothing but true knowledge and love, no sorrow, nor pain, nor grief, nor shame nor fear (Dresser, 1969). Love or True Mind heals all."

Mind Cure often advocated "entering the silence" to make Mind impressions, self-love, or autosuggestion imprint more effectively (Fuller, 1982; Meyers, 1965). Almost 100 years ago William James (1842-1910) described a phenomenon that still is current when he said that the "mind-cure principles are beginning to so pervade. . . . One hears of the Gospel of Relaxation of the Don't Worry Movement or people who repeat to themselves Youth, Health, Vigor" (James, 1961). Mind Cure's meditation, relaxation, and breathing techniques (which partially derive from somnambulistic or mesmeric trance states [cf. Davis, 1885]) were some of the indigenous Western practices that prepared the way for Asian-style meditations that are so influential in the alternative health movement (see following).

CHRISTIAN SCIENCE

Quimby's most famous legacy to unconventional healing is through his student and patient who later became known under the name Mary Baker Eddy (1821-1919). She went on to establish Christian Science, radically declaring that all disease, pain, misfortune, and evil are illusion. Knowing Divine Truth and Divine Science allows perception of the underlying perfection. Divine Mind is the only reality. Rigid, doctrinaire, exclusive, and sectarian, Mrs. Eddy denied any relationship with Mind Cure, mesmerism, or alternative healing, but her venomous denunciations of Quimby and malicious animal magnetism revealed her origins only too clearly and assured Christian Science a place in the history of vital energy (Feldman, 1963; Fox, 1984; Schoepflin, 1988).

CHIROPRACTIC, OSTEOPATHY, AND MASSAGE

Mesmeric vital energy took a somatic and even mechanical twist in the creation of chiropractic, the largest contemporary alternative health care profession in North America, licensed in 50 states (Wardwell, 1992). Discovered in 1895 by D.D. Palmer (1845-1913), chiropractic's origin is a unique marriage of the indigenous healing craft of bonesetting (Cooter, 1987; Schiotz & Cyriax, 1975) and the American tradition of mesmeric healing (Beck, 1991). For 10 years before his discovery of chiropractic, Palmer worked as a magnetic healer. Like Quimby, he occasionally used hand passes and magnetic rubbings of the spine (Fuller, 1982). In an intuitive flash (or, some say, clairvoyant communication [Beck, 1982]), he realized that "putting down your hands" worked better than an esoteric "laying on of hands." Mechanical adjustment was more precise than magnetic activity administered from a distance. Yet even 20 years after abandoning his magnetic clinical work, Palmer's mesmeric heritage is readily evident in his writings: "Disease is a manifestation of too much or not enough energy. Energy is liberated force; in the living being it is known as vital force. . . . It is an intelligent force, which I saw fit to name Innate, usually known as spirit" (Beck, 1991).

Disease is disruption in what Palmer calls *innate intelligence.* The nervous system is the conduit for this force. By aligning the spine, one frees the nerves so that this force can move without interference and produce healing. The vital energy is guided and shaped by the structure of the body. The noncorporeal agency of life is housed in the nerves and guarded by the spinal vertebrae. Chiropractic and spinal manipulation, despite its alternative associations, recently has generated considerable interest from researchers, both in terms of basic science (Goldstein 1975), controlled clinical trials (Anderson et al., 1992; Shekelle et al., 1992), and comparative health care outcome trials (Meade et al., 1990). Official government reports, such as the Manga Report in Canada (Manga et al., 1993) and a recommendation from the Agency for Health Care Policy and Research (Bigos et al., 1994) on chiropractic for acute low back pain, have blurred the demarcation between alternative and mainstream medicine and encouraged wider acceptance of chiropractic.

Osteopathy, chiropractic's older cousin, was developed by Andrew Still (1828-1917), who was also a magnetic healer for many years. In 1874 he discovered that misaligned bones impeded the flow of fluids and blood, and he developed the system of osteopathy. In addition to having episodes of clairvoyance and channelling, Still also had connections to metaphysical,

Mind Cure, and spiritualist groups (Gevitz, 1988; Terrett, 1991). Obviously, osteopathy has taken a different trajectory from chiropractic. By breeding out its mesmeric influence, it has become practically indistinguishable from mainstream medicine (Baer, 1987; Gevitz, 1982).

Massage is one of the earliest and most pervasive forms of healing (Sigerist, 1961). Yet in the last 100 years many unconventional massage therapies have increasingly found their rationale in vital energy theory. Many styles of massage therapies exist (Knapp & Antonucci, 1990) with different theories and therapeutic goals, including Rolfing (Rolf, 1977), reflexology (Carter 1969), Aston-Patterning (Low, 1988), Hellerwork, and shiatsu (Namikoshi, 1969). The multiplicity of forms, the fact that anyone can give a massage, and constant introduction of new methods have hampered the regulation, licensing, and professional development that is analogous to chiropractic. Nonetheless, "bodywork" provides an extensive and important network of much energy work (Good & Good, 1981).

HOMEOPATHY

Although mesmerism dominated the vital energy tradition, the mainstream vitalist hypothesis also continued to survive and remained operational in the alternative medical world. Often this survival was made possible by an explicit or implicit strategic union with mesmerism. Homeopathy is the most important system of medicine to derive from this tradition.

For a considerable period of time during the last century, homeopathy was the most serious challenge to conventional medicine (Rothstein, 1985) and currently is enjoying a serious revival (Kaufman, 1988). Discovered by Samuel Hahnemann (1755-1843), homeopathy espouses the belief that whatever symptom-complex a substance can cause in a healthy person, infinitesimally small amounts of the same substance can cure diseases with the same symptom configuration. The small dosage has the capacity to evoke the spiritual, self-acting (automatic) vital force, everywhere present in his organism (Hahnemann, 1980). *Sililia similibus curentur*—like cures like. The tiny dosage enhances the spiritual essence of the bodily response to disease. The alchemical homeopathic remedy was to rescue the insufficient self-help mechanisms of the physical body and supply a corrective to nature (Neuburger, 1933). Hahnemann's idea of vital energy derived from early German romantic sources (from Paracelsus and van Helmont) and the later academic tradition of G.E. Stahl (Coulter, 1977). Yet, even from its inception, an alliance with mesmerism was discernible. Hahnemann himself ascribed mesmeric healing as a marvelous, priceless gift of God to mankind (Hahnemann, 1980). Today it is virtually impossible to distinguish homeopathy's vital force from other conceptions rooted in mesmerism. Despite its alternative status, however, homeopathy has generated considerable conventional biomedical research and debate (Hill & Doyon, 1990; Kliejnen et al., 1991a; Linde et al., 1994).

HERBALISM AND THE "VIS MATECATRIX NATURAE"

Another energy in alternative medicine is the healing force of nature, which has a long history independent of mesmerism or the vitalist hypothesis (Neuburger, 1933). In 1772 William Cullen (1710-1790), a professor at the University of Edinburgh—himself no friend of this approach in medicine—proposed the term *vis matecatrix naturae* to describe this power (Neuburger, 1933). Again, like the academic vitalist hypothesis, the natural force became more important in the alternative world and eventually was indistinguishable from the whole concept of vital energy.

The rise of the market economy and industrialization allowed for nostalgia and a romantic view of nature, which made possible the natural healing movements that date from the early nineteenth century. Alternative healing movements "irregulars" launched crusades to overthrow the orthodox medicine "regulars," who used "contaminated unnatural poisonous" drugs and bleeding (Warner, 1987). The earliest American natural healing movement was Thomsonian herbalism. The history of herbal medicaments lies deep in antiquity (Wheelwright, 1974), but Samuel Thomson (1769-1843), a native of New Hampshire, initiated the first herbal social reform movement in the 1820s and 1830s. Borrowing from indigenous colonial and Indian treatments, Thomsonians substituted herbal purges and soporifics for mainstream minerals, chemicals, and bloodletting. This movement developed into the profession of eclectic medicine, which mounted a challenge to conventional medicine with a systematic herbal approach, its own medical schools (Berman,

1951), and eventually a strong following in Europe (Griggs, 1981). Somewhere in this history, herbalism formed an alliance with mesmerism. The two languages fused. Herbalists insisted that treatment must be in harmony with nature and the vital force and must assist the vital force instead of destroying it (Brown, 1985). The last eclectic medical school closed in Ohio in 1939 (Rothstein, 1988), and herbalism as a professional system of healing had practically disappeared in the United States, although it survived in Great Britain (Sharma, 1992). In the United States, vestiges of the herbal movement remain in popular self-help manuals, and the concept of medicinal herbs remains an important symbol for alternative medicine. Some scientific research continues into popular herbal remedies (Ernst, 1995; Johnson et al., 1985; Melchart et al., 1994), but much of the conventional biomedical discussion is in terms of potential adverse effects (Huxtable, 1992).

HYDROPATHY AND NATUROPATHY

Water cure, or hydropathy, is another healing movement that relied on a natural force. Like herbalism, hydrotherapy has early roots but became a health reform movement only in the nineteenth century (Donegan, 1986). It has practically disappeared, except for spas and in physical therapy. Nevertheless, its legacy has important ramifications for contemporary alternative healing.

Originally, hydropathy was imported to the United States from Germany in the 1840s as the Priessnitz method and later reimported in the 1890s as the Kneipp method. In these systems water was the pure force of healing. Often combined with massage, exercise, and health food, water could purify the body of "morbid matter" (toxins), stimulate nervous energy, and promote natural healing (Cayleff, 1988). Quickly, the water cure movement became a catchall for other methods and by 1850 associated with dietary regimens, dress reform, home doctor, and, finally, with all natural methods including herbs, mesmeric energies, electropathy, and manipulation. This natural healing movement took on many forms and names, such as drugless healing, sanipractic, vita-o-pathy, sagliftopathy, panpathy, and physculopathy (Fishbein, 1932; Whorton, 1986), but the most enduring one is the name associated with Benedict Lust

(1872-1945), a water cure therapist who trained under the Bavarian hydropath Father Kneipp.

In 1895 Lust purchased the term *naturopathy* to describe his eclectic water cure system, and the term was used publicly for the first time in 1902 in association with Lust's New York–based American School of Naturopathy (Baer, 1992; Cody, 1985). His naturopathy was a nature cure system, defined as "the art of natural healing and the science of physical and mental regeneration on the basis of self-reform, natural life, clean and normal diet, hydropathy (Priessnitz, Kneipp, Lehmann, and Just systems), osteopathy, chiropractic, naturopathy [sic], electrotherapy, sun and air cult, diet, physiotherapy, physical and mental culture to the exclusion of poisonous drugs and non-adjustable surgery" (Fishbein, 1932). Naturopathy, whose eclecticism resembles the current holistic movement, was common practice in many states during the 1920s and 1930s under the name "drugless practitioner" (Gort & Coburn, 1988; Whorton, 1986), but now functions legally only in eight states, the stronghold being the Pacific Northwest (Baer, 1992). Legal constraint prevents its widespread adoption as a unifying ideology for all natural therapies. Nevertheless, naturopathy is a potent concept in the alternative health movement and sometimes is used as a synonym for alternative health.

ACUPUNCTURE AND ASIAN MEDICAL SYSTEMS

The vital energy of alternative medicine received a dramatic infusion of credibility and possibility with the introduction of acupuncture and other Asian medicines into the United States in the 1960s after several unsuccessful introductions (Haller, 1973).

The Chinese notion of "qi" (as well as the Indian and Tibetan equivalents) obviously developed before any Western Cartesian detachment of mind from matter. Qi was not so much an entity added to lifeless matter, but the state of being—either animate or inanimate (Chiu, 1986; Kuriyama, 1986; Sivin, 1987). It was more akin to pneuma than any other Western idea (Needham, 1956). Asian medical systems, similar to archaic Western systems, relied on hierarchies and gradations of organizations to explain differences between organic and inorganic forms of being (Yoke, 1985). Qi was characteristic of rocks, plants, and even human rationality. It was the common thread that al-

lowed for "ladders of the soul" that extended from minerals to human life (Yoke, 1985).

The qi of acupuncture or the prana of India have been swept in the undertow of Western vitalistic ideas. Contemporary Western literature generally translates qi as vital energy. Ancient Chinese notions, which defy severing of mind-body, have been discarded from modern Asian medical dialogue (both in Asia and the West) in favor of vital energy. Nonphysician acupuncturists have gained licensing, registration, or certification in 27 states plus the District of Columbia between 1977 and 1993 (Lytle, 1993; McRae, 1982). Although still small, acupuncture is one of the most rapidly growing health care professions, and its success provides an important ideological boost to alternative health care. The excitement of acupuncture has generated basic scientific investigations (Pomeranz & Stux, 1988) and more than 200 controlled clinical biomedical research studies (Eisenberg, 1995; Kleijnen et al., 1991b; Riet et al., 1990).

The Eastern opening also brought new massage (shiatsu, anmo, tui na, acupressure, jin shin jyutsu), new esoteric psychic energies (reiki johrei, qi gong), and countless new forms of meditation to supplement and supplant indigenous American forms. Again, they usually are formulated in nineteenth century vitalist terms (Miura, 1989).

PSYCHOLOGICAL INTERVENTIONS

Of all the mesmeric forces, the most complex, prolific, and hidden ones lie concealed in psychology, which deals with mind (with a small *m*). Significant aspects of clinical psychology's origins are connected with attempts to legitimize, mainstream, or find the real source of mesmerism and vital energy. In 1843 James Braid (1795-1860), an English physician, sought to clean up mesmerism's tainted reputation by postulating that its effects were due to a mental force, not a mysterious fluid. He changed its name to hypnosis, after the Greek god for sleep (Kaplan, 1974). Hypnosis became a major concern in psychology—dependent on perspective, even a legitimate mesmerism—and retains its importance in some areas of conventional medicine (Hall & Crasilneck, 1978). Hypnosis was taken seriously by such figures as Jean Martin Charcot (1825-1893) and Hippolyte Bernheim (1840-1919) and is a crucial ingredient of Sigmund Freud's

(1856-1939) early development of psychodynamic psychiatry (Ellenberger, 1970). Hypnosis became less critical after Freud, becoming simply a porthole to the unconscious. Vital energy transforms into various forms of dynamic tensions that are thought to have potent psychological and physiological consequences. A clinical research agenda has also become a companion for psychotherapies (Strupp & Howard, 1992).

Hypnosis and such forms of passive volitional intention as autogenic training and guided imagery also later interact with the academic behavioral psychology developed by I.P. Pavlov (1849-1936), J.B. Watson's (1878-1958) rigorous investigations of classic conditioning, and E.L. Thorndike's (1874-1949) work in operant conditioning (Thorndike, 1931). This cross-fertilization of disciplines and ideas eventually contributed to the formation of such modern cognitive behavioral mind-body interventions as biofeedback (Basmajian, 1981), modern autogenic training (Linden, 1990), visualization and guided imagery (Sheikh, 1983), the relaxation response (Benson, 1975), and the reexamination of older self-control practices such as meditation (West, 1991). These cognitive behavioral interventions, along with the psychosomatic movement, began as academic pursuits but have become valuable intellectual and clinical resources for alternative medicine. The vital force now can be conceptualized in psychosomatic terms or in the current mind-body framework. These mind-body techniques shift between conventional and nonconventional. They are less on the fringe, almost accepted, and often wholly accepted aspects of vitalist ideology. They are the lowest, most scientific aspects of the mesmeric legacy, a kind of legitimate mesmerism. Because of their university connections, these mind-body interventions have generated much research (Eisenberg et al., 1993; Holroyd & Penzien, 1990; Turner & Chapman, 1982). The vital energy has gone psychological. This has lent significant credibility to alternative medicine. Psychology has been a rich source of new interventions and theory for both conventional and alternative medicine. Occasionally, these efforts have been used to support more outlandish alternative healing ideas, to the discomfort of more scientifically inclined researchers. In any case the mesmeric force has become a hyphenated mind-body connection between the invisible mind (small *m*) and the visible body. in the last 50 years there probably have been more new psychological interventions and names developed—between 250 (Herink, 1980) and 400 (Karasu, 1986) types, depending on who counts and when—than in the entire history of mesmeric forces.

HOLISTIC MEDICINE

Vital energy and vitalism regrouped and reorganized itself during its post-1960s renaissance. Holism or holistic medicine has become the new family name, coined to avoid the tarnished image of older discredited medical ideas. The term originates within conventional medical debates of the early twentieth century over vitalism and reductionism.

Reductionism has been the corollary of the ascendancy of physicochemical mechanistic viewpoint. The trajectory of reductionism is roughly described by Morgagni's situation of life-activity and pathology in organs (1761), followed by Bichat's focus on tissue (1800), leading to Broussais's attention to lesions in tissues (1830s), to Virchow's localization in cells (1848), to Koch's germ theory (1882), all the way to modern dissection of genes. Obviously, this process is complex and not linear (cf. Mendelsohn, 1965). Emphasis on a mechanical physicochemical agency leads to progressively smaller analytical pieces. Yet again, within academic medicine there have been important antidotes to reductionism; organismic tendencies try to counterbalance or prevail over excessive reductionism. Antireductionist tendencies within conventional medicine emphasize homeostasis, predisposition, susceptibility, and psychosocial factors as opposed to those tendencies that emphasize an idea of disease that Tauber calls ontologic, autonomous, well-circumscribed states (Tauber, 1994). A few of the many names associated with nonreductionism within biomedicine include Claude Bernard, Walter Cannon, L.J. Henderson, George Draper, Charles Sherrington, Hans Selye, Helen Dunbar, George Engels, and Arthur Kleinman (Tracy, 1992).

One antireductionist position developed in the philosophy of biology was by J.C. Smuts, the Cambridge-educated, South African statesman who in 1926 coined the word *holism* (Smuts, 1926). Holism was meant to be both antivitalist and antimechanistic and argued that the entirety of an organism necessarily implied a teleologic purpose that could not be exhaustively explained by the laws governing component parts. The idea and word were appropriated by a few conventional scientists (Needham, 1955) and were later used positively by conventional medicine to imply humanistic, psychosocial, or systemic approaches in health care. For example, a December 18, 1948, editorial in the *Journal of the American Medical Association* speaks of the holistic concept as being "an integrated approach to the sick person as a being in a state of mental, moral, and physiological imbalance with his environment" (Editorial, 1948). In the 1970s holistic partially changed its association. A 1979 *New England Journal of Medicine* editorial criticized holistic medicine, saying, "patients must be dealt with as whole people. But this worthwhile philosophy is ill served by those who seek quick solutions to all the ills of mankind through the abandonment of science and rationality in favor of mystic cults" (Relman, 1979). The word *holism* is adopted by many unconventional health practitioners, most of whom are seemingly unaware of Smuts or his philosophy (Whorton, 1989), causing confusion; holism has become an amorphous label often glibly used or made trivial (Kopelman & Moskop, 1981) for any perspective that sees biomedicine as too reductionist or materialist. It also has become a generic name for any therapy that does not consider its clinical perspective to be reductionist. And, finally, it has become the new family name for any intervention—no matter how reductionist, such as chiropractic or crystals—that is informed, knowingly or unknowingly, by some form of a nineteenth century vitalist perspective. Recently the word *complementary* has been introduced, often replacing the word *holistic,* first in the United Kingdom in the 1980s and then in the United States in the 1990s.

VITALISM'S ATTRACTION

Vitalism can be attractive. Life is more than chemicals and mechanism. Agency is more than chemistry and physics. Mind, ideas, volition, intentions, spiritual entities, beliefs, innate intelligence, feelings, and mysterious vital forces can all become critical phenomena. The multivalent possibilities of vital energy—its lower, higher, natural, psychological, or supernatural forms—allow practitioners and patients to customize explanations and treatment options. Its very imprecision allows for enormous flexibility and adaptibility.

In conventional medicine it is sometimes too easy for a person to become an irrelevant spectator, over-

whelmed by a mechanical world of technology, tests, and surgery. The vitalist perspective, on the other hand, aligns itself with coherent, life-affirming principles. The vitalist universe is not random, detached, or mindless; it is benign, coherent, and extremely hospitable for people. Instead of a medicine whose central issues can seem coldly mechanical and buried in unaccessible physiology, vitalism instinctively invites a person to experience a unifying, transcendent, and reassuring ontological presence. Whatever the outcome of the recent scientific investigations of vitalist medical traditions, vitalism's attractiveness for practitioners and patients is likely to remain a growing presence in health care.

References

Anderson R, Meeker WC, Wirick BE, et al. 1992. A meta-analysis of clinical trials of spinal manipulation. J Manipulative Physiol Ther 15

Baer HA. 1987. Divergence and convergence in two systems of manual medicine: osteopathy and chiropractic in the United States. Med Anthro Q 1:2176-2193

Baer HA. 1992. The potential rejuvenation of American naturopathy as a consequence of the holistic health movement. Med Anthropol 13:369-383

Basmajian JV (ed). 1981. Biofeedback Principles and Practice for Clinicians. Institute for Psychosomatic Research, New York

Beck BL. 1991. Magnetic healing, spiritualism and chiropractic: Palmer's union of methodologies, 1886-1895. Chiro Hist 11(2):11-16

Beckford JA. 1984. Holistic imagery and ethics in new religious and healing movements. Social Compass 21(2-3):259-272

Benor DJ. 1990. Survey of spiritual healing research. Comp Med Res 4(3):9-33

Benson H. 1975. The Relaxation Response. Morrow, New York

Benton E. 1975. Vitalism in nineteenth-century scientific thought: a typology and reassessment. Stud Hist Phil Sci 5:1

Berman A. 1951. The Thomsonian movement and its relation to American pharmacy and medicine. Bull Hist Med 25:5

Beutler JJ, Attenvelt JT, Schooten SA, et al. 1988. Paranormal healing and hypertension. BMJ 296:1491-1494

Bigos SJ, Bowyer OR, Braen GR, et al. 1994. Clinical Practice Guideline #14. Acute Low Back Problems in Adults. U.S. Department of Health and Human Services, PHS Agency for Health Care Policy and Research. Rockville, Maryland

Braden CS. 1987. Spirits in Rebellion: The Rise and Development of New Thought. Southern Methodist University Press, Dallas

Braude A. 1989. Radical Spirits. Beacon Press, Boston

Brown PS. 1985. The vicissitudes of herbalism in late nineteenth- and early twentieth-century Britain. Med Hist 29:71-92

Campbell BF. 1980. Ancient Wisdom Revived: A History of the Theosophical Movement. University of California Press, Berkeley, California

Carter M. 1969. Helping Yourself With Reflexology. Parker, West Nyack, New York

Carter ME. 1972. My Years with Edgar Cayce. Harper & Row, New York

Cayleff SE. 1988. Gender, ideology and the water-cure movement, in Other Healers: Unorthodox Medicine in America. The Johns Hopkins University Press, Baltimore

Chiu ML. 1986. Mind, Body and Illness in Chinese Medical Tradition. Unpublished Ph.D. thesis. Harvard University

Chopra D. 1993. Creating Affluence. New World Press, New York

Coddington M. 1990. Seekers of the Healing Energy. Healing Arts Press. Rochester, Vermont

Cody G. 1985. History of naturopathic medicine, in Pizzorno JE, Murray MJ (eds). A Textbook of Natural Medicine. John Bastyr College Publications, Seattle

Cole-Whittaker T. 1983. How to Have More in a Have-Not World. Fawcett Crest, New York

Cooter R. 1987. Bones of contention? Orthodox medicine and the mystery of the bone-setter's craft, in Bynum WF, Porter R (eds). Medical Fringe & Medical Orthodoxy 1750-1859, Croom Helm, London: pp. 158-173

Coulter HL. 1977. Divided Legacy: A History of the Schism in Medical Thought, Vol II. Wehawaken Books, Washington, D.C.

Darton R. 1968. Mesmerism and the End of the Enlightenment in France. Harvard University Press, Cambridge, Massachusetts

Davis AJ. 1885. The Harbinger of Health. Colby and Rich, Banner Publishing, Boston

Donegan JB. 1986. Hydropathic Highway to Health. Greenwood Press, Westport, Connecticut

Dresser HW (ed). 1969. The Quimby Manuscripts. Citadel Press, Secaucus, New Jersey

Easthope G. 1986. Healers and Alternative Medicine. Gover, Aldershot, England

Editorial. 1948. Holistic Medicine. JAMA December 18, 1948

Eisenberg D. 1985. Encounters with Qi: Exploring Chinese Medicine. W.W. Norton, New York

Eisnberg D. 1995. Traditional Chinese Medicine, in Alternative Medicine: Implications for Clinical Practice. Harvard Medical School, Department of Continuing Education, Boston

Eisenberg D, Delbanco TL, Berkey CS, et al. 1993. Cognitive behavioral techniques for hypertension: are they effective? Ann Intern Med 118:964-972

Ellenberger HF. 1970. The Discovery of the Unconscious. Basic Books, New York: pp. 53-60

Ernst E. 1995. St. John's wort, an anti-depressant? a systematic, criteria-based review. PhytoMed 2(1):67-71

Feldman AB. 1963. Animal magnetism and the mother of Christian Science. Psychoanal Rev 50:153-160

Fishbein M. 1932. Fads and Quackery in Healing. Blue Ribbon, New York

Forber TR. 1972. Lapis Bufonis: the growth and decline of a medical superstition. Yale J Biol Med 45:139-149

Fox M. 1984. Conflict to coexistence: Christian Science and medicine. Med Anthro Fall 292-300

Fuller R. 1982. Mesmerism and the American Cure of Souls. University of Pennsylvania Press, Philadelphia

Fuller R. 1989. Alternative Medicine and American Religious Life. Oxford University Press, New York: p. 104

Galbreath R. 1971. The history of modern occultism: A bibliographical survey. J Pop Cult 5:726-754

Gevitz N. 1982. The D.O.'s: Osteopathic Medicine in America. The Johns Hopkins University Press, Baltimore

Gevitz N. 1988. Andrew Taylor Still and the social origins of osteopathy, in Studies in the History of Alternative Medicine. St. Martin's Press, New York

Gilson E. 1940. The Spirit of Medieval Philosophy. Charles Scribner's Sons, New York

Glick DC. 1988. Symbolic, ritual and social dynamics of spiritual healing. Soc Sci Med 27(11):1197-1206

Goldstein M. 1975. The Research Status of Spinal Manipulative Therapy. U.S. Department of Health, Education and Welfare, PHS, NIH, Bethesda, Maryland

Good BJ, Good MJ. 1981. Alternative health care in one California community. Public Regulation of Health Care Occupations in California, Sacramento

Gort EH, Coburn D. 1986. Naturopathy in Canada: changing relationships to medicine, chiropractic and the state. Soc Sci Med 26(10):1061-1072

Griggs B. 1981. Green Pharmacy: A History of Herbal Medicine. Jill Norman & Hobhouse, London

Hahnemann S. 1980. Organon of Medicine, 6th ed., W Boericke trans. B. Jain Publishers, New Delhi: p. 97

Haight E. 1975. The roots of the vitalism of Xavier Bichet. Bull Hist Med 49:72-86

Hall JA, Crasilneck HB. 1978. Hypnosis. JAMA 239(8):760-761

Hall TS. 1975. History of General Physiology, Vol 1. University of Chicago Press, Chicago

Haller JS. 1973. Acupuncture in nineteenth century western medicine. N Y State J Med May:1213-1221

Hartman E. 1977. Substance, Body and Soul: Aristotelian Investigations. Princeton University Press, Princeton, New Jersey

Herink R (ed). 1980. The Psychotherapy Handbook. New American Library, New York

Hill C, Doyon F. 1990. Review of randomized trials of homeopathy. Rev Epidemiol Sante Publique 38:139-147

Holroyd KA, Penzien DB. 1990. Pharmacological versus non-pharmacological prophylaxis of recurrent migraine headache: a meta-analytic review of clinical trials. Pain 42:1-13

Huxtable RJ. 1992. The myth of beneficent nature: the risks of herbal preparations. Ann Intern Med 117(2):165-166

James W. 1961. The Varieties of Religious Experience. Collier, New York

Johnson ES et al. 1985. Efficacy of feverfew as prophylactic treatment of migraine. BMJ 291:569-573

Judah JS. 1967. The History and Philosophy of the Metaphysical Movements in America. Westminster Press, Philadelphia

Kaplan F. 1974. `The Mesmeric Mania': The early Victorians and animal magnetism. J Hist Ideas 35:4

Karasu TB. 1986. The specificity vs. non-specificity dilemma: towards identifying therapeutic change agents. Am J Psychiatry 14:3-6

Kaufman M. 1988. Homeopathy in America: The Rise and Fall and Persistence of a Medical Heresy. The Johns Hopkins University Press, Baltimore

Kemp S. 1990. Medieval Psychology. Greenwood Press, New York

Keyes K. 1989. Discovering the Secrets of Happiness. Love Line Books, Coos Bay, Oregon

Kleijnen J, Knipschild P, ter Riet G. 1991a. Clinical trials of homeopathy. BMJ 302:316-323

Kleijnen J, ter Riet G, Knipschild P. 1991b. Acupuncture and asthma: a review of controlled trials. Thorax 46:799-802

Knapp JE, Antonucci EJ. 1990. A National Study of the Profession of Massage Therapy/Bodywork. Knapp and Associates, Princeton, New Jersey

Kopelman L, Moskop J. 1981. The holistic health movement: a survey and critique. J Med Philosophy May 6 (2):209-235

Krieger D, Peper E, Ancoli S. 1979. Therapeutic touch: searching for evidence of physiological change. Am J Nur April, 660-662

Kuriyama S. 1986. Varieties of Haptic Experience: A Comparative Study of Greek and Chinese Pulse Diagnosis. Unpublished Ph.D. thesis, Harvard University

Lad V. 1984. Ayuraveda. Lotus Press, Sante Fe, New Mexico

Lain Entralgo P. 1948. Sensualism and vitalism in Bichat's 'Anotomie Generale.' J Hist Med 3

Larson JL. 1979. Vital forces: regulative principles or constitutive agents? Isis 70

Ledermann EK. 1989. Philosophy and Medicine. Gower, Aldershot, England

Levin JS, Coreil J. 1986. 'New Age' healing in the U.S. Soc Sci Med 23:9

Linde K, Jonas WB, Melchart D, et al. 1994. Critical review and meta-analysis of serial agitated dilutions in experimental toxicology. Hum Exp Toxicol 13:481-492

Linden W. 1990. Autogenic Training. A Clinical Guide. Guilford Press, New York

Lipman TO. 1967. Vitalism and reductionism in Liebig's physiological thought. Isis 58:167-185

Low J. 1988. The modern body therapies: Aston-Patterning. Massage Magazine 16:48-55

Lytle CD. 1993. An Overview of Acupuncture. U.S. Department of Health and Human Services, PHS, FDA, Washington, D.C.

Macklin RM. 1993. Magnetic healing, quackery and the debate about the health effects of electromagnetic fields Ann Intern Med 118(5):376-383

Manga P, Angus DE, Papadopoulos C, et al. 1993. A Study to Examine the Effectiveness and Cost-Effectiveness of Chiropractic Management of Low-Back Pain. Pran Managa & Associates, Ottawa

Marvin C. 1988. When Old Technologies Were New: Thinking About Electric Communication in the Late Nineteenth Century, Oxford, New York

McClenon J. 1984. Deviant Science: The Case of Parapsychology. University of Pennsylvania Press, Philadelphia

McRae G. 1982. A critical overview of U.S. acupuncture regulation. J Health Polit Policy Law 1:163-196

McVaugh M, Mauskupf JD. 1976. Rhine's extra-sensory perception and its background in psychical research. Isis 67:161-189

Meade TW, Dyer S, Browne W, et al. 1990. Low back pain of mechanical origin: randomized comparison of chiropractic and hospital outpatient treatment. BMJ 300

Melchart D et al. 1994. Immunodulation with Echinacea—a systematic review of controlled clinical trials. Phytomedicine 1:245-254

Melton JG. 1988. A history of the New Age movement, in Basil B (ed). Not Necessarily the New Age: Critical Essays. Prometheus Books, Buffalo, New York

Mendelsohn E. 1965. Physical models of physiological concepts: explanation in nineteenth-century biology. Br J Hist Sci 2:7

Meyers D. 1965. The Positive Thinkers: A Study of the American Quest for Health, Wealth, and Personal Power from Mary Baker Eddy to Norman Vincent Peale. Doubleday, Garden City, New Jersey

Mesmer FA. 1980. Dissertation on the Discovery of Animal Magnetism in Bloch GJ (ed). trans. Mesmerism: A Translation of the Original Medical and Scientific Writings of F.A. Mesmer, M.D. William Kaufmann, Los Altos, California

Miura K. 1989. The revival of qi gong in contemporary China in Taoist Meditation and Longevity Techniques. Center for Chinese Studies, University of Michigan, Ann Arbor, Michigan

Moore RL. 1977. In Search of White Crows: Spiritualism Parapsychology and American Cult. Oxford University Press, New York

Namikoshi T. 1969. Shiatsu. Japan Publications, New York

Needham J. 1955. Mechanistic Biology and the Religious Consciousness in Science, Religion & Reality. George Brazziler, New York

Needham J. 1956. Science & Civilization in China. vol 2. Cambridge University Press, Cambridge

Netherton M, Shiffrin N. 1978. Past Lives Therapy. William Morrow, New York

Neuburger M. 1933. The Doctrine of the Healing Power of Nature. New York Homeopathic College, New York

Oppenheim J. 1988. The Other World: Spiritualism and Psychical Research in England, 1850-1914. Cambridge University Press, Cambridge

Palmer DD. 1910. Chiropractic Portland Printing House, Portland: p. 691

Perry R. 1987. An Introduction to a Course in Miracles. Miracle Distribution Center. Fullerton, California

Pomeranz B, Stux G (eds). 1988. Scientific Basis of Acupuncture. Springer-Verlag, Berlin

Rather LJ. 1961. G.E. Stahl's Psychological Physiology. Bull Hist Med 35:27-49

Relman AS. 1979. Holistic Medicine. N Engl J Med 300(6):312-313

Reyner JH. 1982. Psionic Medicine. Routledge & Kegan Paul, London

Roger J. 1986. The mechanistic conception of life, in God and Nature. University of California Press, Berkeley

Rolf IP. 1977. Rolfing: The Integration of Human Structure. Harper & Row, New York

Rose L. 1954. Some aspects of paranormal healing. BMJ Dec 4:1329-1332

Rothstein WG. 1985. American Physicians in the 19th Century. The Johns Hopkins University Press, Baltimore

Rothstein WG. 1988. The botanical movements and orthodox medicine, in Other Healers: Unorthodox Medicine in America. The Johns Hopkins University Press, Baltimore

Schaller WE, Caroll CR. 1976. Health, Quackery and the Consumer. W.B. Saunders, Philadelphia

Schoepflin RB. 1988. Christian Science Healing in America, in Other Healers: Unorthodox Medicine in America. The Johns Hopkins University Press, Baltimore

Schotz EH, Cyriax J. 1975. Manipulation: Past and Present. William Heinemann Medical Books, London

Sharma U. 1992. Complementary Medicine Today: Practitioners and Patients. Tavistock/Routledge, London

Sheikh AA. 1983. Imagery. Current Theory, Research and Application. John Wiley, New York

Shekelle P, Adams AH, Chassin MR, et al. 1992. Spinal manipulation for low-back pain. Ann Intern Med 117:7

Siegel BS. 1986. Love, Medicine & Miracles. Harper & Row, New York

Sigerist HE. 1961. A History of Medicine. Oxford University Press, New York

Sivin N. 1987. Traditional Medicine in Contemporary China. Center of Chinese Studies, University of Michigan, Ann Arbor, Michigan

Smuts JC. 1926. Holism and Evolution. Macmillan, New York

Strupp HH, Howard KI. 1992. A brief history of psychotherapy research, in Frehen DK (ed). History of Psychotherapy, American Psychological Association, Washington, D.C.

Sutton G. 1981. Electric medicine and mesmerism. Isis 72(253):375-392

Tauber AT. 1994. Darwinian aftershocks: repercussions in late twentieth century medicine. J R Soc Med 87:27-31

ter Riet G, Kleijnen, Knipschild P, et al. 1990. Acupuncture and chronic pain: a criteria-based meta-analysis. J Clin Epidemiol 43:1191-1199

Terrett AJ. 1991. The genius of D.D. Palmer: an exploration of the origin of chiropractic in his time. Chir Hist 11:1

Thorndike EL. 1931. Human Learning. Century, New York

Toulmin S, Goodfield J. 1962. The Architecture of Matter. Harper & Row, New York: pp. 322-330

Tracy SW. 1992. George Draper and the American constitutional medicine, 1916-1946: reinventing the sick man. Bull Hist Med 66:53-89

Turner JA, Chapman CR. 1982. Psychological interventions for chronic pain: a critical review. I. Relaxation training and biofeedback. Pain 12:1-21

Turner RW. 1990. Naturopathic Medicine. Wellingborought, Northamptonshire, England: p. 21

Vlamis G. 1978. Polarity therapy. Alternatives. 2:4(April) 23-26

Wardwell WI. 1992. Chiropractic: History and Evolution of a New Profession. Mosby–Year Book, St. Louis

Warner JH. 1987. Medical sectarianism, therapeutic conflict, and the shaping of orthodox professional identity in antebellum American medicine, in Bynum WF, Porter R (eds). Medical Fringe & Medical Orthodoxy 1750-1850 London: Croom Helm

West AM (ed). 1991. The Psychology of Meditation. Clarendon Press, Oxford

Wheeler R. 1939. Vitalism. H.F. & G. Witherby, London

Wheelwright EG. 1974. Medicinal Plants and Their History. Dover, New York

Whorton, JC. 1986. Drugless healing in the 1920's: the therapeutic cult of sanipractic Phar Hist 28:14-24

Whorton JC. 1989. The first holistic revolution: alternative medicine in the nineteenth century, in Stalker D, Glymour C (eds). Examining Holistic Medicine, Prometheus Books, Buffalo, New York

Yoke HP. 1985. Li, Qi, and Shu: An Introduction to Science and Civilization in China. Hong Kong University Press, Hong Kong

Suggested Readings

Carlson CJ. 1979. Holism and reductionism as perspectives in medicine and patient care. West J Med 131(6):466-470

Gardner M. 1988. Isness is her business: Shirley MacLaine, in Basil R (ed). Not Necessarily the New Age: Critical Essays. Prometheus Books, Buffalo, New York: p. 193

Kaufman M. 1971. Homeopathy in America: The Rise and Fall of a Medical Heresy. The Johns Hopkins University Press, Baltimore

Pavlov IP. 1928. Lectures on Conditioned Reflexes. International Publishers, New York

Zefron LJ. 1975. The history of the laying-on of hands in nursing. Nursing Forum XIV(4):350-363

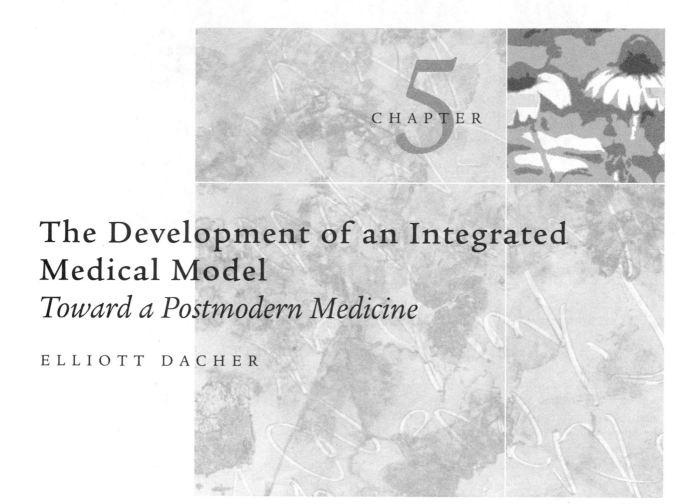

CHAPTER 5

The Development of an Integrated Medical Model
Toward a Postmodern Medicine

ELLIOTT DACHER

oday we find ourselves living in an extraordinary in-between time—a gap in history between two sets of values. This gap has been created by the decline of our previously unquestioned optimism and faith in modernism, its values and institutions, and the slow and as yet uncertain emergence of a new postmodern worldview. Disillusionment with the limitations and excesses of biomedicine and efforts to revitalize our approach to health and healing emerge from this pregnant historical moment. To understand this circumstance is to understand that the changes that we now envision are fundamental rather than cosmetic and as much compelled as chosen. Because of the highly personal nature of health, this shift in worldview is most publicly and passionately played out in the arena of health and healing.

THE DEVELOPMENT OF THE BIOMEDICAL MODEL

The practice of American medicine has been slowly maturing for the past 150 years of the modern era. We can readily identify four distinct phases in its development: its inception as a frontier medicine in the eighteenth and early nineteenth centuries; the rise of the institutions of scientific medicine in the late nineteenth and early twentieth centuries (Figure 5-1); the recognition of the high costs of scientific medicine and the resulting cost sharing and cost containment initiatives of the past 60 years; and the current emergence of a postmodern medicine based on an expanded set of assumptions and values. To accurately understand the maturation of American medicine we must begin by

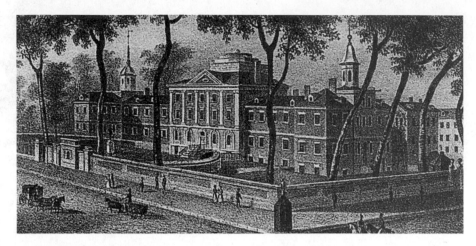

Figure 5-1 Pennsylvania hospital, circa 1800, America's first hospital. (Courtesy The Pennsylvania Hospital, Philadelphia, Pennsylvania.)

examining the forces that have shaped our current approach to health and healing.

Scientific medicine as it is known today was nonexistent before the late nineteenth century. With a few notable exceptions, medical schools were free-standing commercial ventures unaffiliated with universities and lacking the bare essentials of an educational curriculum. For a moderate fee any individual, regardless of the presence or absence of previous educational achievement, could attend a brief 3- to 6-month course of study conducted by local physicians who shared the tuition as personal income. Written examinations were not possible because of the lack of writing skills, licensing procedures were minimal, clinical training with actual patients was nonexistent, and the general status of physicians was fairly low. In 1869 Harvard Medical School, one of the best in the nation, had 300 students, of whom no more than 20% had a college degree and fewer than 50% were said to be able to write English (Harrington, 1905).

This situation began to change toward the end of the nineteenth century as universities slowly improved their undergraduate programs and then focused their attention on professional training. The changes were initiated at Harvard in 1870 by the new and dynamic president Charles Eliot, who strongly supported the German university model that emphasized the scientific and laboratory-based teaching methods that had proved highly successful in identifying the microbial causes of the infectious diseases that had devastated Europe for millennia. The new

medical program at Harvard created more stringent admission criteria, a longer course of study, written examinations, a full-time faculty, a complete integration of the medical school into the university, and a laboratory-based teaching method. In summary, as the study of disease shifted from the context of the individual within his or her family and community to the laboratory, the patient's disease became the doctor's disease, and the unique human story line gave way to generic diagnostic coding.

Over a period of decades, an increasing number of medical schools embraced these ideas, a movement that culminated in the opening of the Johns Hopkins medical school in 1893 (Gilman, 1969 [1906]). As a result of the philanthropy of Johns Hopkins, the medical faculty, under the guidance of Daniel Coit Gilman, William Welch, John Shaw Billings, Sir William Osler, Howard Kelly, and William Halsted, were able to fully develop the new model of medical education unencumbered by the traditions and politics of an existing institution. Yet irrespective of these new approaches, by the turn of the century most of the more than 100 existing commercial medical schools had failed to undertake these changes.

As a result, in 1907 Andrew Carnegie, through his newly formed Carnegie Foundation, funded a study of medical education by Abraham Flexner (Figure 5-2), an aggressive and highly capable educator. The study was designed to document the sorry state of medical education that continued in most medical schools (Flexner, 1910). In this famous report, Flexner insisted that all medical schools comply with

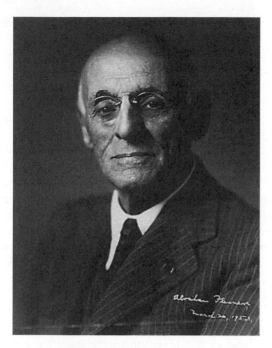

Figure 5-2 Abraham Flexner. (Courtesy National Library of Medicine, Bethesda, Maryland.)

the Hopkins approach or shut down. He, as the medical reformers preceding him, promoted a university-based scientifically trained practitioner.

These efforts were readily accepted by a general public immersed in the spirit of progressivism and, by the 1900s, increasingly aware of the practical results of medical science (the identification of the bacterial causes of specific disease; the use of antisepsis and asepsis; the use of the x-ray; the development of vaccines against rabies, typhoid, and the bubonic plague; and the discovery of Salvarsan, the first effective antibacterial drug). The general public sought an educated, skillful, modern-day medical practitioner. Flexner, subsequently serving as general secretary of the General Education Board, a Rockefeller philanthropy, directed extensive funds (estimated at $1.7 billion in today's dollars) toward the promotion of his report (Ludmerer, 1985). The result of these efforts, as well as those of others, led to the complete transformation of medical education and practice into a disciplined, highly structured applied science, what is now called biomedicine.

As faith in the possibilities of scientific medicine expanded, research blossomed, medical centers emerged, new technologies evolved, and by the 1930s the high costs of scientific medicine became evident.

Slowly, over a period of decades, third parties began to take over the funding of medical services with the goal of distributing their cost among large groups of the sick and well. A lengthy process took place that was in the end to determine the ultimate third party, the federal government or private industry. At the beginning of the 21st century it appears that private industry has won this competition, although not completely free from federal regulatory efforts. Health care has become a commodity subject to market forces and values. The changes promoted by Eliot, Gilman, Welsh, Flexner, and others had unexpectedly resulted in a cascade of changes, many of which would have been unimaginable and unacceptable to these great innovators.

A considered analysis of the development of biomedicine during the period of 1870-1920 demonstrates that it was an appropriate and highly successful response to the *circumstances and needs of that era*. Today, our circumstances and needs are different. They are different because of the success of the biomedical model, changing social conditions accompanied by a shift in the burden of disease from acute to chronic, and the rapid expansion over the past century of our understanding of the relations of consciousness, health, and disease. Our task must be to facilitate the further evolution of medicine in a manner that responds to the imperatives of the new millennium.

NEW INITIATIVES

Much as the escalating costs of scientific medicine became apparent by the 1930s, by the 1960s its effectiveness, given the needs and temperament of our time, and its more covert iatrogenic effects became further causes for concern. Rene Dubos in his book *Mirage of Health* (1961) and Thomas McKeown in his book *The Role of Medicine: Dream, Mirage, or Nemesis* (1976) expressed an emerging skepticism about the ability of scientific medicine to resolve contemporary medical problems. Ivan Illich in *Medical Nemesis* (1976) articulated a growing concern for the clinical and social iatrogenic consequences of scientific medicine. And a recognition of the shift in the burden of disease from infectious diseases to stress-related illness, chronic disease, emotional disorders, and lifestyle and environmentally related disorders further highlighted the limitations of biomedicine when confronted with the complexities of modern existence.

Simultaneously, other developments were occurring in the field of psychology and consciousness research. These included an expanded understanding of the interactions of mind and body (Dacher, 1996; Locke, 1986), the impact of personal relationships (Berkman & Syme, 1979) and socioeconomic status (Adler et al., 1993; Hause et al., 1982) on health and disease, and a renewed interest in the healing powers of the spirit (Benor, 1992). The turn outward in biomedicine to science, manipulative interventions, and technology led to the constellation of a complementary force—the turn inward toward self-care, mind-body resources, holism, and psychological and spiritual development as counterpoints to the limitations and excesses of scientific medicine.

Today's emerging social and personal forces have given rise to four major new initiatives in the arena of health and healing: the wellness, holistic, mind-body, and alternative therapies movements. Beginning in the 1970s, these initiatives began to confront the dominant medical model with a new set of values and perspectives, perspectives that at their core were inconsistent with those of biomedicine. They heralded the potential for a revitalization of health and healing, and the infusion of these new ideas was well received by a culture that no longer held an unquestioned faith in the values and practices of biomedicine.

A study completed by Paul Ray, *The Integral Culture Survey*, shed further light on these developments (1996). He identified the recent emergence of three coexisting subcultures: traditional, modern, and cultural creatives. Each had its unique value system, perspectives, and language. The traditionalists were most clearly identified by their religious and traditional values; the modernists by their focus on materialism; and the most recently emerging group, the cultural creatives, by their emphasis on community, ecology, and self-actualization. It is this group, which Ray suggests may comprise as many as 44 million Americans, that is most challenging the values and perspectives of contemporary medicine.

However, it is the invariable tendency of an existing perspective to sustain itself. Thomas Kuhn suggests in his book *The Structure of Scientific Revolutions* that, when challenged from without, those invested in the dominant perspective, individuals and institutions, first deny the significance of new initiatives, then characterize them as "fringe," and finally attempt to co-opt them by incorporating these initiatives into the mainstream of existing culture, reshaping them in a way that conforms to the old rather than supporting the new (1970). This is largely the fate of each of the movements previously mentioned. The wellness movement, a rich blend of psychological, social, and spiritual perspectives, was reduced to its most physical elements: nutrition, exercise, smoking cessation, and relaxation training. The rich philosophical vision of holism, often mistaken for humanism and a multiplicity of practices, became a commodity to be labeled, bottled, and sold. The mind-body movement has failed to be significantly integrated into the biomedical model. And the alternative and complementary movements in their urgency for licensure, social legitimization, and reimbursement are in danger of losing the essential uniqueness of their traditions as they become mainstreamed and increasingly perceived as merely one more set of therapeutic tools (Duggan, 1995).

These initiatives may expand our therapeutic options and open up the dominant medical system, but once exposed to the system and its unchanged worldview and core values, they cannot prosper. A school that trains students in oriental medicine and instills within them a broader set of values must then release these students into the world of contemporary practice and managed care. A well-designed clinical research program that is inclusive of a broader set of values is unlikely to have its research accepted by the dominant medical model, and well-meaning practitioners may change the character of their practice but not the cultural context within which it is embedded. Much the same can be said for any effort that does not address in a more global sense the fundamental issue of values, particularly the values that are emerging in our current time as a counterforce to the limits and excesses of biomedicine. As a result, what seems hopeful in the beginning turns out to be far less innovative than originally imagined. Although these movements have managed to shake up the system and to catalyze the dissolution of the existing worldview, they have not served to transform it. This failure can be directly attributed to the absence of a guiding dialogue focused on values and vision.

VALUE-CENTERED DECISION MAKING

Values are not addressed in the modern worldview. They are considered soft issues, subjective ones that cannot be seen, touched, or measured through our senses. The objectivistic worldview maps, categorizes, and models the surface of reality. It neither legitimizes nor allows for any discussion about the *context* in which physical reality is embedded: the human and cultural experience. When new initiatives arise, they are seen only in terms of their physical and external aspects: nutrition, exercise, smoking cessation, objectified models of holism, techniques, and therapies. The underside is simply not seen; human meaning, significance, and values are excluded from discussion—the map maker is lost from view. Where there appears to be change there is none.

Although value-centered decision making is an ongoing and natural part of the human experience, we are generally unaware of its occurrence. The choices we make and the actions that we take are too often unconsciously compelled by our personal and collective value systems. For example, in a culture that values objectivism (i.e., sensory-based knowledge) our actions are exclusively based on factual information and data, and intuitive, nonrational knowledge is treated with skepticism and disregard. Our values and actions are predetermined by hidden cultural assumptions. They are not freely chosen. They are neither conscious nor intentional.

Lawrence Kohlberg enhanced our understanding of this issue with his theory of moral development and its three stages: (1) preconventional, the undeveloped perspective of the child; (2) conventional, the unconscious assimilation of enculturated values; and (3) postconventional, the evolution of an authentic individual value system (Kohlberg, 1984). Only in the postconventional level of development is the individual capable of participating in conscious and intentional value-centered decision making.

At any one moment in time individuals are spread throughout each of these three stages of development, but with the maturing of a culture and the expansion of consciousness an increasing number of individuals develop a postconventional capacity to consciously choose and assert their unique value system. The term *value-centered decision making* refers to a manner of decision making that occurs when an individual, community, and culture are capable of consciously reflecting on their values within a context of moral development and then freely choosing from among these values ones that are consistent with the needs of the individual within the framework of the imperatives of the historical age.

Consider the following. When caring for the severely ill individual, physicians and families are called on to make critical decisions. In the usual scenario the underlying yet covert conventional assumption is that a goal of rational medicine is the prolongation of life, the effort to eradicate or deter disease, aging, and death. Our medical expertise and technology are used to promote the value we attribute to this assumption. But what would happen if we made this value explicit to the individuals involved and offered a competing value: for example, the goal of medicine and medical science is to support the individual in living through the natural cycles of life. Now we have two values to consider and choose from, and when we choose that which we value most, it will serve as a compass that guides our actions. This is an example of conscious and intentional value-centered decision making.

So it is apparent that value-centered decision making is an ongoing process. The issue is whether it is conscious or unconscious. In the latter instance, we are automatically chained to the past; in the former we are free to consider the imperatives of our present lives and to choose with a fully informed and aware mind. *Consciousness* and *intention* are the two qualities that distinguish conscious decision making from conditioned decision making. They can allow us to engage each other in the communal effort of choosing what is *good* for us as individuals and as a culture. Existing assumptions can be made explicit so that we may choose to continue to value them or not, and the full range of alternative assumptions can become available for us to examine. In this process we become involved in consciously envisioning the future, and as a result of this process the power over our lives that has been inexorably compelled by covert assumptions is brought to an end.

To bring the process of conscious and intentional value-centered decision making into the arena of health and healing requires that we become familiar with the underlying assumptions of the existing medical model, biomedicine, and of an alternative set of assumptions. With these choices in mind we can attribute value in the direction that seems most appropriate to our current needs and to our vision of the future.

To address this issue we recently completed a study for the Institute of Noetic Sciences in which we examined, from a value-centered perspective, the full range of issues involved in an expanded, comprehensive, and fully integrated approach to health and disease. We undertook a series of targeted interviews with individuals who are working toward a postmodern approach to health care, convened a series of focused group meetings, and completed a qualitative analysis of the patterns that emerged from these discussions.

This dialogue included representatives from diverse groups that share a common interest in the outcome of the health care debate. This included health care providers of various types of practices, consumer groups, policy makers, and key leaders in the reconceptualization of health care. This study considered a variety of issues including the influence of social and cultural perspectives on health care; the epistemological assumptions of various health care systems; the impact of the expanding accessibility of health information; the role of consciousness, intentionality, and spiritual dimensions in health and healing; the changing role of the practitioner and patient; the education of the health care practitioner; the scope and character of related health care research; and the role of public policy and health care financing.

In individual interviews and small group discussions there was a remarkable similarity in the articulation of values on which a postmodern medicine can be formulated. In analyzing this research we identified a specific set of values that could form the basis of a postmodern medicine and the recurrence of several general themes related to the enculturation of these values.

From Encounter to Relationship

Our study participants uniformly focused on the importance of renewing and revitalizing the relationship between physician and patient. The content and character of this relationship continue to hold value and meaning to them. There is general agreement that the proper relationship should be one that emphasizes mutuality, empathy, compassion, caring, authenticity, integrity, and trust. Stated briefly, the practitioner-patient relationship, which currently focuses on efficiently "doing" the standardized activities of diagnosis and therapy, should reconfigure itself toward "being," the process of sharing a relationship, one that is characterized by some as a partnership. This is a shift in emphasis from data collection to human interaction. There is an awareness among both the practitioners and the lay individuals who were interviewed that the character and quality of the healer-healee relationship can itself become a potent healing force.

The recent Pew-Fetzer Task Force report on *Advancing Psychosocial Health Education* focused on "relationship-centered care" (Tresolini & Pew-Fetzer Task Force, 1994). To work effectively in the patient-practitioner relationship it defined the essential knowledge, skills, and values that must be developed in four areas: (1) self-awareness and continuing self-growth; (2) the patient's experience of health and illness; (3) developing and maintaining a relationship with patients; and (4) communicating clearly and effectively. Self-awareness is seen as serving as the foundation for an empathic understanding of another's circumstance, and a sustained healing relationship is seen as based on honest, open, and trusting communication. These views were mirrored in our participant comments.

From Disease Centered to Person Centered

Our study participants went beyond their emphasis on the importance of the quality of the physician-patient relationship to speak about the focal point of the interaction. They expressed a dissatisfaction with the disease-centered orientation of the medical encounter, preferring it to be person centered and individualized. A disease-centered perspective collapses the uniqueness and intactness of an individual and the context that his or her life is embedded in, substituting instead the generic search for data, normative or nonnormative, the sole intent of which is to define the presence or absence of disease categories. Individuals appear to want to be seen, particularly by their healers, as the unique and complex individuals that they are, and similarly, healers express the desire for the time, opportunity, and support that is necessary to hold their patients in this manner. As stated by one participant, ". . . there should be a radical emphasis on the individuality of each person."

The shift from a focus on disease categories to a focus on the individual addresses two further values raised by our participants: wholeness (the appreciation of context) and integrity. To be seen and known as an individual whose experiences constitute a dynamic unity requires the practitioner to expand his or her worldview so as to be large enough to contain both a reductionistic and integrated view of the individual, a perspective that is both analytic and synthetic at the same time. To be seen in a reductionistic manner confirms the observation that for specific purposes the body may potentially be seen as a closed mechanical system. To be seen from an integrative perspective affirms an individual's wholeness, integrity, uniqueness, complexity, and sense of coherence, allowing for empathic understanding. One cannot have empathy for a body part. To be seen as a whole acknowledges the centrality of the individual in the healing process.

From Practitioner and Corporate Empowerment to Personal Empowerment

The power relationships in contemporary medicine derive from the conditions of their historical development. The shift to a science-centered medicine resulted from the simultaneous choice of and extraordinary financial investment in the expansion of medical science and its research facilities, the reinvention of the medical school curriculum by basing it in the laboratory sciences, and the integration of medical education into the emerging academic centers. The consequent development of the profession of medicine as an autonomous and authoritative profession granted to it the exclusive rights to practice medicine and to define and manage its domain, a right that was increasingly formalized by state licensing boards in the early part of the twentieth century. The power over the healing process shifted from household family members to an eclectic group of healers and then to the physician and his institutions.

The second shift in power occurred as the financial costs of a scientific-centered medicine became apparent in the 1930s. The high costs of health care, which rapidly became unaffordable to most families, resulted in the development of the third-party payer system and the subsequent decades-long drama that was to decide the central third-party payer—government or private industry—a drama that has been resolved in one direction or another nation-by-nation. This process has resulted in a shift of power, and the accompanying capacity to define the character of health care, from the professional domain of physicians to governmental institution or the board room of the corporation. This can be seen as the shift in health care from a service to a product.

But these shifts in power occurred in an era of expanding social and political citizen activism that has served to create another potentially powerful center of interest: the consumer of health care. The wellness, holistic, mind-body–self-regulation, and complementary and alternative care movements are each a demonstration of this new and growing force. Indi-

viduals are discovering their central role in the healing process, capacities for self-healing, ability to access scientific and other health-related information rapidly and effectively through the Internet, and their right to question the actions of physicians, corporations, and government.

From Illness to Wellness

In the 1970s John Travis, MD, opened the first wellness center in Mill Valley, California. Influenced by Halbert Dunn's book *High Level Wellness,* Travis sought to expand our ideas about health beyond the customary focus on preventing and curing disease to include a concern for the promotion of well-being. Health and healing were seen in a broader context as a psychological-social-spiritual process of education, lifestyle change, and personal growth and development. This concept was rapidly accepted by an increasingly health-conscious self-help culture, resulting in a proliferation of exercise facilities and fitness programs, health food stores, self-help books, corporate employee wellness programs, and wellness workshops and seminars conducted by individuals and institutions. Prevention, usually considered to reside within the domain of public health and population-based interventions, expanded into a social and private activity as it extended its vision toward health promotion.

The shift from an exclusive focus on illness to an emphasis on wellness, even in the context of illness, is related to the values we have already discussed: the emphasis on the practitioner-patient relationship, person-centered care, and personal empowerment. Although the interest in wellness and health promotion, an interest that should be seen as a radical expansion of all previous conceptualizations of health, has been apparent in our culture for 25 years, it has yet to be fully enculturated into our health care system or our popular culture.

GENERAL THEMES

The Absence of a Bridging Language

The language of government and corporate health and market forces is increasingly becoming the dominant language that defines the character of health care. Words and terms like *consumer, provider, payer, capitation, market share, per member per month costs, stream of revenue, managed care, delivery of services, utilization, encounters, purchasers of care,* and *lives covered* reflect a specific set of values applied by the corporate culture to the process of health care. This language relates to a specific view of medicine that emphasizes the economics of disease and curative therapeutics.

In contrast, participants in the new study have been working to develop a very different set of words and terms, ones that define the human dimensions of health care rather than its commodification. Such a language may include words and terms such as *holism, integrity, caring, listening, mind-body, spirituality, consciousness,* and *soul.* This reflects a view of medicine that emphasizes the relational aspects of healing and focuses on health as a broader experience of mind, body, and spirit, one that is ongoing and multidimensional.

The Absence of Enculturation

When values have failed to become enculturated, they are neither *collectively* held nor acknowledged, affirmed, or supported by the culture at large. External social structures that bring tangibility and affirmation through acknowledged social roles, community rituals, and institutional structures are absent. As a result, the emerging values can only be personally embodied (in contrast to enculturated), individually expressed by those who nurture them, and supported by islands of like-minded individuals or institutions.

If one considers the three subcultures defined by Ray—traditionalists, modernists, and cultural creatives—it becomes apparent that the first two subcultures have clear social contexts (enculturation) within which to live out and affirm their core values. In the first instance, traditionalists can look toward their fundamentalist religious affiliations and institutions for ongoing support and validation. In the second instance, modernists need only to turn to the dominant institutions of contemporary culture that readily offer the roles and rituals to support their value system. For both these groups interior values are reflected in external social structures that bring tangibility in the form of community, roles, and institutional structures to what otherwise would remain a set of values that can only be experienced and validated internally or interpersonally. Cultural creatives, the prime proponents of the emerging postmodern values, lack the built-in external social con-

texts within which they can readily live and experience their new value system.

The absence of normalized social contexts (enculturation) within which to "talk and walk" postmodern values appears to impose both a burden and a responsibility on those who hold these values. The burden is the inability to easily and routinely live and affirm these values within the existing cultural roles and models. This will continue until these values become enculturated. The responsibility appears to be a personal sense of importance attributed to finding a way to successfully infuse these values into the normative life of our culture. In the arena of health and healing this effort is to instill into a scientifically and technologically based medicine (education, research, and clinical practice) the emerging postmodern values discussed previously.

AN INTEGRAL MODEL OF HEALING

The following model draws on the values research discussed previously and uses systems theory, a theory that first developed as a modern response to the accumulation of expanding volumes of information and data and an increasing emphasis on microspecialization (Dacher, 1996). Systems, or organizational, theory is an attempt to integrate, to create wholes out of parts. It is in essence a science of wholeness. Its concepts and principles are based on the observation that nature is organized in patterns of increasing complexity and comprehensiveness and that these larger wholes, or units, have characteristics and qualities unique to the whole and cannot be identified or accessed through an analysis of their component parts (van Bertalanffy, 1968; Weiss, 1977). For example, the human organism, composed of cells, tissues, and organ systems, contains qualities and characteristics that cannot be exclusively accounted for through the linear summation of its parts. These include the capacity for self-organization, integrated action and adaptability, will, intention, and creativity.

Each of the subsystems of this model is a complete and distinct whole in itself, yet at the same time it is part of a more comprehensive healing system. As an intact system, each of these component systems has its own frame of reference, operating principles, internal stability, characteristics, and research methodology. As we ascend the hierarchy of healing systems, we expand

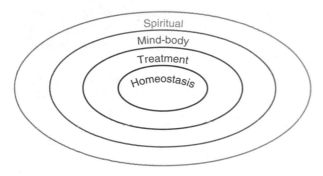

Figure 5-3 An integral model of healing.

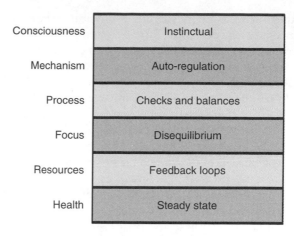

Figure 5-4 Homeostasis.

our conceptualization of healing, adding both complexity and comprehensiveness at each new level. Each component of the systems can be studied separately, and the entire system can be studied both in terms of its system-wide characteristics and the interrelations of its component parts. For the scientific researcher, it is appropriate to selectively study a particular system, applying the research methodology appropriate to the system under study. The practitioner, however, whose focus is always the whole person, must have the dual concern of attending to the individual components of the healing system while considering these components within the context of a more inclusive and comprehensive multisystem approach to healing.

The model is composed of four healing systems: homeostasis, treatment, mind-body, and spiritual. Figure 5-3 illustrates the relation of the component parts to the whole.

The Homeostatic Healing System

Walter Cannon described the most primary and basic healing system available to the human organism, the homeostatic system (Figure 5-4). This built-in instinctual system of internal physiological checks and balances evolved over the millennia of human development, providing the human organism with the potential to automatically respond to internal states of disequilibrium with immediate, reflexlike physiological corrections. This system ensures the maintenance of a steady physiological state, which in turn ensures survival.

However, our homeostatic system is far more suited to the life of early humans than it is to the more recent and dramatic changes in lifestyle and environment that characterize and accompany "civi-

lized" urban life (Weiss, 1977). As a consequence, the homeostatic system is often maladapted to the changing lifestyles, practices, and environments of modern humans: our nutritional choices, exercise patterns, physical environments, and stress levels. This mismatch of primitive adaptive mechanisms and the realities of modern life has resulted in significant limitations and deficiencies in the natural protective mechanisms designed into this system. For example, the maintenance of normal glucose levels and the integrity of the vasculature are undermined by our modern diets and sedentary lifestyles, and the on-and-off mechanism of the stress response and the maintenance of normal levels of blood pressure are distorted by the presence of unrelenting mental stress. To remedy the results of the mismatch between the built-in mechanisms of the homeostatic healing system and the realities of urban life civilized man has developed "treatment" models whose purpose is to step in when homeostasis has failed to restore normal function.

The Treatment Healing System

The treatment system is activated when the patient seeks assistance from a health care practitioner as a reaction to the appearance of a symptom or the presence of overt disease, an indication of the breakdown of the natural homeostatic system. This step is routinely followed by the requisite testing, establishment of a diagnosis, and the prescription of therapy, usually, in the biomedical treatment system, in the form of external agents such as drugs, surgery, or physical therapy. Biomedicine, the dominant form of treatment in Western society, seeks to establish and explain causation by reducing the field of study to a single body system and its associated biochemistry. Its aim is to repair the biophysiological abnormality and reestablish health, which in the biomedical system is defined as the restoration of normal function (Figure 5-5).

The success of biomedicine has resulted in a shift in the burden of illness from acute infectious disease to chronic, often stress-related, degenerative disease, the causes of which are largely a result of personal attitudes and lifestyles. Although biomedicine is well equipped to diagnose and treat these diseases, which are currently the major source of premature death and morbidity, its therapies rarely result in cure. The characteristics that have been responsible for biomedicine's many accomplishments by necessity also define its limits.

The Mind-Body Healing System

The mind-body healing system relies on the assumption of personal responsibility and the self-motivated effort to develop and use the personal skills and capacities (psychological, psychosocial, and physical) that are available to assist in the process of self-regulation and healing (Figure 5-6). Mind-body healing is intentional and preferably proactive. Its focus is on personal attitudes and lifestyle, the central factors in the development of stress-related degenerative dis-

orders. The concern here is with psychological development, individuation, personal transformation, and mastery, to the extent possible, over the activities of the mind and body.

This aspect of healing finds its scientific legitimacy in the emerging research in the field of psychoneuroimmunology (Ader et al., 1991). The discovery of the interconnectedness of psychic and physiological functions mediated by the mobile neuropeptide messenger system has assisted in establishing the biochemical pathways that account for the long-accepted relations between mind and body. Furthermore, we are now able to demonstrate the specific psychological qualities and psychosocial influences that appear to provide enhanced resistance to the detrimental effects of physiological stress (Antonovsky, 1988, 1991; Kobassa, 1979).

The shift in focus from diagnostic categories to issues of personal attitudes, lifestyle, and psychological development alters the relationship of the health practitioner to the patient. The relationship is more of a partnership than the hierarchical relationship that characterizes biomedical healing. The focus is long term, and the treatment modalities, which can more accurately be termed *health promotion practices,* are more internal than external. Examples include meditation, exercise, nutritional practices, psychosocial education, biofeedback, and yoga. The intent is more educational than therapeutic, and the health practitioner serves more as an educator and coach.

As with each of the preceding systems, the defining focus of the mind-body healing system, self-

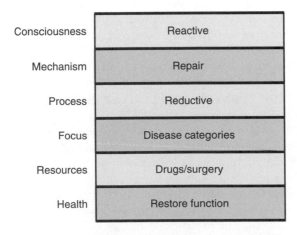

Consciousness	Reactive
Mechanism	Repair
Process	Reductive
Focus	Disease categories
Resources	Drugs/surgery
Health	Restore function

Figure 5-5 Treatment.

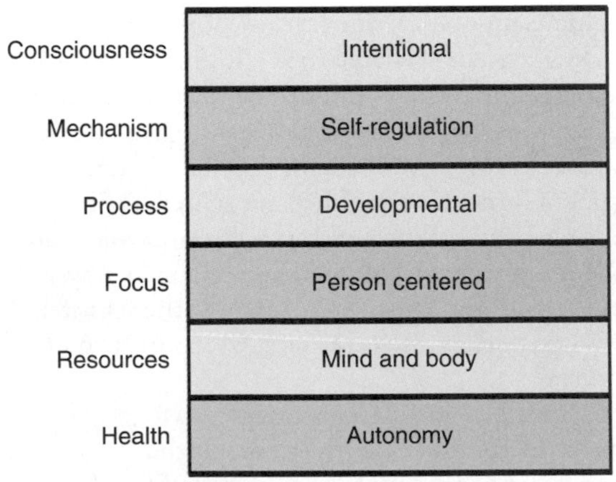

Consciousness	Intentional
Mechanism	Self-regulation
Process	Developmental
Focus	Person centered
Resources	Mind and body
Health	Autonomy

Figure 5-6 Mind-body healing.

regulation, psychological development, and individuation, also accounts for its deficiencies and defines its limits. This system fails to consider the spiritual aspects of the human experience, which transcend and extend the boundaries of personal development, conveying to the individual a more comprehensive and sustaining understanding of the living experience.

The Spiritual Healing System

There are many definitions of spirituality, but for the purposes of this model, I have chosen to define spirituality as an individual's capacity to view the living experience in the context of an organized and unifying perspective that transcends day-to-day experience and provides meaning and purpose to essential human concerns about life and death. A spiritual perspective can have a profound effect on personal attitudes, values, and behaviors, and consequently on biochemistry and physiology. These effects on the mind and the body are termed *spiritual healing* (Figure 5-7).

Characteristics of the Four Systems as a Whole

When these four healing systems are considered as an integrated comprehensive system, certain characteristics appear that are not evident when each is taken separately. We are able to see the evolving characteristics of healing as we approach Figure 5-8 in a horizontal direction—for example, the expansion of consciousness from instinctual to reactive, intentional, and intuitive; the shift in resources from built-in automatic feedback loops to drugs and surgery, mind and body, and finally to an expanded consciousness. Similarly, we can see an increasingly inclusive and comprehensive vision of health as we shift from the goal of maintaining a physiological steady state to restoring function, to individuation, and finally to the attainment of wholeness. Taken as a whole, the movement through each healing system reflects the natural developmental sequence of a human life. We discover that much like this model, we are both parts and wholes—mechanical, interactive, and integrated all at the same time.

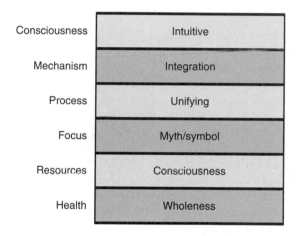

Consciousness	Intuitive
Mechanism	Integration
Process	Unifying
Focus	Myth/symbol
Resources	Consciousness
Health	Wholeness

Figure 5-7 Spiritual healing.

	Homeostasis	Treatment	Mind-body	Spiritual
Consciousness	Instinctual	Reactive	Intentional	Intuitive
Mechanism	Auto-regulation	Repair	Self-regulation	Integration
Process	Checks and balances	Reductive	Developmental	Unifying
Focus	Disequilibrium	Disease categories	Person centered	Myth/symbol
Resources	Feedback loops	Drugs/surgery	Mind/body	Consciousness
Health	Steady state	Restore function	Autonomy	Wholeness

Figure 5-8 Integrative model.

The adversarial distinction between the conventional and the complementary and alternative therapies disappears as we consider the intent, usefulness, and mechanism involved in each form of therapy and properly assign it to one of the four healing systems: homeostasis, treatment, mind-body, and spiritual. This is a more functional way to categorize a therapeutic practice than the current arbitrary and capricious view of its status as "conventional" or "complementary and alternative." To the extent that a practice, conventional or complementary and alternative, fits within a specific system, it then, by necessity, must attain its legitimacy and credibility through the disciplined exploration of its efficacy by means of the research methodology appropriate to that specific system.

This model is inclusive rather than exclusive, honoring and respecting the contributions, independence, and interdependence of each of these healing systems and the integrity and professionalism of the many and varied practitioners whose practices, when proved efficacious through a rigorous system-based research methodology, serve as accepted and valuable resources for one or more of the healing systems. Reductionistic and holistic thinking and conventional and alternative practices are each seen as essential components of a comprehensive intellectual process and a unified approach to health and healing. Of the healing systems discussed in this chapter, the spiritual healing system is the most difficult to define and presents the most significant challenge to our current research methodologies. Yet it conveys an essential completeness and wholeness to this comprehensive healing model by encouraging an existential exploration of the primal human issues of pain and suffering, disease, aging, and death, their meaning and purpose.

In the biomedical system, practitioners-in-training and the active clinician can incorporate these perspectives into the daily practice of healing. In the biomedical system we are accustomed to using a symptom as the "ticket of admission" to the clinical setting and as the basis for the ensuing interview, which begins with a general review of the body systems and progresses, in a reductionistic manner, toward a subsequent focus on the particular single system most directly related to the presenting symptom. This process can be directly applied to the expanded approach proposed here by adding an initial level of triage, which precedes the more detailed interview process. This initial triage decision determines which one or more of the healing systems—homeostatic, treatment, mind-body, or spiritual—is to be applied to the presenting problem.

For example, a minor acute illness is not the basis for a multisystem interview. In contrast, a myocardial infarction requires full attention to the homeostatic, treatment, mind-body, and spiritual healing systems. An individual's age further assists in determining the applicability and usefulness of the mind-body and spiritual healing systems. Mind-body healing cannot be introduced until the attainment of a certain level of maturity, and similarly, a spiritual approach is generally inappropriate for the adolescent or young adult. Mind set is the final indication of which direction to proceed. The latter two healing systems require a certain openness, interest, and intellect as they call on the direct and enthusiastic participation of the patient.

Once made, this triage decision defines the next level of inquiry, which consists of an interview related to the particular healing system(s) that has been selected. If the problem seems most appropriately resolved through the biomedical approach, the traditional review of systems ensues. If an alternative approach is selected, the specific approach-based interview is conducted. If the problem calls for the mind-body or the spiritual system, the inquiry appropriate to one of these systems is inserted. The homeostatic system is concerned with the circumstances (environmental, dietary, and physical) that support the normal autoregulatory functions of the mind and body, the treatment system focuses on the traditional issues of diagnosis and therapy, the mind-body system is concerned with personal attitudes and lifestyle, and the spiritual system considers issues of meaning and purpose. As with the traditional review of systems, an inquiry into each of these aspects of healing proceeds with a series of questions and responses between practitioner and patient.

With the preceding considerations and the appropriate inquiry into the nature of the presenting problem, a comprehensive plan can be agreed on in partnership with the patient. This plan will apply the appropriate range of resources from each of the selected healing systems. In its most complete form, such a plan would aim to support the normal operations of the homeostatic system, restore function where dysfunction has developed (the treatment system), expand personal resources and capacities (the mind-body healing system), and assist the individual in the attainment of a more whole and balanced life (the spiritual healing system). As with any plan, there is a continuing reiterative process that occurs throughout the life cycle.

To better illustrate this process, let us consider the case of an individual who presents for the first time with the symptoms of atherosclerotic heart disease. The initial triage would suggest that the age at which this disease presents itself and the intensity and severity of this particular illness indicate the need to consider, at a minimum, the homeostatic, treatment, and mind-body healing systems (Figure 5-9). Further inquiry, which may continue over weeks, will clarify whether this specific individual is amenable to viewing the implications of his or her disease within the framework of a spiritual perspective. Initially, the appropriate steps related to treatment, diagnosis, and therapy are pursued. Concurrently, an inquiry into personal attitudes and lifestyle is initiated. Finally, if appropriate, a dialogue can be initiated, which is directed toward seeking an understanding of the meaning, purpose, significance, and implications of this disease for the individual's life.

In this case the development of a comprehensive plan would include a mixture of approaches: the use of appropriate diagnostic and therapeutic interventions (the treatment system), the introduction of attitudinal and lifestyle changes in the areas of stress management, nutrition, exercise, and insight-based psychological counseling (the mind-body system), and an ongoing consideration of the impact of this illness on previously held values, beliefs, and priorities (the spiritual system). The goal for the practitioner is to begin to perceive disease and the individual in a larger context. For the individual, the goal is to use disease as a doorway into a more considered and expanded life, one that serves to remedy the problem at hand, reverse the personal factors that have contributed to the development of the illness, and enhance the overall quality of life.

This proposed model has definite implications for practitioners and their patients. If primary care practitioners are to perform the role of triage officers as proposed here, they must be provided with the elements of a comprehensive approach to health and healing. Such a practitioner must be knowledgeable in the dynamics of each of the four healing systems, but the distinctive aspect of his or her education will be an understanding of the principles, concepts, and structural issues that underlie a comprehensive approach to healing. We are not seeking experts in specific domains. The level of data and information available makes that task impossible. Rather, we are seeking practitioners, conventional and "alternative," whose training is expanded to include an understanding of each of the essential aspects of healing complemented by a strong emphasis on integrative studies. The latter is not merely an emphasis on structure and organization but contains a value system that emphasizes synthesis and wholeness, a perspective that is largely absent from current educational programs.

However, it must be remembered that technique, whether it be conventional or alternative, is only one

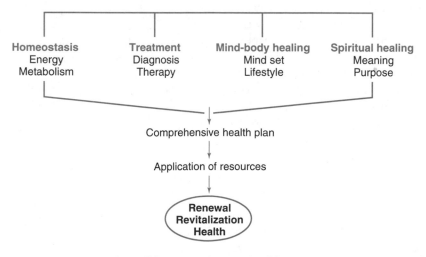

Figure 5-9 Comprehensive health plan.

of two important healing forces Although this force has been the central focus of biomedicine, there is a second healing force that complements technique, the force of personal presence that is marked by active empathic listening, caring, ongoing support, and that certain kind of love that passes through the healing relationship. This traditional aspect of healing is far more subtle than the development and use of technique, and although the source of its healing power is, in a mechanistic sense, largely unknown, it is in fact known to most of us through a personal and direct experience of it. It is in part acknowledged and termed the *placebo effect* by modern science. The development of this healing capacity requires the shift from an emphasis on disease categories toward the consideration of the unique contextual elements of the individual story line; a rediscovery of the art of tending to the patient as a corrective balance to the current overemphasis on treatment; an understanding, appreciation, and patience with suffering, disease, aging, and death, which in part characterize and mature human life; and a commitment by the practitioner to a lifetime process of personal development that parallels the process of professional development.

Our patients must also review their monotheistic and fragmented approach to health care and their incessant conditioned demand for professionals and treatments. It will be increasingly necessary to view health as an artistic creative act, one that is engaged for the duration of the life cycle. The expansion of consciousness, self-knowledge, capacities, resources, and skills is the very process of health itself. In these terms health becomes more a verb than a noun, an intentional and proactive orientation to life that values personal growth and development. Health is then viewed as a lifetime journey rather than as a response to illness. In this context, a consciously lived life cycle will engage an individual in exploring each of the healing systems and in this manner maximize its contributions toward enhancing the quality and duration of life while compressing morbidity into the final years of life.

CONCLUSION

In summary, the development of a postmodern integral medicine can be best accomplished by a full discussion of the values and perspectives that can appropriately underlie an expanded approach to health and healing. On the basis of these values and perspectives it is then possible to create one or more comprehensive healing models that reflect the needs of our time and provide a framework for practitioner education, clinical practice, and research.

References

Ader R, Felten DL, Cohen N. Psychoneuroimmunology. 2nd ed. New York. Academic Press. 1991.

Adler NE, Boyce WT, et al. Socioeconomic Inequalities in Health. JAMA 1993;269:3140-3145.

Antonovsky A. Unraveling the Mystery of Health. San Francisco. Jossey-Bass. 1988.

Antonovsky A. Health, Stress, and Coping. San Francisco. Jossey-Bass. 1991.

Benor DJ. Healing Research: Holistic Energy Medicine and Spirituality. Volume #1: Research in Healing. Munich, Germany. Helix. 1992.

Berkman LF, Syme SL. Social Networks, Host Resistance, and Mortality: A Nine Year Follow up Study of Alameda County Residents. American Journal of Epidemiology. 1979;109:186-204.

Dacher ES. Intentional Healing. New York. Marlowe. 1996.

Dacher ES. Whole Healing. New York. Dutton. 1996.

Dubos R. Mirage of Health. Garden City, New York. Doubleday. 1961.

Duggan RM. Complementary Medicine: Transforming Influence or Footnote to History? Alternative Therapies. 1995;1(2):28-31.

Flexner A. Medical Education in the United States and Canada. Bulletin #4. New York. Carnegie Foundation. 1910.

Gilman DC. The Launching of a University. New York. Garrett Press, Inc. 1969. (original publication 1906).

Harrington TF. The Harvard Medical School: A History, Narrative, and Documentary. Volume III. New York. Lewis Publishing Company, 1905.

House JS, Robbins C, Metzner HL. The Association of Social Relationships with Mortality: Prospective Evidence From the Tecumseh Community Health Study. The American Journal of Epidemiology. 1982;116:123-140.

Illich I. Medical Nemesis. New York. Pantheon Books. 1976.

Kobassa SC. Stressful Life Events, Personality, and Health: An Inquiry Into Hardiness. Journal of Personality and Social Psychology. 1979;37:1-11.

Kohlberg L. The Psychology of Moral Development. San Francisco. Harper & Row. 1984.

Kuhn TS. The Structure of Scientific Revolutions. Chicago. University of Chicago Press. 1970.

Locke S. The Healer Within. New York. Dutton. 1986.

Ludmerer KM. Learning to Heal. Baltimore. The Johns Hopkins University Press. 1985.

McKeown T. The Role of Medicine: Dream, Mirage, Nemesis. London. The Neuffeld Provincial Hospitals Trust. 1976.

Tresolini CP and the Pew-Fetzer Task Force. Health Professions Education and Relationship-Centered Care. San Francisco, California. Pew Health Professions Commission. 1994.

von Bertalanffy L. General Systems Theory. New York. Braziller. 1968.

Weiss P. The System of Nature and the Nature of Systems: Empirical Holism and Practical Reductionism Harmonized. In Schaeffer KE, Hensel H. Brody R. eds. Toward a Man-Centered Medical Science. Mount Kisco, NY. Futura Publishing Company. 1977.

Williams GC, Neese RM. The Dawn of Darwinian Medicine. Quarterly Review of Biology. 1991;66:1-22.

Ray PH. The Integral Culture Survey. The Institute of Noetic Sciences: Research Report 96-A. Sausalito. 1996.

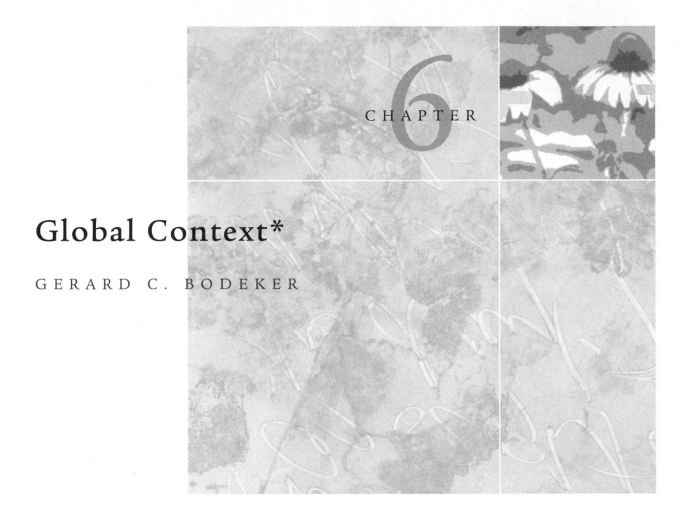

CHAPTER 6

Global Context*

GERARD C. BODEKER

At the basis of the global concern about the ever-increasing cost of health care lies the issue of sustainability. Developing countries recognize that their health care systems are based on expensive, imported medicines and technologies, and that continued reliance on these systems will result in health care costs consuming national finances and stifling national economic growth.

Basic questions are now being asked about priorities in health expenditures and national economic development: How can countries address the health needs of their people without continuing to rely on

expensive, imported medicines? Furthermore, how can local, existing systems of health care be utilized to provide basic health services to rural and poor communities? Increased attention is being paid to the potential of locally available medicinal plants and inexpensive herbal medicines in providing effective primary health care. This in turn has raised concerns about the sustainable use of wild sources of medicinal plants, the conservation of biodiversity, appropriate forms of local cultivation and production, the safety and effectiveness of natural medicines, and the regulatory environment that should accompany the incorporation of traditional systems of health into national health care.

In this chapter, some of these recent trends will be discussed and illustrated with experiences from countries and communities in Africa, the Americas, and

*This article was published originally as "Traditional health knowledge and public policy" in Nature & Resources, 30 (2), UNESCO, 1994. Reprinted by permission.

Asia. We will consider economic, cultural, environmental, and other factors that have led to the resurgence of interest in traditional systems of health. We will conclude with a review of several myths about traditional systems of health care, and a discussion of policy options for incorporating traditional ecological and medicinal knowledge into national and international environmental, health, and economic policy and planning.

BACKGROUND

The terms *traditional medicine* and *traditional systems of health* refer to the long-standing indigenous systems of health care found in developing countries and among the indigenous populations of industrialized countries. The paradigms of these traditional medical systems view humanity as being linked intimately with the wider dimensions of nature. Long relegated to marginal status in the health care plans of developing countries, traditional medicine—or more appropriately, traditional systems of health care, since they provide comprehensive approaches to prevention and treatment that are beyond the scope of medicine alone—has undergone a major renewal in the past decade or more.

The World Health Organization (WHO) has referred to these systems as *holistic,* meaning, "that of viewing man in his totality within a wide ecological spectrum, and of emphasizing the view that ill health or disease is brought about by an imbalance, or disequilibrium, of man in his total ecological system and not only by the causative agent and pathogenic evolution" (WHO, 1978). Traditional medicine has been described as "one of the surest means to achieve total health care coverage of the world population, using acceptable, safe, and economically feasible methods."

The treatment strategies utilized by traditional systems of health include the use of herbal medicines; mind-body approaches such as meditation; physical therapies including massage, acupuncture, and exercise programs; and approaches that address both physical and spiritual well-being. These methods incur limited costs, are available locally, and, according to WHO, are utilized as the primary source of health care by 80 percent of the world's population.

An essential feature of traditional systems of health is that they are based in cosmologies or paradigms that take into account mental, spiritual, physical, and ecological dimensions in the conceptualization and evaluation of health and well-being. Assumptions of causality frequently differ from those of Western medicine, and treatments are designed to reflect those underlying theories of causality. Indeed, classification of diseases, medicinal plants, and ecosystems in traditional knowledge systems may vary substantially from those of Western taxonomies.

A fundamental concept found in many systems is that of balance: the balance between mind and body; between different dimensions of individual bodily functioning and need; between individual and community; individual, community, and environment; and individual and the universe. Disease is understood to arise from a breakdown in the state of balance in one or more of these areas. Treatments are designed not only to address the locus of the disease, but to restore a state of systemic balance to the individual and his or her inner and outer environment.

Historically, the paradigms of traditional knowledge systems have been considered "primitive" by modern or Western science. However, recent advances in environmental sciences, immunology, medical botany, and pharmacognosy have led to a new appreciation for the precise descriptive nature and efficacy of many traditional taxonomies, as well as for the efficacy of the treatments employed. There is an emerging awareness that any meaningful appraisal of a traditional system of health and its contribution to health care must take into account the paradigm or cosmology that underlies diagnosis and treatment.

ORGANIZATIONAL RELATIONSHIPS BETWEEN MODERN AND TRADITIONAL MEDICINE

Under colonial influence, traditional medical systems were frequently outlawed by authorities. In the postcolonial era, the attitudes of Western medical practitioners and health officials have maintained the marginal status of traditional health care providers, despite the role that these practitioners play in providing basic health care to the rural majority, developing countries and within indigenous communities.

Traditional medicine and modern medicine have interfaced with each other in four broad ways (Stepan, 1983):

1. Monopolistic: Modern medical doctors have the sole right to practice medicine.
2. Tolerant: Traditional medical practitioners are not officially recognized, but are free to practice on the condition that they do not claim to be registered medical doctors.
3. Parallel: Practitioners of both modern and traditional systems are officially recognized. They serve their patients through separate but equal systems, such as India.
4. Integrated: Modern and traditional medicine merged in medical education and jointly practiced within a unique health service, such as in China and Vietnam.

FACTORS INFLUENCING POLICY DEVELOPMENT

Despite the historic suppression of traditional medicine by modern medical interests, an increasing number of developing countries are displaying policy interest in traditional approaches to health care that has led to a resurgence of interest in research, investment, and program development in this field. Several factors underlie this new interest.

Economic Factors

The majority of the rural populations of developing countries cannot afford Western medical health care. In Vietnamese peasant communities, there is a common saying that traditional medicine costs one chicken, modern medicine costs one cow, and modern hospital treatment costs many cows. Rural people may have to travel for a day or more to reach a modern medical clinic or pharmacy. This results in lost wages, which is compounded by the cost of transport and the relatively high cost of medicines themselves.

Typically, more than 80 percent of health budgets in developing countries are directed to services that reach approximately 20 percent of the population. Of this, 30 percent of the total health budget is spent on the national pharmaceutical bill.

In Asia, traditional systems of health have been incorporated as formal components of national health care for approximately 20 years. The Indian Medicine Central Council Act of 1970 gave an official place in national health programs to the Ayurvedic and Unani medical systems of India. India now has over 200,000 registered traditional medical practitioners, the majority of whom have received their training in government colleges of Ayurvedic or Unani medicine. China has had a policy of integrating traditional medicine into national health care for more than three decades, and has an extensive national program in which modern and traditional medicine are combined as formal components of health care provision. In both India and China the traditional health sector provides the majority of health care to the poor and rural communities.

In recent years, other countries have begun to provide increased support for their long-standing traditional medical systems, recognizing that they cannot afford Western medicine. In Thailand, for example, the Ministry of Health promotes the use of 66 traditional medicinal plants in primary health care, based on scientific evidence of the efficacy of these plants, as well as on traditional patterns of utilization. The Fourth Public Health Development Plan of Thailand (1977-1981) stated the country's general policy to promote the use of traditional medicinal plants in primary health care. The Seventh Plan (1992 to 1996) promoted the integration of traditional Thai medicine into community health care and prioritized research on medicinal plants. The Thai Ministry of Public Health also promotes the use of medicinal plants in state-run hospitals and health service centers (Koysooko & Chuthaputti, 1993). A study by the Royal Tropical Institute of the Netherlands found that traditional herbal medicines were used most effectively in primary health care in Thailand when self-administered. Since most rural people treat themselves before seeking help from either modern or traditional medical practitioners, herbal medicines offer a low-cost intervention in the early treatment of disease, and provide a safe alternative to the growing problem of self-medication with inappropriate doses and harmful combinations of over-the-counter drugs (Le Grand & Wondergem, 1990).

In Korea, between 15 and 20 percent of the national health budget is directed to traditional medical services, and government reports indicate that traditional medicine is favored equally by all levels of society. Health insurance coverage is available for Oriental medical treatments. In Japan, where physicians have been authorized to prescribe and dispense medications, over two thirds of all physicians reportedly prescribe herbal medications (Norbeck & Lock, 1987).

Cultural Factors

Cultural factors play a significant role in the continued reliance on traditional medicine. Often villagers seek symptomatic relief with modern medicine, and turn to traditional medicine for treatment of what may be perceived as the "true cause of the condition" (Kleinman, 1980). Traditional medical knowledge typically is coded into household cooking practices, home remedies, and health prevention and health maintenance beliefs and routines. The advice of family members or other significant members of a community has a strong influence on health behavior, including the type of treatment that is sought (Nichter, 1978).

Decolonization and increased self-determination for indigenous groups has led some countries to reevaluate and promote their traditional medical systems. At a 1993 Pan American Health Organization conference on indigenous peoples and health, representatives from South America reported increasing activity and interest in traditional medicine in their countries (Zoll, 1993). Several Latin American countries have departments or divisions of traditional medicine within their health ministries.

Mexico has undertaken an extensive program of revitalizing its indigenous medical traditions: over 1000 traditional medicines have been identified as a result of a program of ethnomedical and pharmacognostic research; training centers have been established by the government to pass traditional medical knowledge on to new generations of health care workers; and hospitals of traditional medicine have been established in a number of rural areas. The Mexican Constitution is currently being revised to include traditional medicine in the provision to national health care (Argueta, 1993). Nongovernment organizations (NGOs) have played a strong role in revitalizing traditional health in Mexico, organizing national and international meetings on traditional approaches to health care. More than 50 different traditional medicine associations were represented at a 1992 meeting of the Instituto Nacional Indigenista.

Native North American communities have been incorporating traditional forms of treatment into health programs for some years. In the United States, Indian Health Service (IHS) alcohol rehabilitation programs include traditional approaches to the treatment of alcoholism. An analysis of 190 IHS contract programs revealed that 50 percent of these programs offered a traditional sweat lodge at their site or encouraged the use of sweat lodges (Hall, 1986). Treatment outcomes improved when a sweat lodge was available. Often these sweat lodges include the presence of medicine men or healers, and the presence of a traditional healer greatly improved the outcome when used in combination with the sweat lodge. In northern Canada, The Inuit Women's Association developed a program to revitalize traditional birth practices (Flaherty, 1993). Women who were midwives in their own communities for many years were interviewed and recorded on videotape, and these tapes are being used to train young midwives in the use of traditional methods.

National Crises

In addition to economic and cultural factors, national crises have spurred governments to evaluate their indigenous medical traditions as a means of providing affordable and available health care to their citizens. War and national epidemics are two common crises faced by these nations.

War

During the recent war in Nicaragua, there was an acute shortage of pharmaceutical supplies. In 1985, out of necessity, the country turned to its herbal traditions as a means of fulfilling the country's medical needs. A department was established within the health ministry to develop "popular and traditional medicine as a strategy in the search for a self-determined response to a difficult economic, military and political situation" (Castellon, 1992).

The new department of traditional medicine initiated a program of ethnobotanical research in the midst of war. More than 20,000 people nationwide were interviewed regarding their use of traditional and popular remedies, the methods of preparing these remedies, and the sources of plant ingredients. Previously, nurses and health workers in rural areas frequently manned outposts without medical supplies. They often were surrounded by medicinal herbs of which they knew nothing.

A national toxicology program was begun, based on the extensive survey. Over a period of six to seven years, pharmacognostic studies attempted to determine the chemistry and medicinal properties of commonly used plants. As a result of this effort, inexpensive medicines were produced locally and sustainably in rural areas to treat a wide range of conditions including respiratory ailments, skin problems, nervous disorders, diarrhea, and diabetes.

Following Vietnam's war of independence from France, an official policy was articulated by President Ho Chi Minh in 1954, asserting the importance of preserving and developing traditional medicine as a basic component of health care throughout the country, because a significant proportion of the population could not afford modern medicine.

A national heritage program in traditional medicine was established to ensure that the medical knowledge of experienced practitioners was gathered, recorded, and passed on to future generations through formal training programs. Simultaneously, a policy was developed to promote the modernization of traditional medicine and to incorporate it into health service provision integrated with modern medicine. This policy was expanded and strengthened during the 1960s and 1970s, during the war between the North and the South. Emergency medical strategies were generated, including the development of a traditional medical program for the treatment of burns.

After several decades of pharmacognostic and toxicological research, the National Institute of Materia Medica in Hanoi has developed a list of 1863 plants of known safety and efficacy in the treatment of common medical conditions. Traditional medicine now accounts for one third of all medical treatments provided (Institute of Materia Medica, Hanoi, 1990).

Epidemics

In Africa, governments face huge drug bills for the growing AIDS crisis and are looking to their indigenous medical traditions and medicinal plants for inexpensive and effective methods of at least alleviating the suffering of AIDS victims. The Health Ministry of Uganda has been active in generating research into the role of traditional medical practitioners in treating people with AIDS. The Uganda AIDS Commission and the Joint Clinical Research Centre in Kampala have worked with traditional healers' associations to evaluate several traditional treatments for opportunistic infections associated with HIV/AIDS. An official of the Uganda AIDS Commission commented on research findings, saying that traditional medicine is better suited to the treatment of some AIDS symptoms such as herpes zoster, chronic diarrhea, shingles, and weight loss (Kogozi, 1994).

International support also has been provided for a project in Ethiopia, which has resulted in the development of a cultivated and produced molusciscide that has proven to be effective against the endemic water-borne disease schistosomiasis. Support for this project has included investments from IDRC of Canada, the Rockefeller Foundation, and the World Bank. Linking traditional medicine to biodiversity conservation and economic factors such as affordable health care appears to have attracted a new form of international investment in traditional medicine.

The outbreak of chloroquine-resistant malaria also has inspired a number of countries to reexamine traditional methods of treating malaria. Artemisinin programs, based on an extract of the traditional Chinese antimalarial plant *artemisia annua*, are being used in Africa, China, and Vietnam.

With approximately 30 percent of the health budgets of developing countries being directed to the cost of drugs produced in industrialized countries, the prospect of dealing with epidemics such as AIDS, malaria, and tuberculosis is forcing many governments to look to their indigenous systems of medicine and medicinal flora for low-cost solutions.

International Pressure to Conserve Biodiversity

Traditional health systems intersect with areas of the national economy other than health care: They interface with environmental concerns as well.

Environmental factors such as land degradation through erosion or development have contributed to the loss of natural habitats. Loss of natural habitats can affect the availability of medicinal plants, hence, local health standards. In countries where this has occurred, herb gatherers must walk increasingly longer distances to find herbs that previously grew nearby. This contributes to increasing the cost, availability, and sustainability of naturally occurring sources of medicines that traditionally provided basic health care to rural communities.

National economic development may be linked to the cultivation and use of traditional medicines. Wild harvesting of medicinal plants can provide an additional source of family income and also saves expenditure on other forms of medicine. However, overharvesting constitutes a serious threat to biodiversity. Overharvesting of medicinal plants occurs in China, where approximately 80 percent of the raw materials (animal and plant) for traditional medicines come from wild sources, raising the need for new policies to integrate health, environmental, and economic perspectives. Investments are needed to develop appropriate cultivation and harvesting strategies that will meet the demand for inexpensive and accessible medicines while ensuring the conservation of diverse biologic resources.

Most developing countries lack the information and resources to apply the contemporary methods of studying the inventory of flora and fauna. It has not been possible to track resource depletion systematically in medicinal plants or in animal species that are used in traditional formulae. International collaboration in developing taxonomic capabilities of environmental and forestry departments is one means by which donor agencies can protect diverse medicinal plant species, thus influencing the long-term health of local populations in developing countries.

Although local health needs have constituted the primary beneficiary of the world's medicinal plant resources, there has been a recent growth of interest in traditional medicine from the international pharmaceutical industry, as well as from the natural product industry in Europe and America. Traditional medicine has come to be viewed by the pharmaceutical industry as a source of "qualified leads" in the identification of bioactive agents for use in the production of synthetic, modern drugs. The National Institutes of Health (NIH) in the United States initiated two drug discovery projects along these lines.

The 1992 NIH Biodiversity Project was developed by a consortium of United States government agencies, including the National Cancer Institute, the National Science Foundation, and the United States Agency for International Development. The project was designed to develop partnerships among the agencies, pharmaceutical companies, and the governments of developing countries. It has three main goals: drug discovery, economic development in developing countries through the establishment of economic programs related to the pharmaceutical production process, and conservation of diverse biologic resources in developing countries.

These projects promote the conservation of biodiversity through a model of drug discovery. This model has several important components. First, the local plant knowledge of traditional medical practitioners is made accessible through the use of ethnobotanists. Second, samples of plant materials are tested in laboratories for bioactive properties. If a plant contains molecules that are found to have initial effects, further laboratory research is undertaken, including the modeling of apparently active molecules for synthetic reproduction. Once a molecule is reproduced, it can be patented and commercial production is protected.

The other source of interest in traditional medicine is the natural products industry in Europe and the United States. In Europe, where there is a large industry in phytomedicines, extracts of medicinal plants are sold in purified form to treat and prevent a wide variety of conditions.

These trends have led to a situation where traditional medicine is viewed as a source for the production of other medicines, rather than in terms of its intrinsic value. These concerns have been expressed by the traditional medicine community. A prevailing view is that this trend does not contribute to the development of traditional medicine as a health care system for poor or rural communities, the main constituency of traditional medical care. Rather, the international drug development initiative is seen to take medicinal knowledge from these communities to serve the demand for new drugs in industrial countries. The drugs that are being developed are for the treatment of cancer and heart disease, which are the major killers in industrialized societies, rather than for the treatment of malaria and other endemic diseases that decimate the populations of the developing countries from which the knowledge derives.

There has been no attempt, to date, to develop a scientific understanding of the efficacy of medicinal plants in addressing the primary health care needs of the populations in the areas from which the plants derive. Some projects, however, have recognized this imbalance, the New York Botanical Garden's ethnobotany program in Belize, for example, and are addressing the situation through community-based projects to produce natural medicines for local consumption. They also are working to include knowledge of medicinal plants in school curricula as a means of conserving endangered traditional medical knowledge, as well as to conserve medicinal plants and rain forest areas. In a recent international initiative, the NIH has funded research and policy evaluation on the role of traditional medicine in the provision of cost-effective primary health care in developing countries.

MYTHS CONTRIBUTING TO THE MARGINALIZATION OF TRADITIONAL HEALTH CARE

Myth 1

Traditional medicines are of value only when their active ingredient is known and they are purified for mass production.

The reductionism of Western science leads to the search for a single element that can be identified as the sole or the primary cause of an effect. In pharmacology, this has led to an emphasis on identifying one chemical or compound as the cause of a plant's medicinal properties. This "active ingredient" approach to medicinal plants and traditional medicines reflects a particular paradigm, rather than a particular truth about the way in which natural medicines work. This approach also reflects commercial considerations. For commercial purposes a single ingredient can be replicated in a laboratory easily, synthesized, patented, and mass-produced. In the United States, however, a drug company cannot obtain a patent on a natural product; without patent protection, drug companies have no commercial incentive for producing medicines.

Practitioners of traditional medicine view the active ingredient approach as reductionistic and oversimplified. In the Ayurvedic tradition of natural health care of India, there is an expression that this approach takes the knowledge from the plant and throws away the wisdom. The multiple ingredients in a traditional prescription might include some plant materials that have been selected to address the particular site of pathology, others to stimulate a general immune response, and still others to offset side effects or to increase cellular uptake. This complex approach to pharmacology is based on the concept of "synergistic activity."

Traditional pharmacologies emphasize a principle of synergistic activity among the components of plant ingredients of herbal mixtures. This assumes that just as the body is designed to extract multiple components from food, it is also designed to do so from medicinal plant materials. Traditional medicines typically use complex mixtures of plants, which are prepared through a process that might include drying, crushing, heating, boiling, and even burning. Consequently, the chemical structure of the plant materials is transformed, producing a set of compounds that may differ from that of each plant in the prescription.

The principle that enduring effectiveness can be found in a complex mixture of chemicals rather than in a single molecule is best demonstrated in the case of malaria. In recent years, new strains of the parasite have developed that are resistant to the antimalarial drugs, chloroquine and mefloquine. However, these are still not resistant to the antimalarial activity of the original cinchona bark—the natural source of quinine—on which the synthetic antimalarials were modeled (Wyler, 1992).

In conclusion, it is interesting to note that the principle of synergistic activity also serves as the basis for Western pharmacology's use of multiple drug treatments in cancer chemotherapy. Here, there is a principle that a single compound is not sufficient to produce an overall systemic change, and that a complex of chemical inputs are required to fight the disease. Although the types of chemicals used clearly differ from those traditional medicines, there is a common principle that multiple ingredients produce a greater effect than the sum of the effects of individual components.

Myth 2

Based on findings from the plant screening programs of the pharmaceutical industry and national drug development programs, the therapeutic benefit of traditional medicines is limited.

This view sometimes is espoused by those familiar with plant screening programs, such as those run by the National Cancer Institute in America, where tens of thousands of medicinal plants have been screened for anticancer effects, and only a handful have been identified as having therapeutic potential. It is important to note, however, that the screens used test only for cytotoxicity, the ability of a chemical to kill cancer cells. Any plant or plant-based compound that does not show a cytotoxic effect—that does not kill cancer cells—is considered to have no anticancer properties.

The mechanisms by which natural medicines work might be more sophisticated than a simple mechanism of killing wayward cells. This has been illustrated by a series of experimental studies on Ayurvedic herbal preparations Maharishi Amrit Kalash 4 and 5, which have looked at the effect of these preparations on a range of cancers. The studies (which include research conducted by a different division of the National Cancer Institute) have found that Maharishi Amrit Kalash 4 and 5 have marked anticancer effects. Cancer prevention effects have been shown with experimental breast cancer (Sharma et al., 1990), lung cancer (Patel et al., 1992), and liver cancer. There has been no evidence of cytotoxicity in these effects. A study on the effects of these herbal preparations on neurological cancer cells found that there was a transformation, or morphological differentiation, of the neurological cancer cells (neuroblastoma) into normal healthy nerve cells (Prasad et al., 1994). These herbal preparations did not kill cancer; rather, they produced a process of transformation in cancer cells that some researchers have proposed may be activated at the molecular level.

These examples illustrate that the methodologies utilized in modern medical science completely overlook the effects by which natural medicines produce their effect, due to a fixed and limited view of what constitutes therapeutic action. To address this neglect, the new, Congressionally mandated NIH Office of Alternative Medicine is working to develop a series of methodologies appropriate for the evaluation of non-Western or complementary medical therapeutic approaches.

The conventional view is that traditional health care is best used for chronic, low-level conditions, rather than for the treatment of acute conditions. However, in some countries, traditional medicine is used in the treatment of trauma and major diseases.

In Vietnam the National Institute of Burns conducts an active program of research to evaluate traditional medicinal formulae in the treatment of burns (Institute of Burns, 1993). Traditional medicines now are utilized in combination with modern medicine, widely and effectively, in the treatment of burns. This direction was developed as a matter of necessity during the war with South Vietnam and the United States, when burn treatments needed to be available immediately in remote jungle locations. Traditional medicinal plants were utilized, and resulted in a national program of research and the development of over 60 medicines for use in different aspects of burn therapy. These medications are effective in generating membrane formation, inhibiting bacterial growth, and stimulating the formation of scar tissue on burn lesions. The treatment time with traditional medicine is markedly shorter than that of conventional burn medication (The Trungh et al., 1993).

The Vietnamese Institute of Acupuncture in Hanoi uses acupuncture analgesia in place of general anesthesia for major surgery. The Institute for Burns also uses this approach. Both institutes report that with perioperative acupuncture, patients experience minimal or no pain and have fewer postoperative complications, and their wounds heal more quickly than when general anesthesia is used (Tai Thu, 1993).

In April 1991 the National Council of Ministers in Hanoi renamed the Institute of Burns after an early Vietnamese physician, Le Huu Trac. According to Vietnamese health officials, this is the first time that a national institute has been named after a prominent figure in traditional medicine—a development that reflects a commitment to integrating traditional medicine into national health care, including emergency treatment.

Myth 3

Traditional health systems may have some use in the provision of care for chronic, low-level conditions, but they are of no value in providing acute or emergency care. ❧

Myth 4

Little scientific knowledge is available on the safety and efficacy of traditional medicine, and all international efforts regarding traditional medicine should be directed to toxicity and efficacy research. ❧

It is not correct to state that there has been little or no research done on traditional approaches to health care; studies have been done in many countries. However, the level of research sophistication, the language in which studies are published, the focus of this research, and the bias of the scientific establishment as to what constitutes a published study—all have contributed to these studies being overlooked or, on occasion, rejected by the wider scientific community.

In some countries—India, China, Korea, Vietnam, Mexico, to name a few—a substantial body of toxicity data has been gathered on medicinal plants and traditional medicines. In addition, international botanical research has identified the chemistry, including the toxicity, of many plants used in traditional medicines. Entire journals are dedicated to research on the chemistry of medicinal plants, and studies are referenced in databases such as NAPRALERT, a natural products research database located at the University of Illinois. Other databases contain collections of studies in the area of "complementary" medicine, a term that includes many traditional systems of medicine as they are utilized in industrial countries. These include the British Library's Complementary Medicine Index and the research database of the British Research Council for Complementary Medicine. On review, this collective body of data may well satisfy questions regarding the safety of commonly used herbal treatments.

More data may ultimately be needed on a country by country basis, in order for lending or donor agencies to be able to determine the extent of utilization and treatment, the preventive efficacy, and the suitability and form of investment in this sector. However, existing data need to be evaluated for safety and efficacy.

Regarding the question of efficacy: as noted above, many countries have a body of scientific research on the medical properties of many plants utilized in traditional medicine. It is important to give credit to the countries and the scientists involved in this undertaking, which is partly necessitated by the lack of available Western medicines. Research has been conducted under such circumstances as lack of equipment and chemical supplies, which are far from conducive to the production of Western-style research. However, it would be unscientific to dismiss these studies in making a determination of the availability of effectiveness data of traditional herbal medicines. Although much of this research is not available in English, scientists familiar with Chinese, Hindi, Korean, Vietnamese, Spanish, or Portuguese languages could be called on to evaluate this body of research as a means of supporting international investment. In addition, abstracts could be translated into English for a first level of review.

Finally, to place the Western concern about potential toxicity of herbal medicines in perspective: in the United States, where one in three people report using some form of alternative medicine (Eisenberg et al., 1993), plant poisonings in 1989 were due almost exclusively to consumption of toxic ornamental plants, not herbs. Such poisonings resulted in only one fatality. In the same year, fatal, nonsuicidal poisonings by antidepressants, analgesics, sedatives, and heart drugs totaled 414 (Fugh-Berman, 1993).

Myth 5

The global value of traditional medical knowledge is twofold: it serves as a source of leads for the development of new Western drugs, and the potential medicinal value of tropical rain forest species provides a basis for generating international support to preserve the world's rain forest areas and to conserve regional biodiversity.

Early colonial views construed developing countries in terms of the commodities that would benefit colonial interests, such as minerals, timber, spices, rubber, copra, farm lands, and people. Prospecting for treasure—including silver and gold in the Americas, gems in the Far East, and gold and diamonds in Africa—contributed to the widespread exploitation of local peoples and the loss of their resources.

The term *biodiversity prospecting* has appeared recently in the lexicon of conservation and drug development. It refers to the search for commercially useful medicinal plants in the world's rain forest areas. Using the analogy of gold prospecting, this model looks at methods of harnessing the biological treasures of forest areas for the medicinal needs of the world (Reid et al., 1993).

The gene is behind the growth of the biotechnology industry and the race to patent life forms with new chemicals and new genetic structures. The increase of activity in this field is illustrated by the fact that, although very few international companies and "no U.S. company was working on higher plants" in 1980 (Farnsworth & Soejarto, 1985), in 1990, 223 companies worldwide were investigating medicinal plants as the source of new pharmaceutical leads (Fellows, 1991).

A widely publicized ethnobotanical program in Costa Rica involves a partnership between Merck Pharmaceutical and a local nongovernment organization, INBio, to develop drugs from traditional sources. In this agreement, $1.135 million was provided to Costa Rica by Merck for rain forest conservation activities, and a certain percentage of profits from drugs developed through this program will be returned to the country.

There were large public demonstrations on the streets of Costa Rica in protest of the government forming this kind of relationship with Merck. While this project, and others using this model, may recognize the intellectual property rights of traditional custodians of medical knowledge, concern has been expressed by indigenous organizations about the priorities involved in strategies of this kind. Some critics view this as a form of neocolonialism in which the wealthy countries are still looking at the poorer countries as a source of raw materials to be used to develop products for industrialized societies. These critics argue that, as in other colonial initiatives, the real profits will go elsewhere, rather than to the countries from where the initial material and knowledge originated. Representatives of the biotechnology industry argue that life forms, including medicinal plants, are part of a global commons and are thus available for exploitation.

The traditional perspective is that biotechnology skews public understanding of the importance of preserving tropical rain forest areas. The emphasis on preserving forests for their potential in producing new pharmaceuticals induces governments to focus on pharmaceutical development rather than on developing sustainable, affordable, and locally available medicines from their own indigenous medical traditions. This is a loss both for the present and the future.

Domestic garden and community-based cultivation programs have been developed in several countries; these offer a viable solution to the need for locally accessible and affordable medicines. Research mentioned earlier by the Royal Tropical Institute of the Netherlands concluded that countries focus too much on the role of health care providers, includ-

ing traditional practitioners, whereas studies show that the majority of health activities involve self-medication. People treat themselves and their family members with medicines that they grow, produce, or buy locally, before they seek help from a health care practitioner. In this light, the domestic garden programs of countries such as Vietnam and Nepal and the community garden programs of Belize offer an important model for conservation and sustainable medicinal plant use. In these programs the use of wild sources of plants is reduced, self-sufficiency in health care is strengthened, and each family or communal garden can serve as a miniature conservatory of medicinal plants that otherwise might be endangered. Thus, biodiversity issues can be addressed through community development initiatives that encourage sustainable and effective health care.

To reiterate, then, the "biodiversity prospecting" argument overlooks the role of traditional medical knowledge in addressing the health needs of the communities from where the medicinal plants and the knowledge about their appropriate use and harvesting derive. As has been noted in recent press reports, "the rush of interest in prospecting for new chemicals is taking place in a policy vacuum" (Vidal, 1993). With no clear national or international policies or regulations, the marketplace becomes the final arbiter of procedure. Inevitably, the most powerful players prevail.

A broader economic perspective would recognize that the health status of developing countries is central to the economic health of those countries and thus to the world economy. Traditional medicine and medicinal plants play an important role in meeting the basic health needs of the majority of the world's population. This is an equally if not more potent argument than the biotechnological case for preservation of the world's medicinal plant species.

CONCLUSION

Currently, there is wide variability in the consideration given by health planners to traditional health systems. In some countries, traditional medicine is incorporated routinely into health planning. However, this occurs in only a minority of cases, primarily in Asia. In most cases, the revival has come from nongovernment organizations, particularly in Latin America. Most health ministries continue to overlook

TABLE 6-1

Old and New Perspectives on Traditional Systems of Health Care

Old	New
Primitive	Holistic
Ineffective	Cost-effective
Marginalized	Locally available
Becoming extinct	Undergoing renewal
Need to be regulated	Need to be promoted
Source of leads for pharmaceutical industry	Valid in their own right, with local economic value
Active ingredient model	Synergistic activity concepts

the fact that basic health care is provided to the majority of the population by traditional practitioners and budgets and that national health plans lack any reference to traditional medicine.

National and international funding currently is directed to the provision of Western-style health services in developing countries and indigenous communities. Research consistently links reductions in morbidity and morality rates to economic conditions, educational levels, particularly to years of female education and large scale public health measures such as sanitation and water supply (World Bank, 1993). While these factors—rather than the availability of Western medicines—have been found to lead to improved levels of health, health planners continue to operate under the view that Western medicine provides the primary means of improving health in these communities. This belief is not based in a scientific appraisal of the world's natural systems of health. Some traditional treatments are still more effective than modern treatments, as is the case with South American indigenous preparations of cinchona bark against new strains of malaria, the use of traditional burn medications in Vietnam, and the powerful cancer-prevention effects of Ayurvedic herbal preparations.

While old and limited views of traditional systems of health continue to exist, there is an emerging intellectual and policy climate that is giving expression to a fresh perspective. Whereas the old view favors the marginalization of traditional systems of health, the new view looks to them to provide complementary

therapy, and in some cases, new solutions to major health crises.

The scientific paradigm for evaluating traditional systems of health has been called into question, and a search has begun, including an important endeavor by the United States National Institutes of Health, to identify and develop methodologies that, according to the mission statement of NIH's Office of Alternative Medicine, "respect the paradigms" of traditional systems. The paradigm of health and medicine that has prevailed in this century, namely that of a molecular approach to human biology and the treatment of disease, also is being called into question by new findings from mind-body medicine and environmental health that promote a more integrated and holistic view of human health. This new view is consonant with the ancient or traditional concepts of health and human potential that underlie many of the world's traditional systems of health. Table 6-1 presents an outline of how this shift affects perspectives of traditional health care systems.

References

Argueta A. 1993. Presentation to World Bank Conference on Indigenous Knowledge and Sustainable Development. Washington DC. September 28

Balick M. 1995. Conservation in today's world. Proceedings of WHO Symposium on the Utilization of Medicinal Plants, Philadelphia, April 19-21, 1993. University of Pennsylvania Press, Philadelphia

Castellon U. 1992. Report of the fundacion centro nacional de medicina popular tradicional. Dr. Alejandro Davila Bolanos. Nicaragua

Eisenberg D, et al. 1993. Unconventional medicine in the United States: prevalence, costs, and patterns of use. N Engl J Med 328:4

Farnsworth N, Soejarto D. 1985. Potential consequences of plant extinction in the United States on the current and future availability of prescription drugs. Economic Botany 39:231-240

Fellows LE. 1991. Pharmaceuticals from traditional medicine plants and others: future prospects. A paper presented at the New Drugs from Natural Sources Symposium. London, June 13-14

Flaherty M. 1993. Proceedings of Conference on Indigenous Peoples and Health. Winnipeg, Canada, April 13-18, pp.1-72

Fugh-Berman. 1993. The case for natural medicine, The Nation, September 6 and 13

Hall RL. 1986. Alcohol treatment in American Indian communities: an indigenous treatment modality compared with traditional approaches. Ann NY Acad Sci 472: 168-178

Institute of Burns. 1993. Establishment of a new scientific center of Vietnam—The National Institute of Burns, named Le Huu Trac—that needs much support. Institute of Burns, Hanoi

Institute of Materia Medica, Hanoi. 1990. Medicinal Plants in Viet Nam, WHO Regional Publications. Western Pacific Series No. 3, Manila

Kleinman A. 1980. Patients and Healers in the Context of Cultures. University of California Press, Berkeley

Kogozi J. 1994. Herbalists open hospital. The NEW VISION, Kampala, February 4, 14

Koysooko R, Chuthaputti A. 1993. Promising practices in the use of medicinal plants in Thailand. Presented at The WHO Symposium on the Utilization of Medicinal Plants, Philadelphia, April 19-21

Le Grand A, Wondergem P. 1990. Herbal Medicine and Promotion. KIT Press Royal Tropical Institute, Amsterdam

Nichter M. 1978. Patterns of curative resort and their significance for health planning in south Asia. Med Anthropol 2:29-58

Norbeck E, Lock M. 1987. Health, Illness and Medical Care in Japan. Honolulu, University of Hawaii Press

Patel V, Wang J, Shen RN, et al. 1992. Reduction of mouse Lewis lung carcinoma (LLC) by M-4 rasayana. Nutr Res 12:667-676

Prasad KN, Edwards-Prasad J, Kentrotti S. 1992. Ayurvedic (Science of Life) herbal agents induced differentiation in murine neuroblastoma cells in culture, Neuropharmacol 31:6;599-607

Reid W, et al. 1993. Biodiversity Prospecting. World Resources Institute, Washington DC

Sharma H, et al. 1990. Effect of MAK (M4 & M5) on DMBA-induced mammary tumors. Eur J Pharmacol 183:2;193

Sok CW. 1995. Country report, In Proceedings of WHO Symposium on the Utilization of Medicinal Plants, Philadelphia, April 19-21, 1993. University of Pennsylvania Press, Philadelphia

Stepan J. 1983. Patterns of legislation concerning traditional medicine. In: Bannerman R (ed.) Traditional Medicine. WHO Publication, Geneva

Tai Thu, N. 1993. Personal communication with the director of the Vietnamese Institute of Acupuncture. July

The Trungh L, et al. 1993. Personal communication with the director of the Le Huu Trac Institute for Burns. July

Vidal J. 1993. Whose new lease on life? The Guardian, May 21

World Bank. 1993. World development report on health: World Bank, Washington DC, July

WHO Traditional Medicine. 1978. WHO Publications, Geneva

Wyler DJ. 1992. Editorial: bark, weeds and iron chelators—drugs for malaria. N Engl J Med, Nov. 19

Zoll AC. 1993. Proceedings of Conference on Indigenous Peoples and Health, Winnipeg, Canada, April 13-18

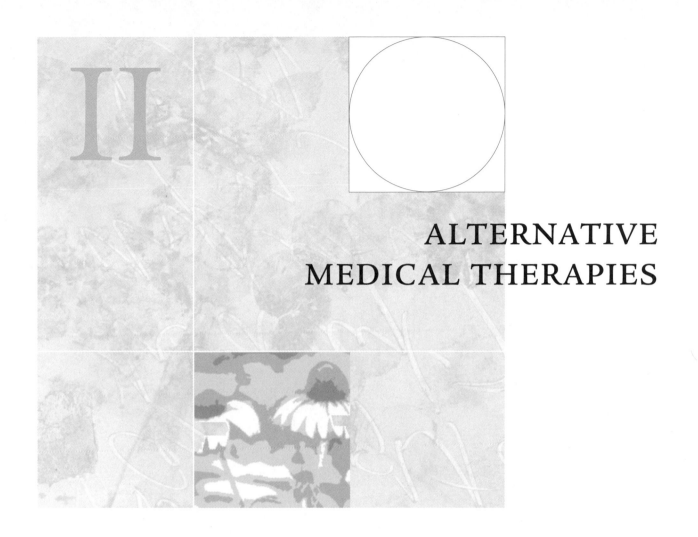

II

ALTERNATIVE
MEDICAL THERAPIES

This section describes the background, context, and clinical approaches of a
selective variety of alternative therapeutic systems as they have developed
throughout European and American history and of individual approaches
that are suggested from contemporary Western research, both within and beyond the
biomedical paradigm. Where these systems and approaches can be understood in
light of the contemporary biomedical paradigm, this view is examined; where they
cannot be, this paradox is pointed out. It is made clear when and how medical systems are embedded in nature and ecology and when they are embedded in technology. In each case these medical practices are presented as products of history that
make sense in terms of that history. ∾

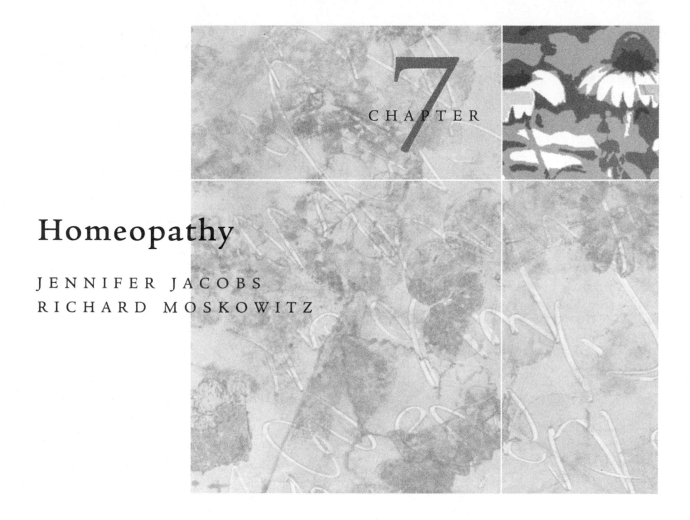

CHAPTER 7

Homeopathy

JENNIFER JACOBS
RICHARD MOSKOWITZ

Homeopathy is a method of self-healing assisted by small doses of medicinal substances and practiced by licensed physicians and other health care professionals throughout the world. In the United States homeopathic medicines are protected by federal law, and most are available over the counter.

HISTORY

The homeopathic method was developed by Samuel Hahnemann, MD (1755-1843), a German physician, chemist, and author of a well-known textbook on the preparation and use of contemporary medicines (Figure 7-1). In a series of experiments from 1790 to 1810, Hahnemann demonstrated (1) that medicinal substances elicit a standard array of signs and symptoms in healthy people and (2) that the medicine whose symptom-picture most closely resembles the illness being treated is the one most likely to initiate a curative response for that patient (Hahnemann, 1833).

Hahnemann understood these experiments to mean that the outward manifestations of illness represent the concerted attempt of an organism to heal itself and that the corresponding remedy reinforces that attempt in some way. He coined the term *homeopathy* to describe his method of using remedies with the power to resonate with the illness as a whole, in contrast with the more conventional method of opposing symptoms with superior force.

*T*he word *homeopathy* is derived from the Greek roots *omoios*, meaning "similar," and *pathos*, meaning "feeling." Hahnemann also began using *allopathy* from the Greek *alloios*, meaning "other" to denote the standard practice of using medicines either to counteract symptoms or to produce an action unrelated to symptoms, such as purging, bloodletting, or blistering of the skin. ∾

Although Hippocrates, Celsus, and Paracelsus advocated treatment with similars for some patients and Stahl in the eighteenth century had proposed giving medicines to healthy people (Hahnemann, 1833), Hahnemann understood that the detailed correspondence between the clinical symptoms of patients and the experimental pathogenesis of remedies indicated a universal law of healing with medicinal substances. He developed a systematic philosophy of medicine and a rigorous method for diagnosis and treatment that were and still remain wholly unique in the history of medicine.

With the old model of self-healing effectively supplanted by the modern idea of technological control, the Hahnemannian law of similars—*similia similibus curentur*, or "Let likes be cured by likes"—never gained general acceptance in medicine and is even consid-

ered implausible to most physicians. Even committed homeopaths regard it as a mystery not yet explained or proven, and Hahnemann taught that it could not be deduced *a priori* or independently of experience and would have to be evaluated, as every other healing practice, by how well it works in the treatment of the sick.

THEORETICAL BASIS

Essentially a methodology for treating the sick rather than a set of hypotheses about the nature of health and disease, homeopathy begins and ends as a radical innovation in the experimental investigation of medicinal substances. Its cardinal principles follow logically from the law of similars and the conceptual transformations required to accommodate it.

Provings

In 1790, while experimenting with cinchona (Peruvian bark), Hahnemann decided to ingest a therapeutic dose. He soon felt cold, numb, drowsy, thirsty, and anxious and experienced palpitations, prostration, and aching bones; he recognized these symptoms as those of *ague,* or intermittent fever, the syndrome that was then being treated with cinchona (Bradford, 1895). He allowed the dose to wear off before taking a second and a third dose that confirmed his original results.

Stunned by the implications of this finding, Hahnemann devoted the rest of his life to ascertaining the therapeutic properties of medicinal substances by administering them to healthy people—himself, his colleagues, and his students. His *Materia Medica Pura* records the detailed symptoms of more than 90 medicines, a truly monumental achievement that represents 20 years of painstaking labor (Hahnemann, 1833, 1880).

In these *provings,* as he called them, Hahnemann administered the substance in question to a group of reasonably healthy people in doses sufficient to elicit symptoms without provoking irreversible toxicity, anatomical changes, or organic damage. A unique composite portrait, or symptom-picture, was assembled for each substance, differentiating it from every other. Therefore homeopathic remedy is a shorthand for the sum of observable responses of all people who

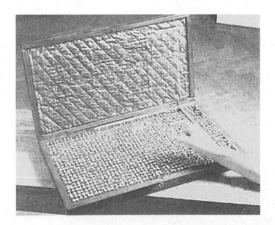

Figure 7-1 Samuel Hahnemann's remedy box. Many homeopaths kept their remedies in a similar box, but few had one that was so splendid. (From Richardson S: Homeopathy, The Illustrated Guide.)

have taken that remedy, a distinctive totality that must be studied as a whole and for its own sake rather than simply as a weapon against a particular disease or a group of symptoms.

THE HOMEOPATHIC *MATERIA MEDICA*

The Hahnemannian concept of medicinal action remains the most distinctive contribution of homeopathy to medical science, with important implications for pharmacology, ethnobotany, and industrial medicine and toxicology. Without recourse to pathological models or unconsenting animal subjects, provings offer a purely experimental technique for investigating the medicinal action of any substance whatsoever.

The homeopathic pharmacopeia currently recognizes more than 2000 remedies, with more being added all the time. Most are of plant origin, including flowers, leaves, roots, barks, fruits, and resins. Although many are poisonous in their crude state (e.g., aconite, belladonna, digitalis, ergot, hellebore, and nux vomica), others are common medicinal herbs (comfrey, eyebright, mullein, yellow dock); foods and spices (cayenne, garlic, mustard, onion); fragrances, resins, and residues (amber, petroleum, charcoal, kreosote); and mushrooms, lichens, and mosses.

Mineral remedies include metals (copper, gold, lead, tin, zinc); metalloids (antimony, arsenic, selenium); salts (calcium sulfate, potassium carbonate, sodium chloride); alkalis; acids (hydrochloric, nitric, phosphoric, sulfuric); elemental substances (carbon, hydrogen, iodine, phosphorus, sulfur); and constituents of the earth's crust (silica, aluminum oxide, ores, rocks, lavas, mineral waters).

Remedies from the animal kingdom include venoms (of jellyfish, insects, spiders, molluscs, crustaceans, fish, amphibians, snakes); secretions (ambergris, cuttlefish ink, musk); milks, hormones, glandular and tissue extracts (sarcodes); and nosodes or disease products (tuberculosis, gonorrhea, syphilis, abscesses, vaccines).

The investigative method of provings is applicable equally to the study of conventional drugs, unproven folk remedies, toxic or laboratory chemicals, pollutants, and commercial or industrial products (dyes, insecticides, paints, solvents). The homeopathic materia medica is as boundless as the creation of the earth and as inexhaustible as its transformation by human or environmental forces.

Finally, the richness and diversity of the materia medica database increases the likelihood that some degree of medicinal help can be found for most people, while its basic principles are simple enough that even a novice can achieve some results with a small number of remedies. As long as a few commonsense guidelines are observed, the method is perfectly safe for laypeople of average intelligence to learn at their own pace and to use for first aid and for the treatment of common domestic ailments. Considerable study and experience are required, however, to take full advantage of this enormous tool.

The Vital Force

Like acupuncture, herbalism, and other natural methods, homeopathy belongs to the vitalist tradition in medicine, based on the old *vis medicatrix naturae*, the natural healing capacity, and summarized in the aphorisms of Paracelsus.

The art of healing comes from Nature, not the physician. . . . Every illness has its own remedy within itself. . . . A man could not be born alive and healthy were there not already a Physician hidden in him.

PARACELSUS, 1958

Underlying these approaches is the following coherent philosophy of ancient lineage (traced elsewhere in this volume) whose precepts still ring true despite modern efforts to ignore or surpass them (Box 7-1).

BOX 7-1

Precepts of Healing

- Healing is a concerted effort of the entire organism and cannot be achieved by any part in isolation from the whole.
- All healing is essentially self-healing, which is a basic property of all living beings.
- Healing applies only to individuals and therefore is inherently problematic, even risky, and never reducible to any technique or formula, however scientific its foundation.

Within homeopathy the fact that curative remedies imitate and therefore resonate with manifested signs and symptoms make sense. Illness is viewed as the organisms attempt to heal itself. Hahnemann identified the life energy itself (the vital force) as the ultimate source of health and illness alike, ending only with the death of the organism. Whatever we wish to call it, some version of the vital force is required to refer to the obvious bioenergetic integrity of living beings.

The Totality of Symptoms

Just as provings include the full range of symptoms elicited by each remedy, homeopathy teaches that illness is primarily a disturbance of the vital force and manifests itself as a totality of physical, mental, and emotional responses that is unique to each patient and cannot be adequately understood as a mere specimen of any disease process. Without including every symptom or assuming that mental symptoms and physical symptoms instigate each other, the Hahnemannian totality of symptoms simply describes the principal signs and symptoms as they appear in the patient and is complete as soon as a reasonable sense of the illness as a whole is discernible.

To the practicing homeopath, this composite totality or psychophysical style—far more than any abstract disease category or printout of laboratory abnormalities—furnishes the truest picture of the health and illness of the patient as a whole, as well as of the particular condition for which treatment is being sought.

In practice the totality of the symptoms demands that the remedy take into account the living experience of the patient, including the full range of thoughts and feelings. It by no means rejects or ignores the technical expertise of the physician and does not hesitate to make use of pathological diagnosis or of conventional drugs or surgery. Homeopathy uses the technical language of abnormalities to educate the patient, allowing the patient to retain control and to participate at every step. The diagnosis also is important in predicting patient response to homeopathic treatment, as well as the prognosis.

The totality of symptoms also explains why mental and emotional symptoms sometimes weigh heavily in choosing the remedy. Whereas most physical symptoms refer to a certain part of the body (e.g.,

arm, nose, back, or stomach), psychological states describe how patients feel as a whole (e.g., afraid, depressed, happy, or confused). The totality of symptoms gives special importance to describing the condition of the patient as a whole.

The Single Remedy

Based on the materia medica, the Hahnemannian method uses one remedy at a time for the whole patient, comparing the totality of symptoms of the individual with those of various remedies until the closest possible match is found. The reason is that single remedies have the capacity to match the totalities with the individuality of each patient. Their power and effectiveness are proportional to the ability of patients to respond to them as a whole by virtue of that resemblance.

On the other hand, its encyclopedic scale ensures that the homeopathic materia medica can never be grasped in its entirety; some have tried to abbreviate and simplify it, and competent and reputable physicians use two, three, or more remedies simultaneously. Over-the-counter combination remedies also are available in many pharmacies and health food stores and are safe and effective if used properly.

The totality of symptoms enables the serious student to accumulate detailed personal experience with remedies and generates much of the excitement while learning how to use them. Administering different remedies to each part of a patient makes it difficult to know which remedy has acted; as such, remedies would have to be selected according to the rough indications of folk medicine or the technical language of abnormalities, much like conventional drug treatment. Under these conditions, what is learned will not yield an experience that can build on itself or a method that can be taught. The revival of American homeopathy in recent years has been achieved largely on the strength of the single remedy concept. Only the totality of symptoms can display remedies, and patients are unique individuals worthy of study for their own sake.

The Minimum Dose

Because homeopathic remedies stimulate an ailing self-healing mechanism rather than correcting a specific abnormality, large or prolonged doses are seldom required and even might spoil the effect. Homeopaths use the smallest possible doses and only repeat them if necessary, allowing remedies to complete their action without further interference. Indeed the remedy will not work unless it fits the illness so closely as to render the patient uniquely susceptible to its action. The minuteness of the dose makes it exceedingly unlikely that any untoward or dangerous side effects will occur.

In a series of experiments, Hahnemann discovered that remedies are still effective in concentrations that are too small to be detected chemically and that mechanical shaking or "succussion" of diluted remedies actually enhances their healing effect in a way that has never been fully understood. Assuming that dilute remedies act by energizing the organism, he theorized that succussion liberates that energy from its chemical bonds and releases it into the solution, thus foreshadowing the discovery of subatomic forces in the twentieth century (Hahnemann, 1833, 1880).

Hahnemann's advocacy of infinitesimal doses remains one of the most controversial aspects of his work. No one has explained satisfactorily how medicines diluted beyond the molecular threshold of Avogadro's number could possibly have any effect, let alone a curative one. But the standard argument that the remedies are simply placebos cuts both ways. People do, in fact, heal themselves of serious illnesses without drugs or surgery. With its dilutions now detectable by laser spectroscopy and bioassay (Boiron, 1976; Noiret, 1976), homeopathy envisions a new bioenergetic science that is still in its infancy.

The Laws of Cure

The totality of symptoms also makes clear why drugs that successfully lower the blood pressure, kill bacteria, or correct physiological abnormality may leave the patient feeling as bad or worse than before. Judgments about improvement, worsening, and the effectiveness of treatment are difficult to interpret apart from the totality of symptoms, from how patients feel as a whole, and from how they function according to their own individual standards. Perhaps the greatest shortcoming of the biomedical model is its failure to comprehend patients as integrated energy systems and to follow them throughout their lifetime.

Since the era of Hahnemann, classical homeopathy has addressed this critical issue by attempting to track the order in which symptoms and illnesses appear, the grouping of symptoms that appear and disappear together, and the relation of each group to the overall health and functioning of the patient. Constantine Hering proposed four general directions in which symptoms tend to move or redistribute themselves during the recovery process (Box 7-2).

Although the fourth principle has proved most reliable for case management, and the relative importance of organs and tissues often is difficult to assess, some approximation of the totality of symptoms over time remains indispensable to the general assessment of the patient as a whole, for clinician and researcher alike.

METHODOLOGY

Pharmacy

The Homeopathic Pharmacopoeia of the United States (American Institute of Homeopathy, 1989) is the official standard for the preparation of homeopathic medicines. Crude medicinal substances are made into remedies by serial dilution and succussion in a liquid or solid medium. First crushed and dissolved in a specified volume of 95 percent grain alcohol, crude plant materials are shaken and stored, and the supernatant liquid is kept as the "mother tincture." The same procedure is used for animal products, nosodes, and any other substances that are soluble in alcohol. Metals, ores, and other insoluble remedies

BOX 7-2

Symptom Movement in the Cure and Recovery Process

- From above downward, from the head toward the feet
- From inside outward, from interior to peripheral parts
- From more vital to less vital organs, from more visceral to less essential structures
- From the most recent to the oldest, in the reverse order of their appearance in the life history of the patient (Hering, 1865, 1875)

are pulverized with mortar and pestle and diluted with lactose, succussing until they become soluble.

Tinctures are further diluted with alcohol or lactose, either 1:10 (the decimal scale, written "X") or 1:100 (the centesimal, written "C") and succussed vigorously, yielding the 1X or 1C dilution. The process is repeated for the 2X, 3X, 4X (or 2C, 3C, 4C), and on up as desired.

In clinical practice any dilution may be used, but the most popular for self-care are the 6th, 12th, and 30th (X or C). Higher dilutions for professional work are in the centesimal scale, namely, the 200th, 1000th, 10,000th, and 50,000th, written 200C, 1M, 10M, and 50M, and representing dilutions of 10^{-400}, 10^{-2000}, $10^{-20,000}$, and $10^{-100,000}$, respectively.

The general skepticism about diluted remedies—as expressed by Oliver Wendell Holmes and modern critics—is readily understandable because even the 12C and 30C are well beyond the Avogadro limit and therefore out of the realm of conventional chemistry entirely (Holmes, 1842).

Case-Taking

As in general medicine, seeing patients requires more than simply taking down information or selecting remedies. Allowing patients to tell their story, in its entirety, relieves their burden of pain and suffering, making the homeopathic interview a powerful healing experience in its own right. It even might suggest a path of recovery, allowing remedies to continue the process.

Patients are invited to speak and allowed to continue for as long a time as possible without interruption, while homeopaths ask "What else?" as often as necessary, to elicit more symptoms and to remind the patient that no one disease is being sought but rather the totality of symptoms. Symptoms are written down verbatim whenever possible, leaving space in the right-hand margin for the homeopath's own observations.

After the patient finishes his or her story and the principal symptoms have been noted, the homeopath must investigate further to characterize symptoms in detail. Conventional diagnosis is based on common symptoms such as fever, pain, cough, and bleeding, whereas homeopaths look for unusual or idiosyncratic features that tend to be ignored or discarded by conventional physicians (Box 7-3).

BOX 7-3

Fully Characterized Symptoms Described in a Homeopathic Interview

- Subjective sensations such as pain, vertigo, fatigue, and anger
- Localization of symptoms (one-sided, wandering, radiating, circumscribed, or diffuse)
- Modalities, that is, factors by which symptoms are modified (intensified or relieved) according to changes in the time of day, the weather, diet, or emotional state
- Concomitants or symptoms that appear simultaneously or in sequence (nausea with headache, fever after chill)

The interview also includes physical examination and laboratory work as needed to establish a diagnosis.

Selecting the Remedy

As the case is taken, symptoms are graded in importance by the extent to which information is freely volunteered and clearly delineated and by how severely limiting they are to the overall health and well-being of the patient. Homeopathic prescribing lays bare the incredible correspondence that exists between the database of the materia medica and the details of each patient's case record. Each of these great texts continually illuminates the other, but an encyclopedic memory or a computer with a similar capacity would be necessary to allow proper study on use of the wealth of remedies and symptoms properly.

For professional homeopaths to gain access to as many remedies as possible, they need help in proceeding from the clinical totality to a menu of possible remedies that they can study and choose from. This is the purpose of the *repertory,* an index of symptoms and the remedies that either have elicited them in provings or that cured them clinically. By finding the remedies that match the leading symptoms in a case, the search for a cure can be narrowed down.

Whether in the form of a book or computer software, the largest, most comprehensive repertories (Archimed, 1993; Warkentin, 1991) include all types of symptoms from every anatomical region and physiological system, as well as mental and emotional symptoms, "generalities" (physical symptoms or modalities attributable to the patient as a whole), and rare symptoms whose very oddity points directly to the remedy. The repertory is only a tool for locating remedies; these remedies must then be studied in the materia medica, and the final selection is based on a total or qualitative fit, more than on any narrow, technical calculation.

Regimen and Precautions

Although they remain stable in the cold and across a wide range of temperatures, dilute remedies are inactivated by direct sunlight and should be stored in a dark, dry place and shielded from X rays. Patients are instructed to put nothing in the mouth for at least 30 minutes before and after each dose. Coffee and camphorated products might reverse the effects of the remedy and should be avoided throughout the treatment period, even when no remedies are actually being taken. The use of medicinal herbs and exposure to mothballs and other aromatic substances also should be curtailed.

Although conventional drugs often interfere and should be avoided when possible, severely ill patients should not stop taking medications. Because of their potentially synergistic effect, acupuncture and chiropractic should not be started concurrently with homeopathic remedies but, if already in progress, may be continued. Relapse might also follow dental work that includes drilling and local anesthesia.

Administration and Dosage

Remedies are dispensed in the form of tablets or pellets of sucrose or lactose that are taken dry on the tongue or dissolved in water. Lower dilutions are preferred in acute situations because they can be repeated as often as necessary and will be somewhat effective even if only broadly similar to the totality of the case. Higher dilutions are used mostly by professionals for chronic treatment; more care must be taken in their selection, and they should not be repeated while their action is in progress.

In homeopathy the term *dosage* refers primarily to the number and frequency of repetitions, which must be tailored to fit the patient, very much like the choice of the remedy itself. In both acute and chronic cases the rule is to stop the remedy once the reaction is apparent, repeating only when the reaction has subsided.

Pros and Cons

There are few, if any, absolute contraindications to homeopathic treatment. Although patients with severely disabling illnesses or chronic drug dependence are difficult to help—by any method—homeopathy at least might be considered before resorting to more drastic measures or after conventional methods have failed. Homeopathic remedies are wonderfully safe, economical, simple to administer, and gentle in their action, with very few serious or prolonged adverse effects. Although subtle at first, the effects of treatment are prompt, thorough, and long lasting.

On the other hand, homeopathy is far from a panacea for all ills. It is a difficult and exacting art. Even after years of study and practice, a skilled prescriber might need to try several remedies before any benefit is obtained. Some cases might show little or no improvement, despite the most conscientious efforts. Remedies are rather delicate and easily inactivated, so certain precautions must be observed. Finally, we do not understand how dilute remedies act and cannot predict how a patient will respond, or which symptoms will change and in what order. Like all medicine, homeopathy is an art dependent on the life energy of individual human beings.

HISTORICAL DEVELOPMENT

Early Controversies

Although his successful treatment and prophylaxis of a scarlet fever epidemic brought fame to homeopathy widely throughout Europe, Hahnemann was ridiculed and persecuted for his heresies until 1822, when he was awarded a stipend to publish his writings (Bradford, 1895). In addition to his *Organon of Medicine* and *Materia Medica Pura,* he wrote many technical and expository works, maintained a busy correspondence, and continued to practice and conduct experimental research. Hahnemann died secure in the knowledge that his students were practicing homeopathy throughout Europe and America. Fired by ambition and gifted with intellect, he left a body of work and a method that have stood the test of time.

Homeopathy in America

In the latter half of the nineteenth century the United States became the center of the homeopathy movement and produced some of its greatest masters, whose works still enjoy international use. Several factors contributed to the rapid growth and development of American homeopathy.

The first was the absence of laws or bureaucracy to license the practice of medicine, a tolerant attitude born of the hope to break free from the oppressive social and economic constraints of Europe. When the first school of homeopathy opened in Pennsylvania during the 1830s, American physicians were organized on a voluntary basis, and state legislatures were reluctant to prevent uneducated or lay healers from helping anyone who wanted to use their services (Starr, 1982).

The second factor was the great migration of those seeking land and fortune in the west, where doctors were scarce and people were forced to heal themselves and their families. Homeopathy was well suited for self-care, and popular manuals on first aid and the treatment of common domestic ailments began to appear during this period (Hering, 1844).

Finally, the concept of the materia medica itself was easily adapted to Native American medicine. Introducing dozens of Native American herbs into the pharmacopeia, American homeopathy was enriched by the botanical lore of midwives, medicine men, eclectics, and other herbalists whose recipes are still in use today (Hale, 1867).

Under these conditions homeopathy flourished in the United States, inspiring the creation of hospitals, medical schools, and insane asylums that scored notable triumphs that attracted public attention (Coulter, 1973). During epidemics of cholera, typhus, and scarlet fever, homeopathy consistently proved its superiority over the punishing treatments then in vogue (Bradford, 1900). Physicians practicing this new method quickly rose to social prominence, treating such rich and famous patients as President Lincoln and the members of his Cabinet (Coulter, 1973). By the turn of the century, 10 percent of all physicians used homeopathy in their practices (Ullman, 1991).

During and after the Civil War, however, the tremendous expansion of American industry transformed the nature of medicine. American homeopathy—with its use of minimal doses at rare intervals—never created a large or profitable industrial base capable of financing large educational or research institutions. Experimental medicine, based on rigorous physicochemical causality, generated such unprecedented technical achievements as anesthesia, antisepsis, surgery, microbiology, vaccines, and antibiotics (Bernard, 1957).

The American Medical Association (AMA) and its state societies forbade its members to consult or fraternize with homeopaths (Coulter, 1973). Such persecution had little effect until state legislatures began to license physicians and accredit medical schools and the pharmaceutical industry won control of the process (Starr, 1982). Thereafter the AMA invited homeopaths and physicians of all schools to become members in exchange for licensing, creating a monopoly against lay healers, midwives, and herbalists. The Flexner Report, published in 1914, proposed a uniform standard of medical education for all physicians and used the power of accreditation to phase out homeopathic colleges that fell short of these standards (Starr, 1982).

The AMA strategy succeeded. By the 1920s the homeopathic schools either had closed or conformed to the new model, and homeopathy was reduced to a postgraduate specialty for the few physicians who were prepared to swim against the tide. Although some fine homeopathic physicians continued to practice, the movement declined rapidly over the next 40 years. By 1970 homeopathy appeared to be moribund, its teachers aged or dead (Kaufman, 1971).

American homeopathy has begun to flourish once more, thanks largely to the rebirth of the self-care movement, the health care crisis, and the overmedicalization that provoked these events (Illich, 1976). By eliminating lay healers and aspiring to control every abnormality by purely technical means, American medicine has become a colossus that thrives on great cost and great risk (Moskowitz, 1988), generating a more iatrogenic illness (Steel, 1981) and consuming a greater share of the gross national product than anywhere else in the world. Facing crises in health insurance, malpractice litigation, and the doctor-patient relationship (Moskowitz, 1988), the public—and now the medical profession itself—have turned to alternatives like those described in this text.

Safe, effective, and inexpensive enough to sustain busy practices even without third-party reimbursement, homeopathy has become increasingly popular with young family physicians, whose instant waiting lists approximate the virtually limitless demand for their services. As in frontier days, the renaissance of American homeopathy would not be occurring were it not for the devotion of laypeople—not only for self-care but also for organizing study groups in their communities and teaching these methods to their friends and neighbors.

RESEARCH

Hahnemann's system of provings—using individuals to determine the symptoms that a medicine could produce—was the first research in homeopathy. Indeed, the whole field is based on this experimental work, which was unprecedented both in method and in scope. Provings are still used on many herbal medicines that have been used by traditional healers for centuries, particularly in Asia and in South America. The proving method also is being modernized; statistical methods are used to determine the significance of various symptoms.

Modern homeopathic research focuses on three basic questions: (1) Do highly dilute substances affect physical and biological systems? (2) Can homeopathic medicines be proven to be effective clinically? and (3) What is the mechanism of action of homeopathic medicines?

Basic Science Research

Basic scientific research in homeopathy primarily has investigated the chemical and biological activity of highly diluted substances. As discussed previously, Hahnemann found that if the homeopathic remedies were highly diluted to concentrations as low as 10^{-30} to $10^{-20,000}$, there would still be a medicinal effect with minimal side effects. Most scientists reject homeopathic theory because of this extreme dilution of the medicine beyond Avogadro's number of 10^{-24}, beyond which point molecules theoretically cease to exist.

In the mid-1950s a review of 25 investigations of microdoses was published, citing their effects on such widely variant systems as paramecia, the Schick test, growth of *Aspergillus mycelia*, germination of wheat germ, and blood flow in the ears of rabbits (Stephenson, 1955). More recent European laboratory studies have demonstrated the effects of homeopathically prepared microdoses on mouse macrophages (Davenas et al., 1987), arsenic mobilization in the rat (Cazin et al., 1987), bleeding time with aspirin (Doutremepuich et al., 1987), and degranulation of human basophils (Poitevin et al., 1988). There also have been studies that showed the insignificant effects of microdoses, such as on the excretion kinetics of lead in rats (Fisher, 1987).

More than 100 studies have researched the effects of high dilutions in the fields of immunology, toxicology, and pharmacology (Bastide, 1994; Belon, 1987). One of the most intriguing studies revealed that highly dilute preparations of thyroid hormone introduced into an aquarium had a statistically significant effect on the climbing behavior of frogs, even when the preparation was completely encased in a glass vial (Endler et al., 1994).

The most well-known study of the effects of high dilutions was published in 1988, showing degranulation of human basophils by IgE antibodies diluted as high as 10^{-120} (Davenas et al., 1988). This article was highly criticized in Europe because it challenged the basic tenets of biomedicine, and its findings were later challenged (Maddox et al., 1988). The controversy over this study continues, with attempts to repeat the experiment reporting success and failure (Benveniste et al., 1991).

Clinical Research

Before the mid-1980s, little clinical research in homeopathy was published outside of homeopathic journals. The first double-blind experiment published in a peer-review medical journal showed statistically significant results in treating rheumatoid arthritis with individualized prescribing of remedies (Gibson et al., 1980). A later study on arthritis showed no effect using homeopathic treatment (Shipley et al., 1983); however, all the patients had been given the same medicine, *Rhus-toxicodendron*. This study illustrates the difficulty in doing clinical research in homeopathy. Homeopathic medicines are individualized, by definition, based on the basis of the totality of symptoms. Most conventional clinical research involves administering the same medicine to all patients.

Recent clinical trials in Europe have suggested a positive treatment association between homeopathic medicines and the treatment of allergic rhinitis (Reilly et al., 1986), fibrositis (Fisher et al., 1989), influenza (Ferley et al., 1989), and asthma (Reilly et al., 1994). A trial of childhood respiratory illnesses had equivocal results (de Lange de Klerk et al., 1995). The *British Medical Journal* published a meta-analysis of homeopathic clinical trials in 1992, which found that 15 of 22 well-designed studies showed positive results and concluded that more methodologically rigorous trials should be done to evaluate the efficacy of homeopathic treatment (Kleijnen et al., 1991). A recent study comparing homeopathic treatment with placebo in the treatment of acute childhood diarrhea demonstrated improvement in the homeopathy group (Jacob et al., 1994).

Mechanism of Action

There is no scientific explanation for the mechanism of action of homeopathic medicines, although there are several theories. Recent developments in quantum physics have led some scientists to suggest that electromagnetic energy in the medicines interact with the body on some level (Delinick, 1991). Researchers in physical chemistry have proposed the *memory of water* theory, whereby the structure of the water-alcohol solution is altered by the medicine during the process of dilution and retains its new structure even after the medicine dissolves (Resch, 1987). Recent developments in chaos theory support these answers because a basic tenet of this theory is that very small changes can affect large systems (Shepperd, 1994).

Cost-Effectiveness and Outcomes

Another relevant area of research in homeopathy is cost-effectiveness and outcomes. In France the annual cost to the Social Security System for a homeopathic physician is 15 percent less than that of a conventional physician, and the price of the average homeopathic medicine is one third that of standard drugs (CNAM, 1991). Many believe that outcomes research will prove to be the most important area of homeopathic research over the next 5 years (Jacobs, 1994). Such indicators as overall health status (for which there are several widely accepted scales), patient satisfaction, days missed from school or work, and the cost of treatment are used to compare the outcomes of different types of treatment. This approach would be particularly useful in looking at the homeopathic treatment of chronic illnesses, which do not lend themselves to the double-blind method.

HOMEOPATHY TODAY

The use of homeopathy is increasing rapidly throughout the world, particularly in Europe, Latin America, and Asia. In Germany 25 percent of all physicians use homeopathy (Ullman, 1991), in France 32 percent of general practice physicians use it (Bouchayer, 1990), and in Great Britain 42 percent of physicians refer patients to homeopaths (Wharton & Lewith, 1986). In India homeopathy is practiced in the national health service, at several hundred homeopathic medical schools, and by more than 100,000 homeopaths (Kishore, 1983).

Other developing countries have turned to homeopathy as the cost of conventional, Western medicine grows out of reach. In both Argentina and Brazil several thousand physicians use homeopathy, and Mexico has five medical colleges that provide homeopathic training. South Africa has homeopathic medical colleges in several major cities, and the health ministry in Israel recently approved the importation of homeopathic preparations for sale in pharmacies.

The use of homeopathy by the United States has increased tremendously in the last 20 years. A survey showed that 1 percent of the American population used homeopathy in 1989 (Eisenberg et al., 1993). Sales of homeopathic remedies increased by 1000 percent during the 1980s (Food and Drug Administration, 1985) and were reported to be $200 million in 1992, climbing at the rate of 25 percent per year (Swander, 1994).

Appropriate Use

Homeopathic remedies are most likely to be successful and to optimize overall health for several types of conditions as described in Box 7-4.

Homeopathy is not appropriate for the treatment of chronic diseases involving advanced tissue damage, such as cirrhosis of the liver or severe cardiovascular disease; for people with prolonged dependence

BOX 7-4

Uses of Homeopathic Remedies

- Functional complaints with little or no tissue damage, such as headache, insomnia, chronic fatigue, and premenstrual syndrome
- Conditions for which no effective conventional treatment is available, such as viral illnesses, traumatic injuries, surgical wounds, multiple sclerosis, and acquired immunodeficiency
- Conditions that require chronic use of conventional drugs, such as allergies, recurring infections, arthritis, skin conditions, and digestive problems
- Conditions for which elective surgery has been proposed, but immediate attention is unnecessary, such as fibroid tumors, gallstones, and hemorrhoids
- Conditions that have not been cured by conventional treatments, either because of the inappropriateness of the medication, the determined nature of the disease, or patient's noncompliance

on conventional medication such as corticosteroids, anticonvulsants, and antipsychotics; or as a substitute for appropriate conventional treatments such as emergency surgery or reduction of fractures.

Practice Patterns

A recent survey of American physicians documented interesting differences between those using homeopathic medicines in their practices and those using more conventional remedies (American Institute of Homeopathy, 1992). Physicians using homeopathy saw fewer patients and spent more than twice as much time with each patient, averaging 30 minutes per visit, as opposed to the 12.5 minutes spent with each patient by conventional physicians. In addition, homeopathic physicians ordered half as many diagnostic procedures and laboratory tests than conventional physicians and prescribed fewer standard medications.

This survey also polled the most common diagnoses seen by these physicians. Asthma, headaches, depression, allergies, psychological problems, and skin problems were among the top 10 conditions treated most frequently by homeopathic physicians.

Conventional physicians, on the other hand, saw more hypertension, upper respiratory tract infections, diabetes, sore throats, bronchitis, back disorders, and acute sprains and strains. These practice patterns suggest that patients seek homeopathic care mostly for chronic conditions that are not managed adequately by conventional medicine. The low number of acute problems seen by homeopaths might be due to patients treating these conditions at home.

References

American Institute of Homeopathy. 1989. The Homeopathic Pharmacopoeia of the United States. Falls Church, Virginia

American Institute of Homeopathy. 1992. Unpublished Survey Data

Archimed, Inc. 1993. RADAR Version 3.0. Namur, Belgium

Bastide M. 1994. Immunological examples of UHD research. In Endler PC (ed): Ultra High Dilution: Physiology and Physics. Kleuwer Academic Publishers, Dordrecht, Germany

Belon P. 1987. Homeopathy and immunology. Proceedings of the 42nd Congress of the LMHI. Arlington, Virginia, pp. 265-270

Benveniste J, Davenas E, Ducot B, et al. 1991. L'agitation de solutions hautement diluees n'induit pas d'activite specifique. Comptes Rendus Acad Sci Paris 312(II): 461-466

Bernard C. 1957. An Introduction to the Study of Experimental Medicine. Greene HC (transl). Dover, New York, pp. 65-67

Boiron J. 1976. Studies of the Physical Structure of Homeopathic Dilutions Utilizing the Raman Laser Effect Proceedings, 31st Congress of the International Homeopathic Medical League, Athens, pp. 459-474

Bouchayer F. 1990. Alternative medicines: a general approach to the French situation. Complem Med Res 4:4-8

Bradford TL. 1895. The Life and Letters of Samuel Hahnemann. Boericke and Tafel, Philadelphia, pp. 37, 124-126

Bradford TL. 1900. The Logic of Figures, or Comparative Results of Homeopathic and Other Treatments. Boericke and Tafel, Philadelphia, pp. 141-145

Cazin J, Cazin M, Gaborit JL, et al. 1987. A study of the effect of decimal and centesimal dilutions of arsenic on the retention and mobilization of arsenic in the rat. Hum Toxicol 6:315-320

CNAM. 1991. Healthcare professionals in private practice in 1990. Social Security Statistics. CNAM publication no 61, Paris

Coulter H. 1973. Divided Legacy. McGrath, Washington, pp. 140-238, 285-316

Davenas E, Beauvais F, Amara J. 1988. Human basophil degranulation triggered by very dilute antiserum against IgE. Nature 333:816-818

Davenas E, Poitevan B, Benveniste J. 1987. Effect on mouse peritoneal macrophages of orally administered very high dilutions of silica. Eur J Pharmacol 135:313-319

de Lange de Klerk ESM, Blommers J, Kuik DJ, et al. 1995. Effect of homeopathic medicines on daily burden of symptoms in children with recurrent upper respiratory tract infections. BMJ 309:1329-1332

Delinick AN. 1991. A hypothesis on how homeopathic remedies work on the organism. Berl J Res Homeopath 1:249-253

Doutremepuich C, et al. 1987. Template bleeding time after ingestion of ultra low dosages of acetyl salicylic acid in healthy subjects. Thromb Res 48:501-504

Eisenberg DM, Kessler RC, Foster C, et al. 1993. Unconventional medicine in the United States. N Engl J Med 328:246-252

Endler PC, Pongratz W, Kastberger G, et al. 1994. The effect of highly diluted thyroxine on the climbing activity of frogs. Vet Hum Toxicol 36:56-59

Ferley JP, Smirou D, D'Adhemar D, Balducci F. 1989. A controlled evaluation of a homeopathic preparation in the treatment of influenza-like syndromes. Br J Clin Pharmacol 27:329-335

Fisher P. 1987. The influence of the homeopathic remedy Plumbum Metallicum on the excretion kinetics of lead in rats. Hum Toxicol 6:321-324

Fisher P, Greenwood A, Huskisson EC, et al. 1989. Effect of homeopathic treatment on fibrositis (primary fibromyalgia). BMJ 299:365-366

Food and Drug Administration. 1985. Riding the coattails of homeopathy. Food and Drug Administration Consumer. p. 31

Gibson RG, Gibson SL, MacNeill AD, Buchanan WW. 1980. Homoeopathic therapy in rheumatoid arthritis: evaluation by double-blind clinical therapeutic trial. Br J Clin Pharmacol 9:453-459

Hahnemann S. 1833. Organon of Medicine, 5th Ed., Boericke W. and Dudgeon E. (transl). Roy, Calcutta, pp. 45, 53-70, 269-270

Hahnemann S. 1880. Materia Medica Pura, Dudgeon E. (trans). Hahnemann Publishing Society, Liverpool

Hale EM. 1867. Homeopathic Materia Medica of the New Remedies. Lodge, Detroit

Hering C. 1844. The Homeopathist or Domestic Physician. Philadelphia

Hering C. 1865. Hahnemann's three rules concerning the rank of symptoms. Hahnemannian Monthly 1:5-12

Hering C. 1875. Analytical Therapeutics. Boericke and Tafel, Philadelphia, p. 24

Holmes OW, Sr. 1842. Homeopathy and its Kindred Delusions. Ticknor, Boston

Illich I. 1976. Medical Nemesis. Pantheon, New York

Jacobs J. 1994. Future directions in homeopathic research. J Am Inst Homeopat 87:155-159

Jacobs J, Jiménez LM, Gloyd SS, et al. 1994. Treatment of acute childhood diarrhea with homeopathic medicine: a randomized clinical trial in Nicaragua. Pediatrics 93:719-725

Kaufman M. 1971. Homeopathy in America: the Rise and Fall of a Medical Heresy. Johns Hopkins, Baltimore

Kishore J. 1983. Homeopathy: the Indian experience. World Health Forum 4:105-107

Kleijnen J, Knipschild P, ter Riet G. 1991. Clinical trials of homoeopathy. BMJ 302:316-323

Maddox J, Randi J, Stewart J. 1988. "High-dilution" experiments a delusion. Lancet 334:287-290

Moskowitz R. 1988. Some thoughts on the malpractice crisis. Br Homeopat J 77:17

Noiret R. 1976. Activity of Several Homeopathic Dilutions of Copper Sulfate in Different Microbial Species, Proceedings, 31st Congress of the International Homeopathic Medical League, Athens, pp. 137-147

Paracelsus PATB. 1958. Selected Writings, Guterman N. (transl). Jacobi J. (ed). Pantheon, New York, pp. 50, 76

Poitevin B, Davenas E, Benveniste J. 1988. In vitro immunological degranulation of human basophils is modulated by lung histamine and apis mellifica. Br J Clin Pharmacol 25:439-444

Reilly DT, Taylor MA, Beattie NGM, et al. 1994. Is evidence of homeopathy reproducible? Lancet 344:1601-1606

Reilly DT, Taylor MA, McSharry C, Aitchison T. 1986. Is homoeopathy a placebo response? Controlled trial of homoeopathic potency, with pollen in hayfever as model. Lancet ii:881-885

Resch G. 1987. Physical Chemistry of Highly Attenuated Remedies. Proceedings, 42nd Congress of the International Homeopathic League, Washington, pp. 300-304

Shepperd J. 1994. Chaos theory: implications for homeopathy, J Am Inst Homeopat 87:22-29

Shipley M, Berry H, Broster G, et al. 1983. Controlled trial of homeopathic treatment of osteoarthritis. Lancet i:97-98

Starr P. 1982. The Social Transformation of American Medicine. Basic Books, New York, pp. 30-59, 99-123

Stephenson J. 1955. A review of investigations in the action of substances in dilutions greater than 1×10^{-24} (microdilutions). J Am Inst Homeopat 48:327-335

Swander H. 1994. Homcopathy: medical enigma attracts renewed attention. Am Acad Fam Pract Rep XXI(6):1-2

Ullman D. 1991. Discovering Homeopathy. North Atlantic Books, Berkeley, California

Ullman D. 1991. The international homeopathic renaissance. Berl J Homeopat 1(2):118-120

Warkentin D. 1991. MacRepertory, Version 3.41. Kent Homeopathic Associates, San Anselmo, California

Wharton R, Lewith G. 1986. Complementary medicine and the general practitioner. BMJ 292:1498-1500

Suggested Readings

Clarke JH. 1962. Dictionary of Practical Materia Medica, 3 vols., Health Science Press, Rustington, United Kingdom

Hering C. 1891. Guiding Symptoms. Hering Estate, Philadelphia

Resch G, Gutmann V. 1987. Scientific Foundations of Homeopathy, English ed. Barthel & Barthel, Germany

Steel K. 1981. Iatrogenic Illness on a General Medical Service at a University Hospital. N Engl J Med 304:638

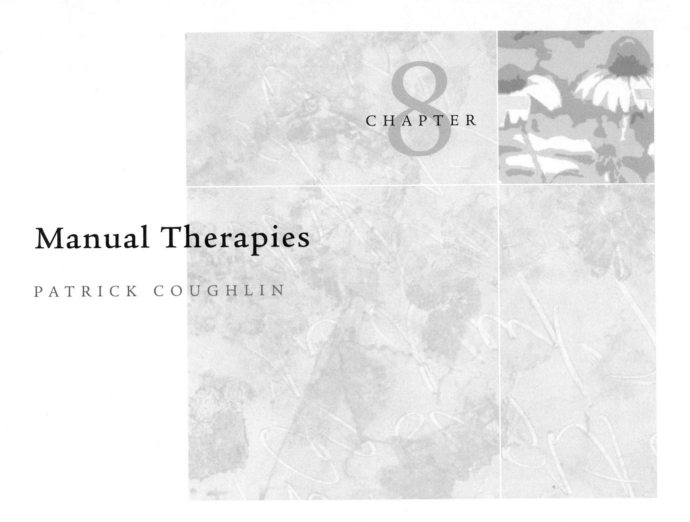

CHAPTER 8

Manual Therapies

PATRICK COUGHLIN

anipulation as a therapeutic practice has existed for thousands of years, and the exact date of origin of the earliest forms of manipulative therapy is unknown. It has been recorded that Hippocrates was skilled in the use of manipulation and taught it in his school of medicine. In China the history of manual therapy (tui na, Figure 8-1) predates the development of the technology necessary to produce the needles used for acupuncture (see Chapter 18). Virtually all of the world's cultures demonstrate the use of manipulation as a form of therapy. However, much of this information has been passed on in oral rather than written tradition, so documentation is difficult if not impossible to obtain in many instances. Consequently the styles of manipulation presented here will be confined to those about which information is readily available. In addition, the basic principles and theories of manipulative practice are presented.

Like other "complementary" therapies, manipulation espouses a holistic philosophy that has several outstanding tenets:

1. The body is a unit.
2. Structure and function are interrelated.
3. The body has an inherent ability to heal itself.
4. When normal adaptability is disrupted, disease may ensue.

Based on these defining principles, manipulation seeks to correct structural imbalances to optimize the body's ability to self-correct or repair itself, which includes the defense against invasion from foreign substances or organisms.

100

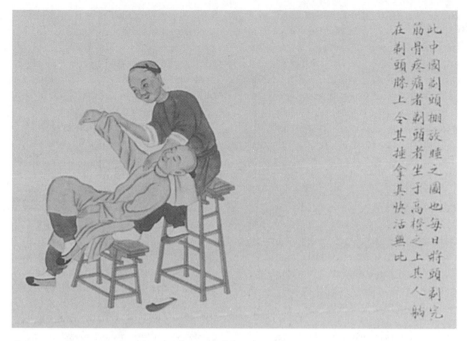

Figure 8-1 A patient receiving manipulation of the shoulder. Joint manipulation has always been an important feature of Chinese medical treatment. (Courtesy The Wellcome Trustees, London.)

CONCEPTS APPLICABLE TO ALL MANIPULATION PRACTICES

Several concepts should be borne in mind when one is dealing with the principles of manipulation. These concepts, based on physical laws and anatomical principles, are universal and thus apply to all manipulation practices. They are briefly described so that they then can be associated with the various forms (styles) of manipulative therapy and hopefully produce for the reader a greater understanding of the reasons for applying or seeking this type of treatment.

Bilateral Symmetry

The musculoskeletal system is usually described as being bilaterally symmetrical. That is, if the body is divided in half by a slice made from top to bottom and front to back along the midline (midsagittal), the right side should be an exact mirror image of the left side. This of course is an idealized assumption because few, if any, human bodies are in reality symmetrical. Certain behaviors that we engage in both

consciously and unconsciously are specifically designed to compensate for a lack of bilateral symmetry.

Gravity

The human organism is similar to all other organisms in that we are subject to the laws of physics. As such, the way we interact with planet earth is governed by the pull of the earth on our bodies—the force of gravity. This constant force and the fact that our bodies have mass give us the weight we are obliged to carry with us as we go about our activities.

Postural Maintenance and Coordinated Movement

As we evolved from a quadrupedal (four-legged) to a bipedal (two-legged) stance, we became at once able to manipulate our environment (pun intended) by freeing up our hands but also more unstable (visualize the result of removing two legs of a four-legged table). From an architectural point of view, we became a buttressed arch system (the feet, legs, and pelvic girdle), supporting an elongated tower (the spine and head), with two appendages (the arms) that can at times assist with balance. However, we are designed for movement and are rarely stationary, even when seated. Consider the act of walking. For about 40% of the time allotted to the normal gait cycle (the period of two strides), we are moving with only one foot on the ground. Because we do move around quite a bit, we are constantly adapting to our position relative to the earth, which exerts its gravitational pull. As such we have programmed into our system a device that lets us know what that position is at all times and directs the constant physical adjustments that we make. This is commonly referred to as the *equilibrial triad,* which consists of the proprioceptive system, the vestibular system, and the visual system.

The proprioceptive system gives us positional information based on the state of contraction of each muscle in the body, and the position of each joint. The vestibular system is our "gyroscope," which gives us information as to the position of the head and how it and the rest of the body are rotating or accelerating in space. The visual system is self-explanatory because we are all well aware of our surroundings and position if we can see where we are. In fact, because the visual system is so important in our normal range of activity, the other two parts of the triad act to support it. This is done by sensing the position of the head relative to the body and adjusting the posture so that the head is situated with the eyes aligned parallel to the horizon. Together these three systems act with the motor system to produce coordinated movement, balanced posture, and a properly aligned head.

Fascia

Connective tissue can be highly organized, as in the case of joint capsules, ligaments, tendons, the meninges of the central nervous system (CNS), intervertebral discs, and articular cartilage, or more diffuse and seemingly less organized. *Fascia* is another name for the connective tissue that surrounds and gives form to the tissues and organs of the body.

Fascia can be divided into two major components: superficial fascia and deep fascia. The superficial fascia resides just under the skin (the hypodermis) and serves as a staging center for the immune system (large quantities of antigens from the skin are presented to immune cells in this layer) and as a fat stor-

age depot (this fact is the cause of significant human attention). The deep fascia is far more extensive and exists throughout the body, serving to "connect" virtually all tissues and organs. Skeletal muscles are surrounded by capsules of deep fascia, as are nerves and blood vessels (the neurovascular bundles alluded to later are wrapped in the deep fascia). In this sense the deep fascia forms compartments that separate these tissues but also forms a structural continuum, where, if physical stress is applied to one area of fascia, this continuity will result in effects being "felt" in other areas or fascial layers as well. The compartmentalization of tissues by the deep fascia also results in specific pathways for and/or limits to the spread of infection (i.e., along fascial planes) and for the accumulation of fluid. Both superficial and deep fascia are richly supplied by blood and lymphatic vessels and nerves (especially pain fibers).

On the molecular level fascia is composed of a fibrous component (primarily the macromolecular proteins collagen and elastin) and a soluble, gel-like component, mostly water. Cells also reside in the fascia (the fat and immune cells in the superficial fascia). Connective tissue cells (fibroblasts) are responsible for the secretion of fibrous proteins that make up the scaffold of the fascia, whereas immune cells constantly patrol the fascia, seeking out foreign antigens and ingesting and destroying extracellular debris, including old constituents of the fibrous matrix. This creates a significant turnover in the components of the fascia and contributes to its innate adaptability to changing body conditions. The cellular component of the fascia can be significantly altered by a state of inflammation, in which large numbers of immune cells migrate into the area in response to tissue damage or antigenic challenge. Inflammation also stimulates fibroblasts to secrete larger amounts of collagen to reseal any breaches in the continuum, which on a large scale results in scar formation.

The fascia not only is adaptable to the everchanging internal environment but also is significantly affected by the aging process. As the human body ages, the chemical bonds that bind collagen molecules together, known as *cross-links,* become more prevalent. As this occurs the amount of space in the fascia can be occupied by water and the other soluble components of the fascia becomes less and less. The result is a loss of tissue water and an increase in the fibrous component, which decreases the relative elasticity and physical adaptability of the tissue. To put it bluntly, we dry up and become more brittle. This leaves the musculoskeletal system in particular significantly more susceptible to microtrauma and macrotrauma.

The physical properties of fascia have stimulated manual therapy practitioners to devise specific techniques to address these properties and the relationship between the fascia and the tissue it surrounds. Because the fascial matrix can become distorted as a result of the forces brought to bear on it, so too can it be restored to its original structural relationships by manual means. In addition, because of the continuity of the fascia throughout the body, local fascial distortions can (and do) produce distant effects. This is especially true in the case of muscle-associated deep fascia, which, if distorted, can alter the vector and function of that muscle.

The gel-like consistency of the soluble component of the fascia enables it to behave like a colloid, which resists force in direct proportion to its velocity. Conversely, because of this property, fascia, like a colloid, will respond much more readily if force is applied slowly and gently. In addition, gentle application of force results in gradual yet sustained realignment of the fibrous component of the fascia, which can be palpated in the form of a "release." This is the rationale behind the development of myofascial, craniosacral, and other low-velocity techniques.

Segmentation or the Functional Spinal Unit

Anatomically the human body is arranged lengthwise as a series of building blocks or segments. This can be observed most directly by looking at the individual vertebrae that make up the spinal column, which extends from the base of the skull to the "tailbone," the coccyx. Just above the coccyx is the sacrum, which is a single bone resulting from the fusion of five vertebrae. This fusion is significant because the sacrum articulates with the pelvic bones, which articulate with the femurs. This relationship produces an arch that has the sacrum as its keystone.

Passing between the vertebrae and going from the spinal cord to the periphery are 31 pairs of spinal nerves (one for each side, with the exception of the coccygeal nerve, which is fused at the midline). Each of these spinal nerves contains sensory and motor nerve fibers that are distributed around the body (Figure 8-2). In most cases the nerves are accompanied by arteries that supply blood to the same region supplied by the spinal nerve. In addition, the *neurovascular bundle,* as it is called, contains veins and lymphatic vessels, which serve to drain away waste products from the same territory. Thus each segment of the body receives information (and is sending information back to the CNS) and nourishment and is being drained of waste products. It might appear that each segment functions as a separate entity, but this is not the case. Because of significant overlap both inside and outside the CNS, in a sense each segment is "aware" of what is transpiring in the segments adjacent to it.

The individual spinal nerve and all of the tissues that it innervates has another name in addition to *the segment,* or *the spinal segment.* It is also referred to as the *functional spinal unit* (FSU). The FSU thus includes two adjacent vertebrae, the spinal nerves, skeletal muscles, and fascia between them, other bones, muscles, and fascia associated with the segment (e.g., ribs and intercostal muscles), the blood and lymphatic vessels that supply these tissues, and visceral structures within the body cavities that receive innervation from the autonomic portion of the spinal nerves.

Reflexes or the Autonomic Nervous System

The CNS, consisting of the brain and spinal cord, can be compared with a computer insofar as it is designed to integrate and process information. This information basically takes two forms: sensory (input) and motor (output). The most fundamental unit of information processing is the reflex. Information enters the CNS through a sensory neuron and is processed in the spinal cord through an interaction between the sensory neuron and the motor neuron known as a *synapse;* motor information then leaves the CNS directly through a motor neuron to effect a response in a skeletal muscle. The most common example of this type of reflex (called *somatic* for the type of tissue involved) is the withdrawal response when a painful stimulus is encountered, a hand on a hot burner, for example. The painful information is relayed through the spinal cord and out to the muscles, which effect the removal before the sensation reaches the brain and is perceived.

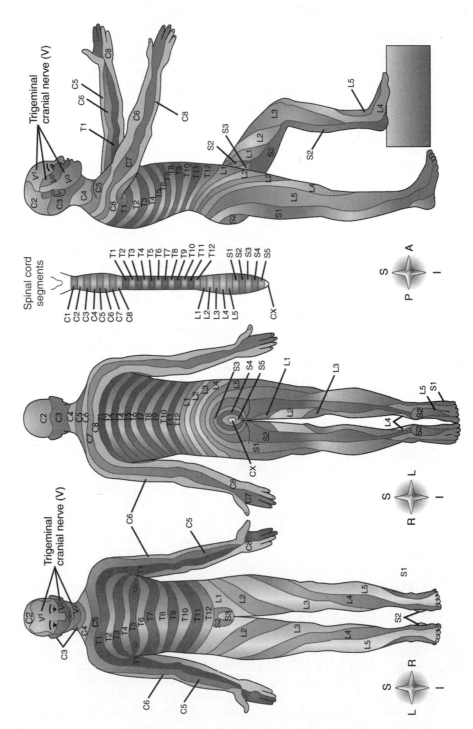

Figure 8-2 Diagram of dermatome man. (From Thibodeau GA: *Anatomy and physiology*, ed 4, St Louis, 1999, Mosby.)

Although much of the sensory information coming into the CNS reaches consciousness (i.e., is perceived), a great deal does not, and we go about our business neither knowing nor feeling what is happening. The same is true of motor activity, which can be voluntary or involuntary (see autonomic nervous system) [ANS] later). An example of this involuntary phenomenon is the digestive system, which under normal circumstances functions without our knowledge (with an important daily exception). With respect to postural maintenance, if we are asked to attend to our position, we are usually able to do so (a test of this system [conscious proprioception] is to ask the subject to close his or her eyes and to state the location and position of different parts such as the hands and feet). However, we usually are not particularly attentive to our position (unless of course, we lose our balance), and indeed there is an entire division of the proprioceptive system (unconscious proprioception) that is never perceived. In short we are constantly adjusting ourselves to adapt to the gravitational pull of the earth and our position relative to it, and most of this activity takes place at the level of the reflex.

The ANS is responsible for the unconscious control of visceral structures. These structures include smooth muscle (as found surrounding blood vessels and the bronchial tubes), cardiac (heart) muscle, glands, and lymphoid (immune) tissue. There are two divisions that act opposite one another: the sympathetic or thoracolumbar division, responsible for arousal, or the "fight or flight" reaction, and the parasympathetic or craniosacral division, responsible (among other things) for stimulating the activity of the digestive system, the "rest and digest" function. Although each division predominates in certain situations, the divisions normally coexist in balance with one another to maintain a state of homeostasis, which is a form of internal equilibrium. The names *thoracolumbar* and *craniosacral* indicate the origin of the motor nerves of each division. Therefore the spinal nerves of the thoracolumbar region contain both somatic and sympathetic nerve fibers, whereas some of the cranial nerves and sacral nerves contain both somatic and parasympathetic nerve fibers.

Within the CNS, interactions between sensory and motor nerves are constantly taking place through reflexes. Although it has long been known that somatic and visceral reflexes occur, it has only recently been discovered that the two types of reflex loops overlap with one another. That is to say, stimulation of a visceral structure can produce a somatic response, and stimulation of a somatic structure can elicit a visceral response. This discovery is of extreme importance to the practitioners of manipulation because it essentially validates the claim that manipulation has global effects on the body, especially when it comes to the maintenance or reestablishment of proper blood and lymphatic flow. In fact, it is quite arguable that manipulation of somatic structures (the musculoskeletal system) is entirely capable of restoring proper blood flow to visceral structures through reflexes mediated through the CNS.

Pain and Guarding, Muscle Spasm, and Facilitation

Pain is the result of a noxious stimulus, one that produces tissue damage. This of course can come from outside the body, such as a thermal or chemical burn, which is perceived at the skin, producing a classic withdrawal response. Or it can also come from inside the body, such as a sprained ankle, where the damage is perceived at a muscle, joint, or ligament.

If pain occurs as a result of damage to a bone, joint, or ligament, a natural response is for the surrounding muscles to contract reflexly, producing a natural splint of the area. This is also known as *guarding*. Of course, another result of this kind of damage is an altered gait pattern (a limp), which is merely an attempt to "get off" the affected joint if weight bearing causes additional pain. This can also happen when a paravertebral muscle is overstretched because of a bending or lifting maneuver. Proprioceptors in that muscle would report the stretch, causing a reflex contraction of that muscle. If the amount of damage is sufficient, the reflex contraction becomes stronger, and other muscles in the area are recruited to "guard" against further stretching and damage. The involved muscles are now in spasm. This reaction can spread (through reflex spread within the CNS) until a great deal of the back musculature is involved. This is what happens when the back "goes out" and one has back spasms. Because of the altered position of the body away from the norm and the prolonged spastic contraction, the involved muscles are required to do a great deal more work than they normally do, which results in fatigue. When this occurs, there is a resultant buildup of lactic acid in the tissues, which causes soreness (i.e., more pain). As can be seen, a downward spiral of pain leading to spasm leading to more pain can result.

As time goes on and more and more sensory input is being fed to the CNS, a situation develops in which the nerves that are reporting this information and the nerves that are reacting (the motor neurons) become more sensitive; that is, their threshold for activity becomes significantly reduced. This situation, known as *facilitation,* is responsible to a large extent for the downward spiral just mentioned.

Muscle spasm presumably lasts until the injury is healed and the surrounding muscles are allowed to release their grip on the area. This is why most allopathic physicians prescribe bed rest for back pain. Sooner or later it will resolve on its own. However, this is not always the case, and the spasm can persist at a reduced level. This can cause the vertebrae, which are normally moved by that muscle, to become fixed in a certain position. The vertebrae may remain in that fixed position even when the muscle spasm is completely resolved. This also creates a need for a compensatory reaction or altered behavior to prevent the generation of more pain, just like a limp (see the following discussion). It is possible in many cases to break the cycle of pain leading to spasm leading to pain by the application of manipulative therapy.

Compensation and Decompensation

As mentioned previously, the proprioceptive system is constantly reporting sensory information to the CNS regarding body position. This is so that postural adjustments can be made primarily to maintain the eyes parallel to the horizon (horizontal gaze). Unfortunately a situation may arise in which such compensatory behavior becomes more prolonged. As an example, visualize a person with one leg longer than the other (asymmetry). If this is the case the pelvis on the "longer" side would be elevated relative to the other side. Because the sacrum is strongly connected to the pelvic bones, the base on which the fifth lumbar vertebra rests would be tilted toward the short side. This information would be reported by the proprioceptive system, and the FSU above (L4-L5) would begin a compensatory reaction (via muscular contraction) to move the spine back into vertical alignment, creating a scoliotic curve. These compensatory reactions can

occur all the way up the spine, as long as the result is a level head. This creates an overall increased load on the system as a whole and significantly increases the amount of work needed just to maintain proper alignment.

In most cases these reactions work well and no pain or damage is produced. This is especially true in younger people. However, as we age, changes in our body tissues occur (most notably the loss of water and reduced elasticity), which alter the mechanical properties of the body as a whole. Sooner or later the system fails and begins to decompensate. This results in a rise in the amount and number of compensatory reactions as the system gets further out of whack, eventually leading to tissue damage (usually on the microscopic level), which ultimately leads to pain, sometimes chronic. This scenario explains, in part, the preponderance of complaints of low back and neck pain in the general population. In fact, musculoskeletal complaints cause about one third of all the office visits to physicians in the United States. On a holistic or preventive level intervention to correct a musculoskeletal problem or dysfunction before its becoming chronic or debilitating would be sensible and cost-effective in the long run. This is where manipulative therapy is indicated and most effective.

Range of Motion and the Barrier Concept

Each joint of the body has a normal direction and amount of motion associated with it. This is referred to as *range of motion* (ROM). When motion is outside this normal range (this of course is a statistical norm and can vary considerably), that joint is said to be *hypermobile* or *hypomobile.* In addition, joints with a greater ROM generally are less stable than those with less ROM (visualize the hip and shoulder joints, for example). In the case of the spine the lumbar and cervical areas have the greatest ROM, which establishes an increased probability of instability and injury, especially in the lumbar spine, where significantly greater weight is being borne. This is the principal reason for the relative frequency of lumbar and cervical spine problems in the general population.

Typically, if there is pain around a joint for any reason, ROM will be decreased or limited, and in this case motion is said to be restricted. The restriction of motion in a particular direction or plane of space produces a "barrier" to normal motion. Motion barriers may not necessarily be accompanied by or be the result of pain, however. In fact, under normal circumstances there are barriers to motion. These can be "anatomical" barriers, "physiological" barriers, or both. A good example of an anatomical barrier is the elbow joint, where the olecranon process of the ulna locks into the olecranon fossa of the humerus, thus preventing overextension of the joint. Therefore the bones themselves present a motion barrier. Joint capsules and ligaments also create anatomical barriers. Physiological barriers are produced by the normal tone of the muscles around a joint, which also act in balance with one another, so that no individual muscle becomes too taut or stretched, producing damage. The proprioceptive system plays an important role in maintaining physiological barriers. If a guarding reaction is present or if a muscle is in spasm, a temporary physiological motion barrier can be established, in this case referred to as a *restrictive barrier*. As noted previously, this situation is where manipulation can be effective in reducing or eliminating musculoskeletal dysfunction and restoring normal motion.

Active versus Passive and Direct versus Indirect

In treating musculoskeletal ailments with manipulation, two approaches can be used with the variety of techniques. *Active* versus *passive* refers to the activity level of the patient (i.e., is he or she actively participating in the treatment or is the practitioner doing the mechanical work?).

Direct versus *indirect* refers to the motion barrier and the practitioner's approach to it. Recall that a motion barrier is a decrease in normal ROM as a result of an increase in the normal physiological motion barrier. The practitioner seeks to remove or release this barrier and restore normal motion. The technique used can either move the affected joint toward the motion barrier (direct) or away from the barrier (indirect). A simple example of this is as follows: The flexors of the elbow joint are in spasm, thus holding the elbow in flexion (bent) and creating a barrier to extension (straightening). A direct technique would be an attempt to move the joint into extension (i.e., into or toward the motion barrier). An indirect technique would move the elbow joint further into flexion, producing a change in the position of the

joint, which would be reported by the muscle and joint proprioceptors. This, over a short period, causes a reflex release of the spastic contraction of the flexor muscles, thereby eliminating the motion barrier.

In summary, the practitioner of manual therapy seeks to restore proper anatomical and physiological balance in the patient. At least three types of balance are potential targets of the various styles and techniques used:

1. The restoration of proper joint range of motion and body symmetry
2. The restoration of balance of nervous activity between the sensory and motor systems, between the somatic and autonomic nerves, and between the sympathetic and parasympathetic divisions of the autonomic nervous system
3. The restoration of proper arterial flow and venous and lymphatic drainage for proper nutrition of all tissues of the body

OSTEOPATHIC MEDICINE

Osteopathy was founded by Andrew Taylor Still (1828-1917), a practicing physician and ordained Methodist minister (Figure 8-3). Trained in both disciplines by his father, Still acted as an itinerant preacher and physician, ministering principally to the settlers and Indian tribes then living in the state of Missouri and the Kansas territory. He received additional "training" as a surgeon for the Union army during the Civil War.

In 1864 an outbreak of meningitis claimed the lives of three of his children. This tragic event and his helplessness to affect its outcome, coupled with the method of medicine practiced at the time (including the application of leeches, bleeding, purging, and treatments with such toxic elements as mercury and arsenic), sowed the seeds of his discontent with his (inherited) profession. During this period Oliver Wendell Holmes, Sr., the renowned physician, declared, "If the whole *materia medica* as now used could be sunk to the bottom of the sea, it would be better for mankind—and all the worse for the fishes." Still began to search for a better way.

Still's search led him to a prolonged and detailed study of human anatomy, the bones in particular. He ultimately came to the conclusion that if the bones of the body were not in the proper relation to one another and could not move properly, then other

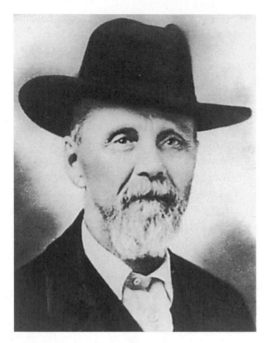

Figure 8-3 A.T. Still, the founder of osteopathy. (Courtesy Still National Museum of Osteopathy, Kirksville, Missouri.)

systems of the body would become affected and disease could develop. He strongly espoused the theory of holism, in which all body systems are considered both structurally and functionally interrelated. Still was also a strong advocate of the importance of balance (homeostasis) within the body, with a specific emphasis on the unimpeded arterial flow and venous and lymphatic drainage to and from the organs. He also believed in the inherent ability of the body to defend and repair itself. Bearing in mind that these observations were made before the discovery by Western science of the immune and endocrine systems, Still's ideas were at the time considered quite radical.

In 1892 Still founded the American School of Osteopathy in Kirksville, Missouri, where he remained until his death. Between the time he "discovered" osteopathy and the establishment of the American Society of Osteopathy (ASO), Still was developing his osteopathic technique and billed himself as a "Lightning Bonesetter." The ASO has evolved into the Kirksville College of Osteopathic Medicine (sometimes euphemistically referred to as *the mecca*). The success of the ASO was such that the founding of os-

teopathic colleges in Des Moines, Chicago, Philadelphia, and Kansas City followed within the next 15 years. After Still's death, osteopathy sought to gain legal if not philosophical equality with the allopathic profession, which had established itself as the gold standard of medical practice. Through the American Medical Association (AMA), allopathic physicians were making a concerted effort to eradicate perceived competition (see Chiropractic).

The first step toward parity for the osteopaths was to provide equivalent education for their students, which was based on the Flexner model of medical education (2 years of basic science, followed by 2 years of such things as clinical rotations, internship, and residency). The unity stimulated by persecution by the AMA and the loyalty of its patients provided for the slow yet steady growth of the osteopathic profession until after World War II. Hospitals were built, legal battles for practice rights were fought on a state-by-state basis, and the profession developed on a "separate but equal" basis (doctors of osteopathy [DOs] prescribe all manner of drugs, perform surgery, and practice OB-GYN, emergency medicine, and other types of medicine).

The postwar period brought accelerated growth caused in large part by the commissioning of DOs into the U.S. armed services. New colleges were established, and full practice rights were finally granted in all 50 states in the 1960s (osteopathic physicians are still not fully licensed in Canada). The struggle for equality was won, but not without a price. The push for equivalence with MDs created a desire to shed what originally made osteopathy unique. As a result the DOs began to deemphasize manipulation as the benchmark of their clinical practice, and many today view it as archaic and an embarrassment. In fact, most DOs in the United States, although having learned manipulative theory and technique in their student days, do not use it at all, or use it only sparingly. This has become especially true with the advent of managed care. Manipulation is not cost-effective for physicians because reimbursements by insurance companies are insufficient. This is the rationale for using the term *osteopathic medicine* as the title of this section, rather than the more traditional term *osteopathy*. As a result, there is a distinct danger that manipulation will become the lost art of osteopathic practice. This and the fact that there are currently fewer than 40,000 DOs in the United States compared with more than 600,000 MDs would indicate that osteopathic medicine's days as a distinct profession are numbered.

Despite these developments, the American Academy of Osteopathy (AAO), a subgroup of the American Osteopathic Association (AOA), has dedicated itself to the preservation and nurturing of osteopathic manipulation and philosophy. Through the efforts of this association and the paradigm shift in medicine brought on by the complementary medicine movement, osteopathic manipulation may yet surge again within the profession. In addition, there are growing osteopathic movements in Europe and Asia, but in each country licensing and scope of practice issues must be resolved separately.

Osteopathic manipulative treatment (OMT) is based on the diagnosis of somatic dysfunction. This term was coined by Rumney when the coding system (ICD) was developed for insurance reimbursement. Until then, the more provincial term *osteopathic lesion* was used. Several criteria must be met for a diagnosis:

1. *Asymmetry:* This can be observed while the patient is standing (e.g., uneven shoulder height, pelvic tilt, scoliosis, kyphosis, genu valgum [knock knees], foot pronation), walking (e.g., limp, pelvic tilt, uneven arm swing), lying supine (e.g., pelvic rotation, leg length discrepancy), prone (e.g., scoliosis, abnormal bony prominence), or in other positions or during other movements.
2. *Restriction:* Motion restriction is diagnosed with ROM testing, usually passive, by attempting to move the affected joint through normal range and observing restrictions, changes in motion characteristics, or when discomfort is encountered. In the case of the spine ROM can be analyzed regionally (e.g., thoracic spine) or intersegmentally (e.g., T4-T5). ROM testing also extends to the fascial system, which is assessed by a variety of techniques.
3. *Tissue texture changes:* These changes can include excessive dryness or oiliness, redness or pallor, a feeling of "ropiness," or excessive hardness or softness compared with the surrounding tissues. The tissues involved can be skin, fascia, muscles, joint capsules, or visceral structures.
4. *Tenderness:* Pain can be elicited on active motion, on passive motion, or by palpation with light to deep pressure. Occasionally tenderness is not observed by the patient until the operator points it out.

Diagnosis is usually made on the basis of combining observation and palpation, with palpation being by far the more important of the two elements (see Cranial Osteopathy).

As with other forms of manual therapy, the discretion of the practitioner is operative when selecting specific techniques to be used with individual patients. Different combinations and sequences are observed, depending on the preference of the physician and his or her observations of the tolerance level of the patient. Because DOs are fully licensed, drugs and injections may also accompany manipulative treatment when considered necessary or beneficial. Some of the more commonly used osteopathic techniques follow.

Muscle Energy

Muscle energy technique can be applied directly or indirectly. When applied directly (i.e., toward the motion barrier or in an attempt to lengthen a shortened or spastic muscle), it is based on the principle of reciprocal inhibition, which states that as a muscle contracts (e.g., flexion), its antagonist (the associated extensor) reflexively relaxes. If a muscle in spasm is contracted against resistance and then relaxed, the effect is to break the reflex spasm cycle, resulting in increased ROM (reduction of the motion barrier). When applied indirectly, it is based on the principle of postisometric relaxation (also known as *postcontraction relaxation*). This technique is one of the few active techniques in manual therapy (i.e., where the patient does the work). Individual muscles can be treated, as well as muscle groups. A distinction of muscle energy technique is the amount of effort exerted by the patient. Usually less than 20% of the total strength of the muscle is brought to bear during the interval of contraction. Another way of putting this is the "one finger rule," in which the amount of force necessary is that to move a single finger of the therapist, lightly resisting the contraction. This is in contradistinction to the proprioceptive neuromuscular facilitation (PNF) technique, which uses a maximum muscle contraction (exposing the patient to the risk of injury). A thorough knowledge of muscle attachments and their motion vectors is necessary to apply this technique effectively and efficiently.

High-Velocity, Low-Amplitude Technique

The high-velocity, low-amplitude (HVLA) technique, although by no means the only one available to the osteopath (or chiropractor for that matter), is probably the single most publicly recognized technique of the two professions. This is a thrust-oriented technique designed to aggressively break through a motion barrier. More often than not an audible pop is heard, the result of a brief cavitation of the involved joint. HVLA can be applied directly (toward the barrier) or indirectly (away from the barrier), using short or long levers. Although commonly associated with manipulation of the spine, HVLA is also performed on the extremities. This technique is *not* indicated in patients with osteoporosis, bone tumors, severe atherosclerosis, or vertebrobasilar arterial insufficiency.

Strain and Counterstrain

The strain and counterstrain technique is a gentle, passive technique, developed by L. Jones. The operator palpates a muscle in spasm, and the patient is brought into a position that shortens the muscle (counterstrain), thereby exaggerating the motion restriction. This position is held usually for 90 to 120 seconds, and the patient is slowly returned to the original position. The technique is designed to interrupt the reflex spasm loop by changing and holding altered proprioceptive input into the CNS. This technique can also be done directly (strain), that is, gently stretching the involved muscle, with the same result. Tender points are also treated in this manner, where the patient is brought to a position of ease, held in the position until a "softening" or change in tissue texture is felt, then slowly returned to the original position.

Myofascial Release

Myofascial release is a gentle technique that uses a knowledge of the physical properties of the fascia as it relates to muscles. A high level of palpatory skill is necessary to apply this technique effectively. The operator uses light or deep pressure to palpate motion restriction and either moves toward or away from the restriction. The position is held until a "release," or softening, is felt; the tissues are then slowly returned to their original position. The release can be the relaxation of muscle, the slow breaking of fascial adhesions, or the realignment of fascia to its correct orientation.

Myofasciae–Soft Tissue Technique

The myofascial-soft tissue technique is a combination direct and indirect massage technique for reducing muscle spasm and fascial tension. It is similar to petrissage (see Massage) except that more parts of the hand are typically used. This technique can be used as a prelude to HVLA.

Lymphatic Drainage Techniques (Pumps)

Lymphatic drainage techniques are similar to effleurage (see Massage) in that light pressure is applied to the skin or superficial fascia in the direction of the heart to increase the venous and lymphatic drainage of the involved structure(s). Lymphatic pumps are rhythmic techniques applied over organs such as the liver and spleen to increase drainage. The thoracic diaphragm is also sometimes used as a lymphatic pump.

Cranial Osteopathy

Cranial osteopathy was developed by W.G. Sutherland. His work was based on the observation that the joints between the skull bones are meant to permit motion just as they do in other areas of the body. While palpating these bones and joints, he discovered the existence of a very subtle rhythm in the body unrelated to respiration or cardiovascular rhythms. Sutherland named this rhythm the *cranial rhythmic impulse* (CRI). This impulse, he learned, was capable of moving the cranial bones through a very small ROM—small yet palpable to well-trained hands. Cranial theory posits that there is inherent motility of the CNS, resulting in fluctuations of the cerebrospinal fluid (the fluid that bathes the brain and spinal cord). This fluctuation in turn moves the cranial bones through their small yet palpable ROM, primarily at the sutural joints. Motion is not restricted to the cranial bones by means of this rhythm, though. Through the dural membranes, which cover the CNS, the sacrum is linked to the cranium, and motion is palpable there as well. Through the fascia-fluid system of the body, the CRI has effects all over the body. Motion restrictions in this system can be palpated and corrected (either directly or indirectly) through very gentle manipulation, also with global effects (see Fascia). Because releases are produced in this fascial system and throughout the body, and perhaps because of its proximity to the brain, memories—sometimes painful—can be reawakened, producing what is referred to as the somatoemotional release, a form of mind-body connection.

Evidence of the effectiveness of cranial osteopathy comes almost exclusively in the form of clinical case reports and testimonials. Successes have been reported for many conditions. Cranial osteopathy has been reported to result in improvements in such conditions as chronic headache, cerebral palsy, autism, and behavioral disturbances.

Cranial osteopathy has been controversial from its inception because of the lack of definitive experimental evidence (although workers in the field would dispute this). However, data are being gathered, and outcomes-based studies are being conducted that lend credence to its effectiveness. Because of the time and effort necessary to develop this skill, relatively few osteopaths practice cranial osteopathy. However, training in cranial osteopathy (or CranioSacral Therapy) is now being offered to other practitioners of manual therapies by the Upledger Institute.

Visceral Manipulation

Visceral manipulation generally involves gentle massage of the accessible internal organs (abdominopelvic organs). Although not indicated in patients with tumors or inflammatory disease, visceral manipulation can be useful in stabilizing and balancing blood flow and autonomic innervation and can even dislodge certain obstructions of the gastrointestinal system. This form of manipulation, along with cranial osteopathy, is practiced extensively by European osteopaths.

Articulatory Technique

When using the articulatory technique, the operator moves the affected joint through its ROM in all planes, gently encountering motion barriers and gradually moving through them to establish normal motion. This would be considered a passive, direct-indirect, oscillatory technique.

Functional Technique (Facilitated Positional Release)

In the functional technique the patient is positioned such as to produce a "position of ease" or comfort. The operator typically places a hand or finger over a tender area and positions the patient until the discomfort is significantly reduced; this position is held for a certain time period. The patient is then brought slowly back to the original position. The position of ease reduces nociceptive and aberrant proprioceptive input to the CNS, thus breaking the cycle of pain and spasm. Realignment of fascia is also a result of this technique.

CHIROPRACTIC

During the mid-1890s, Daniel David Palmer, a practicing magnetic healer, relieved a man of his longstanding deafness by administering an adjustment to his thoracic vertebrae. This was his first experience with what he began to call *chiropractic*. Within 2 years he had established the Palmer School of Chiropractic in Davenport, Iowa. It is interesting to note that at approximately the same time and within 200 miles of one another, the professions of chiropractic and osteopathy grew up together. It has been rumored (by the osteopaths) that Palmer was a patient of Still's at Kirksville and carefully observed his technique and its results, but this is not confirmed. It is, though, a statement regarding the atmosphere of intellectual freedom at that period of time and in that part of the United States.

Palmer was a devotee of vitalism, which states that the universe and its inhabitants are imbued with an innate intelligence. He believed that this intelligence accounted for the self-healing capacity of the body. Using vitalism as a foundation, he developed the "one cause, one cure" theory, which posits that all disease can be traced to subluxations of the vertebral column. Therefore, he stated, all disease can be cured by chiropractic adjustment (Figure 8-4). Vertebral subluxation was explained by the "bone out of place," or static, model. This model stated that the malpositioned vertebra entrapped the spinal nerve at the neural foramen, thereby affecting normal body tonus and causing disease. The treatment involved a thrusting technique to put the bone back in its proper alignment. Palmer took great pains to explain the technique, which used the spinous and transverse processes of the vertebra as short levers, thereby distinguishing himself from Still and the osteopaths, who taught both short and long lever techniques.

In 1906 Palmer spent 3 months in the Scott County (Iowa) jail for practicing medicine without a license. This event marked the beginning of a long period of conflict between the chiropractic and medical professions. It has been estimated that by 1930 more than 30,000 such jail terms had been served.

Over the next few years several additional chiropractic schools were established. In contrast to the early growth in the number of osteopathic colleges (to expand and promote the profession), the outgrowth of chiropractic colleges was primarily due to intractable philosophical conflicts between their founders and Palmer. One of these, Solon M. Langworthy, established the American School of Chiropractic and Nature Cure (1903). Langworthy, along with Oakley Smith and Minora Paxson, published a textbook that delineated what would later become the dynamic model of spinal subluxation, proposing that vertebral subluxation is a result of motion restriction or "fixation." Palmer also had serious differences of opinion with his son, B.J., who took over the administration of the Palmer school after his father's death. B.J. believed that the upper cervical vertebrae were the seat of all spinal subluxations and treated his patients accordingly. Treating all patients with the same technique gave rise to the term *hole in one* to describe the procedure.

As a defender of the profession, B.J. was tireless. In 1907 he retained lawyers in the defense of Shegatoro Morikobu, another chiropractor accused of practicing medicine without a license. Using the Langworthy et al. textbook in the defense, it was pointed out that chiropractic is not medicine and that the profession was separate and distinct from the allopathic profession. Therefore Dr. Morikobu was not in fact practicing "medicine" without a license, he was practicing chiropractic. The case was won, and the "separate and distinct" concept was publicly established.

B.J. Palmer was also enamored of technology. He purchased and extensively used the first available

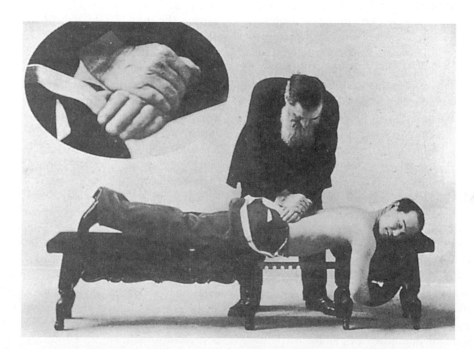

Figure 8-4 One of the few photographs of D.D. Palmer giving an adjustment. (From Palmer DD, Palmer BJ: *The science of chiropractic: its principles and adjustments,* 1906.)

X-ray equipment and advocated its use in documenting subluxations. As a means of earning additional money to support the college, he became involved in the wireless communication business, eventually starting World of Chiropractic (WOC) in Davenport. One of WOC's more famous alumni was Ronald Reagan.

By the 1930s the rift between the Palmer philosophy (one cause, one cure/bone out of place/hole in one) and that of the rationalists came to a critical point when Henri Gillet, a Belgian chiropractor, put forth the dynamic model, based in part on Langworthy's earlier work. Gillet stated that subluxations were due to vertebral fixations, which could be muscular, articular, ligamentous, or bony in nature. The fixation, in turn, caused a nerve entrapment, causing symptoms associated with that segment. This theory is by far the most widely espoused today and is the origin of the commonly used terms *vertebral subluxation complex* (VSC) and *segmental dysfunction* (SDF). By the 1940s the chiropractors falling on the side of the Langworthy-Gillet theory, disavowing the one cause, one cure theory of Palmer, became known as the *Mixers,* whereas those adhering to the Palmer theory were referred to as *Straights.*

In conjunction with the split in the profession, the persecution at the hands of the allopaths continued. In the 1960s and 1970s MDs were forbidden by the AMA to have any professional association with DCs. This led to an antitrust suit brought against the AMA *(Wilk vs AMA).* That lawsuit was won in the early 1990s, a major victory for the profession.

At the time of the original schism, the National Chiropractic Association had been established for more than 10 years. Claude O. Watkins, the NCA's chairman, strongly advocated embracing the scientific method and establishing educational standards. He believed that the greatest hope for the profession was through the validation of chiropractic theory through research. The NCA eventually became the American Chiropractic Association (ACA), and from this grew the Foundation for Chiropractic Research (FCER) and the Council on Chiropractic Education (CCE). The CCE now accredits all chiropractic colleges in the United States, including those that continue to profess the one cause, one cure philosophy (the "Straights").

Most chiropractors today treat primarily musculoskeletal complaints and restrict their manipulation to the spine and pelvis, although occasionally treatment may be given to the cranium and extremities. Because of research conducted by Korr, Patterson, Sato, and others on the effects of somatovisceral reflexes and the research that continues today on many questions related to manual therapy in general, the impact of spinal manipulation on other ailments may yet be more clearly explained.

The hallmarks of the VSC or SDF are similar if not identical to the osteopathic somatic dysfunction. Motion restriction in the form of a fixation is present; that is, something is restricting movement of the vertebra in one of the three planes of space. Possibilities include a joint (articulatory), usually a facet joint; a ligament; a muscle (in spasm); or a bone (as a result of arthritis or other pathological condition). Tenderness is also present, along with texture changes in the surrounding tissues.

The disorders commonly treated by chiropractors are classified in three groups.

1. *Type M (musculoskeletal):* This group is fairly self-evident and includes such complaints as facet syndrome, sacroiliac joint dysfunction, tension headache, myositis, fibromyalgia, trigger points, strain and sprain injuries, torticollis (wry neck), some forms of sciatica, and undifferentiated low back and neck pain. Successes have been reported in cases of herniated discs, but treating this ailment with high-velocity technique is somewhat controversial.

2. *Type N (neurogenic):* Some successes have been reported in cases of nystagmus, migraine, Bell's palsy, Tourette's syndrome, and other neurogenic complaints, but these reports are anecdotal and no controlled studies have as yet been conducted to confirm the results.

3. *Type O (organic, stress related):* These disorders include hypertension, headache, bowel and bladder dysfunction, dysmenorrhea, infantile colic, gastritis, angina, and asthma. As noted previously, reports of success using chiropractic manipulative therapy (CMT) are anecdotal and research is needed to confirm these claims.

As mentioned previously, chiropractic technique is primarily thrust (HVLA)-oriented, using a short lever approach. The classic joint "pop" or "crack" is a hallmark of chiropractic treatment. Four types of thrusts are presented here, although variations on each exist. They are used to increase joint mobility and decrease or eliminate muscle spasm.

Impulse: In this thrust the motion barrier is engaged with the hands and a quick, short thrust is applied.

Recoil: The thrust is delivered with force generated from the chest, arms, and hands of the operator. After it is delivered, the hands recoil from the spinous process of the vertebra.

Body drop: The operator's arms are fully extended and the elbows are locked in performing this thrust. The weight of the operator is quickly brought to bear on the vertebra to be manipulated.

Leverage: This thrust is performed with counter-stabilization applied to prevent the loss of force during the thrust.

Thrusts can be applied singly or in groups (multiple thrust) with gradually increasing force. The direction of the thrust and selection of fulcrum depend on the type of fixation and direction of motion restriction.

Over the years many different models for the analysis and treatment of the VSC/SDF have been developed. Almost all are HVLA-oriented, and all are passive.

Diversified: This is by far the most common of the chiropractic approaches. HVLA is delivered to individual segments and/or groups of segments, as determined by motion analysis and palpatory diagnosis.

Gonstead: This approach uses direct HVLA to thrust in a direction opposite of that of the motion restriction (i.e., directly into the motion barrier). X-ray analysis is commonly used, with lines drawn on the films to aid in the diagnosis.

Cox/flexion-distraction: This approach uses a traction-mobilization technique. It is used primarily in cases of intervertebral disc pathosis and is one of the few non-HVLA techniques in the chiropractic armamentarium.

Activator: This technique is applied with a device that delivers a very high-velocity impulse. It is used with muscles and other soft tissues, as well as joints.

Thompson: In this approach HVLA is applied primarily to the pelvis to correct dysfunction there and as a result of leg length discrepancy. The legs and pelvis are regarded as a support-

ive arch system for the body and the seat of dysfunction.

Sacro-occipital technique (SOT): Modeled after cranial osteopathy, SOT attempts to balance the cerebrospinal fluid system through gentle, direct technique.

Nimmo/tonus receptor: This technique is designed to treat trigger points (see Neuromuscular Therapy) with direct pressure for a period of approximately 7 to 8 seconds. When one trigger point releases, the next is treated in the same manner.

Applied kinesiology (AK): AK is one of the most controversial of the chiropractic techniques. Promulgated by G. Goodheart, AK theory states that the VSC creates weakness in specific muscle groups. Therefore, when a muscle group is found to be weak when pressure is applied to a particular segment, that segment is expressing a spinal dysfunction. This system is also applied to various points on the body that, when pressure is applied, will induce weakness in specific muscle groups. When the point is treated with pressure, the weakness subsides and the dysfunction is corrected. The points identified in AK are similar to acupuncture points and correspond to visceral and somatic dysfunction.

Logan basic: The sacrum is the center of this theory, with the focus on the sacrotuberous ligament. Sacral dysfunctions are relieved by means of a fascial release–oriented treatment.

Palmer upper cervical (HIO): As described earlier, B.J. Palmer proposed that all vertebral subluxations were secondary to the first two cervicals. As such, he devised the hole in one technique, in which a lateral thrust is applied to C1-C2.

Meric: In this system it is believed that the third thoracic vertebra is the primary center of subluxation. HVLA is applied.

Pierce-Stillwagon: This approach targets the cervical spine and pelvis with an HVLA thrust.

Along with manipulative treatment, chiropractors also commonly use treatment modalities typically associated with physical therapy. Hot packs, ultrasonography, transcutaneous electronic nerve stimulation (TENS), and others can be found in the contemporary chiropractic office.

Despite the philosophical departure from the original theories of the Palmers, the chiropractic profession has never, in contrast to the osteopaths, attempted to attain equivalency with allopathic medicine, a fact that would please B.J. Palmer were he alive today. Even though intramural disagreements still exist, the chiropractors have remained essentially true to their roots as separate and distinct health care professionals.

MASSAGE

Massage, like other manipulative forms, predates written history. The Greek physician Aesculapus became perhaps the first practitioner of the one cause, one cure approach when he abandoned the other forms of contemporary medical treatment in favor of massage to restore the free movement of body fluids and return the patient to a state of health. During the Renaissance the physician Paré, author of a widely used surgery text, espoused the application of massage and manipulation and was reportedly the first to use the term *subluxation.* In 1813 Henrik Ling, a gymnastics instructor, founded the Central Royal Institute of Gymnastics, where his theory of massage as passive gymnastics was developed. This work was the genesis of what is now referred to as *Swedish massage,* and Ling is considered the father of massage. The classification of massage techniques was accomplished by Berghmann and Helleday, students of Metzger, a Dutch physician and student of Ling. In the late nineteenth century the prominent French physician Lucas-Champonnière advocated the use of massage therapy in the treatment of fractures, arguing the case for consideration of soft tissue union in the healing process. His students, the English physicians William Bennett and Robert Jones, effectively brought massage to England. Bennett incorporated the use of massage at St. George's Hospital in London around 1899, while Jones used massage therapy at the Southern Hospital in Liverpool. Both James Mennell, author of the text *Physical Treatment by Movement, Manipulation, and Massage* (1917) and a tireless advocate of massage, and Mary McMillan, who was very influential in the introduction and promotion of massage in the United States, were taught by Jones. As awareness of this form of treatment grew, so did the science of physiology, and the two entities became intertwined with the growth of the scientific

basis of medicine. Some authors attribute the development of the physical therapy profession as an outgrowth of massage and its incorporation into the Euro-American therapeutic armamentarium. Many other forms of so-called bodywork are also outgrowths of massage and its various techniques and styles.

The essential theory of massage therapy is based on the principle that the tissues of the body will function at optimal levels when arterial supply and venous and lymphatic drainage are unimpeded (see Osteopathic Medicine). When this flow becomes unbalanced for any reason, muscle tightness and changes in the nearby skin and fascia will ensue, which may produce pain. The basic techniques of massage are designed to reestablish proper fluid dynamics and are directed at the skin, muscles, and fascia, although occasionally nerve pathways are included. In general, articulations are not directly addressed in this form of therapy. Contraindications to massage or areas to avoid during the application of massage include skin infections or melanoma, bleeding (especially within 48 hours of a traumatic event causing bleeding into the tissues), or the existence of acute inflammation (e.g., rheumatoid, appendicitis), thrombophlebitis, atherosclerosis, varicose veins, or an immunocompromised state of the patient (to avoid transmission of infection from massage therapist to patient).

The techniques of massage are generally applied in the direction of the heart to stimulate increased venous and lymphatic drainage from the involved tissues. Muscles are treated in groups, with one group being treated before advancing to the next. Different combinations of techniques are used, depending on the objectives of treatment. Treatment ordinarily begins with more gentle techniques before progressing to deeper, more aggressive applications. Massage is usually performed with a powder, oil, or other type of lubricant applied to the skin of the patient, who lies prone, supine, or laterally on a table or may be seated in a massage chair. Verbal communication between the operator and patient is important because the operator will use the cues given by the patient as a guide to treatment.

The visceral effects of massage of course include the general vasoactivity in somatic tissues as regulated by the ANS, but effects also can be observed on blood pressure and/or heart rate (usually decreases in both) as the patient relaxes into the treatment.

There are five basic techniques of massage, and all are of the passive variety (i.e., the operator does the work). They include effleurage, petrissage, friction, tapotement, and vibration.

Effleurage

Effleurage is the most commonly used massage technique and typically begins a treatment session to introduce the patient to the process of touching. Effleurage is a stroking technique applied with light to moderate pressure (superficial or deep), serving to modulate the arterial supply and venous/lymphatic drainage of the tissues contacted. The amount of pressure applied determines the layer of the body contacted (e.g., a very light pressure would affect only the skin, deeper pressure the superficial fascia, still deeper pressure the deep fascia, and so on). Either the entire palmar surface of the hand is used, or a "knuckling" technique may be used (after Hoffa, see later). When used during the initial stages of treatment, effleurage is also used as a palpatory diagnostic tool as the operator "looks" for areas of altered texture, asymmetry, or tenderness. Specific long strokes are also used at the conclusion of treatment, especially if sleep induction is desired.

Petrissage

Petrissage is somewhat more aggressive, with the thumb and fingers working together to lift and "milk" the underlying fascia and muscles in a kneading type of motion. Care is taken not to pinch or produce bruising. The effect of petrissage is to increase venous and lymphatic drainage of the muscles and to break up adhesions that may be present in the fascia. Depending on the direction of application and vector of motion restriction (if any), this technique could be considered either direct or indirect.

Friction

Friction can be the most deeply applied of the massage techniques. The tips of the fingers or thumb are used in a circular or back-and-forth movement. If deeper pressure is desired or if the operator is easily fatigued, the heel of the hand can be used or sometimes even the elbow. Friction can be used in cases of tenosynovitis, where adhesions are present, or where the target tissue is too deep for petrissage. James Cyriax developed the technique of transverse friction massage, which is widely used by physical therapists. As in the preceding technique, the direction of the applied technique, relative to any motion restriction, will determine whether the application is direct or indirect.

Tapotement

Often seen in classic fight films, tapotement involves rapid, repeated blows of varying strength done with the sides or palms of the hands, with the hands cupped, or with the fists. Occasionally rapid pinching of the skin is done. The purpose of tapotement is to stimulate arterial circulation to the area. Again, the technique should not produce bruising and is not applied over the area of the kidneys or on the chest (nor of course over any recent incisions or areas of inflammation or contusion).

Vibration

Usually considered to be one of the more difficult of the massage techniques to master or to perform without becoming fatigued, the application of vibration typically uses a mechanical vibrator of some type. When the hands are used, a light, rhythmic, quivering effect is achieved.

Some Other Styles of Massage

Albert Hoffa

Albert Hoffa's text, *Technik der Massage,* was published in 1900, and the techniques described therein are still in use today. He advocated the limitation of massage to 15-minute treatments with no pain experienced by the patient. Like Ling, Hoffa stated that massage should be applied from distal to proximal, with the point of reference being the heart. His adaptations included knuckling and circular effleurage and two-finger petrissage.

Mary McMillan

Mary McMillan is also credited with the categorization of massage into its five basic techniques. In each of those categories she introduced innovative variations. She advocated the use of olive oil as a lubricant for its nutritive capability when absorbed through the skin. Her influence in the development of massage is universally recognized, and her techniques have been widely adopted by massage therapists in the United States.

Bindgewebmassage (Dicke)

Elisabeth Dicke was a student of Hoffa's who described massage based on the connective tissue system of the body. She described areas of referred pain on the back that indicate internal pathological conditions but do not necessarily correspond to segmental distribution. Areas of tenderness do correspond to certain acupuncture points. Treatment is given with the middle finger in a series of sequenced strokes without lubricant.

James Cyriax

James Cyriax was a strong advocate of friction as the most effective technique in massage. He developed the transverse friction massage technique, which is widely used by manual therapists. Deep friction massage is used to stimulate increased circulation to the affected area. It can be applied to muscles, tendons, ligaments, and bones. Cyriax's methods are described in detail in his book *Textbook of Orthopedic Medicine, Volume II.*

Massage is used in a variety of clinical scenarios. The expertise of the operator is essential in determining which techniques may or may not be indicated and how the massage may be delivered. Application may be based on the motion restrictions that may be present in the patient or in the environment, such as in a hospital. Massage is routinely applied to pediatric and geriatric patients (infant massage is a burgeoning field). Massage therapists often expand their therapeutic horizons by taking postgraduate study in other forms of bodywork, some of which are described in the following discussion. It is not uncommon to find a therapist who not only does Swedish massage but who also uses Trager work, Feldenkrais, and CranioSacral Therapy.

OTHER FORMS OF BODYWORK

Neuromuscular Therapy

Neuromuscular therapy (NMT) was pioneered by Lief and Chaitow in Europe and Nimmo in the United States. It continues its development today through St. John, Walker and others. Like osteopaths, neuro-

muscular therapists also use the term *somatic dysfunction* when describing what was formerly referred to as the *neuromuscular lesion.* It is characterized by an area of tenderness and limited motion. Causes of these lesions include connective tissue changes, ischemia, nerve compression, and postural disturbances that are due to things such as trauma, stress, and repetitive microtrauma, (stress from work and/or recreationally related activities).

The concept of reflex points (Chapman's points, Jones's tender points, Bennett's points), especially trigger points, is also emphasized and treated in NMT. Trigger points, as named by Janet Travell, are areas of tenderness within a muscle that radiate in a defined zone when pressure is applied. Reflex and trigger points (like the connective tissue zones described by Dicke) may or may not correspond to the distribution of a segmental nerve (i.e., common referred pain patterns) and appear to be associated with acupuncture points.

NMT is generally applied with a combination of effleurage or gliding, petrissage (for specific muscles) or grasping, friction (especially transverse friction), muscle energy, and strain and counterstrain techniques. Lubricants may be used, depending on the technique used, and the therapist may use the fingers, thumbs, forearms, elbows, or pressure bars to apply force. When deep muscles or muscle groups are treated, some discomfort may be felt, followed by pain relief.

Trager Method (Psychophysical Integration and Mentastics)

Milton Trager, MD, originally a boxer and gymnast, developed (almost by accident) his technique of psychophysical integration more than 50 years ago. To obtain the credentials he believed were necessary to bring his technique to the medical community, he obtained a medical degree from the University of Guadalajara in 1955. While there he was able to demonstrate his technique and treat polio patients with a relatively high degree of success. After developing the technique over many years afterward in his medical practice, he began to teach the method in 1975. The Trager Institute (Mill Valley, California) was founded shortly thereafter and is responsible for dissemination of information and certification programs.

Trager method is a two-tiered approach along the lines of Feldenkrais (see discussion later). The psychophysical integration phase is otherwise known as *table work* and consists of a single treatment or series of treatments. Mentastics is an exercise taught to the patient so that he or she may continue the work on his or her own.

Psychophysical integration is essentially an indirect/functional technique. The patient lies on a table, and the practitioner applies a gentle rocking motion to explore the body for areas of tissue tension and motion restriction. No force, stroking, or thrust is used in this technique, merely a light rhythmic contact. The purpose is to produce a specific sensory experience for the patient, one that is positive and pleasurable. Any discomfort breaks the continuum of "teaching" and "learning."

The focus of the treatment, though, is not on any specific anatomical structure or physiological process, rather it is on the psyche of the patient. An attempt is made to bring the patient into a position (or motion) of ease, where a sensation of lightness or freedom is experienced. This sensation is "learned" by the patient during the process of sensorimotor repatterning. In the words of Dr. Trager, the patient learns "how the tissue should feel when everything is right." This mind-body interaction is the core of the treatment, where the patient's psyche is brought to bear on the CNS to break the feedback loop of pain/guarding/muscle spasm and induce a change. The result is deep relaxation and increased range of motion (i.e., the sense of lightness).

Many patterns, such as those relating to behavior and posture, are learned during the course of a person's life, in part, as reactions to trauma or withdrawal from pain, either physical or emotional (see Structural Integration or "Rolfing"). Initially the body may be able to compensate for such reactions, but it will eventually decompensate, resulting in various somatic or visceral symptoms. The Trager method "allows" the patient to reexperience the norm through this exploratory process.

The practitioner seeks to integrate with the patient by entering a quasimeditative state of awareness referred to as the *hookup*. This allows the operator to acutely attend to the work at hand and feel very subtle changes in tissue texture and movement, not unlike the level of attention necessary to practice cranial osteopathy (see preceding discussion). Without any specific anatomical protocol, the work is intuitive and "letting go" is necessary on the part of both parties. The practitioner maintains a position of "neutrality" and makes no attempt to "make anything happen"

because it is actually the patient who is sensing and learning. The practitioner's role is one of a facilitator, in which he or she seeks to provide a safe and nurturing environment for the patient to explore new and pain-free patterns of motion (see Feldenkrais [Awareness Through Movement, Functional Integration]).

Mentastics, the continuing phase of the Trager method, is short for "mental gymnastics" and follows table work. A basic exercise set is taught, and the patient instructed to practice on his or her own. This consists of repetitive and sequential movements of all the joints, designed to relieve tension from the body. These movements are meant to be performed in an effortless, relaxed state of awareness, where the individual "hooks up" with himself or herself. The basic principles of Hatha-Yoga and tai chi are used in these exercises. Once the set is learned, the individual can then continue to explore independently, creating his or her own custom-designed series.

Trager work practitioners have reported success (not necessarily cures) in patients with multiple sclerosis, muscular dystrophy, and other debilitating diseases. Athletes have also reported significant improvements in performance as a result of Trager techniques.

Feldenkrais (Awareness Through Movement, Functional Integration)

Moshe Feldenkrais (1904-1985) was an Israeli physicist who developed a system of movement and manipulation over a period of several decades. The Feldenkrais method is divided into two "educational" processes. The first, *awareness through movement,* is a sensorimotor balancing technique that is taught to "students" as active participants in the process. The students are verbally guided through a series of very slow movements designed to create a heightened awareness of motion patterns and to reeducate the CNS as to new patterns, approaches, and possibilities (not at all unlike learning tai chi).

The second process is referred to as *functional integration.* This is a passive technique, using a didactic approach. The operator acts as a "teacher" and the patient as "student." The teacher brings the student through a series of manipulons (a manipulative sequence consisting of information, action [as initiated by the operator], and response) to reestablish proper neuromotor patterning and balance. Manipulons are gentle and are treated as exploratory, with the therapist introducing new motion patterns to the patient.

Manipulons are referred to as *positioning, confining, single,* or *repetitive.* They can also be oscillating. In all cases the teacher plays a supportive and guiding role while creating a nonthreatening environment for change. Functional integration could be considered a combination of passive, articulatory, or functional techniques.

Structural Integration or "Rolfing"

Structural integration was developed by Ida Rolf. A PhD in biochemistry, she was treated for pneumonia by an osteopath whom she sought out, being dissatisfied with conventional medical treatment. After this experience Dr. Rolf embarked on a lengthy period of study, including yoga, which resulted in the manipulative system that now bears her name. In 1971 she founded the Rolf Institute in Boulder, Colorado, which now trains and certifies practitioners of this style.

The theory of rolfing is based primarily on physical consideration of the interaction of the human body with the gravitational field of the earth. As a dynamic entity, the human body moves around and through this field in a state of equilibrium, storing potential energy and releasing that kinetic energy. In this system, form (potential energy) is in direct proportion to function (kinetic energy), and the balance between the two is equivalent to the amount of energy the body has available to it. In simple terms, the worse the posture, the more energy we consume on a baseline level, and thus the less we have available for normal activity. Furthermore, the physical energy of the body is in direct proportion to the "vital energy" of the person. Ideally the body is always in a position of "equipoise" (Box 8-1), but of course this is seldom, if ever, the case.

Rolfing involves a 10-session treatment protocol designed to integrate the entire myofascial system of the body. Photographs are taken of each patient before and after each session to evaluate progress.

The body is treated as a system of integrated segments consolidated by the myofascial system (see Segmentation or the Functional Spinal Movement).

BOX 8-1

Equipoise

Balance ⟷ Energy
Form ⟷ Function

Attempts are made through "processing," as the treatment is called, to lengthen and center through the connective tissue system by a series of direct myofascial release techniques. As distortions in the system are released, the patient may experience pain. The pain experienced is not merely structural, though. It is thought that emotions are expressed through the musculoskeletal system as behavior, which is reflected in various postures and movement patterns (i.e., the widely accepted psychological concepts of Pavlovian conditioning and body language). In other words, the musculoskeletal system is viewed as a link between the body and mind. Emotional or physical traumas are stored in the body as postures that mirror a withdrawal response from the offending or painful agent. Over time, compensatory reactions occur, but the body ultimately decompensates, resulting in somatic or visceral dysfunction (see Compensation and Decompensation). The direct technique seeks to put the energy of the operator into the system of the patient in an attempt to overcome the resistance to change affected in the withdrawal response. As releases are affected through the treatment, the emotional component may also be expressed (i.e., the somatoemotional release) (see Cranial Osteopathy).

The result of the treatment is a feeling of balance and "lightness" experienced by the patient. In addition, the patient should experience a heightened sense of well-being as the treatment releases the effects of emotional trauma. So the feeling of "lightness" is greater than simply an increase in the basal physical energy in the body but a raising of the body's vital energy as well.

Acupressure/Jin Shin Do

Acupressure is the application of the fingers to acupuncture points on the body, or "acupuncture without needles." It is based on the meridian or channel system, which permeates Asian medical arts and philosophy. According to this system there are 12 major channels through which the body's energy, or *qi,* flows. Although most of the channels are named for specific organs, they do not necessarily correspond to the anatomical body part but are more functional in nature. Interruptions in the flow of qi (prana, ki, vital energy) cause functional aberrations associated with that particular channel. These interruptions can be released by the application of needles or fingers.

Jin Shin Do, or the "way of compassionate spirit," was developed by psychotherapist I. Teeguarden. It is a form of acupressure in which the fingers are used to apply deep pressure to *hypersensitive acupuncture points*. Jin Shin Do represents a synthesis of Taoist philosophy, psychology, breathing, and acupressure techniques. In accordance with this philosophy the body is linked to the mind and spirit, and tender points found in the body can represent expressions of emotional trauma or locked memories (i.e., the somatoemotional component).

The theory of Jin Shin Do states that various stimuli cause energy to accumulate in acupuncture points. Repeated stress in turn causes a layering of tension at the point known as *armoring*. The most painful point is termed the *local point* as a frame of reference. Other related tender points are referred to as *distal points*. Deep pressure applied to the point ultimately causes a release, and the tension dissipates. The overall effect is to reestablish flow in the channel and balance body energy.

During the treatment session the operator identifies a local point and asks permission nonverbally to treat it. A finger is placed on the local point while another finger is applied to a distal point. Gradually increasing pressure is applied to the local point. After 1 or 2 minutes the operator feels the muscle relaxing, followed by a pulsation. When the pulsing stops, the patient usually reports a decreased sensitivity at the point, indicating a successful treatment.

Myofascial releases are sometimes accompanied by emotional releases as painful memories are brought to consciousness. The context of the Jin Shin Do treatment is as much psychological as physical and reiterates the importance of the body-mind-spirit philosophy of this treatment form.

Shiatsu (Zen Shiatsu)

Shiatsu means "finger pressure" in Japanese. It originally developed as a synthesis of acupuncture and Anma, traditional Japanese massage. During the eighteenth and nineteenth centuries Anma became more associated with carnal pleasure and subsequently lost its place as a therapeutic practice. Shiatsu further diverged and became systematized in the twentieth century, with the Nippon Shiatsu School opening in the 1940s.

As with other Asian-derived systems, shiatsu uses the meridian or channel concept of the human body. The points along the channels are referred to as *tsubos* (Japanese for "vase"). Shiatsu theory states that when a channel becomes blocked, the tsubos along it can express a "kyo" state (weak energy, low vibration, cold, open) or a "jitsu" state (strong energy, high vibration, heat, closed). The hands are used for three purposes: to diagnose, to treat, and for maintenance (to strengthen the newly attained balance).

During a shiatsu treatment the practitioner (or "giver") uses acupressure to open or close jitsu or kyo tsubos, respectively. The technique is applied with the thumb, elbow, or knee, perpendicular to the skin of the "receiver." The body part applied and the duration of application depend on the state of the tsubo. Acupressure is combined systematically with passive stretching and rotation of the joints to stimulate flow of ki through the channels. Treatments are described for the whole body (basic) and for each of the 12 major meridians.

Several issues are raised in observing the Asian styles of manual therapy. The intertwining of body-mind-spirit becomes evident as a holistic method of treatment born of an ancient philosophy. The practitioner-patient (giver-receiver) relationship is one of partnership because each is a participant in the healing process. This is born of the yin-yang principle (*giver* = yang, *receiver* = yin). The intention of the practitioner plays a major role in the effectiveness of the treatment: the giver is a nonjudgmental observer or plays an empathetic role. As opposed to the more neutral "do no harm" principle of Western caregivers, there appears to be more of a natural expression of love as a defined part of these systems (see Reiki). Intuition is also an important part of the treatment because each session is an exploration of the process of healing and of the individuals involved.

Reflexology

In the Asian meridian system of the body all of the major meridians or channels are represented in the hands and feet. Because acupuncture is usually not done on the feet because of their sensitivity, a system of foot massage was developed in China. This system was brought to the United States in 1913 by Fitzgerald, who called it *zone therapy*. Now referred to as *reflexology*, the technique involves deep pressure on various points on the hands and feet (the feet receive the preponderance of attention in this method) applied with the thumbs and fingers of the operator. The various identified points not only correspond to the energy channels of the body but also to specific organs and systems. When treatment is given, areas of tenderness or texture change are identified and pressure is applied. This has the effect of opening that channel and allowing body energy to flow unimpeded through its entirety. When all points are successfully treated, the energy system is flowing and balanced.

TUI NA

Tui na is the manipulative practice within traditional Chinese medicine (TCM). The literal translation is "pushing and grasping." As mentioned at the beginning of this chapter, it is more than 4000 years old and predates the manufacture of acupuncture needles. It was the forerunner of shiatsu in Japan (see the preceding discussion). Tui na may be practiced by TCM physicians as part of their general practice, or they may specialize in it like members of the osteopathic profession.

As with the other Chinese medical arts, tui na is based on the meridian or channel view of the human body, the yin-yang principle, and the five elements theory. The organs of the body exist not only as anatomical structures but also in a functional context (e.g., the triple burner), as well as in relation to one another. Yin and yang, as opposite forces, coexist in equilibrium with one another. Of the 12 major meridians of the body that correspond to the organs, 6 are yin, the others yang.

Qi, or vital energy, is a universal force that permeates everything. It is manifest as five separate elements: fire, wood, metal, water, and earth. The organs of the body are categorized accordingly. Qi flows through all the meridians once each day in 2-hour cycles. Thus each meridian, and hence its associated organ, has its daily strong and weak periods. When the flow of qi is impeded in any channel, that organ/function may become dysfunctional, resulting in disease.

Tui na can be applied to virtually anyone and has few contraindications. Those that do exist are similar to those found for massage, including skin lesions or infection, skin or lymphatic cancer, and osteoporosis. In addition, it is recommended that the low back and abdomen be avoided during pregnancy.

Anatomically tui na is applied to the musculoskeletal system and viscera, with attention being paid to the meridians and flow of qi (as specific meridians flow through specific joints, muscle groups, and visceral structures). Like other forms of manipulative treatment, tui na seeks to produce a feeling of well-being and health in the patient. In addition, as the emotional and spiritual components of the patient are addressed, emotional release can also be produced.

The techniques of tui na combine soft tissue, visceral, and joint manipulation. The patient typically is lying on a table or is seated. Soft tissue techniques, which are applied to the limbs, trunk, and head, precede joint mobilization to prepare the joint for movement and to relax the surrounding musculature. They are designed to stimulate local blood flow, venous and lymphatic drainage, and the flow of qi (see Shiatsu [Zen Shiatsu]). These soft tissue techniques include the following:

- Pressing: using the thumbs, elbows, or palms
- Squeezing: using the whole hand or finger-thumb combination
- Kneading: a circular pressing technique, using the thumbs, heel of the hand, elbow, or forearm
- Rubbing: a high-frequency technique, using the palms, heels of the hands (chafing), or forearms
- Stroking (see Effleurage): moving the hand over the skin in a long stroke, in one direction only
- Vibration: similar to that used in massage
- Thumb rocking: for deep penetration of acupuncture points
- Plucking: a transverse friction-type technique (see James Cyriax) applying deep pressure with the palm of the hand to the thumb of the opposite hand and moving across individual muscles or muscle groups
- Rolling: using the back of the hand to roll over the skin and underlying tissue
- Percussion (see Tapotement): includes pummeling with the fists, hacking with the heels of the hands, and cupping the hands

Included in the joint manipulative techniques are the following:

- Shaking is a technique in which traction is applied to the limb and it is shaken with low-amplitude movements (HVLA) 10 to 20 times.
- Flexion/extension is applied primarily to the elbow and knee joints (i.e., the hinge joints). These

are both high- and low-velocity techniques designed to engage a motion barrier but not to challenge it. In addition, in some of these techniques a thumb is simultaneously applied to an acupuncture point to open a meridian.

- Rotation is an articulatory technique used for the ankles, wrists, hips, and shoulders. This technique is not applied to the neck by practitioners of tui na.
- Pushing and pulling is a low-velocity technique designed to directly engage a motion barrier. A counterforce is applied by the opposing hand in the opposite direction.
- Stretching is a general, low-velocity flexion-extension technique used to loosen the joints of the spine.
- Thrust is used in a similar manner as with osteopathic and chiropractic methods on the spinal joints.

AYURVEDIC MANIPULATION

Ayurveda, in Sanskrit, means "the study of life." As a healing art, it is one of the world's oldest and like the Indian culture probably predates TCM. Like TCM, Ayurveda has many concepts and components and is far too complex to be described here with anything other than the very basics (see Chapters 19 and 20). However, several principles pervade Ayurveda (as also do TCM) and apply to the manual component of Ayurvedic treatment.

Both Ayurvedic theory and Chinese theory present five basic elements. However, in contrast to those of Chinese theory (fire, water, earth, wood, metal), Ayurveda defines space (ether), air, fire, water, and earth as the five basic elements. These elements flow through the body with one or more predominating in certain areas, corresponding to such things as specific organs and emotions. *Prana*, or the life force (qi, ki), also flows through the body, permeating the organs and tissues, and is especially concentrated at various points along the midline of the body known as *chakras*.

The unity and balance of body, mind, and spirit has deep cultural roots in Ayurveda. Body structure and a person's actions, feelings, and beliefs are all reflections of his or her constitution. The constitution of the human being is based on the relative proportions and strengths of these three constituents and the five elements. Three basic types of constitutions

(doshas) are recognized, which are based on different combinations of the five elements. The first, *vata*, is a combination of air and space and is reflected in kinetic energy. The second, *pitta*, combines fire and water and reflects a balance between kinetic and potential (stored) energy, which is expressed in the third constitution, *kapha*, a combination of earth and water.

The manipulative treatment developed within the Ayurvedic tradition offers three types of touch. *Tamasic* is strong and solid, firmly rooted in the earth (and might be well suited for a kapha constitution). The application is fast, and time is needed for the mind and spirit to "catch up." In other terminology presented earlier in this chapter, tamasic might correspond to HVLA (osteopathy, chiropractic), tapotement (massage), or rubbing and thumb rocking (TCM). The second type of touch, *rajasic*, is slower and is used to expand and integrate initial manual explorations and findings. It is more in resonance with the mind and spirit. As mentioned earlier, greater depth can be achieved with less tissue resistance because of the makeup of the body fascia. Effleurage (massage) and myofascial release might correspond with this type of touch, which in turn might be more suited to a pitta constitution. The vata constitution might benefit from the third type of touch, *satvic*, in which the application is very slow and gentle and can follow the intention of the mind and spirit. This might correspond to cranial (osteopathy), SOT (chiropractic), counterstrain (osteopathy), Trager work, Feldenkrais, or healing/therapeutic touch.

In a massage-oriented treatment different oils are used as lubricants according to the constitution of the individual and the problem to be treated. The patient is prone or supine, lying on either side, or sitting up, the positions arranged in a specific sequence. Strokes are applied either toward or away from the heart, also in a specific sequence. Another technique, which is rarely encountered, uses the feet to perform the manipulation. The operator stands above the patient, who is lying prone on a reed mat, and applies the technique with his or her feet. Oils again are used as lubricants, and to maintain balance the operator holds onto a cord strung lengthwise above the patient. The strokes go from the sacrum up the spine and out to the fingers, then back down to the feet. One side is done, then the other. The patient then lies supine and the process is repeated.

Techniques can be direct or indirect relative to motion barriers. They can also be active or passive. Both the patient and practitioner act as partners during treatment, exploring tissue and motion in an attempt to unlock the body and restore the unimpeded flow of prana and constitutional balance. Visualization, non-verbal communication, and mind intent are elements of treatment, regardless of the technique used.

ENERGY WORK

Energy work refers to the techniques that have developed as either part of ancient traditions (Qigong) or as recently "discovered" methods in which the operator manipulates the bioenergy of the patient. The theory of bioenergy basically states that a life force, or vital energy, permeates the entire universe. This energy flows through all living things in distinct patterns. These patterns of flow are reflected in the meridian system (where *qi,* or *chi,* is the name of the life force) originally conceived by the Chinese, and the chakra system of Hindu tradition (where the word *prana* is used to indicate this force). Various exercise forms have been developed for the cultivation of bioenergy (yoga, internal Qigong, tai chi).

Three basic concepts are important in understanding energy work: intention, cooperation, and the tripartite nature of the human being. Intent is important in that the practitioner projects his or her mind-intent to heal into the patient. As such, that intent must go one step further than the "do no harm" doctrine of Western therapeutics to an attitude of love and concern. Intent also assumes a high level of visualization. Cooperation implies the partnership between the practitioner and patient as participants in the healing process, neither being exclusively active or passive. The tripartite concept refers to the acceptance of three parts of the human being: body, mind, and spirit. This concept is imbued in the far older Asian cultures as to go beyond religion, whereas Western cultures rely on belief systems driven by faith. In addition, the "scientific," reductionist approach to conventional Western medicine is rather dismissive of spiritual aspects and has only recently acknowledged the mind-body connection.

Qigong (China)

The term *qigong* refers to the manipulation on bioenergy and loosely translated means "chi work." Qigong can be internal, in which an individual can strengthen and balance the flow of qi within himself or herself, or external, in which a trained practitioner can project his or her chi into a patient to induce a therapeutic effect.

Although most of the vital energy of an organism is contained within the body, some of it radiates off the skin, the "aura," which can be visualized with Kirlian photography. The qigong practitioner is able to palpate the meridian system through this aura, locate points of blockage, and free these blockages by projecting his or her qi into the patient, using intent and visualization. Like Trager work, Feldenkrais, and yoga, specific "external qigong" exercises have been developed, which, when performed by an individual, serve to cultivate qi within himself or herself. Qigong is also a natural result of long-term "internal" martial arts training, in which practitioners are capable of seemingly superhuman feats of strength and balance.

Reiki

Reiki (literally "universal energy") was "rediscovered" by Dr. Mikao Usui in the mid nineteenth century. Usui was interested in exploring the nature of spiritually oriented healing power, as expressed through healers such as Jesus Christ, the Gautama Buddha, and others. After much study, including a doctorate from the University of Chicago, he began an extended period of fasting and meditation. At the end of this period he reportedly received a vision and the ability to channel "reiki" through his body to affect healing in others. From that point he continued healing, eventually training others in his method. Usui handed the title of Grand Master to Dr. Hiyashi Chugiro, who in turn passed it to Hawayo Takata, a Hawaiian woman of Japanese descent. In this way, reiki was exported from Japan to the West.

For practitioners, reiki must be received from a master or teacher. Only then is an individual able to effect healing. There are three degrees of reiki training. The first-degree practitioner is capable of giving a basic treatment with the hands on the patient, or about 1 inch away from the skin if touching is not possible. The second-degree practitioner can effect healing with the hands removed from the body (see qigong), and treatments can be given at a faster rate. The third-degree practitioner is referred to as a master, and is qualified to teach reiki.

The five principles of reiki are as follows:
1. Today I give thanks for my many blessings.
2. Just for today, I will not worry.
3. Today I will not be angry.
4. Today I will do my work honestly.
5. Today I will be kind to my neighbor and to every living thing.

The objective of reiki treatment is to restore internal harmony to the body and to release any blockages that may reside therein. These may be physical or emotional in nature.

During a reiki treatment the practitioner's hands are placed with the fingers together on the patient. As energy is transferred from giver to receiver, the hands and the area treated become warm, indicating a release of tension in the area and an increase in the blood flow. The head of the patient is treated first (four locations or positions), followed by the front (five positions) and back of the body (five positions). Each position is held for 8 to 10 minutes (or less, if the practitioner is above first degree). Problem areas may be "held" longer until a result is sensed. The hand positions correspond to the energy points or chakras, identified in Hindu tradition, as well as other points. The treatment is completed with a series of general myofascial techniques, including kneading, counterforce, and stroking (effleurage) to close the energy channels.

As with other energy-oriented manipulative techniques, reiki requires significant verbal and nonverbal communication between the giver and receiver, who act in partnership. Permission must be granted both consciously and subconsciously for healing to be successful. Somatoemotional release is quite possible in this treatment.

It is likely that from a historical and practical standpoint, the reiki method was originally derived from qigong as practiced by the Chinese Taoists and Buddhists. It probably disappeared from practice in Japan at some point, only to be rediscovered by Usui hundreds of years later.

Therapeutic or Healing Touch

Therapeutic touch was developed by Dr. Dolores Krieger and by Dora Kunz in the late 1960s and early 1970s. In this style of energy work, energy is directed through the hands (either on or off the body, usually off) of the giver to activate the healing process of the receiver. The therapist essentially acts as a support system to facilitate the process. Therapeutic touch treatments typically last 20 to 25 minutes and are accompanied by a relaxation response and a decrease in perceived pain. Although skeptics have claimed that this technique merely elicits a placebo effect (an interesting concept in itself), successes have been reported with comatose patients, patients under anesthesia, and premature infants. A major research project is currently under way in New York analyzing the effects of therapeutic touch on coronary bypass patients (see Chapter 15).

Therapeutic touch posits that humans are open energy systems, that humans are bilaterally symmetrical (see previous discussion), and that illness is the result of an imbalance in the patient's energy field. The healer places himself or herself between the patient's illness and his or her energy field to effect the healing process. The receiver, or healee, must accept the energy of the healer and the necessity of change for the healing to occur. This should happen both consciously and subconsciously.

There are two phases of the treatment: assessment and balancing. Before balancing, the practitioner "centers" himself or herself, entering a state of relaxation and awareness. The hands are moved around the patient's body at a distance of 2 to 3 inches. The patient's energy field is encountered and assessed by feeling for changes in temperature, pressure, rhythm, or a tingling sensation. Simultaneously the practitioner nonverbally requests the permission of the patient to enter his or her field and effect a change. During the balancing phase the healer (sometimes referred to as the *sender*) then attempts to bring the two energy fields into a harmonic resonance by means of intent and visualization.

The attitude of the sender is one of empathy and compassion. The intent of the treatment is to facilitate the flow of vital energy, to stimulate it, to dissipate areas of congestion, and to dampen any areas of increased activity. In addition, the concept of rhythm and vibration is used, with color observed as a product of different frequencies within the field. Either at the beginning of the treatment, the end of the treatment, or both, the practitioner "smoothes" out the patient's energy field by running the hands from head to toe. This sometimes has a cooling effect and is referred to as *unruffling*.

Healing touch, as developed by Barbara Brennan, is somewhat similar to therapeutic touch in that the healer seeks to balance the energy field of the patient. A specific sequence of techniques is used in which the healer encounters, assesses, and treats different layers of the patient's visible "aura," again correcting any imbalances and smoothing out the field. This technique is more spiritually oriented than therapeutic touch, using techniques such as channeling, and uses colors and crystals to assist in the process.

The successful application of these "energy-based" techniques (in addition to many of the other styles mentioned) underscores the importance of psychoemotional cooperation or participation on the part of the patient (i.e., the mind-body connection). In addition, the mind-intent of the manipulator comes into play as the director of his or her internal energy outward and into the patient. This concept, as might be imagined, is quite controversial by Western standards of scientific analysis.

Although critics refer to these (and other manipulative) techniques as pseudoscience because of a lack of empirically supportive evidence, clinical outcomes studies have indicated that the intent of both the patient and clinician has a demonstrable effect in determining treatment outcome. This evidence sheds new and interesting light on the placebo effect as a real phenomenon. It also indicates that treatment of the somatic component of disease can be approached effectively through acknowledgment of the "three-legged stool" model of the human being, (i.e., body, mind, and spirit).

CONCLUSION

It is important to note the preventive aspect of manipulation as a holistic practice. Manipulative treatment can be used for proactive general maintenance, as well as for reactive treatment of dysfunction. I like to use the automobile analogy in describing how we as Americans think nothing of periodically getting our cars tuned up and paying considerable sums for the privilege. Why do we fail to do the same for our own bodies? In addition, the concept of manual treatment for the young cannot be overstated. Structural corrections can be made before fascial distortions become relatively locked in; or before continuous aberrant sensory input results in facilitated sensorimotor patterning; or before compensatory reactions in muscles, fascia, and behavior can create unbalanced anatomy and physiology that function poorly and

eventually lead to a decreased resistance to disease. As Alexander Pope once proclaimed, "Just as the twig is bent, the tree's inclined."

Suggested Readings

Osteopathic Medicine

The D.O.'s: Osteopathic Medicine in America
Norman Gevitz/Johns Hopkins University Press/October 1991
Appropriate for general reading

Foundations for Osteopathic Medicine
Robert C. Ward, John A. Jerome, John M. Jones, Robert E. Kappler (Editors)/Williams & Wilkins/October 1996
Appropriate for professional reading

Dr. Fulford's Touch of Life: The Healing Power of the Natural Life Force
Robert C. Fulford, Gene Stone/Simon & Schuster Trade/July 1997
Appropriate for general reading

An Osteopathic Approach to Diagnosis and Management, 2nd Edition
Stanley Schiowitz, Eileen L. Digiovanna (Editors)/Lippincott-Raven/December 1996
Appropriate for professional reading

Chiropractic

Chiropractic First: The Fastest Growing Healthcare Choice . . . Before Drugs or Surgery
Terry A. Rondberg, World Chiropractic Alliance/February 1996
Appropriate for general reading

Contemporary Chiropractic
Daniel Redwood (Editor)/August 1997, Churchill Livingstone; ISBN: 0443078092
Appropriate for general and professional reading

The Chiropractor's Health Book: Simple, Natural Exercises for Relieving Headaches, Tension, and Back Pain
Leonard McGill/Crown Publishing Group/January 1997
Appropriate for general and professional reading

Therapeutic Exercise for Spinal Segmental Stabilization in Low Back Pain: Scientific Basis and Clinical Approach
Carolyn Richardson, Paul Hodges, Gwendolen Jull, Julie Hides, Foreword by Monohar M. Panjabi/Harcourt Brace/February 1999
Appropriate for chiropractic students, medical and chiropractic professionals

Chiropractic Technique: Principles and Procedures
Thomas F. Bergmann, Dana J. Lawrence, David H. Peterson, Nicholas Lang (Illustrator), Foreword by Herbert J. Vear/Churchill Livingstone, Inc./August 1993
Appropriate for chiropractic students, medical and chiropractic professionals

Foundations of Chiropractic: Subluxation
Meridel I. Gatterman/Mosby/April 1995
Appropriate for chiropractic students, medical and chiropractic professionals

Dare to Break Through the Pain! A Guide to Eliminating Back and Neck Pain Naturally Without Drugs or Surgery!
Rick, Dr. Barrett (January 1998), Brockton; ISBN: 1887918205
Appropriate for general reading

The 12 Stages of Healing: A Network Approach to Wholeness
Donald M. Epstein, With Nathaniel Altman/Amber-Allen Publishing/September 1994
Appropriate for general reading

Massage
Tappan's Handbook of Healing Massage Techniques: Classic, Holistic, and Emerging Methods
Frances M. Tappan, Patricia J. Benjamin/Appleton and Lange/October 1997
Appropriate for general and professional reading

Massage for Common Ailments
Sara Thomas/Barnes & Noble Books/December 1998
Appropriate for general reading

Mosby's Fundamentals of Therapeutic Massage
Sandy Fritz/Harcourt Brace/January 1999
Appropriate for therapeutic massage student, therapeutic massage practitioners

The Healing Art of Sports Massage
Joan Johnson (May 1995), Rodale Pr; ISBN: 087596186X
Appropriate for general reading

Shiatsu
The Book of Shiatsu
Paul Lundberg, Fausto Dorelli (Photographer)/Simon & Schuster/January 1992
Appropriate for general reading

The Complete Book of Shiatsu Therapy: Health and Vitality at Your Fingertips
Toru Namikoshi/Japan Publications (USA), Incorporated/November 1979
Appropriate for general reading

The Complete Illustrated Guide to Shiatsu: The Japanese Healing Art of Touch for Health and Fitness
Elaine Liechti/Element Books/January 1998
Appropriate for general and professional reading

Trager
Movement as a Way to Agelessness: A Guide to Trager Mentastics
Milton Trager, with Cathy Hammond/Station Hill Press/March 1994
Appropriate for general reading

Moving Medicine: The Life Work of Milton Trager, MD
Jack Liskin/Station Hill Press/October 1995
Appropriate for general reading

Feldenkrais
Awareness Through Movement: Easy-to-Do Health Exercises to Improve Your Posture, Vision, Imagination, and Personal Growth
Moshe Feldenkrais/Harper San Francisco/April 1991
Appropriate for general and professional reading

The Feldenkrais Method
Yochanan Rywerant, Daniela Mohor (Illustrator), foreword by Moshe Feldenkrais, preface by Thomas Hanna/Keats Publishing/July 1991
Appropriate for general and professional reading

Neuromuscular Therapy (NMT)
Modern Neuromuscular Techniques
Leon Chaitow/WB Saunders/August 1996
Appropriate for general and professional reading

Soft-Tissue Manipulation: A Practitioner's Guide to the Diagnosis & Treatment of Soft Tissue Dysfunction & Reflex Activity
Leon Chaitow/Inner Traditions International, Limited/April 1991
Appropriate for professional reading

Fibromyalgia and Muscle Pain: What Causes It, How It Feels and What to Do about It
Leon Chaitow/HarperCollins Pub/January 1999
Appropriate for general reading

Structural Integration or "Rolfing"
Rolfing: Reestablishing the Natural Alignment & Structural Integration of the Human Body for Vitality and Well-Being
Ida P. Rolf, Ron Thompson/Inner Traditions International, Limited/September 1989
Appropriate for general and professional reading

Rolfing: The Integration of Human Structures
Ida P. Rolf/Dennis-Landman Publishers/June 1977
Appropriate for general reading

What in the World Is Rolfing?
Ida P. Rolf/Dennis-Landman Publishers/November 1975
Appropriate for general reading

Acupressure/Jin Shin Do
Acupressure Way of Health, Jin Shin Do: Jin Shin Do
Iona Teeguard/Japan Publications (USA), Incorporated/
    March 1978
Appropriate for general and professional reading

Reflexology
The Complete Illustrated Guide to Reflexology:
    Therapeutic Foot Massage for Health and Well-Being
Inge Dougan, Anne Townley (Editor), Paul Allen
    (Illustrator), Guy Ryecart (Photographer), Designed by
    Andrew Milne/Barnes & Noble Books/June 1999
Appropriate for general reading

The Reflexology Manual: An Easy-to-Use Illustrated Guide
    to Healing Zones of the Hands & Feet
Pauline Wills, Sue Atkinson (Photographer)/Inner
    Traditions International, Limited/October 1995
Appropriate for general and professional reading

Tui Na
Chinese Massage Manual: The Healing Art of Tui Na
Sarah M. Pritchard, Foreword by Wang Jianmin/Sterling
    Publishing/November 1999
Appropriate for general and professional reading

Ayurvedic Manipulation
Ayurvedic Massage: Traditional Indian Techniques for
    Balancing Body and Mind
Harish Johari/Inner Traditions International, Limited/
    August 1995
Appropriate for general and professional reading

Massage Therapy in AyurVeda
Vaidya B. Dash, Bhagwan Dash/Concept Publishing/
    December 1992
Appropriate for general and professional reading

Massage for Health and Healing: AyurVedic and Spiritual
    Energy Approach
S. V. Govindan/South Asia Books/January 1996
Appropriate for general reading

Qigong
Qi Gong for Health and Longevity: The Ancient
    Chinese Art of Relaxation, Meditation, Physical
    Fitness
Simon Wang, Julius L. Liu/East Health Development
    Group/March 1999
Appropriate for general and professional reading

Qigong for Health and Well-Being
Fa Xiang Hou, H. Wallin, Faxiang Hou/Charles E. Tuttle/
    May 1999
Appropriate for general and professional reading

Mastering Miracles: The Healing Art of Qi Gong as
    Taught by a Master
Hong Liu, with Paul Perry/Brilliance Corporation/
    December 1996
Appropriate for general reading

Reiki
The Complete Reiki Handbook: Basic Introduction and
    Methods of Natural Application, A Complete Guide
    for Reiki Practice
Walter Lubeck/Lotus Light Publications/April 1998
Appropriate for professional reading

Essential Reiki: A Complete Guide to an Ancient
    Healing Art
Diane Stein/The Crossing Press/April 1995
Appropriate for general and professional reading

Reiki: The Healing Touch
William Lee Rand, Susan A. Martin (Editor), Sheryl M.
    Matsko (Illustrator)/Vision Publications/April 1996
Appropriate for general reading

Therapeutic or Healing Touch
The Therapeutic Touch: How to Use Your Hands to Help
    or to Heal
Dolores K. Krieger/Simon & Schuster/January 1992
Appropriate for general and professional reading

Hands of Light: A Guide to Healing through the Human
    Energy Field
Barbara Ann Brennan, Joseph A. Smith (Illustrator)/
    Bantam Doubleday Dell Publishing Group/May 1988
Appropriate for general and professional reading

Job's Body: A Handbook for Bodywork
Deane Juhan, foreword by Ken Dychtwald/Barrytown,
    Ltd./September 1998
Appropriate for general and professional reading

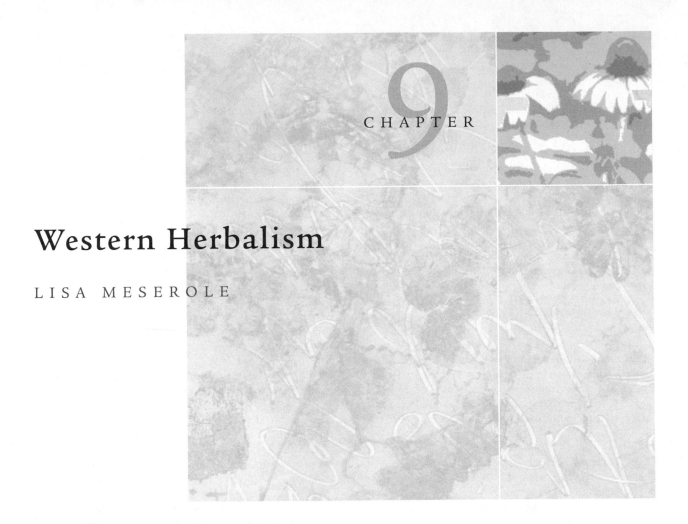

CHAPTER 9

Western Herbalism

LISA MESEROLE

Plants have been used by humans for food, medicine, clothing, and tools, as well as in religious rites, since before recorded history, more than 60,000 years ago (Solecki & Shanidar, 1975). No continent, island, climate, or geography that is home to human culture lacks a formal tradition of incorporating local flora into daily and ceremonial life as a means of enhancing health and welfare. Prehistoric plant life prepared the earth to be a viable and hospitable habitat for *Homo sapiens*, and plant ecology continues to help maintain the oceans, continents, and atmosphere today.

It is the power of the truth that endures.

—IMHOTEP (EGYPTIAN PHYSICIAN, LATER EXALTED AS THE GOD OF MEDICINE, PAPYRUS, 2400 BC)

Through contention all things are made manifest.

—HERAKLEITOS THE DARK

DEFINITION

Herbalism is the study and practice of using plant material for food, medicine, and health promotion. This includes not only treatment of disease but also enhancement of quality of life, physically and spiritually. Although a fundamental principle of herbalism is to promote preventive self-care and guided, simple self-treatment among the general population, an herbalist, or herbal practitioner, is someone who has undertaken specific study and supervised practical training to achieve competence in treating patients.

An herb can be an angiosperm, that is, a flowering plant, shrub, or tree, or a moss, lichen, fern, algae, seaweed, or fungus. The herbalist may use the entire plant or just the flowers, fruits, leaves, twigs, bark, roots, rhizomes, seeds, or exudates (e.g., tapped and purified maple syrup), or a combination of parts. Botany defines an herb as a nonwoody, low-growing plant, but herbalists use the entire plant kingdom. In many herbal traditions nonplants are used as healing agents, including animal parts (organs, bone, tissue), insects, animal and insect secretions, worm castings, shells, rocks, metals, minerals, and gemstones. These examples are recorded in ancient and contemporary materia medicae and formal manuscripts of healing agents and their indication and uses. Egyptian, Chinese, Tibetan, European, American, and other worldwide material medicae are important references for herbal practitioners. This discussion addresses only plant herbal agents.

Herbalism is a misleading term because it implies that a single hidden root gives rise to the diverse ways in which all human cultures across the millennia have used plants for food, medicine, and ritual. The use of herbs by the peoples of the Americas, Europe, Africa, the Middle and Far East, the Pacific Islands, and other regions is specific to each society and paradigm. For example, contemporary Western scientists have been restricted until recently by the Western mechanistic premises of biology and physics (see Chapter 1).

Although there is no single, worldwide system of herbalism, all herbal traditions share certain themes.

"Herb" and Other Words

*H*erb* as a word has an ancient pedigree, originating with the Latin word *herba* that refers to green crops and grasses and that could also mean the same as we mean by *herb* today *(OED)*. The word entered English through Old French. The

English use of *herb* in the sense of a plant whose stem does not become woody and persistent, but which remains more or less soft and succulent, dying down to the ground (or entirely) after flowering, can be traced to the 13th century. The 13th century also understood *herb* (with variant spellings, such as *erbe*) as a plant whose leaves and stems (and sometimes roots) could be used as food or medicine or for scent or flavor.

"Herbarium" in the sense of a collection of dried plants, has its origins in the 18th century. A source that associates "herbarium" with the medicinal properties of plants is that the idea for drying plants for study originated with a professor in the 16th century Italy who also held a chair in "simples," where he studied medicinal and other plants. (*Penn. Heritage*, Summer 1998).

"Herbalist" has shifted meaning. Originally (in the 16th century) an herbalist was one versed in the knowledge of herbs and plants—a collector of and writer about plants, more what we mean by "botanist" today. Usually, however, "herbalist" is now used to refer to early writers about plants—and a person who uses alternative medical therapy, though the *OED* does not mention this.

"Herbal," meaning a book containing names and descriptions of herbs (or other plants in general) which provides properties and virtues, came into use in the early 16th century. "Herbal," meaning belonging to, consisting of, or made from herbs, has its origins in the early 17th century.

Early botanic gardens started in Renaissance Italy. These should properly be called "physic gardens" because they were used to help educated medical students, that is, to teach people—in this case medical students—about medicinal plants. Physic gardens appeared in England in the 16th century, in private hands. The Oxford Physic Garden began in 1621. (Chelsea Physic Garden was begun in 1673 by the Society of Apothecaries.) The Oxford Physic Garden became the Botanic Garden in 1840—an important and representative change. Early on there was no difference to speak of between a "physic garden" and a "botanic garden" because botany and the study of the medicinal properties of plants were not distinct fields. William Turner (1510-1568) was a physician, author of an

Continued

Continued

herbal, and is considered the father of English botany. Taxonomy was not separate from pharmacology in the study of plants for Turner.

Although the process was gradual, by the 19th century the study of plants for their own sake—botany—was a clearly separate field. Pharmacopoeias and botanical atlases grew in importance as the need for herbals waned.

What does this say about the name of our garden? Up front I have to say that we can, with defensible logic, call it a number of names, but there are clear ways to classify types of gardens.

In the 1790s, Dr. Benjamin Rush called for the establishment of a "botanic garden" at the College of Physicians of Philadelphia. In Rush's time this would have meant a garden to study the properties of plants, in this case, of course, medicinal properties. Rush suggests, though, that the garden could also be a *source* of medical preparations, as well as a place to grow plants that might be lost as Europeans settled North America. Although it was not the only purpose of Rush's garden, study was a component, and research lies at the heart of any botanical garden's purpose. (Botanical gardens don't limit themselves strictly to taxonomy.)

"Medical botany" would be the study of the medicinal properties of plants—chemical analysis to find new medically important compounds, for instance. A "medical botanical garden" would be the source of plants for studying their medical properties.

A "medicinal herb garden" would, in a technical sense, be a place that has examples of plants, from which samples could be taken to make medicinal preparations. Also, the garden would contain only herbaceous plants, not plants with woody stems and branches. ❧

Sources:
Oxford English Dictionary
Oxford Companion to Medicine
The College of Physicians of Philadelphia: A Bicentennial History
Pennsylvania Heritage (Summer 1998)
Medicines from the Earth: A Guide to Healing Plants
—Charles Greifenstein

Common Themes of Herbalism

- *Optimization of health and wellness:* Most traditions include specific systems of food, spice, and herb taboos and recommended inclusions; adherence to these protects practitioners and users from undesirable consequences. A pregnant woman in Mexico avoids eggs because they could push her into a state of excess cold that could weaken her (see Chapter 15). During winter flu season, extra ginger and hot peppers are added to curries in Indian cuisine to protect against infection. Similarly, shitake mushrooms (powerful immunomodulators) are used in winter soups in traditional Japanese cooking.

- *Emphasis on the whole person:* This includes body, mind, and soul; past, present, and future; and community.

- *Emphasis on the individual:* In Chinese herbal medicine, 10 patients with high blood pressure might receive 10 different herbal formulas. Furthermore, the same patient might take different hypertension formulas at age 45 and at age 65, and each formula might be adjusted repeatedly according to pulse, tongue, and other readings.

- *Emphasis on the community:* The illness or recovery of a member might influence the community itself, beyond emotional group empathy.

- *Attention to finding and treating the root cause of a problem, not just the manifestations and symptoms:* However, like most healers and medicine suppliers, if the cause remains unidentified or untreatable, symptomatic treatment is offered.

- *Application of the principle of duality between both the healing and the life-threatening forces of nature:* The fundamental assumption of this principle is that natural law is greater than the will of the individual or community and that healing demands that the healer, the patient, and the community align with natural forces.

- *Belief in the reality of the unmeasurable and abstract:* Although dual, the abstract and physical worlds are inseparable. An herbalist who also is a true healer devotes himself or herself to maintaining balance and communication between the visible and invisible. This might be accomplished through communing with ancestors, spiritual forces, nature, or plants and adjusting activities to natural cycles (e.g., in Tibetan medicine, blending a formula during a specific season, moon phase, or auspicious date).

- *Premise of recycling:* Nature is inherently circular and repetitive; generally sequential, but not predominantly linear; and predictable, but seldom certain. This leads to the common traditional practice of offering an object or prayer in return for healing plants and for addressing requests for healing to both the physical and spiritual worlds.
- *Openness to exchange of knowledge:* Most traditions incorporate new medicinal plants and new herbal uses and preparations that have been learned about through trade or travel.
- *Regulation of the herbalist's practice through local accountability to his or her community:* Success and prestige arise primarily from professional reputation that grows by word of mouth, not from image, business acumen, or material wealth.
- *Humility generated from the healer's recognition of his or her own limits and skills:* Because reputation generally depends on treatment efficacy and community standing, an herbalist would be reluctant to take on a case without reasonable confidence that he or she would succeed. Complex or incurable cases would be referred to another, or the patient would be advised that no treatment was available other than minimization of suffering.

CLASSIFICATIONS OF HERBALISTS

Each cultural or medical system has different types of herbal practitioners, all consistent with its paradigm. However, most paradigms identify professional herbalists, lay herbalists, plant gatherers, and medicine makers. (Professional or lay herbalists often collect their own plants and prepare their own medicines.)

Professional Herbalist

A professional herbalist undertakes formalized training or a long apprenticeship in plant and medical studies or alternatively in plant and spiritual or healing studies. This knowledge includes extensive familiarity—often a relationship—with specific plants, which involves their identification, habitat, harvesting criteria, preparation, storage, therapeutic indica-

tions, contraindications, and dosing. A professional herbalist is not necessarily the primary healer (Iwu, 1993). A professional herbalist might follow a family tradition or might be selected at a young age as being endowed with potential mastery of using plants as healing aids. In Europe and the United States, this group includes officially trained medical herbalists, clinical herbalists, licensed naturopathic doctors specializing in botanical medicine, licensed acupuncturists with training in Chinese herbal medicine, licensed Ayurvedic doctors, Native American herbalists and shamans, Latin American curanderos, and other lineage or culturally recognized professional herbalists. The shaman from Madagascar who—although never acknowledged or compensated for his contribution—revealed the usefulness of *Caranthas roseus,* the greater periwinkle developed in the west as vinblastine and vincristine against certain cancers, exemplifies the spirit and expertise of a professional healer and herbalist.

Many herbalists consider the patient's direct involvement in his or her own healing and the summoning of the patient's intellectual, emotional, physical, and spiritual attention to the process as critical. Partly for this reason and because of traditional herbalism's emphasis on "right relationship," social context, and self-responsibility, many herbal practitioners deliberately prescribe elaborate rather than convenient herbal therapies. For example, upon returning home to Ghana, a merchant developed an infected leg ulcer. Instead of being supplied an herbal medicine by the herbalist, he was directed to the nearby live plant source (a local tree bark). He collected and prepared the antimicrobial and vulnery poultice and applied it daily until his wound healed. Although self-collection and medicine preparation is impractical in the United States, self-involvement in the healing process is possible in many ways and parallels the complex lifestyle changes now routinely recommended to patients with chronic ailments such as cardiovascular disease.

Lay Herbalist

A lay herbalist has a broad knowledge of plants useful for health problems but does not have extensive training in medical and spiritual diagnosis and management. He or she may be an herb vendor with a sensitivity to the needs and desires of the market-place, whose livelihood has been passed down as a family business. Evaluation of medicinal plant quality, strength, uses, and dose is included in the lay herbalist's domain. The Irish herbalist who uses specific herbal treatments for certain skin or stomach symptoms is an example.

Plant Gatherer, Plant Grower, and Medicine Maker

Plant gatherers, plant growers, and medicine makers might consider themselves herbalists; actually, they are to the practicing herbalist what the contemporary pharmacist is to the clinical physician. In Chinese medicine there is one specialist who produces and collects plants, one who processes and stores plants, and a clinical herbalist/doctor who prescribes the medicines. In some systems preparing and handling medicines is considered a spiritual privilege and responsibility. Therefore certain herbal medicines are prepared only by the herbalist or healer or a designated assistant.

HERBS AND MEDICINAL PLANTS

Physicians in the United States studied and relied on plant drugs as primary medicines through the 1930s. Until then medical schools taught basic plant taxonomy and pharmacognosy and medicinal plant therapeutics. The term *drug* derives from an ancient word for *root,* and the roots and rhizomes of many medicinal plants continue to provide alkaloids, steroidal saponins, and many active constituents that are clinically useful today. The *United States Pharmacopeia* listed 636 herbal entries in 1870; only 58 were listed in the 1990 edition (Boyle, 1991). Although some plants were dropped because they were found to be weak or unsafe, the majority of clinically useful plants were replaced with pharmaceuticals, which generated profits from patented drugs and helped support the industrialization of medicine.

Characteristics and Composition

In many traditional systems the characteristics of a medicinal plant are emphasized without attention to its composition because techniques and equipment for plant analysis are new. Preanalytical, chemical knowledge of medicinal and food plants is derived from direct perception through the five senses; from the herbalist's attentive, empirical observation of plants' effects on animals and humans; and in some traditions, from sacred teachings and sixth sense intuition. Plants' healing uses and properties are paradigm specific. In Chinese and Tibetan medicine the "five tastes" are sweet, sour, salty, pungent, and bitter. Each flavor is associated with certain qualities and corresponding physiological actions. For example, cinnamon *(Cinnamomum cassia)* bark is warm, sweet, and pungent and is used to warm the channels and disperse cold. It is prescribed for certain infections, correlating with recent pharmacological and clinical research, which demonstrated that aqueous decoctions strongly inhibit *Staphylococcus aureus* and *Salmonella typhi* (Bensky & Gamble, 1986).

Knowledge of the chemical composition of food and medicinal plants is growing worldwide as access to analytical technology improves. Perhaps the only disadvantage to identifying, categorizing, and researching molecular constituents from plants is the risk of equating the plant's therapeutic efficacy to its composition; analysis is reductionist in paradigm, and data cannot exist beyond the limits of the technology (and available funding to apply it) or the paradigm from which it arises.

Food, medicinal, and healing plants contain digestible fiber (carbohydrates and hemicellulose) and indigestible fiber (cellulose and lignins), nutritives (calories, vitamins, minerals, trace elements, amino acids, essential fatty acids, and water), and inert and active constituents.

Adhering to a western paradigm, plant constituents can be classified according to their morphology, source plant taxonomy, therapeutic (pharmacological) applications, or chemical constituents (Tyler et al., 1988). A classical organization of the active chemical constituents includes the following:

1. *Carbohydrates:* sugars, starches, aldehydes, gums, and pectins
2. *Glycosides:* cardiac glycosides in *Digitalis purpurea* leaf, anthraquinone glycosides in *Aloe* species latex, and rhubarb, *(Rheum officinale)* root and rhizome, flavinol glycosides (rutin and hesperidin used to reduce capillary bleeding), and other glycoside types
3. *Tannins:* present in coffee and tea

4. *Lipids:* fixed oils and waxes
5. *Volatile oils:* essential oils such as peppermint and eucalyptus
6. *Resins*
7. *Steroids:* including the steroidal saponins from Mexican yam (*Diocorea* species), the original source of early oral contraceptives
8. *Alkaloids:* atropine from *Atropa belladona,* quinine from chinchona, morphine from *Papaver somniferum*
9. *Peptide hormones*
10. *Enzymes:* bromelain from pineapple

Activities

Activities and correspondent indications for the use of plants are, again, paradigm specific (Box 9-1). In the United States alone, opinions vary regarding a particular plant's full spectrum of physiological action because of the complex nature of plants and their uses.

The many influences on plant activities and their therapeutic properties might threaten the confidence of the researcher, herbalist, or patient that the desired effect will be produced. However, every factor listed is present in the human food supply, which has supported human life since prehistory. A true scientist might agree that there is no way to control all variables, although identifying, controlling, or tracking those most suspected of producing specific outcomes is the tedious and honorable responsibility of all healers and researchers. Plant actions are recorded in the pharamacopeia through the first half of this century in archaic terminology. Many terms are similarly used to describe the actions of contemporary pharmaceuticals.

A sample of some classic plant actions—often associated with identifiable nutritives or active constituents—are as follows:

- *Respiratory system:* stimulating expectorant (*Marrubium vulgaris,* hoarhound), relaxing expectorant (*Prunus serotina,* black cherry bark), antitussive *(P. serotina),* and immunomodulator for upper respiratory tract infection (*Echinacea purpurea* and other species)
- *Gastrointestinal system:* emetic (*Cephaelis ipecacuanha),* antiemetic (*Zingiber officinale,* ginger), laxative (*Plantago ovata,* psyllium seed), and spasmolytic (*Papaver somniferum,* opium poppy)

BOX 9-1

Influences on Plant Activities and Their Therapeutic Properties

- Specific plant species, variety, and sometimes individual plant itself
- Habitat, including latitude, longitude, exposure, humidity, rainfall, sun, shade, wind, temperature and daily and seasonal variation, soil, soil microorganisms, insects, birds, animals, companion plants, pests, plant diseases, and interaction with humans (damage, cultivation, harvesting, and pollution)
- Composition and constituents (presence of active and inert ingredients)
- How and when the plant is collected, stored, processed; how the herb is dispensed and dosed
- Presence of adulterants, pests, or disease
- The prescriber—many traditional systems in Africa and Asia ascribe the ability to potentiate the plant's healing properties only to initiated healers or shamans
- The patient's health status, disease, age, and receptivity to healing
- The symbolic or cultural significance of the plant
- The placebo effect

- *Nervous system:* sedative (*Valeriana officinalis),* stimulant (*Piper myristicum,* kava kava), cardiotonic (*Crataegus oxycantha* or monogyna, hawthorne), and antidepressant (*Hypericum perforatum,* St. John's Wort)

These examples illustrate a few of the many actions ascribed to classical western paradigm herbs. Often, contemporary research explains the constituents, mechanisms of action, and clinical responses that justify traditional uses. Occasionally, some plants are found to be inactive or ineffective or to contain potential toxins, resulting in their discontinuance or requiring special methods of preparation and dosing. Like most prescription medications today, some strong herbs must be dosed carefully to render them safe and effective. However, to provide a realistic perspective, casava root—one of the leading sources of calories and carbohydrates for people worldwide—contains cyanide-like compounds that produce permanent neurotoxicity, paralysis, and death if improperly prepared; traditional preparation involves cooking, which renders the toxins inert.

Other complications to the direct association of active constituents to in vivo and clinical medicinal actions are that many times the active compounds remain unidentified, or the physiological response to the medicinal part of the whole plant is distinct from the actions of the individual active constituents (as in the cases of *Valeriana* and *Echinacea*). In addition, ingredients that appear inert are sometimes later found to be active when a more accurate mechanism of action or bioassay associated with the plant's effects is discovered. This occurred in the National Cancer Institute's screening program, when inactive plants were rescreened decades later with advanced methods and found to contain biologically active compounds.

From a nonreductionist paradigm, plant composition alone offers an incomplete explanation of the full scope of the properties and actions of food and healing plants. Traditional herbalists, turn-of-the-century vitalists, naturopathic doctors, and many contemporary medical doctors and practitioners share a belief in a "life force" that is yet to be fully understood. Many herbalists hold that healing energy is inherent to plants; it is primarily this energy, rather than nutritive or chemical constituents, that promotes healing. Shamans, traditional healers, and alchemists use their skills, knowledge, and power to instill certain plants with special healing properties in this view.

Herbal Therapeutics

Different cultural paradigms use plants for healing in a manner founded on each paradigm's premises. Herbal practitioners in the United States may rely primarily on the plant's pharmacological actions (in some cases enhanced by specific processing and extractive solvents and techniques or formulating plant medicines into standardized extract products to concentrate and guarantee unit doses of active constituents), individual plant pharmacokinetics (best preserved by using single, whole plants or their extracts), synergistic formulating (blending a number of medicinal plants together to achieve specific therapeutic effects unachievable by using a single herb alone), nutritive value (as when *Urtica repens,* or nettles, are recommended as a tea rich in absorbable iron), energetics, or a combination of these.

Case Study

A 35-year-old patient in the United States consults with a Western naturopathic doctor or medical herbalist about experiencing mild anxiety. The patient's family history and personal and psychological health history are "unremarkable."

A health screening and physical examination within the last 6 months identified no health problems. The patient is evaluated for a "constitutional" physiological profile, a personal and social profile, and a lifestyle profile (stress, diet, exercise, recreation, and spiritual values). Treatment for her simple, circumstantial, stress-induced anxiety is to increase exercise and gardening (time outdoors), make some minor adjustments to her diet and lifestyle, soak her feet each evening in a lavender (*Lavandula officinalus*) foot bath (mildly relaxing) for 10 days, and use *Passiflora incarnata* tincture (specifically dosed) twice daily for 2 weeks, and then consult with the practitioner on her progress and symptoms. *P. incarnata* is listed in Martindale's *Extra Pharmacopeia* (Martindale, 1994) and in the Pharmacopeia's of Egypt, France, Germany, Switzerland, and Brazil, although it is not listed in the United States *Pharmacopeia.*

It acts as a mild sedative and antispasmodic. Among its constituents are a volatile oil (sedating on inhalation but of unknown composition), cyanogenic flavinoids 5-7-dihydroxyflavone ("chrysin," a monflavinoid shown to act as a partial agonist, displacing three H flunitrazepam from central benzodiazepine receptors from mice), and passiflorine (a hormone alkaloid).

Food and medicinal plants have multiple actions, caused at least in part by their multiple constituents. This is in relative contrasts to many pharmaceuticals, which typically have a single or few specific therapeutic actions. However, pharmaceutical side effects demonstrate how uncommon a true single action is physiologically—whether because of minor but concurrent nontherapeutic pharmacological actions or because a single action provokes the desired therapeutic physiological response along with unintended, nontherapeutic responses.

The multiple actions of plants—although a challenge to the isolation of single active constituents or primary single pharmacological or physiological actions—are only a problem if plants are classified as highly potent, synthetic pharmaceuticals. However, because most medicinal plants are much less potent than pharmaceuticals and because humans have evolved on plant-based diets (each individual plant or animal food a complex chemical soup of unknown formula), it seems appropriate to assume that humans are probably better adapted to plants as food and medicine than to strong pharmaceutical drugs that have 50 years or less of use in the population worldwide.

Herbal medicines can be delivered in many forms. Some plants are best used fresh but are seldom marketed fresh because they are highly perishable. Dried, whole, or chopped herbs can be prepared as infusions (steeped as tea) or decoctions (simmered over low heat). Flowers, leaves, and powdered herbs are infused (chamomile or peppermint), whereas fruits, seeds, barks, and roots require decocting (rose hips, cinnamon bark, licorice root). Many fresh and dried herbs can be tinctured as preserved medicines in alcohol; some plants are suited to acetracts (vinegar extracts), whereas others are active and well preserved as syrups, glycerites (in vegetable glycerine), or miels (in honey). Powered or freeze-dried herbs are available in bulk, tablets, troches, pastes, and capsules. Fluid and solid extracts strong concentrates (four to six times the crude herb strength)—and fresh plant juices preserved in approximately 25 percent alcohol (as in the fresh plant echinacea succus) are other forms.

Nonoral delivery forms include herbal pessaries, suppositories, creams, ointments, gels, linaments, oils, distilled waters, washes, enemas, baths, poultices, compresses, moxa, snuffs, steams, and inhaled smokes and aromatics (volatile oils). The predominant plant delivery forms vary among different herbal traditions. Tinctures are widely used in Britain and the United States; tablets of standardized extracts of certain herbs (e.g., ginko biloba) are popular in Germany and the United States; decoctions are common in Tibetan, Chinese, and African traditions; therapeutic oils are used topically and internally in Ayurvedic treatments; and teas, smokes, and compresses are used in the Native American tradition.

There is another point to be made regarding herbal therapeutics as distinct from contemporary over-the-counter and prescription pharmaceuticals. Herbal therapies have never been used as intended, nor do they show high efficacy when used as pharmaceutical substitutes. Crude or processed plant foods and medicines tend to work best preventively or therapeutically as slow-acting, gradual, healing agents. They must be taken consistently in the correct form and dose. (Some medicinal plants work rapidly.) In addition, the herbal practitioner's familiarity with each medicinal plant or herbal formula usually is much greater than the medical doctor's familiarity with each individual pharmaceutical, and this permits the herbalist to precisely select a particular plant or formula for each patient. Three different patients each with a chief complaint of headache would each receive a different herbal prescription. The approach an herbalist uses to arrive at which herbs to prescribe is distinct from how a conventional Western physician prescribes a pharmaceutical.

HERBS IN PREVENTIVE HEALTH AND PATIENT SELF-CARE

What is more respectable than to take care of oneself within one's own means?

—WORLD HEALTH ORGANIZATION

This discussion would be incomplete if it were not reemphasized that herbs are essentially "people's medicine." Traditional systems of herbalism generally make little distinction between food and medicinal plants, and local accessibility to food, spice, and therapeutic herbs was a given in nonindustrialized societies.

Before the twentieth century, people everywhere had closer personal contact with food and medicinal plants. The modern era has brought many advantages to human health and sanitation, but one potential disadvantage of economic and occupational specialization is the loss of this contact with the source of plant medicines. The marketplace has become multileveled, so the consumer usually has no direct or personal relationship with the herb producer. Sometimes, because of costs of production, taxes, and marketing, the packaged herbal product costs 20 times the price of the crude herb. There are undeniable advantages to certain prepackaged or concentrated herbal products, but two disadvantages are accountability and economic access. If fresh or bulk crude herbs are abandoned in the marketplace for less perishable and higher-return products, the patient has access to only highly processed products and the cash-poor patient loses access altogether. This is particularly ironic in the case of medicinal plants; most traditional systems considered healing plants a gift of nature or God and access to them a basic human right.

A partial solution to ensure access to high-quality herbs is to support the renewed national interest in home gardens and urban "pea patches," thus embracing herbalism's unwritten dictum of self-responsibility and direct individual contact in the cycles of nature. Many culinary herbs such as thyme, oregano, and rosemary contain antioxidants and antimicrobial volatile oils and are digestive stimulants and antiseptics. Although specific herbs may vary depending on climate and region, such kitchen gardens could serve as preventive and therapeutic medicines for minor ailments.

In contemporary America, the context for using medicinal plants for preventive and therapeutic purposes already has been lost—except for subcultures in which it has been preserved, such as among the Amish and Native Americans. A restoration of the personal and symbolic relationship to food and medicine plants could be linked with contemporary scientific knowledge of herbal applications. Appropriate self-care could be encouraged with public education, access to consultation with professional herbalists and physicians, and access to fresh herbs and high-quality, processed herbal medicines when needed. This improved patient involvement in the self-care of the body and its signals might then improve the use of professional medical care.

RESEARCH IN FOOD AND MEDICINAL PLANTS

Although there is a relatively extensive contemporary literature on medicinal and healing plants, most of it exists outside of the United States and often in languages other than English. In addition, there is little consistency in standard research designs and protocols among various countries.

The need for more research on food, spice, and medicinal plants, especially for their potential use in syndromes and diseases poorly treated by conventional Western medicine, is great. The challenge is to conduct the research in the holistic spirit. This requires creative funding of research unlikely to provide high-profit returns to a single source. Fortunately, research on crude or extracted traditional plant remedies is relatively inexpensive compared with the astronomical costs of new drug development by pharmaceutical companies. Many medicinal plants eliminated from the *United States Pharmacopeia* over the years were dropped because they lacked contemporary research documentation of efficacy, not because they were proven to be ineffective (although some plants proved less useful clinically than newly developed drugs).

Retaining a holistic context in medicinal plant research also involves addressing differences in paradigm. Involving traditional herbalists as research design consultants would protect against inadvertently eliminating a critical element of the paradigm in which the herb is used. In the past plant collection for research has sometimes proved an environmental threat (habitats, species, or traditional knowledge were lost or threatened). The holistic approach to contemporary plant collection and research must be conducted in a way to conserve the traditional knowledge and ecology of the source plant to avoid transgression of intellectual property rights, destruction of the plant habitat, or an imbalance of economic or intellectual returns to the source habitat and community.

There is a need for simple, well-documented analysis and outcomes research of crude and whole plant medicines to determine their greatest potential applications and benefit to human health. British sailors were cured of scurvy with limes, originally presumed to be therapeutic against the disease solely because of their vitamin C content. However, limes and citrus proved more effective against scurvy than vitamin C supplementation; this was largely explained by the presence of bioflavonoids, later isolated and discovered to be prevalent in citrus pulp. The desirability of performing bioassays and clinical efficacy studies on whole herbs and herbal formulas, as well as on identified active constituents within the plants, is clear.

Increasing contemporary research on medicinal plants is critical, but the importance of documenting and incorporating the empirical knowledge of healing plants cannot be overemphasized. One of the greatest disadvantages of modern research is its highly selected—often single sex age group, ethnicity, or locality—human cohort; its relatively brief treatment and monitoring intervals; and its failure to fully document subclinical or seemingly irrelevant symptoms of the participating individuals. Sample populations are relatively tiny compared with the worldwide population. However, if information gleaned from research is linked with empirical knowledge (usually derived from hundreds of years of human use across many generations and ethnic groups), along with contemporary clinical reporting from patients and practitioners on tolerance and efficacy, then herbal therapeutics and preventive protocols can reach the threshold of the twenty-first century positioned to enhance the health of future generations.

CHALLENGES FOR CONTEMPORARY HERBALISM

The greatest opportunity for human benefit from food, spice, and healing plants will be afforded only if at least some elements of the traditional contexts and paradigms in which herbs have been used are preserved. The special relationship of humankind to the plant world is one of these traditions.

Challenges for the future include the preservation of germ plasm; the conservation of biodiversity and plant habitat; training professional and other herbalists, exchanging information with traditional healers; providing physicians and other health care professionals with a familiarity with plant medicines; educating the public in the appropriate use of herbs for self-care; ensuring the funding of medicinal plant research that focuses on public health, clinical therapeutics, and wellness—not just drug development; and preserving public access to inexpensive, tonic, and therapeutic herbs through economic, environmental, market, legislative, and health policy.

In a recent study the most trusted professional chosen by a sample of the American public was the pharmacist. This survey reveals the value and need of many people to have a personal, face-to-face relationship with the one who prepares and provides them with medicine. Traditionally, this was the role of the herbalist and healer, as well as the turn-of-the-century medical doctor. Today, many pharmacists are becoming interested in learning about herbal medicines, and students in herbal training and naturopathic medical schools are becoming more interested in natural products chemistry. This appears to be a timely example of nature's principle of reciprocity.

The reemergence of herbalism in the West might have been predicted by traditional herbalists and healers centuries ago, who believed in the recycling patterns of nature. All herbal traditions rely predominantly on an ecological relationship between the natural environment, the community, the herbal practitioner, and the individual. Self-sufficiency and personal responsibility are emphasized amid the irrevocable interdependence of human society with nature. The role of "herbalism" in contemporary Western society is not to serve as a substitute for the pharmaceutical advances of the last decades but to serve as an ancient paradigm that was less mechanistic and more holistic and humane in scope and that, if responsibly reclaimed and integrated, could greatly benefit future health care worldwide. This is illustrated in the following quote by Paiakan, a contemporary Kayapo Indian leader. "I am trying to save the knowledge that the forest and this planet are alive, to give it back to you who have lost the understanding" (Odum, 1971).

References

Bensky D, Gamble A. 1986. Chinese Herbal Medicine Materia Medica. Eastland Press, Seattle, pp. 34-35

Boyle W. 1991. Official Herbs in the United States Pharmacopoeias 1820-1990. Buckeye Naturopathic Press, East Palestine

Iwu MM. 1993. Handbook of African Medicinal Plants, CRC Press, Boca Raton, Florida, pp. 343-349

Martindale, 1994.

Odum H. 1971. Environment, Power and Society. John Wiley & Sons, New York, p. 8

Solecki RS, Shanidar IV. 1975. A neanderthal flower burial in northern Iraq. Science 190:880-889

Tyler VE, Brady LR, Robbers JE. 1988. Pharmacognosy. Lea & Febiger, Philadelphia

Suggested Readings

DeFeudis FV. 1991. Ginkgo biloba extract (Egb 761): Parmacological Activities and Clinical Applications. Elsevier, Paris

Donden Y. 1986. Health Through Balance: An Introduction to Tibetan Medicine. Snow Lion Publications, Ithaca, New York

Farnsworth NR, Bunyapraphatsara N. 1992. Thai Medicinal Plants Recommended for Primary Health Care Systems. Medicinal Plant Information Center, Bangkok

Hoffmann DL. 1987. The Herb User's Guide: The Basic Skills of Medical Herbalism. Thorsons Publishing Group, Wellingborough

Junius MM. 1993. The Practical Handbook of Plant Alchemy. Healing Arts Press, Rochester, New York

Scudder JM. 1874. Specific Diagnosis: A Study of Disease with Special Reference to the Administration of Remedies. Wilstach, Baldwin and Co, Cincinnati

Stetter C. 1993. The Secret Medicine of the Pharaohs—Ancient Egyptian Healing, Edition Q, Chicago

Suzuki D, Knudtson P. 1992. Wisdom of the Elders: Sacred Native Stories of Nature. Bantam Books, New York

Wood M. 1986. Seven Herbs: Plants as Teachers. North Atlantic Books, Berkely.

Top Twenty Herbs for Primary Care

VICTOR S. SIERPINA

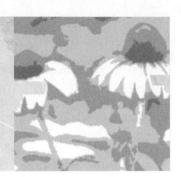

erbal treatments for common problems are increasingly popular. Until the twentieth century, herbal medicines were the primary method of administering medicinally active compounds. In many countries herbal medicine remains the core of healing practice.

With the advent of the first purified plant extracts of morphine from the opium poppy in 1805 to the highly sophisticated chemical laboratories of Europe and the United States in the present century, herbal use fell into disfavor. Home remedies offered by a family member seemed quaint and old-fashioned compared with the allure of scientific medical treatments. This trend was certainly emphasized by the marvelous success of antibiotics and their single-cause, single-remedy model.

In many countries, however, including the European subcontinent, herbal medicines are the primary form of health care. The World Health Organization has taken the following balanced position: *the traditional, historical use of herbal preparations is evidence of safety and efficacy in the absence of scientific evidence to the contrary.* This means that herbal therapies need not be subjected to double-blind, randomized, controlled studies to be acknowledged as valid medicines.

In the day-to-day practice of modern medicine, however, with the issues of professional liability and standards of care ever in mind, the conventional health practitioner with little or no training in herbal therapy is in a quandary. Should he or she recommend a therapy that the patient has already started or is interested in taking simply because the patient requests it? Are there any scientific studies to support the contemporary use of popular and widely marketed herbal products? Are these products safe? effective? What is their dosage? Are there interactions with currently prescribed pharmaceuticals? What is the mechanism of action?

Physicians interested in the total well-being of their patients acknowledge and encourage patient efforts in self-care and responsible choices for their own health. Herbal medicine seems to offer the patient latitude with choices in self-care and healing that are outside the traditional physician-patient interaction. Many alternative therapies, diets, supplements, and modalities fit into this framework. However, much of the data regarding herbals has been developed in Europe and not published in mainstream American medical journals. This leaves an information gap that requires some learning by the already busy physician.

As a practicing family physician who has worked in urban, suburban, frontier, and university practices with a wide variety of patient populations, this list comprises the herbs I have used or recommended most commonly. More importantly, it represents the bulk of herbs patients ask me about regularly. Others may easily be added to the list and some deleted.

A journey of a thousand plants must begin . . . with something useful!

If you can speak to patients intelligently about these 20 herbs, you are well on your way to learning more about them and other herbs. Patients will trust you because you are willing to listen to their interest in the use of products they can acquire at any health food store without your knowledge or permission. Still, they often would like your involvement and approval of their choices.

TABLE 9-1

Common Uses for Top 20 Herbs

Herb	Common use
1. Aloe	Skin, gastritis
2. Black cohosh	Menstrual, menopause
3. Dong quai	Menstrual, menopause
4. Echinacea	Colds, immunity
5. Ephedra (ma huang)	Asthma, energy, weight loss
6. Evening primrose oil	Eczema, psoriasis, premenstrual syndrome, breast pain
7. Feverfew	Migraine
8. Garlic	Cholesterol, hypertension
9. Ginger	Nausea, arthritis
10. Ginkgo biloba	Cerebrovascular insufficiency, memory
11. Ginseng	Energy, immunity, mentation, libido
12. Goldenseal	Immunity, colds
13. Hawthorne	Cardiac function
14. Kava kava	Anxiety
15. Milk thistle	Liver disease
16. Peppermint	Dyspepsia, irritable bowel syndrome
17. Saw palmetto	Prostate problems
18. St. John's Wort	Depression, anxiety, insomnia
19. Tea tree oil	Skin infections
20. Valerian	Anxiety, insomnia

For simplicity of association, key indications are in bold type.

ALOE

Aloe vera is a common succulent houseplant. Long kept in the kitchen for soothing burns, it is now available in commercial preparations for such indications as sunburn and the treatment of **stomach ulcers.** The solidified gel from the leaves, which extrudes when they are broken, can be used directly on the affected area of the skin and is useful in many **skin conditions** as a *vulnerary* (promotes wound healing). For internal use, it comes in a diluted liquid form.

It can be a powerful *cathartic* and an *emmenagogue* (increases menstrual flow), and it should be avoided during pregnancy and lactation because of its *purgative* effects.

Dosage is simply putting some of the juice from the plants on the affected area and the internal use is 0.1 to 0.3 g. Commercial preparations of the juice are also available for internal use.

BLACK COHOSH

Cimicifuga racemosa is best thought of as a female herb. Its traditional uses include the relief of **menstrual cramps, premenstrual syndrome (PMS),** and **menopausal symptoms.** It has been found to be useful in treating symptoms associated with menopause such as hot flashes, mood and sleep disturbance, and vaginal atrophy. The American Indians used it for these indications and dysmenorrhea. Its active ingredients are triterpenes and flavonoids, some of which act on the pituitary gland to suppress luteinizing hormone. It does not alter the production of follicle-stimulating hormone and prolactin. Stomach upset is the only reported side effect, and no other contraindications or drug interactions are reported. Some experts recommend limiting treatment to 3 to 6 months because long-term safety has not been evaluated.

A contemporary preparation of black cohosh is *Remifemin,* which is provided in a convenient tablet form for both dysmenorrhea (once or twice daily) and menopause (two tablets twice daily). Forty milligrams daily is a therapeutic dose. It can also be taken as a tea made of ½ to 1 tsp of the dried root. This tea is taken three times daily, or 2 to 4 ml of tincture is used three times daily.

DONG QUAI

Angelica sinensis is an Asian herb widely respected as a "women's remedy." It has been widely used for **dysmenorrhea, menopause,** and **metrorrhagia.** It is useful in stabilizing the estrogenic activity and relieving hot flashes. Its imputed mechanism of action is by means of phytoestrogens, and it also contains ferulic acid, ligustilide, vitamin B_{12}, and vitamin E. It has been shown to have both a relaxing and stimulating effect on the uterus.

Some patients may experience hypersensitivity, which can cause excess bleeding and fever. It can also be photosensitizing. It should not be used during pregnancy and lactation, although various sources disagree on this point. There is a potential drug interaction with coumarin.

For PMS the three-times-daily dose is 1 to 2 g of powdered root or as tea, 1 tsp of tincture, or ¼ tsp of fluid extract starting on day 14 of the menstrual cycle. It is also available in teas.

ECHINACEA

Echinacea angustifolia is best known as an **immune stimulant.** Long favored by the American Indians, it is considered an antibiotic, useful against both bacterial and viral infections. It is one of the best-selling herbs in health food stores in the United States.

Its imputed actions are encouraging the swarming of white blood cells to the site of an infection, stimulating phagocytosis, improving lymphocyte production, and increasing interferon production. Some sources discourage its use in autoimmune disease or tuberculosis. It is not recommended during pregnancy. Side effects are not reported.

The dosage is 3 to 4 cups of tea a day or 1 to 4 ml of tincture three times a day during an infectious episode such as the **common cold** and **chronic respiratory tract infections.** Although sources vary on treatment dosing, a cycle of 5 days on and 2 days off during an infection is widely recommended. Taking

it all the time is not considered to be as useful, and in any case it should not be taken for longer than 8 weeks.

EPHEDRA

Ephedra sinica or *ma huang* contains alkaloids, ephedrine, and pseudoephedrine. It is widely used for **asthma, allergy, low blood pressure,** and **cerebral insufficiency;** as a **stimulant;** and for **weight loss.** It has marked sympathomimetic effects and can be overused or even abused. Its effects on the central nervous system have been characterized as stronger than caffeine but less than amphetamines. It is best avoided in patients who are hypertensive or anxious and in those with glaucoma or diabetes.

The dosage is 1 to 2 tsp of dried herb steeped as a tea for 10 to 15 minutes taken three times a day or 1 to 4 ml of the tincture three times a day. It is also found mixed in a number of other preparations.

EVENING PRIMROSE OIL

Oenothera biennis produces seeds that are a source of omega-6 essential fatty acids. It has a fairly long list of indications, but it is most commonly used for **atopic eczema, premenstrual syndrome, psoriasis, cyclical** and **noncyclical mastalgia.** Some trials have used it without benefit in multiple sclerosis. Its actions are thought to be related to antioxidant effects and the replacement of deficiency of the essential fatty acids linoleic acid and gamma-linolenic acid (GLA). It should not be used with phenothiazines because it may precipitate seizures. Side effects are mild gastrointestinal effects and headache.

The dosages based on a standardized GLA content of 8% are 2 to 4 g a day for children and 6 to 8 g for adults for atopic eczema, 3 to 4 g for mastalgia, and 3 g for PMS.

FEVERFEW

Tanacetum parthenium is a primary remedy in the treatment of **migraine headaches** and associated nausea and vomiting. It may also be useful for dizziness, tinnitus, and dysmenorrhea. It should not be used during pregnancy because of the stimulant action on the uterus or during lactation. It may cause mouth ulcers in some people, particularly those chewing the leaves. It treats and prevents migraine by inhibiting the release of blood vessel—dilating substances from platelets, inhibiting inflammatory mediators, and regulating vascular tone. The active ingredient is parthenolide, which should be present in at least a 0.2% concentration in preparations.

The dosage is one fresh leaf one to three times a day, fresh or frozen. The drug equivalent is 0.2 to 0.6 mg of parthenolide, which is equivalent to 50 to 200 mg of dried aerial parts in tablets or capsule. It also is available in a tincture of 1:5 in 25% ethanol with a dose of 5 to 20 drops. Continuous use for at least 4 to 6 weeks is recommended for prophylaxis at a dose of not less than 125 mg of dried feverfew containing a minimum of 0.2% of the parthenolide active ingredient.

GARLIC

Allium sativum is a favorite kitchen herb in many cultures that has many health effects, including its antiplatelet activity (at about 1 clove a day), use as an antibiotic, and immune-enhancing effects. The volatile oil is largely excreted by the lungs and is useful in respiratory infections. Studies have shown its benefit in reducing **blood pressure** and **cholesterol** levels. The active ingredient is allicin. Fresh garlic has compounds such as S-allylcysteines and gamma-glutamylpeptides, which exert beneficial effects as well. Some gastrointestinal side effects, such as nausea, diarrhea, and vomiting or a burning sensation, may occur. It may potentiate the antithrombotic effects of antiinflammatory drugs or coumadin.

Dosages of up to three cloves a day (or in the form of garlic oil capsules) are recommended. The capsules should deliver at least 10 mg of alliin or a total allicin potential of 4000 μg. The German Commission E that reviewed herbal products recommended that commercial preparations contain not less than the equivalent of 4000 mg of fresh garlic. The bottom line is to take fresh garlic or standardized preparations. Cooking removes some of the benefits of garlic.

Preparations of garlic oil, 2 to 5 mg/day, or tincture 1:5 in 45% alcohol 2 to 4 ml three times a day are also available.

GINGER

Zingiber officinale is another favorite among Asians and cooks everywhere. It is useful in a variety of conditions, including use as an **antiinflammatory,** a **digestive aid,** a gargle for sore throats, and a compress for abdominal and gynecological problems. A recently marketed preparation claims effectiveness as a **rheumatological** agent via inhibition of leukotrienes and prostaglandins. It has been widely used as an **antinauseant,** particularly in pregnancy, in which a tea made from fresh grated ginger root, ginger ale, lemon, and a bit of honey or sugar is sipped in the morning. Its antiinflammatory and antiplatelet functions may account for its imputed effectiveness in some kinds of migraine.

The dosage is a standardized capsule three times a day. An infusion is prepared by pouring boiling water over the sliced root or a decoction from using 1½ tsp of dried root powder or finely chopped. It also is available in a tincture 1.5 to 3 ml three times a day (a stronger tincture is available to be taken 0.25 to 0.5 ml tid). The tea or decoction can be drunk as needed. A compress made from fresh grated root in cheesecloth soaked in hot water and applied to the abdomen has long been favored as a stimulant for digestive and gynecological functions.

GINKGO

Ginkgo biloba is the most widely sold herb in Europe where it is used for **cerebral insufficiency, circulatory disorders,** and **memory problems, vertigo** and **tinnitus.** Studies have recently indicated its effectiveness in slowing the progression of Alzheimer's disease and multiinfarct dementia. Its mechanism of action is thought to be from its function as an antioxidant, a free radical scavenger, a membrane stabilizer, and from its inhibition of platelet-activating factor. This later effect makes its use in conjunction with coumarin potentially a problem, as does its use with aspirin. Clotting studies need to be followed carefully in this situation. Rarely stomach or intestinal upsets, headaches, or skin rashes can occur.

Standardized extracts contain 24% mixed flavonoid glycosides and 6% terpene lactones. Dosage is 120 to 240 mg/day taken in two to three doses for memory problems and dementia. A lower dosage of 120 to 160 mg/day in two or three doses is used for vertigo, tinnitus, and peripheral arterial occlusive disease. An initial period of 6 to 8 weeks is recommended to assess the effectiveness of ginkgo.

GINSENG (Figure 9-1)

Panax ginseng, Panax quinquifolius, Panax pseudoginseng, and *Eleutherococcus senticosus* (Oriental, American, Sanchi, and Siberian species) are widely reputed as **tonics for stress** and **fatigue.** A favorite among Orientals for centuries, it is considered an *adaptogen*—a substance that helps restore homeostasis during periods of physiological or psychological stress. Probably the simplest statement about ginseng is that the claims for its effectiveness are contradictory and difficult to verify. Nonetheless, it remains one of the top three best-selling herbs.

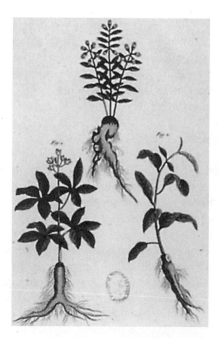

Figure 9-1 The gingseng root was considered in China to have quite miraculous properties to treat a wide range of diseases. (Courtesy Bibliotèque Interuniversitaire de Médecine, Paris.)

Improved athletic performance, sexual potency, memory, immune function, circulation, longevity, and treatment of cancer are all imputed to this panacea (the name *Panax* is derived from the Greek word meaning "all-healing"). Evidence of its effects on the endocrine system has been shown with increases in pituitary and adrenal hormones. Direct effects on potency have not been proven. It may reduce cholesterol levels. Many of the studies are in animal models, and the problems of source, standardization of dosing, and the opposing effects of the active ginsenosides account for the difficulty in studying this herb and proving its wide range of imputed effects.

The ginsenosides belong to a chemical group called *saponins,* which are similar in composition and structure to steroids such as testosterone, estrogen, and adrenocorticotropin hormone. Korean ginseng may raise blood pressure. Caution should be exercised when using ginseng in certain conditions, such as cardiac problems, diabetes, psychosis, and agitation; with steroid therapy or monoamine oxidase inhibitors; and possibly during pregnancy.

A standardized dose is 4% ginsenosides. Daily dosages vary from 0.5 to 1.0 g of root or equivalent preparations for healthy young persons for short-term use. Older and unhealthy people should take about half that amount. Doses can be taken in chronic states continuously. My conclusion on ginseng is that it is a mild stimulant tonic and probably best for older people rather than for the young and healthy, although it is generally safe in both groups.

GOLDENSEAL

Hydrastis candensis is a widely used **immune stimulant** and **natural antibiotic.** It has an astringent effect, and its most common use is for **sore throats.** The berberine alkaloid of goldenseal exerts antibiotic effects and has been shown to inhibit the attachment of group A streptococci to the endothelial lining of the throat. It has effects against other microorganisms such as *Staphylococcus, Candida, Giardia, Escherichia coli, Trichomonas vaginalis,* and *Entamoeba histolytica.* The alkaloid berberine also has been shown to activate phagocytosis. As an external agent, it is used for eczema, ringworm, pruritus, earache, and conjunctivitis. It is also used for infectious diarrhea, gastritis, infection and inflammation of mucous membranes, and digestive disorders. Because of its stimulant effect on the uterus, it should not be used during pregnancy.

The dosage is dried root and rhizome 0.5 to 1 g three times daily; tincture (1:10, 60% ethanol) 2 to 4 ml; liquid extract (1:1, 60% ethanol) 0.3 to 1 ml; or the extract standardized to contain 5% hydrastine, 250 to 500 mg, also three times daily.

HAWTHORNE

Crateaegus laeviagata is best known as a **cardiac tonic.** The hawthorn berries have been used for centuries in the Orient and Europe for their beneficial effects on the cardiovascular system. It is a traditional heart tonic, often used in conjunction with digoxin. Testing has shown that it increases myocardial contractility and coronary blood flow while decreasing heart rate and oxygen consumption. Its active constituents are proanthocyanidins and cardiotonic amines. It also contains antioxidant flavonoids that are produced in highest quantity from the young floral buds and leaves. It also inhibits angiotensin-converting enzyme and acts as a vasodilator and mild diuretic. It is used clinically in angina, congestive heart failure, and hypertension, although it is best used as an adjunctive therapy in severe cases. The extracts are well tolerated, show no drug interaction, and have a wide therapeutic index.

The dosage is 2 tsp of berries and leaves infused for 20 minutes and drunk three times a day over a long period. The tincture is taken 2 to 4 ml three times a day. The capsule dosage is 150 to 300 mg three times daily and should contain 1.8% vitexin-4'-rhamnoside or 10% procyanidins.

KAVA KAVA

Piper methysticum is a Polynesian euphoriant used primarily for **anxiety, depression,** and **insomnia.** The active ingredients are kavalactones, which are potentiated in the crude form and seem to have a gamma-amino butyric acid (GABA) receptor augmentation effect compared with the pure extract. It is a member of the pepper family. Small doses improve mental function, and it is notable that chiefs of Polynesian tribes, when in council, often drank kava (originally prepared by chewing on the root and then expectorating the extract into a large pot for brewing) before serious negotiations. Of note, it should not be used in patients with Parkinson's disease or in those currently taking benzodiazepines because the combination may cause disorientation. According to some sources, it may push limbic system impressions forward. It is safe and nonaddictive according to clinical studies, mainly from Germany. It also has some benefit as a skeletal muscle relaxant such as for nervous tension and stress headaches. High dosages of 400 mg/day or more over long periods may cause a scaly rash that resolves with discontinuance of the herb.

The dosage is 60 to 70 mg three times daily for anxiety or depression. For insomnia, 180 to 210 mg is taken 45 to 60 minutes before retiring. The dosage is based on the kavalactone content in the standardized preparation. The dried rhizome dosage is 1.5 to 3 g/day, and the alcoholic 1:2 extract is taken at a dosage of 3 to 6 ml/day. Kava's effects are potentiated by alcohol, and the standard bowl drunk by a group in its traditional social context has about 250 mg of kavalactones. Several bowls are often consumed at a sitting.

MILK THISTLE

Silybum marianum contains the active constituent silymarin. This herb acts as an antioxidant, inhibits leukotriene formation, stabilizes membranes, and is a choleretic and lipotropic. It has a decongesting effect on the liver and is most well known for preventing fibrosis and **cirrhosis** in **toxic** or **chemical-induced liver damage,** including **viral hepatitis.** No toxicity in animals or humans has been found. Patients with hepatitis C have shown a 30% reduction in abnormal liver enzymes in a 2- to 3-month period. It is also useful for psoriasis. It promotes milk secretion and is safe during lactation. It may also stimulate bile production and may have a cathartic effect as a result.

The standard dosage based on silymarin content is 70 to 120 mg three times daily. A phosphatidylcholine-bound form is available at 100 mg three times daily. The tea is prepared from 1 tsp of the dried herb and leaves infused for 10 to 15 minutes in a cup of boiling water. This is taken three times a day. A tincture of 1 to 2 ml can also be taken three times daily.

PEPPERMINT

Mentha piperita is considered a candy and breath mint, yet it has significant medicinal value. Its presence at the checkout counter of most restaurants has to do not only with its breath-enhancing benefits but also its effects on the lower esophageal sphincter. Peppermint reduces the lower esophageal sphincter tone, allowing for comfortable belching and the improved comfort of restaurant-goers. Herbalists refer to it as a *carminative,* a digestive aid that stimulates peristalsis, relaxes the stomach, and prevents gas. Its volatile oils have been found to be useful for **irritable bowel syndrome** (IBS) in the form of enteric-coated peppermint oil (ECPO), which allows it to reach the small and large intestines. It acts as a smooth muscle relaxant by means of its calcium channel blocking effects. It is an antispasmodic and reduces bile output. A study published in *Gastroenterology* showed it had significant effects in reducing abdominal pain, distension, stool frequency, borborygmi (loud bowel sounds), and flatulence in patients with IBS.

The dosage is 0.2 to 0.4 ml of ECPO three times daily half an hour before meals. A tincture of 1 to 2 ml three times daily is also helpful. The preferred method of taking peppermint for **dyspepsia** is a teaspoon of the herb infused as a tea taken as often as desired. However, keep in mind that gastroesophageal reflux disease (GERD) may be worsened by peppermint because it can increase heartburn. It does this by its effect of relaxing the lower esophageal sphincter tone, especially in those with a hiatal hernia, and thereby encouraging acid reflux.

SAW PALMETTO

Serenoa repens is obtained from the berries of the saw palmetto plant, which contain fatty acids, sterols, and carotenes. These inhibit steroids essential to prostate metabolism such as 5α-reductase and also have a mild α_1-receptor antagonism. These effects result in a clinically beneficial effect on **benign prostatic hypertrophy** (BPH). It can also be used for **prostatitis** along with zinc, echinacea, and bearberry. It has been shown to be more effective than placebo in treating BPH. Some sources claim it does not reduce prostate-specific antigen levels, although others disagree with this point. In any case it is a safe product with a reduced side effect profile compared with the prescription α_1-receptor antagonists, particularly in those who have the side effect of low blood pressure with the latter.

An examination must be performed to rule out more serious problems of the prostate, especially prostate cancer in men older than 50. Saw palmetto is also considered a tonifier of the male reproductive system that boosts male sex hormones. Quality-of-life indicators show marked improvement with saw palmetto use. It is thought that the value of a good night's sleep caused by reduction in nocturia contributes significantly to this.

The dosage is 160 mg twice daily of the extract containing 85% to 95% fatty acids and sterols. Teas are primarily water soluble and have no benefit in prostate conditions. Most patients taking saw palmetto receive relief with a month of treatment.

ST. JOHN'S WORT

Hypericum perforatum is a well-researched herbal product used primarily for mild to moderate **depression.** It has active ingredients in the anthraquinone class such as hypericin and flavonoids. It acts primarily as an antidepressant and is a serotonin reuptake inhibitor (SSRI). It has additional effects on the MAO inhibition pathway and on catecholamine methyl transferase (COMT). Although much has been made of its potential with MAO inhibitor–type drugs, no clinical evidence has been found verifying this concern. Its use with SSRIs is of some concern, however. The potential of a serotonin syndrome with the use of such common antidepressants as paroxetine (Paxil), fluoxetine (Prozac), and sertraline (Zoloft) requires caution in concomitant use. Experts in this area recommend tapering of the SSRI drug while starting St. John's Wort to reduce risk of serotonin syndrome. No other drug interactions are known.

Photosensitivity is a potential concern, especially in fair-skinned individuals, although the sunburn reported with St. John's Wort has primarily been in range animals eating large amounts of the raw herb. Other side effects are mild but include hypersensitivity. It is not recommended during pregnancy or lactation because of lack of toxicity data.

St. John's Wort is the most-prescribed agent for depression in Germany, exceeding fluoxetine sales by a large multiple. It has been tested against tricyclic antidepressants and found to have improved depression scales with a significantly reduced side effect profile. It is also considered to be useful for anxiety, sleep disturbances, acquired immunodeficiency syndrome, and chronic fatigue syndrome.

The dosage is based on the standardized hypericin content of 0.3%. The usual daily dosage is 300 mg three times daily in capsules. For insomnia, 900 mg should be taken an hour before sleep. Tea is prepared by pouring boiling water over 2 to 4 g of the herb and steeping for 5 to 10 minutes; the infusion is also taken three times a day. There is a liquid extract (1:1 in 25% alcohol) taken 2 to 4 ml three times daily. The tincture (1:10 in 45% alcohol) is taken three times daily in a dose of 2 to 4 ml. Perhaps the greatest advantage of St. John's Wort is patient compliance because of lack of side effects. It is also much less expensive than the leading SSRI antidepressants.

TEA TREE OIL

Melaleuca alternifolia is an Australian plant from which an essential oil is extracted. It is considered a useful **dermatological with antibacterial, antiviral, and antifungal properties.** It is used topically in full strength on boils, wound infections, and acne. At least one study showed it improved the healing of boils and reduced scar formation, presumably by its effect on *Staphylococcus aureus.* Another study showed it to be as effective as clotrimazole for treatment of tinea pedis.

It has a minimal tendency to irritate skin despite its penetrating qualities. Occasionally, it can cause contact dermatitis and irritation and will need to be diluted, or even discontinued, for a time.

VALERIAN

Valeriana officinalis yields valerenic acids, flavonoids, and valepotriates from its root; these are used for **nervousness, anxiety,** and **insomnia.** Valerian has been shown to improve the quality of sleep by improving slow waves in those with low baseline values. It is nonaddictive, unlike many of the sleep aids and anxiolytics, particularly those of the benzodiazepine class. It stimulates release of GABA and inhibits its reuptake. Its components bind directly to GABA receptors.

Because of its mechanism of action, it theoretically may potentiate the action of medications that have depressant effects on the central nervous system.

Thus, if taking it with antidepressants or sedatives, it may be prudent to do so under medical supervision. Several studies showed that valerian did not cause daytime drowsiness, reduced concentration, or reduction in physical performance. Nor does it have a synergy with alcohol, unlike many prescription sedatives. Although no evidence shows it to be harmful in pregnancy or lactation, like most herbs, it probably should be avoided during these times. There are no known side effects except occasional mild stomach upset, and there are no known interactions with other drugs.

The dosage of 0.8% valerenic extract for insomnia is 150 to 300 mg before sleep; for anxiety, 150 to 300 mg three times daily. The tea can be taken as needed three times a day or at bedtime and is made from steeping 1 to 2 tsp of the root in boiling water for 10 to 15 minutes. This yields 2 to 3 g of drug per cup. A tincture is available, and 2 to 4 ml is recommended three times daily. Of note is its odorous character likened to dirty socks.

Bibliography for Herbal Medicine

Blumenthal M, Busse WR, Goldberg A, et al. 1998. The Complete German Commission E Monographs: Therapeutic Guide to Herbal Medicines. American Botanical Council, Austin, Texas; Integrative Medicine Communications, Boston, Massachusetts.

Lininger S, Wright J, Austin S, Brown D, Gaby A. 1998. The Natural Pharmacy. Prima Publishing, Rocklin, California. A referenced overview of natural remedies for multiple conditions; refers to herbal, nutritional, homeopathic, and other alternative therapies. They also make a useful CD-ROM, which may be sampled at www.healthnotes.online

Murray M, Pizzorno J. 1998. Encyclopedia of Natural Medicine. Prima Publishing, Rocklin, California. For only $25, an economic and practical guide to naturopathic healing methods, including herbs, nutraceuticals, diet, and lifestyle changes.

PDR for herbal medicines. 1999. Medical Economics Company, Montvale, New Jersey. For their first edition, an effort to give physicians and other health professionals a usable handbook.

Useful Websites for Information about Herbs

www.drweil.com
www.herbs.org
www.herbalgram.org

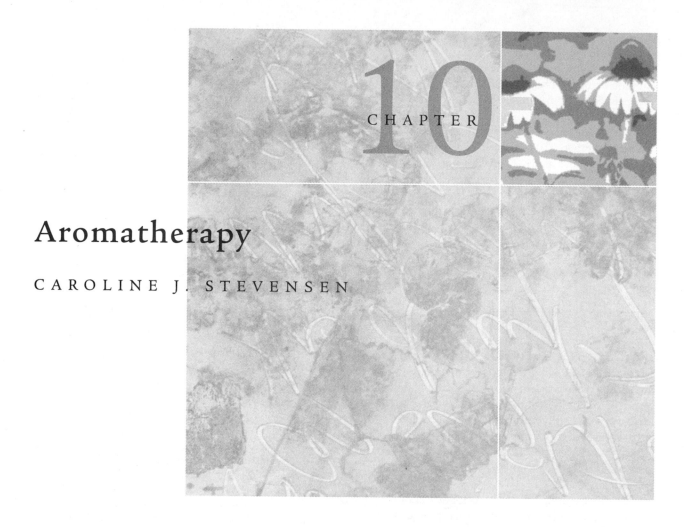

CHAPTER 10

Aromatherapy

CAROLINE J. STEVENSEN

romatherapy is the therapeutic use of essential oils extracted from plants. The term *aromathérapie* was coined by the French chemist René-Maurice Gattefossé in 1928. (His book of the same name was published in 1937.) Gattefossé is considered by many to be the father of the modern-day scientific use of essential oils.

The food and perfume industries are the largest users of essential oils. Some confusion about the therapeutic potential of aromatherapy may be because of this link with the cosmetic industry. The dictionary definition of *aromatherapy* is a method of treating bodily ailments using essential plant oils (Chambers Dictionary, 1988). *Aroma* is defined in chemical terms as belonging to the closed-chain class of organic compounds or benzene derivatives. *Therapy* is defined as a treatment used to combat a disease or

abnormal condition. *Essential oils* are described as oils forming the odiferous part of plants and as ethereal, suggesting not only a chemical constituent but also a heavenly, spiritlike or airy quality. On the basis of these definitions, *aromatherapy* is a treatment using a range of organic compounds of which the odor or fragrance play an important part.

Jean Valnet, the French physician well known for his invaluable work on aromatherapy, speaks of aromatherapy as the medicinal use of aromatic essences derived from plants (Valnet, 1990). Kusmirek, an aromatherapist based in England, describes aromatherapy as an industry combining perfumery, science, psychoaromatherapy, and aromacology, saying that the use of essential oils seeks to influence or change body, mind, or spirit (Kusmirek, 1992). Tisserand, an English aromatherapist, refers to essential oils from

146

plants as the blood of a person. "They are not the whole plant, but are whole organic substances in themselves. Like blood they will die if not properly preserved. The essential oil is like the most ethereal and subtle part of the plant, and its therapeutic action takes place on a higher more subtle level than that of the whole organic plant . . . having in general a more pronounced effect on the mind and emotions than does herbal medicine" (Tisserand, 1988).

Statements such as these are not based in scientific fact, and no trials have been performed to support their validity. It is unfounded, anecdotal comments like this that have helped keep aromatherapy from being considered a serious science. Valnet states that forgotten and ignored for many years, aromatic essences are coming back into their own, for many researchers and for a large section of public opinion, as the stars of medicine. Many patients are now unwilling to be treated except by natural therapies, foremost among which plants and their essences have a rightful place (Valnet, 1990). It is evident that both the scientific and the more subtle qualities of aromatherapy are important to those working with aromatherapy oils.

Essential oils are extracted from different parts of plants such as the roots, bark, stalks, flowers, or leaves. These extracts are mostly distilled, although other methods might be used. Essential oils might be applied to the body via massage with a vegetable oil, inhaled, used as a compress, mixed into an ointment, or inserted internally through the rectum, vagina, or mouth. The latter method is used chiefly by the medical profession in France.

Aromatherapy appears to be one of the fastest growing complementary therapies in the United Kingdom. Aromatherapy was brought to the United Kingdom from France by Madame Marguerite Maury, born in Austria. She was the first layperson to study and use the effects of essential oils absorbed through the skin. Her research was based on that of Gattefossé and her own clinical work with her husband, a French homoeopathic doctor. She promoted the modern-day use of massage with essential oils, the *aromatherapy massage,* and began teaching aromatherapy to beauticians. This training has gradually filtered from the cosmetic into the therapeutic domain and is increasingly being used by nurses, physiotherapists, and other health care professionals.

Modern-day aromatherapy is one of the fastest growing complementary therapies. This growth includes not only training and practice of aromatherapy but also production of essential oils. In the United Kingdom it is difficult to pick up a magazine or watch a program on alternative medicine that does not mention aromatherapy. Trained aromatherapists in the United Kingdom currently number approximately 5,000 without the existence of a central register. In a recent survey more than 21,000 people responded to a questionnaire on alternative medicine. Of the respondents, 7 percent had used aromatherapy, compared with 25 percent for osteopathy, 14 percent for chiropractic, 12 percent for homeopathy, and 9 percent for acupuncture.

Aromatherapy gradually is becoming more accepted in the orthodox medical field as a treatment to enhance both physical and psychological aspects of patient care. Skeptics might reject the therapy because of a lack of clinical trials—a criticism levelled at other branches of complementary medical treatments—as well as concern regarding the safety and quality of essential oils. These issues will be resolved as more research is performed, and aromatherapy will have its full and appropriate place in modern health care.

HISTORY

René-Maurice Gattefossé was a French chemist and scholar who described aromatherapy as a particular branch of science and therapeutics in 1928. He became interested in the study of essential oils after an accident in his laboratory. Gattefossé burnt his hand badly after a chemical explosion. He applied lavender essential oil that was close by. The burn healed with remarkable speed and without infection or scarring. Amazed at this result, Gattefossé began to investigate the properties of essential oils. He was the first person to analyze and record the individual chemical components in each oil, classifying the oils according to their properties (e.g., antitoxic, antiseptic, tonifying, stimulating, calming) (Franchomme & Pénoël, 1990).

Gattefossé carried out experiments in military hospitals during World War I. He claimed to achieve remarkable results using essential oils, preventing gangrene, curing burns, and obtaining cicatrization far more quickly than usual. However, after the war his methods came under professional scrutiny and were largely left behind (Maury, 1964).

Essential oils from aromatic plants were used before 1928. Over what length of time distilled essential oils have been used is uncertain. Popular opinion claims that the Arabs discovered the distilling of plants in the Middle Ages, and Avicenna has been given credit for this achievement in the tenth century AD (Arcier, 1990). However, an Italian research party led by Dr. Paolo Povesti, the director of the International Biocosmetic Research center in Milan, found a perfectly preserved terra-cotta distillation apparatus or still in the museum of Taxila at the foot of the Himalayas. It was used for beauty products and dated back 5000 years to the Indus Valley civilization (Williams, 1989).

Aromatic substances, which may or may not include essential oils as prepared today, were used in the ancient civilizations of Egypt, China, Greece, Rome, and Arab countries; in the Middle Ages; during the scientific revolution; and up to the present day. The importance of this is captured in the comment of Marguerite Maury (1964): "Perfumes and aromatics have their own history and long past. The latter is so bound up in the story of mankind that it is impossible to separate the two."

In Egyptian times Nefertum was the God of perfumes, incense, and fragrant oils. He was the son of Ptah, the creator God, and Sekmet, the Goddess of fiery protection, healing, and alchemical distillation. In a hymn to Nefertum he is described as the "Lord of oils and ungents, the soul of life." Nefertum smells the soul of the lotus and plants and purifies the body. In Egyptian life fragrance was a means of communication between the gods and humanity, offering health to the living and assisting the dead in the next life (Steele, 1992). There was some overlap between the use of aromatic products for spiritual well-being, health, and beauty. King Ramses III reportedly burned 2 million blocks of incense during the 30 years of his reign (Stoddard, 1991). The medicinal properties of aromatic oils were understood by the later Egyptian periods, and a wide range of essential oils was used, including frankincense, myrrh, cedarwood, henna, and juniper. The essence of cedarwood was prepared by heating in clay vessels covered by a layer of woolen fibers. These fibers were then squeezed, allowing the essence to be extracted (Valnet, 1990). When the tomb of Tutenkhamun was discovered in 1922, vases were found in the tomb, which, upon analysis, contained ointments of frankincense in a base of animal fat. The scent was apparently faint but still in evidence (Tisserand, 1988).

The ancient Chinese are well known for their use of herbal medicine, acupuncture, and moxibustion (the burning of mugwort to balance the body's energy), but there seems to be little detail regarding the use of aromatic oils. The Hebrews gained their knowledge of aromatic oils from prisoners held by the Egyptians.

The ancient Greeks used the aromatic essences both for medicine and for perfumes. Hippocrates expounded the virtues of a daily bath and a scented massage to maintain health and well-being. Aristotle argued that pleasant smells contribute to the well-being of humanity. The Roman poet Lucretius described the particles of pleasant smells as being smooth and round, whereas particles of unpleasant smells were barbed and prickly.

Biblical evidence of the use of aromatic substances is present in both the old and new testaments. God commanded Moses to make a holy anointing oil of myrrh, cinnamon, calamus, cassia, and olive oil (Exodus 30:22-25); frankincense and myrrh were brought to the birth of Jesus Christ (Matthew 2:11).

The Middle Ages saw a rise in the use of oils both as perfumes and medicines. Catherine de Medici, married to King Henry II, made the use of aromatic substances for ailments and perfumery fashionable. Her perfumer Cosimo Ruggieri not only assisted her with her health and beauty but was also able to prepare much less pleasant substances to help dispose of her enemies. Aromatic oils also were used to block out the smell of poor hygiene and ward off various plagues; pomanders and the fragrant tops on walking sticks were commonly used for this purpose. In 1589 a German pharmacopeia listed 80 essential oils for treating different conditions, and lavender essence was first prepared in France at this time (Arcier, 1990).

Away from Europe, the Native American shamans were no strangers to the use of herbs and aromatics. The perfumeros, or healers, bathed their patients in scents and, by the skillful use of perfume, could transform the auric field—the energetic or emotional envelope that surrounds a person. The blowing of tobacco smoke over a person, combined with a perfume, also was seen as having curative powers. The use of fragrance enabled transformations in religious, magical, and healing rituals. An ancient connection exists between fumigating and perfuming in this culture (Steele, 1992).

The scientific revolution and the manufacturing of synthetic substances that began in the nineteenth century saw the retreat of essential oils until the work by Gattefossé and his followers during this century. The perfume industry developed separately from the therapeutic field, with the introduction of such names as Coco Chanel, who launched the famous Chanel No. 5 in 1921. It was she who said that the most mysterious, most human thing, is smell. With the subsequent commercial development of the cosmetic industry, the gap between the cosmetic and the therapeutic use of essential oils became evident. Chanel and her scientific advisers successfully used synthetic products to make modern perfumes. This process separated cosmetics completely from the therapeutic use of essential oils, except perhaps for good feelings experienced by people wearing and experiencing the perfumes.

Marguerite Maury's research into the cutaneous application of essential oils began the teaching of aromatherapy in the 1950s as it is used today. Maury was influenced by the work of Valnet, who was an army doctor during World War II. He recognized that essential oils could have been used to alleviate some of the infection experienced by the soldiers rather than the massive amounts of penicillin that were prescribed. He obtained consistent results using essential oils with his wartime patients in Tonkin (Valnet, 1990). Madame Maury identified two uses of aromatherapy in France: (1) as part of allopathy in its use by doctors and (2) as a beauty treatment in the form of massage. She also acknowledged the more subtle aspect of aromatherapy and mentioned its link to vibratory medicine.

DEVELOPMENT

Madame Maury influenced the beginnings of the practice of aromatherapy in the United Kingdom. Micheline Arcier, a well-known aromatherapist in London, met Madame Maury at a beauty conference in 1959. Arcier and three other masseuses asked Maury to run a course for them. Madame Maury had clinics in London, Paris, and Switzerland, and Madame Arcier worked with her in London. Madame Arcier then began working with the oils and teaching small numbers of masseuses in the 1960s and 1970s. She also met Valnet, who worked and consulted from her London clinic.

Aromatherapy was still little known at this time. In fact, this method did not earn widespread popu-

larity until the 1980s. It is interesting to note the recent growth of aromatherapy, and yet, how few people have been responsible for its development over the last few decades.

Since the 1980s numerous schools of massage and aromatherapy have opened. Nearly 5000 aromatherapists are trained in the United Kingdom, although not all practice full-time. The number of people receiving aromatherapy is less than the number of those receiving osteopathy, and there are only 2000 registered osteopaths. Training in aromatherapy has continued in schools for lay massage practitioners but has grown to be included in nursing colleges and universities of higher education where the courses may be taken as part of a diploma or degree program.

The skills of therapeutic massage, usually the Swedish style, were taught to masseuses and physiotherapists as part of their professional training. Massage was part of the curriculum at nursing schools at the turn of the twentieth century but was excluded as their training became more scientific and technically oriented. It is now recognized as a valuable skill in terms of pain management and stress relief and is slowly being reintroduced into their training.

Fifty books were published on the topic of aromatherapy in the United Kingdom in the 7 years before 1995, indicating the rise in its popularity. Unfortunately, these books do not add new research-based information about essential oils. They often are published for commercial benefit rather than to further the science of aromatherapy. Most books are aimed at both lay and professional audiences, indicating the lack of sophistication in this field. Many books offer recipes of essential oils, losing sight of the fundamental principles involved. The exceptional work by Franchomme and Pénoël gives detailed chemical analysis of each oil and conditions, indications, and contraindications for each (Franchomme & Pénoël, 1990). Two new books by Tisserand and Balacs and Vickers address this problem by providing more scientific information, including the available research on essential oils, their chemical constituents, and the clinical practice of aromatherapy (Tisserand & Balacs, 1995; Vickers, 1996). To my knowledge, no books have been published on aromatherapy, and virtually no research has been performed in North America, except for a study on the inhalation of essential oils for the treatment of respiratory conditions (Boyd & Pearson, 1946).

THEORETICAL BASIS

Essential oils are volatile, fragrant, organic constituents that are obtained from plants either by distillation, which is most common, or by cold pressing, which is used for the extraction of citrus oils. Oils may be extracted from leaves (eucalyptus, peppermint), flowers (lavender, rose), blossoms (orange blossom or neroli), fruits (lemon, mandarin), grasses (lemongrass), wood (camphor, sandalwood), barks (cinnamon), gum (frankincense), bulbs (garlic, onion), roots (calamus), or dried flower buds (clove). Varying amounts of essential oil can be extracted from a particular plant; 220 pounds of rose petals will yield less than 2 ounces of the essential oil, whereas other plants, such as lavender, lemon, or eucalyptus, give a much greater proportion. This accounts for the variation in price among essential oils. Essential oils come from sources worldwide—lavender from France, eucalyptus from Australia, and sandalwood from India.

Essential oils are commonly a mixture of more than 100 organic compounds, which may include es-

TABLE 10-1

Chemical Components of Essential Oils and Their Therapeutic Actions

Chemical component	Therapeutic action
Aldehydes	Antiinfectious, litholitic, calming
Ketones	Mucolitic, litholitic, cicatrising, calming
Esters	Antispasmodic, calming
Sesquiterpenes	Antihistamines, antiallergic
Coumarins, lactones	Balancing, calming
C15 and C20 alcohols	Estrogen-like action
Acids, aromatic aldehydes	Antiinfectious, immunostimulants
Phenols, C10 alcohols	Antiinfectious, immunostimulants
Oxides	Expectorant, antiparasitic
Phenyl methyl ethers	Antiinfectious, antispasmodic
C10 terpenes	Antiseptic, cortisone-like action

From Franchomme P, Pénoël D. 1990. L'aromatherapie Exactement. Roger Jallois. Limoges.

ters, alcohols, aldehydes, terpenes, ketones, coumarins, lactones, phenols, oxides, acids, and ethers. Table 10-1 lists the major chemical components and their attributed therapeutic effects. Within the oils there might be more of some active constituents than others, which gives the oil its particular therapeutic value. For example, oils containing large amounts of esters (50 to 70 percent), such as neroli *Citrus aurantium aurantium,* are thought to be calming, whereas other oils, such as tea tree *Melaleuca alternifolia terpineol-4,* are regarded as antibacterial, antiviral, and immune system boosters because of the large amounts of alcohol (45% to 50%) in their composition (Franchomme & Pénoël, 1990). Critics of aromatherapy may say that the idea of an active ingredient goes against the desire for a whole natural substance. There is a question of the naturalness of any oil removed from a plant because immediately after the flower is cut, chemical changes occur; other chemicals may appear in the oil that were not originally in the plant (Dodd, 1991).

Aromatherapy is used for a wide range of physical, mental, and emotional conditions, including burns, severe bacterial infections, insomnia, depression, hypertension, and arrhythmias. Some of the findings that support these claims are discussed in the research section of this chapter.

The process of liquid gas chromatography is used to identify the quantity of each chemical constituent within the oil (Franchomme & Pénoël, 1990). As with grapes grown for wine, the quality of the yield varies according to the climate and other growing conditions of the plant. Lavender oil is popularly thought to be harmless, but according to its chemical type, or chemotype, it might not be suitable for use as a therapeutic oil. True lavender, *Lavandula angustifolia,* grown at approximately 1000 meters in the French Alps, has a high degree of purity and therapeutic constituents, whereas Stoechas lavender, *Lavandula stoechas,* grown at sea level by the Mediterranean, contains high quantities of ketones and therefore may be neurotoxic and abortive and is contraindicated in pregnant women, babies, and children (Franchomme & Pénoël, 1990).

Potential side effects of essential oils include the neurotoxic and abortive qualities already mentioned, as well as dermal toxicity, photosensitivity, allergic reactions, problems with internal use, and liver sensitivity (Franchomme & Pénoël, 1990). Unless oils are labeled with the full botanical data in Latin, it is impossible to tell whether they are dangerous or contraindicated. Lack of legislation over labeling and quality control of essential oils in the United Kingdom has contributed to the unease in some health care settings about their use. The fact that essential oils can be purchased at retail stores also gives the general public a false idea as to the relative safety of these oils.

The quality of essential oils also can be affected by their producers, who might add chemicals to extend the oil's capabilities or pesticides to act as contaminants. Gas chromatography will identify the chemical makeup of any oil, but it is not a complete assurance of quality. A certain degree of adulteration is common in the essential oil world, and it is often impossible for the consumer to detect. Reputable oil suppliers who perform their own quality control are currently the only safeguard.

There are few principles for the treatment of aromatherapy. Many aromatherapists discuss the concept of synergy at some length, that the whole natural essence is more active than its principal constituent. Those constituents that form a smaller percentage of the whole are found to be more active than the principal constituent (Valnet, 1990). As early as 1919, Heurre is noted as saying it is not enough to place side-by-side the principal chemical elements that analysis shows to be present in a particular vegetable essence to obtain a product that, therapeutically speaking, is as active as that of the natural essence (Valnet, 1990).

The basis of the action of aromatherapy is thought to be the same as that of modern pharmacology, using smaller doses. The chemical constituents are absorbed into the body, affecting particular physiological processes. Aromatherapy oils are taken into the body through the oral, dermal, rectal, or vaginal routes, or simply by olfaction.

The cutaneous administration of essential oils mixed in a vegetable carrier oil in the form of an aromatherapy massage is a common method of administration. Benefits can be gained not only from the oils through the skin but also from inhalation of the vapor and from physical therapy in the form of massage. Once the oil reaches the upper dermis, it enters the capillary circulation, where the oil can be transported throughout the body (Hotchkiss, 1994). A massage oil made with lavender penetrated the skin after 10 minutes (Jäger et al., 1992). Blood samples taken at intervals after massage, when analyzed by gas chromatography, showed that two major constituents of lavender oil, linalool and linalyl acetate, reached maximal concentrations 20 minutes after the massage, although traces had been evident at 5 minutes. Levels returned to baseline after 90 minutes, indicating elimination of lavender from the bloodstream (Jäger et al., 1992). Other studies support the passage of aromatic compounds through the skin of humans (Bronough, 1990; Collins et al., 1984).

Oral administration of essential oils carries more potential risks of poisoning or irritation to the gastric mucosa if administered by unqualified persons. It might be useful for qualified medical practitioners to get larger doses of essential oils into the body for the treatment of serious infections. A more detailed knowledge of essential oil toxicology is required for administration via this route than is possessed currently by the average aromatherapist.

A significantly smaller dose is administered to the body through the skin than when given orally (Tisserand & Balacs, 1995). Rectal administration of oils in the form of suppositories may be useful for local problems and to avoid the portal system of the body, thus allowing higher systemic concentrations of the oils to be absorbed (Tisserand & Balacs, 1995). Vaginal administration in the form of pessaries or douches also is used for local problems.

Simple inhalation of the oils is a method used for respiratory conditions, insomnia, and mood elevation and enhancement, or simply for making an environment more pleasant. It is not surprising that essential oils are absorbed through inhalation, considering that conventional medications such as those for asthma are administered in this way. Steam inhalers can be used for respiratory infections, and a variety of electrical and fan-assisted apparatus may be used to scent a room. Locomotor activity in mice increased after the inhalation of rosemary oil (Kovar et al., 1987). A rise in serum levels of 1,8-cineole, a major constituent of rosemary, corresponded with the rise in locomotor activity. Aromatic compounds of sandalwood, rose, neroli, and lavender all were present in the blood of mice after inhalation (Buchbauer et al., 1991). Studies also have demonstrated the absorption of aromatic compounds by humans (Falk, 1990; Falk-Filipsson, 1993). Overexposure to oils absorbed by this method can result in headaches, fatigue, or allergic reactions such as streaming eyes and skin problems.

The influence of touch in the form of massage is a major aspect of aromatherapy treatment when the oils are administered cutaneously. One study was able to show additional psychological benefit, including reduction in anxiety, to cardiac patients who had aromatherapy massage with the essential oil of neroli *(citrus aurantium ssp. aurantium)* compared with those who had massage with a plain vegetable oil (Stevensen, 1994). Other studies have shown positive psychological benefits from massage, including positive subjective response (Madison, 1973), the perceived state of relaxation (Longworth, 1982), reported pleasurable feelings (Bauer & Dracup, 1987), and an improvement in the perceived level of anxiety (Dunn, 1992). Physiological results from massage generally have shown no significant difference in heart rate or arterial blood pressure (Bauer & Dracup, 1987; Dunn, 1992; Kaufmann, 1964; Longworth, 1982; Reed & Held, 1988) or in respiratory rate (Bauer & Dracup, 1987; Dunn, 1992; Kaufman, 1964; Longworth, 1982; Reed & Held, 1988). The importance of massage for both relaxation and release of physical and psychological stress should not be underestimated and can be seen only as a positive aid to the administration of essential oils when administered appropriately.

It is suggested that aromatherapy would not have gained its rapid increase in popularity if the oils were not fragrant, thus affecting mood and emotions. Several references have already been made to the inextricable link between the development of human biology, the sense of smell, and the importance of aromas. Sigmund Freud developed the idea of "organic repression" of the sense of smell. He attributed this to upright gait, which elevates the nose from the ground, where it had enjoyed pleasurable sensations previously (Freud, 1929). This repression may not be complete, but many people have a diminished sense of smell, a sense more vital to the survival of animals than humans. It may be this need to satisfy pleasurable sensations via the sense of smell that is attracting so many people to aromatherapy.

The human response to aromas is associated with olfaction naturally. The neurons of the olfactory system, which are the chemical senses of the body, rest in the section of the midbrain known as the *limbic system*. The structures of the limbic system extend from the midbrain through the hypothalamus into the basal forebrain, which is concerned not only with visceral functions but also with emotional expression. The cortical and medial nuclei of the amygdala, a body situated within this system, receive information from the olfactory system. The basolateral nuclei are involved with the expression of emotion (Shepherd, 1983). Therefore aromatherapy's effect on emotion and psychological state is not surprising (Hardy, 1992; Stevensen, 1994). The emotional and psychological benefit of aromatherapy is important in many clinical situations, including chronic, life-threatening conditions such as cancer, heart disease, and acquired immunodeficiency syndrome.

SETTINGS

Aromatherapy is used in many settings throughout Europe and the United Kingdom. These settings include clinics run by private aromatherapists, clinics attached to general medical practices, and orthodox health care settings used by aromatherapists or other health care professionals who have been trained in aromatherapy. With regard to the practice of aromatherapy, individual member countries of the European Union each have their own regulations.

Under English Common Law a person is innocent until proven guilty. Because there is no law currently stating a minimum level of training and practice in aromatherapy in the United Kingdom, practitioners can perform without attaining a minimum standard of competence. The British Department of Employment has granted funding for a working party to define national occupational standards for aromatherapy, reflexology, homeopathy, and hypnotherapy. A core curriculum for these complementary therapies also is being proposed. Meanwhile, aromatherapists are working toward statutory registration in line with what currently exists for osteopaths since 1993. The Aromatherapy Organisations Council, the governing body for aromatherapy, currently represents 80 percent of the profession, 13 professional associations, and 80 schools and colleges with set minimum standards.

In other European countries legislation on the practice of complementary therapies, including aromatherapy, is different because European law differs from English law. Under the Napoleonic Law developed from the Treaty of Rome, a person is guilty until proven innocent. The practice of complementary therapies in Switzerland, Germany, and France is illegal unless a person is medically qualified, although nonmedical practitioners are tolerated to a certain extent. No therapist in Europe can advertise treatment of any kind or make medical claims except helping stress. *Treatment* is taken to mean a treatment of any physical or mental disorder by medical or physical means. Because of the legal difficulties of calling oneself a therapist in either Switzerland or Germany, practitioners of aromatherapy have coined the term *aromatology* and call themselves *aromatologists* (Ashby, 1993).

Aromatherapists who work in practices with general medical practitioners generally do so on a session-by-session basis. The physician often maintains clinical responsibility for the patient referred to the aromatherapist. Aromatherapy in orthodox health care settings is being provided by lay aromatherapists and increasingly by trained nurses or other health care professionals such as physiotherapists with aromatherapy training. According to the United Kingdom Central Council (UKCC) Code of Professional Conduct, each nurse is accountable for his or her own actions, including standards of training to ensure competence in practice (UKCC, 1992). The use of aromatherapy within nursing practice falls into this category. Professional bodies such as the Royal College of Nursing (RCN) will provide insurance for nurses using aromatherapy within their nursing practice. Chartered physiotherapists in the country have to obtain separate insurance for the use of aromatherapy.

Growth in the use of and interest in aromatherapy has developed so rapidly in recent years that professional legislation has struggled to keep up. Aromatherapy and massage are being taught to professional audiences in Southeast Asia, Australia, and North America, while being reintroduced as a mod-

ern concept with cutaneous application for the use of health care professionals other than doctors in some European countries.

Settings in the United Kingdom where aromatherapy has been adopted are included in Box 10-1. The reasons for the use of aromatherapy in these settings are diverse and may include the reasons mentioned in Box 10-2. These boxes are not conclusive, but research performed to support the use of aromatherapy in some of these settings is discussed later.

The United Kingdom is being used as a model for many other countries with regard to legislation regarding the practice of aromatherapy. In the European Union debate in 1994 focused on the regulation of herbal medicines, including essential oils, in preparation for the single European market. Historically, English practitioners have been able to dispense herbal medicines using special rights afforded them by Henry VIII. In the 1994 debate, no undue pressure was being placed on the United Kingdom to implement the directive, and in line with a discretionary caveat allowing each European member country to amend a directive, Germany chose to exempt herbal medicines from licensing. The British House of Commons tabled a motion on October 27, 1994 (Motion 1672, 1994), to discuss this matter. The British government decided that herbal medicines should continue to be exempt from licensing requirements and not subject to the new regulations required by the European directive. Notice was made of the valuable contribution of herbal medicines over the centuries and concern was raised at the large cost of providing the research data necessary to meet the licensing

---

BOX 10-1

Conventional Medical Settings Where Aromatherapy Is Used in the United Kingdom

Intensive care units	Palliative care settings
Coronary care units	Hospices
Renal units	Pediatric units
Neurologic units	Midwifery units
HIV/AIDS units	Learning disability
Geriatric units	settings
Cancer units	Burns units

HIV, Human immunodeficiency virus; *AIDS,* acquired immunodeficiency syndrome.

BOX 10-2

Reasons to Administer Aromatherapy in Conventional Medical Settings

Relaxation
Stress and anxiety relief
Pain and discomfort relief
Insomnia and restlessness
Infections and wound healing
Burns
Enhancing self-image
Stimulating immune function
Treatment for constipation

requirements, as well as the cost of licensing each product.

RESEARCH

As with many other complementary therapies, the research basis for aromatherapy is incomplete. Problems already have been noted regarding the attributes given to some essential oils that have their basis in herbal medicine rather than aromatherapy research. In fact, much of the research performed on the use of essential oils or their individual constituents has been performed in animal models and isolated tissue cultures. Few trials have been conducted in human subjects under clinical conditions. Kusmirek (1992) identifies the problem with the rapid development of aromatherapy: popular use has outstripped research. Members of the medical profession and those wanting to use aromatherapy in the conventional health care settings have found that this lack of research in essential oils precludes acceptance of aromatherapy in the clinical environment. Little is known about possible interactions with conventional medications or treatments, but it is presumed that because the doses of essential oils absorbed in the body generally are small and because there has been no reported incidence of difficulties, essential oils administered in physiological doses are safe given the contraindications mentioned earlier. However, further research is required. This section presents a brief review of aromatherapy research data, with particular emphasis on the action of the essential oils. A more detailed description may be found in Vickers (1996).

Antimicrobial Activity

The effect of essential oils on a wide variety of pathogens is well known. Their chemical constituents of alcohols and aldehydes, terpenes, and phenyl methyl ethers help explain this action. The antimicrobial aspects of essential oils have been the most widely investigated. Janssen et al. (1987) performed a useful review of the literature in this field from the 1970s to the early 1980s. They concluded that many essential oils do have antimicrobial effects but found this difficult to qualify because of the variation in test methods and the insufficient description of essential oils and microorganisms in some studies. From the different chemotypes or chemical subgroups of *Thymus vulgaris* (common thyme), the strongest antifungal chemotype had eight times the effect of the weakest (Janssen et al., 1987).

Another investigation reported antibacterial activity of a number of oils, including *Artemisia dracunculus* (tarragon), *Salvia officinalis L* (sage), *Salvia sclarea* (clary sage), and *Thymus vulgaris L* (thyme) (Zani, 1991). Other studies support the antimicrobial actions of essential oils (Baylier, 1979; Panizzi et al., 1993). There also is evidence that the constituents of essential oils have antimicrobial properties. The alcohols geraniol, eugenol, menthol, and citral all showed high antibacterial activity in one investigation (Moleyar & Narasimham, 1992).

Animal Models

Buchbauer et al. (1991) performed perhaps the most extensive research on essential oils in animal models. After 1 hour of inhaling an essential oil or fragrance compound, mice became sedated by sandalwood, rose, neroli, and lavender. Some of the constituent compounds found to have a sedative effect on inhalation were anethole, bornyl salicylate, coumarin, 2-phenylethyl acetate, benaldehyde, citronella, and geranyl acetate. Compounds that resulted in stimulation after inhalation include geraniol, isoborneol, isoeugenol, nerol, methylsalicylate, α-pinene, and thymol. Lavender oil was found to be a more effective sedative than either of its major constituents (linalool and linalyl acetate) in isolation (Buchbauer, 1993). Again, this supports aromatherapists' claims of synergy within essential oils (Price, 1995; Tisserand, 1988).

Tissue Cultures

Peppermint, commonly known for its benefit in digestive disorders, has been found to inhibit gastrointestinal smooth muscle in tissue models (Taylor et al., 1983) and affects the flow of calcium across the cell wall of the gastrointestinal smooth muscle (Taylor et al., 1984). Large doses of peppermint might have been found to induce spasm. This idea would support findings that large doses in essential oils may produce opposite effects.

Pharmacological Preparations in Animals

The effects of essential oils with pharmacological preparations in animals have been studied. The concern from the medical profession and aromatherapists alike regarding the lack of information about interaction between aromatherapy oils and conventional drug preparations in humans already has been mentioned. Jori investigated the effects of essential oils on drug metabolism, using pentobarbital, a sedative drug, to induce sleep in rats. 1,8-cineole, an oxide, was found to significantly interfere with pentobarbital. Both the sleeping times and the brain levels of the drug were reduced by about 50 percent after subcutaneous injection and aerosol inhalation. These effects were persistent even when the 1,8-cineole was administered 36 hours before the pentobarbital (Jorich, 1969). Similar results were reported elsewhere (Wade et al., 1986).

Psychological Effects

In Torri et al.'s 1988 study, inhalation of various essential oils was found to lead to a change in brain wave activity. The oils were measured for an increase (+) or decrease (−) of brain wave activity. Table 10-2 summarizes the results of Torri et al.'s study.

This study generally supports the claims of stimulation and relaxation made about essential oils, with particular reference to jasmine as stimulating and lavender as relaxing (Tisserand, 1988). Overstimulation from the oils was found to have a lowering effect on brain waves, which is suggested to be the same effect that oil would have in clinical use. If this is so, dosage of essential oils may need closer examination through further trials.

Analgesic Effects

Analgesic properties are attributed to some oils, although the evidence for this is scarce. One study demonstrated that lemongrass leaves produced a dose-dependent analgesia in rats. Both subplantar and oral doses of the constituent myrcene were administered with similar effect. Myrcene, a constituent of oils, including rosemary, lavender, juniper, and lemongrass to a lesser extent, was credited with the effect (Lorenzetti et al., 1991). Undiluted lavender oil is well known as a first-aid remedy for minor burns, both removing pain and promoting healing, as in Gattefossé's laboratory accident.

Recent Clinical Research

Most of the recent aromatherapy research in the conventional health care settings in the United Kingdom has been undertaken by nurses with a particular interest in the field. A number of studies have been performed in the intensive care setting, with others performed in the field of midwifery, palliative care, and care of the elderly. Some of these trials found psychological benefits to the patients from aromatherapy, in addition to massage. In a randomized controlled trial, 100 cardiac surgery patients in intensive care received the aromatherapy oil of neroli citrus (*aurantium ssp. aurantium*) in foot massage and found anxiety in particular to be further reduced than in patients who were massaged with a plain vegetable oil after 4 days (Stevensen, 1994). Both groups who had the massage with or without the neroli oil scored significantly better statistically on a modified Spielberger state anxiety questionnaire than did the control groups on the day of massage. The only significant physiological difference between the massage and nonmassage groups was transient and related to respiratory rate immediately after the massage. Buckle

TABLE 10-2

Effects of Inhalation of Essential Oils on Brain Wave Activity

Oil	Effect	Oil	Effect
Basil	++	Marjoram	−
Bergamot	−	Neroli	+++
Rosewood	+/−	Patchouli	+
Camomile	−	Peppermint	+++
Clove	+++	Rose	++
Geranium	+/−	Sage	+
Jasmine	++	Sandalwood	−
Lavender	−	Valerian	+/−
Lemon	−	Ylang ylang	+++
Lemongrass	+		

+, Increase in brain wave activity; *−*, decrease in brain wave activity.

(1993) massaged postcardiotomy patients with two different lavender essential oils, *Lavandula angustifolia* and *Lavandula latifolia,* hoping to show a difference between the effects of the two oils. Although the presentation of the trial lacked detail and the results were insignificant, there was some difference between the two oils, somewhat supporting the conclusion that massage with essential oils proved more beneficial than massage without essential oils (Buckle, 1993). In an unpublished study Dunn (1992) used intensive care as a setting in a randomized trial to measure the effects of massage with lavender oil compared with plain oil massage and rest in 122 patients. Physiological changes were not significant, but positive psychological changes were better for those massaged with essential oil than for those who received the plain oil massage, and that over the period of rest (Dunn, 1992).

Anecdotal reports from mothers that lavender oil helped relieve perineal discomfort after childbirth were followed with a randomized trial involving 635 women. Each woman was given a bottle of either pure lavender oil, a synthetic lavender oil that smelled like the other, or an inert compound, with instructions to add six drops to their bath daily. Results were not significant, but pain was slightly reduced in the pure lavender group. That group also had the highest rates of infection (Dale & Cornwall, 1994). This study may demonstrate that anecdotal reports from patients about essential oils are not reliable.

In a study of 51 patients attending a center for palliative care, the effects of three aromatherapy massages given weekly were examined with or without the essential oil of Roman chamomile, *Chamemalum nobile.* Using the Rotterdam Symptom checklist (RSCL) and State-trait anxiety inventory, posttest scores for all patients improved. These were statistically significant in the aromatherapy group on the RSCL physical symptom subscale, quality-of-life subscale, and state anxiety scale (Wilkinson, 1995). In a small study of four patients on a long-stay elderly care ward, researchers assessed sleep over three consecutive 2-week periods—the first period with night sedation, the second without, and the third with lavender diffused into the air at set intervals. Sleep was poorer in the second week, and in the third week sleep was as good as in the first week (Hardy, 1992). However, this trial was assessed only by observation.

Aromatherapy in clinical research is in its infancy. There are methodological problems with much of the clinical research presented that make results difficult to assess. In the absence of further clinical trials, there also is the problem that aromatherapists are relying on many trials from animal and tissue models for the basis of their practice. There is no guarantee that these results can be replicated in humans. It is likely that, as more and better-quality research is performed in the clinical use of aromatherapy, its appropriate place in the field of complementary medicine will become established. Perhaps because of this history, Europe (including the United Kingdom) is well advanced in aromatherapy. This situation provides another example of the advancement of Europe over the United States in the application and integration of alternative therapies.

CONCLUSION

This chapter has demonstrated the relatively recent development of aromatherapy compared with other areas of complementary medicine. Although aromatic substances and oils have been used throughout history, no sound system has been developed for their use, a fact especially evident when comparing aromatherapy to a system such as Chinese Medicine. Recent interest in essential oils by both aromatherapists and health care professionals should encourage more research into the science of aromatherapy so that understanding may be gained as to the importance and worth of this natural therapy. Until a sound scientific base is ascertained, it is believed that aromatherapy will not take a full place beside the more established complementary health care systems.

Acknowledgments

I would like to acknowledge the information given by Andrew Vickers of the Research Council for Complementary Medicine, London, in completion of the research section in this chapter.

References

Arcier M. 1990. Aromatherapy. Hamlyn, London
Ashby N. 1993. Aromatherapy in the balance: aromatherapy in the UK and Europe—an overview by law. Aromatherapy Q 37:13-14

Bauer WC, Dracup KA. 1987. Physiologic effects of back massage in patients with acute myocardial infarction. Focus Crit Care 14(6):42-46

Baylier MF. 1979. Bacteriostatic activity of some Australian essential oils. Perfumer and Flavourist 4(23):23-25

Boyd EM, Pearson GL. 1946. The expectorant action of volatile oils. Am J Med Sci 211:602-611

Bronough RL. 1990. In vivo percutaneous absorption of fragrance ingredients in rhesus monkeys and humans. Food Chem Toxicol 28(5):369-374

Buchbauer G, et al. 1991. Aromatherapy: Evidence for sedative effects of the essential oil of lavender after inhalation. Z Naturforsch 46:1067-1072

Buckle J. 1993. Aromatherapy: does it matter which lavender oil is used? Nurs Times 89(20):32-35

Chambers Dictionary. 1988. R and W Chambers Ltd and Cambridge University Press, Cambridge

Collins AJ, Notarianni LJ, Ring EF, Seed MP. 1984. Some observations on the pharmacology of 'deep-heat', a topical rubefacient. Ann Rheum Dis 43(3):411-415

Dale A, Cornwall S. 1994. The role of lavender oil in relieving perineal discomfort following childbirth: a blind randomized clinical trial. J Adv Nurs 19:89-96

Dodd GH. 1991. The molecular dimension in perfumery, in Van Toller S, Dodd GH (eds). Perfumery: The Psychology and Biology of Fragrance. Chapman and Hall, London

Dunn C. 1992. A report on a randomized controlled trial to evaluate the use of massage and aromatherapy in an intensive care unit. Unpublished paper. Reading, Battle Hospital

Falk A. 1990. Uptake, distribution and elimination of alpha-pinene in man after exposure by inhalation. Scand J Work Environ Health 16:372-378

Falk-Filipsson A. 1993. d-limonene exposure to humans by inhalation: uptake distribution, elimination and effects on the pulmonary system. Toxicol Environ Health 38:77-88

Franchomme P, Pénoël D. 1990. L'aromatherapie exactement. Roger Jallois, Limoges

Freud S. 1929. The Complete Psychological Works. Vol 21. Civilization and Its Discontents. Strachy J (ed). Hogath Press, London

Hardy M. 1992. Sweet scented dreams. Int J Aromatherapy CW Daniels, Saffron Waldon

Hotchkiss S. 1994. How thin is your skin? New Scientist 141 (1910):24-27

House of Commons Notices of motions 1672 No. 150 27. October 1994

Jäger W, Buckbauer, Jirovetz L, Fritzer M. 1992. Percutaneous absorption of lavender oil from a massage oil. J Soc Cosmetic Chem 43:49-54

Janssen AM, et al. 1987. Antimicrobial activity of essential oils: 1976-1986 literature review. Planta Med 53(5):395-398

Kaufman MA. 1964. Autonomic responses as related to nursing comfort measures. Nurs Res 13:45-55

Kovar KA, Gropper B, Friess D, Ammon HP. 1987. Blood levels of 1,8-cineole and locomotor activity of mice after inhalation and oral administration of rosemary oil. Planta Med 53(4):315-318

Kusmirek J. 1992. Perspectives in aromatherapy, in Van Toller S, Dodd GH (eds). Fragrance: The Psychology and Biology of Perfume. Elsevier Science Pub. Ltd., Barking

Longworth JCD. 1982. Psychophysiological effects of slow stroke back massage in normatensive females. Adv Nurs Sci July:44-61

Lorenzetti BE, Souza GE, Sarti SJ, et al. 1991. Myrcene mimics the peripheral analgesic activity of lemongrass tea. J Ethnopharmacol 34(1):43-48

Madison AS. 1973. Psychophysiological response of female nursing home residents to back massage: an investigation of one type of touch. Doctoral thesis, University of Maryland

Maury M. 1964. The Secret of Life and Youth. Macdonald, London

Moleyar V, Narasimham P. 1992. Antibacterial activity of essential oil components. Int J Food Microbiol 16(4):337-342

Panizzi L, Flamini G, Cioni FL, Morelli I. 1993. Composition and antimicrobial properties of essential oils of four Mediterranean Lamiaceae. J Ethnopharmacol 39(3):167-70

Price S. 1995. Aromatherapy for Health Care Professionals. Churchill Livingstone, Edinburgh

Reed BV, Held JM. 1988. Effects of sequential tissue massage on autonomic nervous system of middle aged and elderly adults. Phys Ther 68(8):1231-1234

Shepherd GM. 1983. Neurobiology. Oxford University Press, Oxford

Steele JJ. 1992. The anthropology of smell and scent in ancient Egypt and South American Shamanism, in Van Toller S, Dodd GH (eds). Fragrance: The Psychology and Biology of Perfume. Elsevier Science Pub. Ltd, Barking

Stevensen CJ. 1994. The psychophysiological effects of aromatherapy massage following cardiac surgery. Comple Ther Med 2:27-35

Stoddart DM. 1991. Human odour culture: a zoological perspective, in Van Toller S, Dodd GH (eds). Perfumery: The Psychology and Biology of Fragrance. Chapman and Hall, London

Taylor BA, Luscombe CK, Duthie HL. 1983. Inhibitory effect of peppermint oil on gastrointestinal smooth muscle. Gut 24:A992

Taylor BA, Luscombe DK, Duthie HL. 1984. Inhibitory effect of peppermint and menthol on human isolated coli. Gut 25:A1168

Tisserand R. 1988. The Art of Aromatherapy. Daniel Co Ltd, Saffron Waldon, United Kingdom

Tisserand R, Balacs T. 1995. Essential Oil Safety. Churchill Livingstone, Edinburgh

Torri S, Fukuda H, Kanemoto H, et al. 1988. Contingent negative variation (CNV) and the psychological effects of odour, in Van Toller S, Dodd GH (eds). Perfumery: The Psychology and Biology of Fragrance. Chapman and Hall, London, pp. 107-121

UKCC. 1992. Code of Professional Practice. United Kingdom Central Council of Nursing, Midwifery and Health Visiting, London

Valnet J. 1990. The Practice of Aromatherapy. Daniel Co Ltd, Saffron Waldon, United Kingdom

Vickers AJ. 1996. Massage and Aromatherapy: A Guide For Health Care Professionals. Chapman and Hall, London

Wade AE, et al. 1986. Alteration of drug metabolism in rats and mice by an environment of cedarwood. Pharmacology 1:317-328

Wilkinson S. 1995. Int J Palliative Nurs 1(1);21-30

Williams D. 1989. Lecture notes on essential oils. Eve Taylor

Suggested Readings

Consumers' Association. 1992. Survey: Alternative Medicine. Which? London. November. pp. 44-49

Davis P. 1990. Aromatherapy: A-Z. CW Daniel, Saffron Waldon

Dodd GH, Van Toller S. 1983. The biology and psychology of perfumery. Perfumer and Flavorist 8:1-14

Van Toller S, Dodd GH. 1992. Fragrance: The Psychology and Biology of Perfume. Elsevier Science Pub. Ltd., Barking, United Kingdom

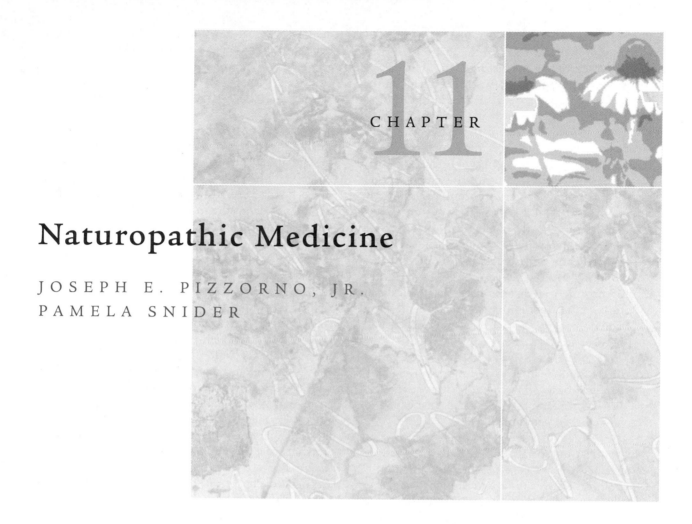

Naturopathic Medicine

JOSEPH E. PIZZORNO, JR.
PAMELA SNIDER

The doctor of the future will give no medicine, but will interest his patient in the care of the human frame, in diet and in the cause and prevention of disease.

—THOMAS EDISON

Thomas Edison's insightful prediction is proving true today, as natural medicine finds itself in the midst of an unprecedented explosion into mainstream health care. Consumers are spending more annually out of pocket for alternative medicine than for conventional care. In particular, naturopathic medicine as the model for integrative primary care natural medicine is undergoing a powerful resurgence. With its unique integration of vitalistic, scientific, academic, and clinical training in medicine, the naturopathic medical model is a potent contributing factor to this health care revolution.

HISTORY*

Although naturopathic medicine traces its philosophical roots to many traditional world medicines, its body of knowledge derives from a rich heritage of writings and practices of Western and non-Western nature doctors since Hippocrates (circa 400 BC). Modern naturopathic medicine grew out of healing systems of the eighteenth and nineteenth centuries. The term *naturopathy* was coined in 1895 by Dr. John

*The author expresses his appreciation to George Cody, whose chapter "History of Naturopathic Medicine," in *A Textbook of Natural Medicine*, JE Pizzorno and MT Murray, eds., John Bastyr College Publications, Seattle, Wash, 1995, provided the basis for much of this section.

Scheel of New York City to describe his method of health care. However, earlier forerunners of these concepts already existed in the history of natural healing, both in America and in the Austro-Germanic European core. Naturopathy became a formal profession after its creation by Benedict Lust in 1896. The profession has now celebrated its 104th birthday. Over the centuries, natural medicine and biomedicine have alternately diverged and converged, shaping each other, often in reaction. During the past hundred years the profession progressed through several fairly distinct phases:

1. Latter part of the nineteenth century: *The Founding By Benedict Lust;* origin in the Germanic hydrotherapy and nature cure traditions.

2. 1900 to 1917: *The Formative Years;* convergence of the American dietetic, hygienic, physical culture, spinal manipulation, mental and emotional healing, Thompsonian/eclectic, and homeopathic systems.

3. 1918 to 1937: *The Halcyon Days;* during a period of great public interest and support, the philosophical basis and scope of therapies diversified to encompass botanical, homeopathic, and environmental medicine.

4. 1938 to 1970: *Suppression and Decline;* growing political and social dominance of the American Medical Association (AMA), lack of internal political unity, and lack of unifying standards, combined with the American love affair with technology and the emergence of "miracle" drugs and effective modern surgical techniques perfected in two world wars, resulted in legal and economic suppression.

5. 1971 to present: *Naturopathic Medicine Reemerges;* reawakened awareness of the American public of the importance of health promotion; prevention of disease; and concern for the environment and the establishment of modern, accredited, physician-level training reestablished public interest in naturopathic medicine, resulting in rapid resurgence. Current projections predict a continuing increase in naturopathic physicians.

The per capita supply of alternative medicine clinicians (chiropractors, naturopaths and practitioners of Oriental medicine) will grow by 88% between 1994 and 2010, while allopathic physician supply will grow by 16%. . . . The total number of naturopathy graduates will double over the next five years. The total number of naturopathic physicians will triple (Cooper & Stoflet, 1996).

The Founding of Naturopathy

Naturopathy, as a generally used term, began with the teachings and concepts of Benedict Lust. In 1892, at the age of 23, Lust came from Germany as a disciple of Father Kneipp (the greatest practitioner of hydrotherapy) to bring Kneipp's hydrotherapy practices to America. Exposure in the United States to a wide range of practitioners and practices of natural healing arts broadened Lust's perspective, and after a decade of study, he purchased the term *naturopathy* from Scheel of New York City (who coined the term in 1895) in 1902 to describe the eclectic compilation of doctrines of natural healing that he envisioned was to be the future of natural medicine. Naturopathy, or "nature cure," was defined by Lust as both a way of life and a concept of healing that used various natural means of treating human infirmities and disease states. The earliest therapies associated with the term involved a combination of American hygienics and Austro-Germanic nature cure and hydrotherapy.

In January of 1902, Lust, who had been publishing the *Kneipp Water Cure Monthly* and its German language counterpart in New York since 1896, changed the name of the journal to *The Naturopathic and Herald of Health* and began promoting a new way of thinking of health care with the following editorial:

We believe in strong, pure, beautiful bodies . . . of radiating health. We want every man, woman and child in this great land to know and embody and feel the truths of right living that mean conscious mastery. We plead for the renouncing of poisons from the coffee, white flour, glucose, lard, and like venom of the American table to patent medicines, tobacco, liquor and the other inevitable recourse of perverted appetite. We long for the time when an eight-hour day may enable every worker to stop existing long enough to live; when the spirit of universal brotherhood shall animate business and society and the church; when every American may have a little cottage of his own, and a bit of ground where he may combine Aerotherapy, Heliotherapy, Geotherapy, Aristophagy and nature's other forces with home and peace and happiness and things forbidden to flat-dwellers; when people may stop doing and thinking and being for others and be for themselves; when true love and divine marriage and prenatal culture and controlled parenthood may fill this world with germ-gods instead of humanized animals.

In a word, Naturopathy stands for the reconciling, harmonizing and unifying of nature, humanity and God.

Fundamentally therapeutic because men need healing; elementary educational because men need teaching; ultimately inspirational because men need empowering.

Benedict Lust

According to his published personal history, Lust had a debilitating condition in his late teens while growing up in Michelbach, Baden, Germany, and had been sent by his father to undergo the Kneipp cure at Woerishofen. He stayed there from mid-1890 to early 1892. Not only was he "cured" of his condition, but he became a protégé of Father Kneipp. He emigrated to America to proselytize the principles of the Kneipp Water-Cure (Figure 11-1).

By making contact in New York with other German Americans who were also becoming aware of the Kneipp principles, Lust participated in the founding of the first "Kneipp Society," which was organized in Jersey City, New Jersey, in 1896. Subsequently, through Lust's organization and contacts, Kneipp Societies were also founded in Brooklyn, Boston, Chicago, Cleveland, Denver, Cincinnati, Philadelphia, Columbus, Buffalo, Rochester, New Haven, San Francisco, the state of New Mexico, and Mineola on Long Island. The members of these organizations were provided with copies of the *Kneipp Blatter* and a companion English publication Lust began to put out called *The Kneipp Water-Cure Monthly*. In 1895 Lust opened the Kneipp Water-Cure Institute on 59th Street in New York City.

Father Kneipp died in Germany, at Woerishofen, on June 17, 1897. With his passing, Lust was no longer bound strictly to the principles of the Kneipp water-cure. He had begun to associate earlier with other German American physicians, principally Dr. Hugo R. Wendel (a German-trained "Naturarzt") who began, in 1897, to practice in New York and New Jersey as a licensed osteopathic physician. In 1896 Lust entered the Universal Osteopathic College of New York and became licensed as an osteopathic physician in 1898.

Once he was licensed to practice as a health care physician in his own right, Lust began the transition toward the concept of "naturopathy." Between 1898 and 1902, when he adopted the term *naturopath,* Lust acquired a chiropractic education; changed the name of his Kneipp Store (which he had opened in 1895) to "Health Food Store" (the first facility to use that name and concept in this country), specializing in providing organically grown foods and the materials

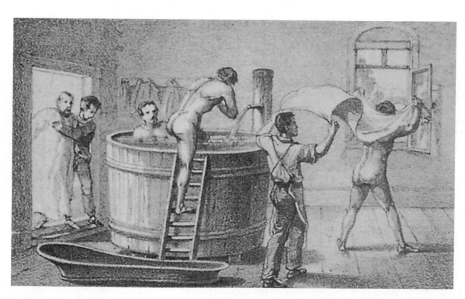

Figure 11-1 Curative baths, one form of hydrotherapy, were a popular form of natural healing in the late nineteenth century. (Courtesy Wellcome Institute Library, London.)

necessary for drugless cures; and founded the New York School of Massage (in 1896) and the American School of Chiropractic.

In 1902, when he purchased and began using the term *naturopathy* and calling himself a "naturopath," Lust, in addition to his New York School of Massage and American School of Chiropractic, his various publications, and his operation of the Health Food Store, began to operate the American School of Naturopathy, all at the same 59th Street address. By 1907 Lust's enterprises had grown sufficiently large that he moved them to a 55-room building. It housed the Naturopathic Institute, Clinic, and Hospital; the American Schools of Naturopathy and Chiropractic; the now entitled "Original Health Food Store"; Lust's publishing enterprises; and New York School of Massage. The operation remained in this four-story building, roughly twice the size of the original facility, from 1907 to 1915.

In the period of 1912 through 1914, Lust took a sabbatical from his operations to further his education. By this time he had founded his large estatelike sanitarium at Butler, New Jersey, known as "Yungborn" after the German sanitarium operation of Adoph Just. In 1912 he attended the Homeopathic Medical College in New York, which, in 1913, granted him a degree in homeopathic medicine and, in 1914, a degree in eclectic medicine. In early 1914 Lust traveled to Florida and obtained an MD's license on the basis of his graduation from the Homeopathic Medical College.

From 1902, when he began to use the term *naturopathy,* until 1918, Lust replaced the Kneipp Societies with the Naturopathic Society of America. Then in December 1919, the Naturopathic Society of America was formally dissolved because of insolvency and Lust founded the "American Naturopathic Association." Thereafter, the association was incorporated in some additional 18 states. Lust claimed to at one time have 40,000 practitioners practicing naturopathy. In 1918, as part of his effort to replace the Naturopathic Society of America (an operation into which he invested a great deal of his funds and resources in an attempt to organize a Naturopathic profession) and replace it with the American Naturopathic Association, Lust published the first *Yearbook of Drugless Therapy.* Annual supplements were published in either *The Naturopath and the Herald of Health* or its companion publication with which *The Naturopath* at one time merged, *Nature's Path* (which began publication

in 1925). *The Naturopath and Herald of Health,* sometimes printed with the two phrases reversed, was published from 1902 through 1927, and from 1934 until after Lust's death in 1945.

Benedict Lust's principles of health are found in the introduction to the first volume of the *Universal Naturopathic Directory and Buyer's Guide,* a portion of which is reproduced in Box 11-1. Although the terminology is almost a century old, the concepts Lust proposed have provided a powerful foundation that has endured despite almost a century of active political suppression by the dominant school of medicine.

The Schools of Thought That Formed the Philosophical Basis of Naturopathy

Because of its eclectic nature, the history of naturopathic medicine is by far the most complex of any healing art, hence the unusually large portion of this chapter devoted to this subject. Although the following discussion is divided into distinct schools of thought, this is somewhat artificial because those that founded and practiced these arts (especially the Americans) were often trained in, influenced by, and practiced several therapeutic modalities. However, it was not until Benedict Lust that the many threads were woven together into a unified professional practice, making naturopathic medicine the first Western system of full-scope integrative natural medicine based on the *vis medicatrix naturae.* The following presents the formative schools of Western thought in natural healing and some of their leading adherents. Although the therapies differ, the philosophical thread of promoting health and supporting the body's own healing processes runs through them all. These threads are derived from centuries of medical scholarship, both Western and non-Western, concerning the self-healing process. After a brief overview of Hippocrates' seminal contribution to the natural medicine way of thought, the basic themes are presented in order: healthful living; natural diet; detoxification; exercise, mechanotherapy and physical therapy; mental, emotional, and spiritual healing; and natural therapeutic agents. Hippocrates and centuries of nature doctors' writings remain empirically rich repositories of observations for future research.

BOX 11-1

The Principles, Aim, and Program of the Nature Cure System

Since the earliest ages, medical science has been of all sciences the most unscientific. Its professors, with few exceptions, have sought to cure disease by the magic of pills and potions and poisons that attacked the ailment with the idea of suppressing the symptoms instead of attacking the real cause of the ailment.

Medical science has always believed in the superstition that the use of chemical substances that are harmful and destructive to human life will prove an efficient substitute for the violation of laws, and in this way encourages the belief that a man may go the limit in self-indulgences that weaken and destroy his physical system, and then hope to be absolved from his physical ailments by swallowing a few pills, or submitting to an injection of a serum or vaccine, that are supposed to act as vicarious redeemers of the physical organism and counteract life-long practices that are poisonous and wholly destructive to the patient's well-being.

The policy of expediency is at the basis of medical drug healing. It is along the lines of self-indulgence, indifference, ignorance and lack of self-control that drug medicine lives, moves and has its being.

The natural system for curing disease is based on a return to nature in regulating the diet, breathing, exercising, bathing and the employment of various forces to eliminate the poisonous products in the system, and so raise the vitality of the patient to a proper standard of health.

Official medicine has, in all ages, simply attacked the symptoms of disease without paying any attention to the causes thereof, but natural healing is concerned far more with removing the causes of disease, than merely curing its symptoms. This is the glory of this new school of medicine that it cures by removing the causes of the ailment, and is the only rational method of practicing medicine. It begins its cures by avoiding the uses of drugs and hence is styled the system of drugless healing.

The Program of Naturopathic Cure

1. ELIMINATION OF EVIL HABITS, or the weeds of life, such as over-eating, alcoholic drinks, drugs, the use of tea, coffee and cocoa that contain poisons, meat eating, improper hours of living, waste of vital forces, lowered vitality, sexual and social aberrations, worry, etc.
2. CORRECTIVE HABITS. Correct breathing, correct exercise, right mental attitude. Moderation in the pursuit of health and wealth.
3. NEW PRINCIPLES OF LIVING. Proper fasting, selection of food, hydropathy, light and air baths, mud baths, osteopathy, chiropractic and other forms of mechano-therapy, mineral salts obtained in organic form, electropathy, heliopathy, steam or Turkish baths, sitz baths, etc.

Natural healing is the most desirable factor in the regeneration of the race. It is a return to nature in methods of living and treatment. It makes use of the elementary forces of nature, of chemical selection of foods that will constitute a correct medical dietary. The diet of civilized man is devitalized, is poor in essential organic salts. The fact that foods are cooked in so many ways and are salted, spiced, sweetened and otherwise made attractive to the palate, induces people to over-eat, and over eating does more harm than under feeding. High protein food and lazy habits are the cause of cancer, Bright's disease, rheumatism and the poisons of autointoxication.

There is really but one healing force in existence and that is Nature herself, which means the inherent restorative power of the organism to overcome disease. Now the question is, can this power be appropriated and guided more readily by extrinsic or intrinsic methods? That is to say, is it more amenable to combat disease by irritating drugs, vaccines and serums employed by superstitious moderns, or by the bland intrinsic congenial forces of Natural Therapeutics, that are employed by this new school of medicine, that is Naturopathy, which is the only orthodox school of medicine? Are not these natural forces much more orthodox than the artificial resources of the druggist?

Benedict Lust's "Principles of Health," Vol. 1, *Universal Naturopathic Directory and Buyer's Guide,* 1918, Lust Publications, Butler, NJ.

Hippocrates

Prehistoric people believed that disease was caused by magic or supernatural forces, such as devils or angry gods. Hippocrates, breaking with this superstitious belief, became the first naturalistic doctor in recorded history. Hippocrates regarded the body as a whole and instructed his students to prescribe only beneficial treatments and refrain from causing harm or hurt.

Hippocratic practitioners assumed that everything in nature had a rational basis; therefore the physician's role was to understand and follow the laws of the intelligible universe. They viewed disease as an effect and looked for its cause in natural phenomena: air, water, food, and so forth. They first used the term *vis medicatrix naturae,* the healing power of nature, to denote the body's ability and drive to heal itself. One of the central tenets is that "there is an order to the process of healing which requires certain things to be done before other things to maximize the effectiveness of the therapeutics" (Zeff, 1997). The step order used by Tibetan medicine is also an example of this tenet represented in traditional world medicines.

Hydrotherapy

The earliest philosophical origins of naturopathy were clearly in the Germanic hydrotherapy movement: the use of hot and cold water for the maintenance of health and the treatment of disease. One of the oldest known therapies (water was used therapeutically by the Romans and Greeks), the modern history of hydrotherapy began with the publication of *The History of Cold Bathing* in 1697 by Sir John Floyer. Probably the strongest impetus for its use came from Central Europe, where it was advocated by such well-known hydropaths as Priessnitz, Schroth, and Father Kneipp. They were able to popularize specific water treatments that quickly became the vogue in Europe during the nineteenth century. *Vincent Preissnitz* (1799-1851), of Graefenberg, Silesia, was a pioneer natural healer. Unfortunately, he was prosecuted by the medical authorities of his day and was actually convicted of using witchcraft because he cured his patients by the use of water, air, diet, and exercise. He took his patients back to nature—to the woods, the streams, the open fields—treated them with nature's own forces, and fed them on natural foods. His cured patients were numbered by the thousands, and his fame spread over the whole of Europe. *Father Sebastian Kneipp* (1821-1897) became the most famous of the hydropaths, with Pope Leo XIII and Ferdinand of Austria (whom he had walking barefoot in new-fallen snow for purposes of hardening his constitution) among his many famous patients. He standardized the practice of hydrotherapy and organized it into a system of practice that was widely emulated through the establishment of health spas or "sanitariums." The first sanitarium in this country, the Kneipp and Nature Cure Sanitarium, was opened in Newark, New Jersey, in 1891.

The best known American hydropath was J.H. Kellogg, a medical doctor who approached hydrotherapy scientifically and performed many experiments trying to understand the physiological effects of hot and cold water. In 1900 he published *Rational Hydrotherapy,* which is still considered a definitive treatise on the physiological and therapeutic effects of water, along with an extensive discussion of hydrotherapeutic techniques. Drs. O.J. Carroll, Harold Dick, and John Bastyr, among others, brought the use of hydrotherapy techniques forward into modern naturopathic practice.

Nature Cure

Natural living, a vegetarian diet, and the use of light and air formed the basis of the Nature Cure movement founded by *Dr. Arnold Rickli* (1823-1926). In 1848 he established at Veldes Krain, Austria, the first institution of light and air cure or as it was called in Europe the *atmospheric cure.* He was an ardent disciple of the vegetarian diet and the founder, and for more than 50 years the president, of the National Austrian Vegetarian Association. In 1891 *Louis Kuhne* (circa 1823-1907) wrote the *New Science of Healing,* which presented the basic principles of "drugless methods." *Dr. Henry Lahman* (circa 1823-1907), who founded the largest Nature Cure institution in the world at Weisser Hirsch, near Dresden, Saxony, constructed the first appliances for the administration of electric light treatment and baths. He was the author of several books on diet, nature cure, and heliotherapy. *Professor F.E. Bilz* (1823-1903) authored the first natural medicine encyclopedia, *The Natural Method of Healing,* which was translated into a dozen languages, and in German alone ran into 150 editions.

Nature Cure became popular in America through the efforts of *Henry Lindlahr,* MD, ND of Chicago, Illinois. Originally a rising businessman in Chicago with all of the bad habits of the "Gay Nineties" era, he became chronically ill while only in his 30s. After receiving no relief from the orthodox practitioners of his day, he learned of Nature Cure, which improved his health. Subsequently, he went to Germany to stay in a sanitarium to be cured and to learn Nature Cure. He went back to Chicago and earned his degrees from the Homeopathic/Eclectic College of Illinois. In 1903 he opened a sanitarium in Elmhurst, Illinois, "Lindlahr's Health Food Store," and shortly thereafter founded the Lindlahr College of Natural Therapeutics. In 1908 he began to publish *Nature Cure Magazine* and began publishing his six-volume series of *Philosophy of Natural Therapeutics*.

One of the chief advantages of training in the early 1900s was the marvelous inpatient facilities that flourished during this time. These facilities provided in-depth training in clinical nature cure and natural hygiene in inpatient settings. Nature cure and natural hygiene are still at the very heart of naturopathic medicine's fundamental principles and approach to health care and disease prevention.

The Hygienic System

Another forerunner of American naturopathy, the "hygienic" school, amalgamated the hydrotherapy and nature cure movements with vegetarianism. It originated as a lay movement of the nineteenth century and had its genesis in the popular teachings of *Sylvester Graham* and *William Alcott*. *Graham* began preaching the doctrines of temperance and hygiene in 1830, and published, in 1839, *Lectures on the Science of Human Life;* two hefty volumes that prescribed healthy dietary habits. He emphasized a moderate lifestyle, a flesh-free diet, and bran bread as an alternative to bolted or white bread. The earliest physician to have a significant impact on the hygienic movement and the later philosophical growth of naturopathy was *Russell Trall, MD.* According to Whorton in his *Crusaders for Fitness:*

The exemplar of the physical educator-hydropath was Russell Thatcher Trall. Still another physician who had lost his faith in regular therapy, Trall opened the second water cure establishment in America, in New York City in 1844. Immediately, he combined the full Priessnitzian armamentarium of baths with regulation of diet, air, exercise and sleep. He would eventually open and or direct any number of other hydropathic institutions around the country, as well as edit the *Water-Cure Journal*, the *Hydropathic Review*, and a temperance journal. He authored several books, including popular sex manuals which perpetuated Graham-like concepts into the 1890's, sold Graham crackers and physiology texts at his New York office, was a charter member (and officer) of the American Vegetarian Society, presided over a short-lived World Health Association, and so on (Whorton, 1982).

Trall founded the first school of natural healing arts in this country to have a 4-year curriculum and the authorization to confer the degree of MD. It was founded in 1852 as a "Hydropathic and Physiological School" and was chartered by the New York State Legislature in 1857 under the name "New York Hygio-Therapeutic College."

He eventually published more than 25 books on the subjects of physiology, hydropathy, hygiene, vegetarianism, and temperance, among many others. The most valuable and enduring of these was his 1851 *Hydropathic Encyclopedia*, a volume of nearly 1000 pages that covered the theory and practice of hydropathy and the philosophy and treatment of diseases advanced by older schools of medicine. The encyclopedia sold more than 40,000 copies.

Martin Luther Holbrook expanded on the work of Graham, Alcott, and Trall and, working with an awareness of the European concepts developed by Preissnitz and Kneipp, laid further groundwork for the concepts later advanced by Lust, Lindlahr, and others. According to Whorton, Holbrook proposed the following:

For disease to result, the latter had to provide a suitable culture medium, had to be susceptible. As yet, most physicians were still so excited at having discovered the causative agents of infection that they were paying less than adequate notice to the host. Radical hygienists, however, were bent just as far in the other direction. They were inclined to see bacteria as merely impotent organisms that throve only in individuals whose hygienic carelessness had made their body compost heaps. Tuberculosis is contagious, Holbrook acknowledged, but "the degree of vital resistance is the real element of protection. When there is no preparation of the soil by heredity, predisposition or lowered health standard, the individual is amply guarded against the attack." A theory favored by many others was that germs were the effect of disease rather than its cause; tissues corrupted by poor hygiene offered microbes, all harmless, an environment in which they could thrive.

The orthodox hygienists of the progressive years were equally enthused by the recent progress of nutrition, of course, and exploited it for their own naturopathic doctors, but their utilization of science hardly stopped with dietetics. Medical bacteriology was another area of remarkable discovery, bacteriologists having provided, in the short space of the last quarter of the nineteenth century, an understanding, at long last, of the nature of infection. This new science's implications for hygienic ideology were profound—when Holbrook locked horns with female fashion, for example, he did not attack the bulky, ground-length skirts still in style with the crude Grahamite objection that the skirt was too heavy. Rather he forced a gasp from his readers with an account of watching a smartly dressed lady unwittingly drag her skirt "over some virulent, revolting looking sputum, which some unfortunate consumptive had expectorated."

Trall and Holbrook both advanced the idea that physicians should teach the maintenance of health rather than simply provide a last resort in times of health crisis. Besides providing a strong editorial voice denouncing the evils of tobacco and drugs, they strongly advanced the value of vegetarianism, bathing and exercise, dietetics and nutrition along with personal hygiene.

John Harvey Kellogg, MD, another medically trained doctor who turned to more nutritionally based natural healing concepts, also greatly influenced Lust. Kellogg was renowned through his connection, beginning in 1876, with the Battle Creek, which was founded in the 1860s as a Seventh Day Adventist institution designed to perpetuate the Grahamite philosophies. Kellogg, born in 1852, was a "sickly child" who, at age 14, after reading the works of Graham, converted to vegetarianism. At the age of 20, he studied for a term at Trall's Hygio-Therapeutic College and then earned a medical degree at New York's Bellevue Medical School. He maintained an affiliation with the regular schools of medicine during

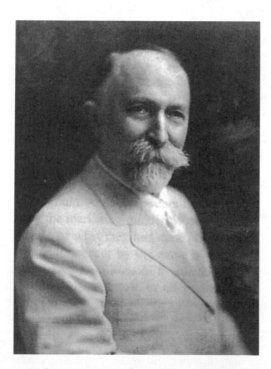

Figure 11-2 A portrait of Dr. John Harvey Kellogg, brother to the Kellogg of breakfast cereal fame and a physical culture movement proponent. (Courtesy Historical Society of Battle Creek, Battle Creek, Michigan.)

his lifetime, owing more to his practice of surgery than his beliefs in that area of health care (Figure 11-2).

Kellogg designated his concepts, which were basically the hygienic system of healthful living, "biologic living." Kellogg expounded vegetarianism, attacked sexual misconduct and the evils of alcohol, and was a prolific writer through the late nineteenth and early twentieth centuries. He produced a popular periodical, *Good Health,* which continued in existence until 1955. When Kellogg died in 1943 at the age of 91, he had had more than 300,000 patients through the Battle Creek Sanitarium, including many celebrities, and the "San" became nationally well known.

Kellogg was also extremely interested in hydrotherapy. In the 1890s he established a laboratory at the San to study the clinical applications of hydrotherapy. This led to his writing of *Rational Hydrotherapy* in 1902. The preface espoused a philosophy of drugless healing that came to be one of the bases of the hydrotherapy school of medical thought in early twentieth-century America.

Influence on Public Health

It is a little known fact that most of our current and accepted public hygiene practices were brought into societal use by the early Hygienic reformers. Before their efforts, neglect of these basic physiological safety measures was rampant. The Hygienists had a great influence on decreasing morbidity and mortality and increasing life span, as well as the adoption of public sanitation. Orthodox medicine is commonly credited with these advances.

Today certified professional Natural Hygienists are the proponents of the highest standards of training and supervised clinical fasting and participate in training naturopathic physicians. Naturopathic medicine uses the precepts of Natural Hygiene in reestablishing the basis of health, the first step in the therapeutic order.

Autotoxicity

Lust was also greatly influenced by the writings of *John H. Tilden, MD* (who published between 1915 and 1925). Tilden became disenchanted with orthodox medicine and began to rely heavily on dietetics and nutrition, formulating his theories of "autointoxication" (the effect of fecal matter remaining too long in the digestive process) and "toxemia." He provided the natural health care literature with a 200-plus page dissertation entitled *Constipation,* with a whole chapter devoted to the evils of not responding when nature called.

Elie Metchnikoff (director of the prestigious Pasteur Institute and winner of the 1908 Nobel Prize for a contribution to immunology) and Kellogg wrote prolifically on the theory of autointoxication. Kellogg, in particular, believed that humans, in the process of digesting meat, produced a variety of intestinal self-poisons that contributed to autointoxication. As a result, Kellogg widely proselytized that people must return to a more healthy natural state by allowing the naturally designed use of the colon. He believed that the average modern colon was devitalized by the combination of a low-fiber diet, sedentary living, the custom of sitting rather than squatting to defecate, and the modern civilized habit of ignoring "nature's call" out of an undue concern for politeness.

Although the concept of toxemia is not a part of the body of knowledge presented in conventional medical schools, all naturopathic students are presented with this concept. Some of that presentation relies on outdated materials, such as the naturopathic texts of 75 and 100 years ago—Lindlahr, Tilden, and so forth. However, modern research and textbooks are beginning to investigate this phenomenon. Drasar and Hill's *Human Intestinal Flora* (1974) demonstrates some of the biochemical pathways of the generation of metabolic toxins in the gut through dysbiotic bacterial action on poorly digested food (Zeff, 1997, 1998). In the last 20 years, our understanding of the concept of toxemia has been significantly updated by practitioners in the newly emerging field of functional medicine, a health care approach that focuses attention on biochemical individuality, metabolic balance, ecological context, and unique personal experience in the dynamics of health. Maldigestion, malabsorption, and abnormal gut flora and ecology are often found to be primary contributing factors not only to gastrointestinal disorders but also to a wide variety of chronic, systemic illnesses. Laboratory assessment tools have been developed that are capable of evaluating the status of many organs, including the gastrointestinal tract. These cutting-edge diagnostic tools provide physicians with an analysis of numerous functional parameters of the individual's digestion and absorption and precisely pinpoint what in the colonic environment is imbalanced, thus promoting dysbiosis.

Thomsonianism

In 1822 *Samuel Thomson* published his *New Guide to Health,* a compilation of his personal view of medical theory and American Indian herbal and medical botanical lore. Thomson espoused the belief that disease had one general cause—derangement of the vital fluids from "cold" influences on the human body—and that disease therefore had one general remedy: animal warmth or "heat." The name of the complaint depended on the part of the body that was affected. Unlike the conventional American "heroic" medical tradition that advocated bloodletting, leeching, and the substantial use of mineral-based purgatives such as antimony and mercury, Thomson believed that minerals were sources of "cold" because they come from the ground and that vegetation, which grew toward the sun, represented "heat" (Figure 11-3).

Thomson's view was that individuals could self-treat if they had an adequate understanding of his philosophy *and* a copy of *New Guide to Health.* The right to sell "family franchises" for use of the Thomsonian method of healing was the basis of a profound lay movement between 1822 and Thomson's death in 1843. Thomson adamantly believed that no professional medical class should exist and that democratic medicine was best practiced by laypersons within

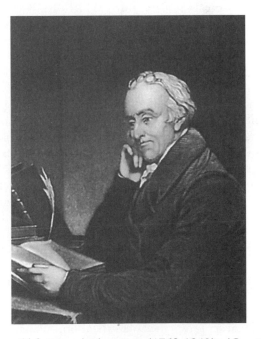

Figure 11-3 Samuel Thomson (1769-1843). (Courtesy National Library of Medicine, Bethesda, Maryland.)

a Thomsonian "family" unit. By 1839 Thomson claimed to have sold some 100,000 of these family franchises called "friendly botanic societies."

Despite his criticism of the early medical movement for their "heroic" tendencies, Thomson's medical theories were "heroic" in their own fashion. Although he did not advocate bloodletting or heavy metal poisoning and leeching, botanic purgatives—particularly *Lobelia inflata* (Indian tobacco)—were a substantial part of the therapy.

The Eclectic School of Medicine

Some of the doctors practicing Thomsonian, called *botanics,* decided to separate themselves from the lay movement. They established a broader range of therapeutic applications of botanical medicines and founded a medical college in Cincinnati. These Thomsonian doctors were later absorbed into the "Eclectic School," which originated with Wooster Beach of New York.

Wooster Beach, from a well-established New England family, started his medical studies at an early age, apprenticing under an old German herbal doctor, Jacob Tidd, until Tidd died. Beach then enrolled in the Barclay Street Medical University in New York. After opening his own practice in New York, Beach set out to win over fellow members of the New York Medical Society (into which he had been warmly introduced by the screening committee) to his point of view that heroic medicine was inherently dangerous and should be reduced to the gentler theories of herbal medicine. He was summarily ostracized from the medical society. He soon founded his own school in New York, calling the clinic and educational facility "The United States Infirmary." However, because of political pressure from the medical society, he was unable to obtain charter authority to issue legitimate diplomas. He then located a financially ailing but legally chartered school, Worthington College, in Worthington, Ohio. There he opened a full-scale medical college, creating the Eclectic school of medical theory based on the European, Native American, and American traditions. The most enduring eclectic herbal textbook is *King's American Dispensary* by *Harvey Wickes Felter* and *John Uri Lloyd.* Published in 1898, this two-volume 2500-page treatise provided the definitive work describing the identification, preparation, pharmacognosy, history of use, and clinical application of more than 1000 botanical medicines. The

eclectic herbal lore formed an integral core of the therapeutic armamentarium of the naturopathic doctor.

Homeopathic Medicine

Homeopathy, the creation of an early German physician, *Samuel Hahnemann* (1755-1843), had four central doctrines: (1) the "law of similars" (that like cures like); (2) that the effect of a medication could be heightened by its administration in minute doses (the more diluted the dose, the greater the "dynamic" effect); (3) that nearly all diseases were the result of a suppressed itch, or "psora"; and (4) Hering's law: healing proceeds from within outward, above downward, from more vital to less vital organs, and in the reverse order of the appearance of symptoms (pathobiography).

Originally, most homeopaths in this country were converted orthodox medical doctors, or *allopaths* (a term coined by Hahnemann). The high rate of conversion made this particular medical sect the archenemy of the rising orthodox medical profession. The first American homeopathic medical school was founded in 1848 in Philadelphia; the last purely homeopathic medical school, based in Philadelphia, survived into the early 1930s (see Chapter 7).

The Manipulative Therapies: Osteopathy and Chiropractic

In Missouri *Andrew Taylor Still,* originally trained as an orthodox practitioner, founded the school of medical thought known as *osteopathy.* He conceived a system of healing that emphasized the primary importance of the structural integrity of the body, especially as it affects the vascular system, in the maintenance of health. In 1892 he opened the American School of Osteopathy in Kirksville, Missouri.

In 1895 Daniel David Palmer, originally a magnetic healer from Davenport, Iowa, performed the first spinal manipulation, which gave rise to the school he termed *chiropractic.* His philosophy was similar to Still's except for a greater emphasis on the importance of proper neurological function. He formally published his findings in 1910, after having founded a chiropractic school in Davenport.

Less well known is "Zone Therapy," originated by *Joe Shelby Riley, DC,* a chiropractor based in Washington, D.C. Zone therapy was an early forerunner of acupressure as it related "pressures and manipulations of the fingers and tongue, and percussion on the spinal column, according to the relation of the fingers to certain zones of the body" (see Chapter 7).

Christian Science and the Role of Belief and Spirituality

Christian Science, formulated by *Mary Baker Eddy* in 1879, comprises a profound belief in the role of systematic religious study (which led to the widespread Christian Science Reading Rooms), spirituality, and prayer in the treatment of disease. In 1875 she published *Science and Health with Key to the Scriptures,* the definitive textbook for the study of Christian Science.

Lust was also influenced by the works of *Sidney Weltmer,* the founder of "Suggestive Therapeutics." Weltmer's work dealt specifically with the psychological process of desiring to be healthy. The theory behind Professor Weltmer's work was that whether it was the mind or the body that first lost its grip on health, the two were inseparably related. When the problem originated in the body, the mind nonetheless lost its ability and desire to overcome the disease because the patient "felt sick" and consequently slid further into the diseased state. Alternatively, if the mind first lost its ability and desire to "be healthy" and some physical infirmity followed, the patient was susceptible to being overcome by disease (see Chapter 8).

Physical Culture

Bernarr McFadden, a close friend of Lust's, founded the "Physical Culture" school of health and healing, also known as *physcultopathy.* This school of healing gave birth across the country to gymnasiums at which exercise programs, designed to allow the individual man and woman to establish and maintain optimal physical health, were developed and taught.

Although many theories exist to explain the rapid dissolution of these diverse healing arts (which at one time made up more than 25% of health care practitioners in the United States) in the early part of the twentieth century, low ratings in the infamous Flexner Report (which rated all these schools of medical thought among the lowest), the self-application of the blessing "scientific" on allopathic medicine and growing political sophistication of the AMA clearly played the most significant role.

All of these healing systems and modalities were naturally unified in the field of naturopathic medicine because they shared one common tenet: respect for and inquiry into the self-healing process and what was necessary to establish health.

The Halcyon Days of Naturopathy

In the early 1920s the "health fad" movement was reaching its peak in terms of public awareness and interest. Conventions were held all over the country, with one attended by several members of Congress, culminating in full legalization of naturopathy as a healing art in the District of Columbia. Not only were the conventions well attended by professionals but the public flocked to them, with more than 10,000 attending the 1924 convention in Los Angeles.

During the 1920s and up until 1937 naturopathy was in its most popular phase. Although the institutions of the orthodox school had gained ascendancy, before 1937 the medical profession had no real solutions to the problems of human disease.

During the 1920s *Gaylord Hauser,* later to become the health food guru of the Hollywood set, came to Lust as a seriously ill young man. Lust, through application of the nature cure, removed Hauser's afflictions and was rewarded by Hauser's lifelong devotion. His regular columns in *Nature's Path* became widely read among the Hollywood set.

The naturopathic journals of the 1920s and 1930s provide much valuable insight into the prevention of disease and the promotion of health. Much of the dietary advice focused on correcting poor eating habits, including the lack of fiber in the diet and an overreliance on red meat as a protein source. In the 1990s and now we are treated to the pronouncements of the orthodox profession, the National Institutes of Health, and the National Cancer Institute that the early assertions of the naturopaths that such dietary habits would lead to degenerative diseases, including cancers associated with the digestive tract and the colon, were true.

The December 1928 volume of *Nature's Path* was the first American publication of the works of Herman J. DeWolff, a Dutch epidemiologist who was one of the first researchers to assert, on the basis of studies of the incidence of cancer in the Netherlands, that there was a correlation between exposure to petrochemicals and various types of cancerous conditions. He saw a connection between chemical fertilizers and their use in some soils (principally clay) that led to their remaining in vegetables after they had arrived at the market and were purchased for consumption. It was almost 50 years before orthodox medicine began to see the wisdom of such assertions.

Suppression and Decline

In 1937 the popularity of naturopathy began to decline. The change came, as both Thomas and Campion note in their works, with the era of "miracle medicine." Lust recognized this and his editorializing became, if anything, even more strident. From the introduction of sulfa drugs in 1937 to the Salk vaccine's release in 1955, the American public became used to annual developments of miracle vaccines and antibiotics. The naturopathic profession adhered to its vitalistic philosophy and a full range of practice but unfortunately was poorly unified at this time on other issues of standards. This made the profession vulnerable to interguild competition.

Lust died in September of 1945 in residence at the Yungborn facility in Butler, New Jersey, preparing to attend the 49th Annual Congress of his American Naturopathic Association. On August 30, 1945, for the official program of that congress, which was held in October of 1945 just after his death, he noted his concerns for the future, especially his frustration with the success of the medical profession in blocking the efforts of the naturopaths to establish state licensing laws that would not only establish appropriate practice rights for NDs but also protect the public from the pretenders (i.e., those who chose to call themselves naturopaths without ever bothering to attain formal training):

Now let us see the type of men and women who are the Naturopaths of today. Many of them are fine, upstanding individuals, believing fully in the effectiveness of their chosen profession—willing to give their all for the sake of alleviating human suffering and ready to fight for their rights to the last ditch. More power to them! But there are others who claim to be Naturopaths who are woeful misfits. Yes, and there are outright fakers and cheats masking as Naturopaths. That is the fate of any science—any profession—which the unjust laws have placed beyond the pale. Where there is no official recognition and regulation, you will find the plotters, the thieves, the charlatans operating on the same basis as the conscientious practitioners. And these riff-raff opportunists bring the whole art into disrepute. Frankly such conditions cannot be remedied until suitable safeguards are erected by law, or by the profession itself, around the practice of Naturopathy. That will come in time.

In the mid-1920s, *Morris Fishbein* came on the scene as editor of the *Journal of the American Medical Association* (JAMA). Fishbein took on a personal vendetta against what he characterized as "quackery." Lust, among others, including McFadden, became Fishbein's epitome of quackery. Unfortunately, he proved to be particularly effective.

The public infatuation with technology, the introduction of "miracle medicine," World War II's stimulation of the development of surgery, the Flexner Report, growing political sophistication of the AMA through the leadership of Fishbein, and the death of Lust in 1945 all combined to cause the decline of naturopathic medicine and natural healing in the United States. In addition, these years, called the *years of the great fear* in Caute's book by that name, were the years during which to be unorthodox was to be un-American.

Across the country, courts began to take the view that naturopaths were not truly doctors because they espoused doctrines from "the dark ages of medicine" (something American medicine had supposedly come out of in 1937) and that drugless healers were intended by law to operate without "drugs" (which became defined as anything a person would ingest or apply externally for any medical purpose). The persistent lack of uniform standards, lack of insurance coverage, lost court battles, a splintered profession, and a hostile legislative perspective progressively restricted practice until the core naturopathic therapies became essentially illegal and practices financially nonviable.

Although it was under considerable public pressure in those years, the American Naturopathic Association (ANA) undertook some of its most scholarly work, coordinating all the systems of naturopathy under commission. This resulted in the 1948 publication of a formal textbook, *Basic Naturopathy*, by Spitler and a significant work compiling all the known theories of botanical medicine, *Naturae Medicina*, by Kuts-Cheraux in 1953. Naturopathic medicine began splintering when Lust's ANA was succeeded by six different organizations in the mid 1950s.

By the early 1970s, the profession's educational institutions had dwindled to one: the National College of Naturopathic Medicine (with branches in Seattle, Washington, and Portland, Oregon).

Naturopathic Medicine Reemerges

The combination of the counterculture years of the late 1960s, the public's growing awareness of the importance of nutrition and the environment, and America's disenchantment with organized institutional medicine (which began after the miracle era faded, and it became apparent that orthodox medicine has its limitations and is prohibitively expensive) resulted in alternative medicine in general gaining new respect and in the rejuvenation of naturopathic medicine. At this time, a new wave of students were attracted to the philosophical precepts of the profession. They brought with them an appreciation for the appropriate use of science, modern college education, and matching expectations for quality education.

It was Dr. John Bastyr (1912-1995) and his firm, efficient, professional leadership that inspired science and research-based training in natural medicine to begin to reach toward its full potential. Dr. Bastyr, whose vision was one of "naturopathy's empirical successes documented and proven by scientific methods," was "himself a prototype for the modern naturopathic doctor, who culls the latest findings from the scientific literature, applies them in ways consistent with naturopathic principles, and verifies the results with appropriate studies. Bastyr also saw "a tremendous expansion in both allopathic and naturopathic medical knowledge, and he played a major role in making sure the best of both were integrated into naturopathic medical education" (Kirchfield & Boyle, 1994).

Responding to the growth in public interest during the late 1970s, naturopathic colleges were established in Arizona (the Arizona College of Naturopathic Medicine, 1977), Oregon (the American College of Naturopathic Medicine, 1980), and California (the Pacific College of Naturopathic Medicine, 1979). None of these three survived. In 1978 the John Bastyr College of Naturopathic Medicine (later renamed Bastyr University) was formed in Seattle, Washington, by Joseph E. Pizzorno, Jr., ND; Lester E. Griffith, ND; William Mitchell, ND; and Sheila Quinn to teach science-based natural medicine. They believed that for the naturopathic profession to move back into the mainstream, it needed to establish accredited institutions, perform credible research, and establish itself as an integral part of the health care system. Bastyr survived and became the first naturopathic college ever to become accredited. In the fall of 1993 Michael Cronin, ND, and Conrad Kail, ND, founded the Southwest College of Naturopathic Medicine and Health Science in Scottsdale, Arizona. In 1997 the University of Bridgeport with the assistance of Jim Sensenig, ND, founded the University of Bridgeport College of Naturopathic Medicine.

With five credible colleges (including the Canadian College of Naturopathic Medicine in Ontario, Canada), active research, an appreciation of the appropriate application of science to natural medicine education, and clinical practice, naturopathic medicine is well on the road to recovery.

Recent Influences

It is now well established that nutritional factors are of major importance in the pathogenesis of both atherosclerosis and cancer, the two leading causes of death in Western countries, and studies validating their importance in the pathogenesis of many other diseases continue to be published. . . . A tremendous amount of scientific support for the principles of naturopathic medicine has been conducted at mainstream research centers. In fact, allopathy is increasingly turning to the use of naturopathic methods in the search for effective prescriptions for today's intractable and expensive diseases (Werbach, 1996).

Although the naturopaths were astute clinical observers and a century ago recognized many of the concepts that are now gaining popularity and the support of scientific data, the scientific tools of the time were inadequate to assess the validity of their concepts. In addition, as a group they seemed to have little inclination to the application of laboratory research, especially because "science" was the bludgeon used by the AMA to suppress the profession. This has now changed. In the past few decades a considerable amount of research is now providing the scientific documentation of many of the concepts of naturopathic medicine, and the new breed of scientifically trained naturopaths is using this research to continue development of the profession. The following are a few of the most important trends.

Therapeutic Nutrition

Since 1929, when Eijkman and Hopkins shared the Nobel Prize in medicine and physiology for the discovery of vitamins, the role of these trace substances in clinical nutrition has been a matter of scientific investigation. The discovery that enzyme systems depended on essential nutrients provided the naturopathic profession with great insights into why an organically grown, whole foods diet is so important for health. Nutritional biochemist Roger Williams' formulation of the concept of "biochemical individuality" in 1955 further developed these ideas and provided great insights into the unique nutritional needs of each individual and how to correct inborn errors of metabolism and even treat specific diseases through the use of nutrient-rich foods or large doses of specific nutrients. Linus Pauling, the two-time Nobel Prize winner, coined the concept of orthomolecular medicine and provided further theoretical substantiation for the use of nutrients as therapeutic agents. Functional medicine is a recent development in the use of therapeutic nutrition in the prevention of illness and promotion of health. Focusing on biochemical individuality, metabolic balance, and the ecological context, functional medicine practitioners avail themselves of recently developed laboratory tests to pinpoint even slight imbalances in an individual's biochemistry that can set into motion a cascade of biological triggers, paving the way to suboptimal function, chronic illness, and degenerative disease. A broad range of functional laboratory assessment tools in the areas of digestion (gastrointestinal), nutrition, detoxification/oxidative stress, immunology/allergy, production and regulation of hormones (endocrinology), and heart and blood vessels (cardiovascular) provide physicians with the information needed to recommend nutritional interventions specific to the individual's needs and to precisely monitor their efficacy.

Environmental Medicine/Clinical Ecology

Although recognition of the clinical impact of environmental toxicity and endogenous toxicity has existed since the earliest days of naturopathy, it was not until the environmental movement and the seminal work of Rachel Carson and others that the scientific basis was established. Clinical research and the development of laboratory methods for assessing toxic load have provided objective tools that have greatly increased the sophistication of clinical practice. Clinical and laboratory methods were developed for the assessment of idiosyncratic reactions to environmental factors and foods.

Spirituality, Health, and Medicine

Naturopathic medicine's philosophy of treating the whole person and enhancing the individual's inherent healing ability is closely aligned with its mission of in-

tegrating spirituality into the healing process. Scientific evidence is growing on how spirituality can play a part in healing. Since Descartes separated mind from body in the seventeenth century, medical science has attempted to explain disease independently of mind, in terms of germs, environmental agents, or wayward genes. Today, however, the evidence is not just clinical observation but chemical fact. An explosion of research in the new and rapidly expanding field of psychoneuroimmunology is revealing physical evidence of the mind-body connection that is changing our understanding of disease. Scientists no longer question whether but *how* our minds have an impact on our health and the implications of the connections uncovered in just the last 20 years are extraordinary.

In his book *Healing Words,* Larry Dossey, MD, pulls together what he describes as "One of the best kept secrets in medical science": the extensive experimental evidence for the beneficial effects of prayer. Dossey reviews studies that provide evidence for a positive effect of prayer on not only humans but mice, chicks, enzymes, fungi, yeast, bacteria, and cells of various sorts. He emphasizes, "We cannot dismiss these outcomes as being due to suggestion or placebo effects, since these so-called lower forms of life do not think in any conventional sense and are presumably not susceptible to suggestion" (Pizzorno, 1995).

Cutting-Edge Laboratory Methods

A final significant influence has been the development of laboratory methods for the objective assessment of nutritional status, metabolic dysfunction, digestive function, bowel flora, endogenous and exogenous toxic load, and liver detoxification function. Each of these has provided ever more effective tools for accurate assessment of patient health status and effective application of naturopathic principles.

PRINCIPLES

Although in many ways, modern medicine resembles a science, it continues to be criticized for its lack of unifying theories, and for this reason alone its claim to being a science has remained suspect.

—BLOIS (1988)

What physicians think medicine is profoundly shapes what they do, how they behave in doing it, and the reasons they use to justify that behavior. . . . Whether conscious of it or not, every physician has an answer to what he thinks medicine is, with real consequences for all whom he attends. . . . The outcome is hardly trivial. . . . It dictates, after all, how we approach patients [and] how we make clinical judgments.

—PELLEGRINO (1979)

Medical philosophy comprises the underlying premises on which a healthcare system is based. Once a system is acknowledged, it is subject to debate. In naturopathic medicine, the philosophical debate is a valuable, ongoing process which helps the understanding that disease evolves in an orderly and truth-revealing fashion.

—BRADLEY (1985)

Naturopathic medicine is a distinct system of health-oriented medicine that, in contrast to the currently dominant disease-treatment system, stresses promotion of health, prevention of disease, patient education, and self responsibility. However, naturopathic medicine symbolizes more than simply a health care system; it is a way of life. Unlike most other health care systems, naturopathy is not identified with any particular therapy but rather a way of thinking about life, health, and disease. It is defined not by the therapies it uses but by the philosophical principles that guide the practitioner.

Six powerful concepts provide the foundation that defines naturopathic medicine and create a unique group of professionals practicing a form of medicine that fundamentally changes the way we think of health care. In 1989 the American Association of Naturopathic Physicians unanimously approved the definition of *naturopathic medicine,* updating and reconfirming in modern terms its core principles as a professional consensus. "The definition and principles of practice provide a steady point of reference for this debate, for our evolving understanding of health and disease, and for all of our decision making processes as a profession" (Snider & Zeff, 1988).

The six core principles of naturopathic medicine are as follows, with one proposed addition:

1. The healing power of nature (*vis medicatrix naturae*)
2. First do no harm (*primum non nocere*)
3. Find the cause (*tolle causam*)
4. Treat the whole person (*holism*)
5. Preventive medicine
6. Wellness (proposed)
7. Doctor as teacher (*docere*)

The Healing Power of Nature (*vis medicatrix naturae*)

Belief in the ability of the body to heal itself—the *vis medicatrix naturae* (the healing power of nature)—if given the proper opportunity, and the importance of living within the laws of nature is the foundation of naturopathic medicine. Although the term *naturopathy* was coined in the late nineteenth century, its philosophical roots can be traced back to Hippocrates and derive from a common wellspring with traditional world medicines: belief in the healing power of nature.

Medicine has long grappled with the question of the existence of the *vis medicatrix naturae* (VMN). As Neuberger stated, "the problem of the healing power of nature is a great, perhaps the greatest of all problems which has occupied the physician for thousands of years. Indeed, the aims and limits of therapeutics are determined by its solution" (Kirchfeld & Boyle, 1994). The fundamental reality of the VMN was a basic tenet of the Hippocratic school of medicine, and "every important medical author since has had to take a position for or against it" (Neuberger, 1932, in Kirchfeld & Boyle, 1994).

When standard medicine soundly rejected the principle of the VMN at the turn of the century, nature doctors, including naturopathic physicians in the United States from 1896 on, diverged from conventional medicine. Naturopathic physicians recognized the clinical importance of the inherent self-healing process; embraced it as their core academic and clinical principle; and developed an entire system of medical practice, training, and research based on it and related principles of clinical medicine.

Naturopathic medicine is therefore "vitalistic" in its approach (i.e., life is viewed as more than just the sum of biochemical processes), and the body is believed to have an innate intelligence or process (the VMN), which is always striving toward health. Vitalism maintains that the symptoms accompanying disease are not typically caused by the morbific agent (e.g., bacteria); rather, they are the result of the organism's intrinsic response or reaction to the agent and the organism's attempt to defend and heal itself (Lindlahr, 1914a; Neuberger, 1932). Symptoms are part of a constructive phenomenon that is the best "choice" the organism can make, given the circumstances. In this construct the physician's role is to understand and aid the body's efforts, not to take over or manipulate the functions of the body, unless the self-healing process has become weak or insufficient.

Although the context and life force of naturopathic medicine is its vitalistic core, both vitalistic and mechanistic approaches are applicable to modern naturopathic medicine. Vitalism has reemerged in today's terms in the body-mind-spirit dialogue. Matter, mind, energy, and spirit are each part of nature and therefore are part of medicine that observes, respects, and works with nature. Much of modern biomedicine and related research is based on the application of the theory of mechanism (defined in Webster's dictionary as the "theory that everything in the universe is produced by matter in motion; materialism") in a highly reductionistic, single-agent, pathology-based, disease-care model. Applied in a vitalistic context, mechanistic and reductionistic interventions provide useful techniques and tools to naturopathic physicians. The Unifying Theory of Naturopathic Medicine (see the following) provides clinical guidance for integrating both approaches.

First Do No Harm
(*primum non nocere*)

Naturopathic physicians prefer noninvasive treatments that minimize the risks of harmful side effects. They are trained to use the lowest force and lowest risk preventive, diagnostic, therapeutic, and comanagement strategies. They are trained to know which patients they can safely treat and which ones they need to refer to other health care practitioners. Naturopathic physicians follow three precepts to avoid harming the patient:

1. Naturopathic physicians use methods and medicinal substances that minimize the risk of harmful effects and apply the least possible force or intervention necessary to diagnose illness and restore health.
2. When possible, the suppression of symptoms is avoided because suppression generally interferes with the healing process.
3. Naturopathic physicians respect and work with the VMN in diagnosis, treatment, and counseling because if this self-healing process is not respected, the patient may be harmed.

Find the Cause (*tolle causam*)

Every illness has an underlying cause or causes, often in aspects of the lifestyle, diet, or habits of the individual. A naturopathic physician is trained to find and remove the underlying cause(s) of disease. The therapeutic order (see the following) helps the physician remove them in the correct "healing order" for the body. As the new science of psychoneuroimmunology is explicitly demonstrating (see Chapter 13), the body is a seamless web with a multiplicity of brain–immune system–gut–liver connections. Not surprisingly, chronic disease typically involves a number of systems, with the most prominent or acute symptoms being those chronologically last in appearance. As the healing process progresses and these symptoms are alleviated, further symptoms then resurface that must then be addressed to restore health. To paraphrase David Jones, MD, "Tack Rules": "If you're sitting on a tack, it takes a lot of aspirin to feel better. If you're sitting on two tacks, removing one does not necessarily lead to a 50% improvement/reductions in symptoms."

Treat the Whole Person (Holism)

As noted in the preceding principle, health or disease comes from a complex interaction of mental, emotional, spiritual, physical, dietary, genetic, environmental, lifestyle, and other factors. Naturopathic physicians treat the whole person, taking all of these factors into account. Naturopathically, the body is viewed as a whole. Naturopathy is often called *holistic medicine* in reference to the term *holism*, coined by philosopher Jan Christian Smuts in 1926, to describe the *gestalt* of a system as greater than the sum of its parts. A change in one part causes a change in every part; therefore the study of one part must be integrated into the whole, including the community and biosphere.

Naturopathic medicine asserts that one cannot be healthy in an unhealthy environment and is committed to the creation of a world in which humanity may thrive. In contrast to the high degree of specialization in the present medical system, which reflects a mechanistic orientation to single organs, the holistic model relegates specialists to an ancillary role. Emphasis is placed on the physical, emotional, social, and spiritual integration of the whole person, including awareness of the impact of the environment on health.

Preventive Medicine

The naturopathic approach to health care helps prevent disease and keeps minor illnesses from developing into more serious or chronic degenerative diseases. Patients are taught the principles with which to live a healthful life, and by following these principles, they can prevent major illness. Health is viewed as more than just the absence of disease; it is considered a dynamic state that enables a person to thrive in, or adapt to, a wide range of environments and stresses. Health and disease are points on a continuum, with death at one end and optimal function at the other. The naturopathic physician believes that a person who goes through life living an unhealthful lifestyle will drift away from optimal function and move relentlessly toward progressively greater dysfunction. Genotype, constitution, maternal influences, and environmental factors all influence individual susceptibility to deterioration, and the organs and physiological systems affected. These and other determinants of health addressed by the naturopathic physician in both treatment and prevention are presented in Box 11-2.

The virulence of morbific agents or insults also plays a central role in disturbance, causing decreasing function and ultimately serious disease.

In our society, although our life span at birth has increased, our health span has not, nor has our health expectancy at age 65. We are living longer but as disabled individuals (Pizzorno, 1997). Although such deterioration is accepted by our society as the normal expectation of aging, it is not common in animals in the wild nor among those fortunate peoples who live in an optimal environment (i.e., no pollution, low stress, regular exercise, and abundant natural, nutritious food).

In the naturopathic model death is inevitable; progressive disability is not. This belief underscores a fundamental difference in philosophy and expectation between the conventional and naturopathic models of health and disease. In contrast to the disease-treatment focus of allopathic medicine, the health-promotion focus of naturopathic medicine emphasizes the means of maximizing health span.

BOX 11-2

Determinants of Health, Disturbances, and Hygienic Lifestyle Factors

Determinants of Health
Inborn
- Genetic makeup (genotype)
- Constitution (determines susceptibility)
- Intrauterine/congenital
- Maternal exposures
  - Drugs
  - Toxins
  - Viruses
  - Psychoemotional
- Maternal and paternal genetic influences
- Maternal nutrition
- Maternal lifestyle

Disturbances
- Illnesses: pathobiography
- Medical interventional (or lack of)
- Physical and emotional exposures, stresses, and trauma
- Toxic and harmful substances

Hygienic/Lifestyle Factors
- Nutrition
- Rest
- Exercise
- Psychoemotional health
- Spiritual health
- Community
- Culture
- Socioeconomic factors
- Fresh air
- Light
- Exposure to nature
- Clean water
- Unadulterated food
- Loving and being loved
- Meaningful work

Wellness (Proposed New Principle)

Establishing and maintaining optimal health and balance is a central clinical goal. Wellness is a state of being healthy, characterized by positive emotion, thought, and action. Wellness is inherent in everyone, no matter what disease is being experienced. The recognition, experience, and support of wellness by the physician and patient will more quickly heal a given disease than treatment of the disease alone.

Doctor as Teacher (*docere*)

The original meaning of the word *docere* is teacher. A principle objective of naturopathic medicine is to educate the patient and emphasize self-responsibility for health. Naturopathic physicians also recognize the therapeutic potential of the doctor-patient relationship. The patient is engaged and respected as an ally and a member of her or his own health care team. Adequate time is spent with patients to thoroughly diagnose, treat, and educate them (see Chapters 1 and 2).

Naturopathic Practice Today

Today's naturopathic physicians are licensed primary care providers of integrative natural medicine and are also recognized for their clinical expertise and effectiveness in preventive medicine. Naturopathic doctors are trained as family physicians, regardless of elective postdoctoral training or clinical emphasis. This is intentional and consistent with naturopathic principles of practice. Naturopathic doctors are trained to assess causes and develop treatment plans from a systems perspective and with systems skills on the basis of naturopathic principles and, specifically, on the principle: Treat the whole person.

"Naturopathy, in fact, is typically *meta-systematic*. . . . The organism [is] always seen in the context of its physical and social environment. . . . Beyond this, naturopathy, ultimately might even be considered *cross-paradigmatic* (Commons et al., 1984), touching inevitably on the economics, politics, history, and sociology of the various healing alternatives (Walters, 1993), ultimately penetrating to the contrasting philosophies underlying naturopathy and allopathy. Naturopathy results from a guiding philosophy at odds with the dominant mechanistic philosophy undergirding Western industrialized society. Allopathy, in contrast, is clearly derived from these same premises. Or in Eisler's (1987) terms, naturopathy embraces a *partnership* model of relationship, while allopathy falls within the *dominator* model. As indicated

below, this partnership/dominator model extends not only to the treatment process but to the healer/patient relationship itself" (Funk, 1995).

Naturopathic doctors (NDs) may also practice as specialists, after postdoctoral training in botanical, homeopathic, nutritional medicine, physical medicine, acupuncture, Ayurvedic medicine, Oriental and Chinese herbal medicine, counseling and health psychology, spirituality and healing, applied behavioral sciences, and midwifery. Some NDs choose to focus their practice on population groups such as children, the elderly, or women, or in clinical areas such as cardiology, gastroenterology, immunology, or environmental medicine. These diverse practices are consistent with the eclectic origins of naturopathic medicine and are part of its strength.

In addition to these specialties, at one end of the spectrum are practitioners who adhere to the nature cure tradition and focus clinically only on diet, detoxification, lifestyle modification, hydrotherapy, and other self-healing modalities. At the other end are those whose practices appear to be similar to the average conventional medical practice with the only apparent difference being the use of pharmaceutical grade botanical medicines instead of synthetic drugs. However, fundamental to all styles of naturopathic practice is a common philosophy and principles of health and disease: the unifying theory in the hierarchy of therapeutics or the therapeutic order described in the following section. The therapeutic order is derived from all of the principles and guides the ND's choice of therapeutic interventions.

UNIFYING THEORY: THE HEALING POWER OF NATURE AND THE THERAPEUTIC ORDER

In facilitating the process of healing, the naturopathic physician seeks to use those therapies which are most efficient and which have the least potential to harm the patient. The concept of harm includes suppression or exhaustion of natural healing processes including inflammation and fever. These precepts, coupled to an understanding of the process of healing, result in a therapeutic hierarchy. This hierarchy (or Therapeutic Order), is a natural consequence of how the organism heals. Therapeutic modalities are applied in a rational order, determined by the nature of the healing process. The natural order of appropriate therapeutic intervention is:

1. Re-establish the basis for health
2. Stimulate the VMN (Vis medicatrix naturae)
3. Tonify and nourish weakened systems
4. Correct structural integrity
5. Prescribe specific substances and/or modalities for specific conditions and biochemical pathways, e.g. botanicals, nutrients, acu-puncture, homeopathy, hydrotherapy, counseling
6. Prescribe pharmaceutical substances
7. Use radiation, chemotherapy, surgery

This appropriate Therapeutic Order proceeds from least to most force. All modalities can be found at various steps, depending on their application. The spiritual aspect of the patient's health is considered to begin with Step 1 (Zeff, 1997; Nos. 5 through 7 added by Snider).

The concepts expressed in the therapeutic order are derived from Hippocrates' writings and those of medical scholars since Hippocrates concerning the function and activation of the self-healing process. Dr. Jared Zeff has summarized and expressed these concepts as the hierarchy of therapeutics in his article "The Process of Healing: A Unifying Theory of Naturopathic Medicine."

The philosophy represented in the therapeutic order does not determine what modalities are good or bad. Rather, it provides a clinical framework for all modalities, used in an order consistent with that of the natural self-healing process. It respects the origins of disease and the applications of care and intervention necessary for health and healing with the least intervention. The therapeutic order schematically directs the ND's therapeutic choices in an efficient order rather than a "shotgun" approach. It is this common philosophy and theory that both distinguishes the field of naturopathic medicine and enables it to consider and incorporate new therapies.

Naturopathic medicine's philosophical approach to health promotion and restoration necessitates a broad range of diagnostic and therapeutic skills and accounts for the eclectic interests of the naturopathic profession. Obviously, at times the body needs more than just supportive help. The goal of the ND in such situations is to first use the lowest force and lowest risk clinical strategies (i.e., the least invasive intervention that will have the most effective therapeutic outcome) or, when necessary, to co-manage or refer to specialists and other health care professionals.

Because the goal of the ND is to restore normal body function rather than to apply a particular therapy, virtually every natural medicine therapy may be used. In addition, to fulfill their role as primary care family physicians, NDs may also administer vaccines and use therapies such as office surgery and prescription drugs when less invasive options have been exhausted or found inappropriate. In the restoration of health, prescription drugs and surgery are a last resort but are used when necessary. As Kirschner and Brinkman (1988) said, "The use of petroleum by products and the removal of body parts is a poor first line of defense against disease."

Naturopathic medical school curricula are continually revised in light of these principles. Curriculum integration is built on the science-based educational structure already in place in these colleges. Basic sciences, ND and non-ND physician faculty are trained in naturopathic philosophy and principles and the therapeutic order as core assumptions that invite scholarly inquiry. Discussion and inquiry concerning the philosophy and theory are stimulated and supported in interdisciplinary faculty teams. The fruits of these endeavors are brought into the classroom to enhance students' critical thinking concerning clinical values and assumptions.

DIAGNOSIS

In the naturopathic medicine program at Bastyr University, for example, these principles and the therapeutic order are translated into a series of questions that drive curriculum development and case analysis and provide guidance to students learning the art and science of naturopathic medicine. These Naturopathic Case Analysis and Management questions (see the following) are integrated with conventional SOAP algorithms as the process of naturopathic case analysis and management, the clinical application of philosophy to patient care. For example, although a conventional pathological diagnosis is made through the use of physical, laboratory, and radiology procedures, it is done in the context of understanding the underlying causes of the pathology and the obstacles to recovery.

NATUROPATHIC CASE ANALYSIS AND MANAGEMENT

 Questions

I. The Healing Power of Nature (Vis Medicatrix Naturae)

1. What is the level of the disease process? What is the direction of the disease process? What is the purpose of the disease process?
2. How is the healing power of nature supported in the case? What therapeutic interventions allow/respect, palliate, facilitate, or augment the self-healing process? How does the therapeutic intervention do this?
3. Is the person in balance with nature?
4. What is being in balance with nature?
5. Is this person in balance with his or her environment?
6. How are you assessing the healing powers of this individual?
7. What is the prognosis for this individual?
8. What is the patient's metaphor for healing? What moves or will move this patient toward healing or recovery?
9. How does the patient see himself or herself healing (the patient process)?
   - Are people helping him or her?
   - Is he or she doing it on his or her own?
   - How long will it take?
   - Is the doctor doing the healing?
   - Is the patient doing the healing?
   - Are the doctor and patient working together?
   - What else is important in this patient's healing process?

II. First Do No Harm (Primum Non Nocere)

1. What is the potential for harm with this particular treatment plan?
2. Are you doing no harm? How?
3. How are you avoiding suppression? Is suppression necessary? Why?
4. What is the appropriate course of action? Is it waiting?
5. What is the appropriate level and force of intervention? Why? How is the least force applied?
6. Identify the appropriate treatment:
   - Level of therapeutic order
   - Modality/substance
   - Dosage
   - Frequency
   - Duration
   Justify the timing of the treatment in terms of short- and long-term management.
7. Are there any obstacles to the patient's recovery? Explain.

8. What referral or comanagement strategies are required to ensure patients' optimal outcome?

III. Find the Cause (Tolle Causam)

1. What level of healing are you aiming toward (i.e., suppression, palliation, cure)?
2. Where and/or what are the limiting factors in this person's life (concept: health is freedom from limitations)?
3. Where is the center of this person's disease (i.e., physical, mental, emotional, spiritual)?
4. What are the causative factors contributing to this patient's condition/state? What is the central cause or etiology? What are other contributing causes? Of these causative factors, which are avoidable or preventable?

IV. Treat the Whole Person (Holism)

1. How are you working holistically?
2. Can you see the person beyond the disease?
3. What aspects of the person are you addressing?
4. What aspects of the person are you not addressing?
5. Would a referral to another health care practitioner assist you in working holistically? When? To whom? If not, why not?
6. What are the patient's goals and expectations in relationship to their health and treatments?
7. What are your goals and expectations for the patient? What are the differences between yours and the patient's? How are they similar?
8. How will the treatment plan help the patient take more responsibility for his or her health and healing?
9. Are you empowering the patient? How?
10. What is the vitality level of this patient?
11. Identify cultural, community, and environmental issues and concerns that need to be included in the assessment.
12. What family/psychological/spiritual/social systems issues need to be included in the assessment?

V. Preventive Medicine

1. What is being done or planned in regard to prevention?
2. Doctor means teacher—what are you teaching this person about his or her health?
3. Have you done a risk factor assessment for this patient? Have all preprimary, primary, secondary, and tertiary interventions and education relevant to life span or gender been identified and addressed?
4. Does this patient do regular health screening self-examinations?

VI. Wellness (Proposed New Principle)

1. What is being done to cultivate wellness?
2. How are you contributing to optimal health in this individual?

3. How can you contribute to optimal health in this individual?
4. What are the patient's goals and expectations in relationship to their own wellness (e.g., creativity, energy, enjoyment, health, balance)?
5. How can these goals be achieved? Are the expectations realistic?
6. How can achievement of these goals be measured?
7. Once achieved, how can the patient maintain an optimal level of wellness?
8. Are you stimulating wellness or treating disease, or both?
9. Is the patient demonstrating positive emotion, thought, and action? If not, why not?
10. Can the patient recall or imagine a state of wellness?
11. Is the patient able to participate in his or her own process toward a state of wellness?

VII. Doctor as Teacher (Docere)

1. What type of patient education are you providing? Assess wellness issues and prevention issues for this person. Identify educational needs of this patient regarding (a) therapeutic goals, (b) prevention, and (c) wellness.
2. How can you determine the level of a patient's responsibility?
3. In what ways do you cultivate and enhance your role as teacher?
4. How have you listened to and respected the patient?
5. In what ways are you working to "draw out" the patient's vital force and vitality through the doctor-patient relationship?

THERAPEUTIC MODALITIES

Naturopathic medicine is a vitalistic system of health care that uses natural medicines and interventionist therapies as needed. Natural medicines and therapies, when properly used, generally have low invasiveness and rarely cause suppression or side effects. This is because, when used properly, they generally support the body's healing mechanisms rather than taking over the body's processes. The ND knows when, why, and with what patient more invasive therapies are needed based on the therapeutic order and appropriate diagnostic measures. He or she also recognizes that the use of natural, low-force therapies; lifestyle changes; and early functional diagnosis and treatment of nonspecific conditions is a form of preprimary prevention. This approach offers one viable solution for cost containment in primary health care.

Traditional health care disciplines such as traditional Chinese medicine (TCM), Unani medicine, and homeopathic medicine each have a philosophy, principles of practice, and clinical theory that form a system for diagnosis, treatment, and case management. A philosophy of medicine is, in essence, the rational investigation of the truth and principles of that medicine. The principles of practice form an outline or guidelines to the main precepts or fundamental tenets of a system of medicine. Clinical theory provides a system of rules or principles explaining that medicine and applying that system to the patient by means of diagnosis, treatment, and management. The specific substances and techniques, as well as when, why, and to whom they are applied and for how long, depend on the system. Modalities (e.g., botanical medicine, physical medicine) are not systems but rather therapeutic approaches used within these systems. One modality may be used by many systems but in different ways.

The importance of systems is that efficacy, safety, and efficiency of diagnostic and treatment approaches depend as much on the system as on the effects of the substance on physiology or biochemical pathways. This is exemplified by data in the TCM Work Force Survey conducted by the Department of Human Services in Victoria, New South Wales, and Queensland, Australia, and published in *Towards A Safer Choice,* November 1996. This study assessed adverse events and length of TCM training for practitioners. "The number of adverse events reported were compared to the length of TCM training undertaken by the practitioner. It appears from these findings that shorter periods of training in TCM (less than one year) carry an adverse event rate double that of practitioners who have studied for four years or more. . . . These practitioners were asked to respond to two questions regarding the theoretical frameworks they used to guide their TCM practice. TCM philosophy is adopted more readily as the basis for practice by primary TCM practitioners than by allied health practitioners using TCM as part of their practice. In answer to the question, 'Do you rely more predominantly on a TCM philosophy and theoretical framework for making your diagnosis and guiding your acupuncture or Chinese herbal medicine treatments?' 90% of primary TCM practitioners answered yes in contrast to 24% of non-primary practitioners." Nonprimary practitioners were typically educated for less than 1 year and were medical doctors (Bensoussan & Myers, 1996).

It is the system used by each of these disciplines that makes it a uniquely effective field of medicine rather than a vague compendium of complementary and alternative medicine (CAM) modalities. Techniques from many systems are used within naturopathic medicine because of its primary care integrative approach and strong philosophical orientation.

Clinical nutrition, or the use of diet as a therapy, serves as the therapeutic foundation of naturopathic medicine. A rapidly increasing body of knowledge supports the use of whole foods, fasting, natural hygiene, and nutritional supplements in the maintenance of health and treatment of disease. The recognition of unique nutritional requirements caused by biochemical individuality has provided a theoretical and practical basis for the appropriate use of megavitamin therapy. Controlled fasting is also used clinically.

Botanical medicines: Plants have been used as medicines since antiquity. The technology now exists to understand the physiological activities of herbs and a tremendous amount of research worldwide, especially in Europe, is demonstrating clinical efficacy. Botanical medicines are used for both vitalistic and pharmacological actions. Pharmacological effects and contraindications, as well as synergetic, energetic, and dilutional uses, are fundamental knowledge in naturopathic medicine (see Chapter 9).

Homeopathic medicine derives etymologically from the Greek word *homeos,* meaning "similar," and *pathos,* meaning "disease." Homeopathy is a system of medicine that treats a patient and his or her condition with a dilute, potentized agent, or drug, that will produce the same symptoms as the disease when given to a healthy individual, the fundamental principle being that *like cures like.* This principle was actually first recognized by Hippocrates, who noticed that herbs and other substances given in small doses tended to cure the same symptoms they produced when given in toxic doses. Prescriptions are based on the totality of all of the patient's symptoms and matched to "provings" of homeopathic medicines. Provings are symptoms produced in healthy people who are unaware of the specific remedy they have received. Large numbers of people are tested, and these symptoms documented. The symptoms are then added to toxicology, symptomatology, and data from cured cases to form the homeopathic materia medica. Homeopathic medicines are derived from a variety of plant, mineral, and chemical substances and are prepared according to the specifications of the *Homeopathic Pharmacopoeia of the United States.* Approximately 100 clinical studies have demonstrated the clinical efficacy of homeopathic therapies (see Chapter 7).

TCM is analogous to naturopathic medicine to the extent that it is a system with principles corollary to working with the self-healing process. According to Bensoussan and Myers (1996),

TCM shares some common ideas with other forms of complementary medicine, including belief in a strong inter-relationship between the environment and bodily function and an understanding of illness as starting with an imbalance of energy. . . . The TCM diagnostic process is . . . particularly holistic in nature [again similar to naturopathic medicine] and is usually contrasted to a reductionistic approach in western medicine. Western medicine often defines disease at an organ level of dysfunction and is increasingly reliant on laboratory findings. In contrast, TCM defines disease as a whole person disturbance.

Quiang Cao, ND, LAC, Bastyr University, explains:

TCM never treats just the symptom, but the individual's whole constitution and environmental conditions; all are considered in a holistic context. The symptom signals constitutional excess or deficiency. The goal is not just to alleviate the symptom but to balance yin and yang, hot and cold, excess and deficiency, internally and externally.

Acupuncture is an ancient Chinese system of medicine involving the stimulation of certain specific points on the body to enhance the flow of vital energy (qi) along pathways called *meridians.* Acupuncture points can be stimulated by the insertion and withdrawing of needles, the application of heat (moxibustion), massage, laser, electrical means, or a combination of these methods. Traditional Chinese acupuncture implies a very specific acupuncture technique and knowledge of the Oriental system of medicine, including yin-yang, the five elements, acupuncture points and meridians, and a method of diagnosis and differentiation of syndromes quite different from that of Western medicine. Although most research in this country has focused on its use for the pain relief and the treatment of addictions, it is a complete system of medicine effective for many diseases (see Chapter 18).

Hydrotherapy is the use of water in any of its forms (e.g., hot, cold, ice, steam) and methods of application (e.g., sitz bath, douche, spa and hot tub, whirlpool, sauna, shower, immersion bath, pack, poultice, foot bath, fomentation, wrap, colonic irrigations) in the maintenance of health or treatment of disease. It is one of the most ancient methods of treatment and has been part of naturopathic medicine since its inception. Nature doctors, before and since Sebastian Kneipp, have used hydrotherapy as a central part of clinical practice. Hydrotherapy has been used to treat disease and injury by many different cultures, including the Egyptians, Assyrians, Persians, Greeks, Hebrews, Hindus, and Chinese. Its most sophisticated applications were developed in eighteenth-century Germany. Naturopathic physicians today use hydrotherapy to stimulate and support healing, for detoxification, and to strengthen immune function for many chronic and acute conditions.

Physical medicine refers to the therapeutic use of touch, heat, cold, electricity, and sound. This includes the use of physiotherapy equipment such as ultrasound, diathermy, and other electromagnetic energy agents; therapeutic exercise; massage; massage energy techniques, joint mobilization (manipulative), and immobilization techniques; and hydrotherapy. In the therapeutic order, correction of structural integrity is a key factor; the hands-on approach of naturopathic physicians through physical medicine is unique in primary care.

Detoxification, the recognition and correction of endogenous and exogenous toxicity, is an important theme in naturopathic medicine. Liver and bowel detoxification, elimination of environmental toxins, correction of the metabolic dysfunction(s) that causes the buildup of non–end-product metabolites—all are important ways of decreasing toxic load. Spiritual and emotional toxicity are also recognized as important factors in restoring health.

Spirituality and health issues are central to naturopathic practice and are based on the individual patient's belief and/or spiritual orientation; simply, what moves the patient toward life and a higher purpose than himself or herself. Because total health also includes spiritual health, naturopathic physicians encourage individuals to pursue their personal spiritual development. As a plethora of studies in the newly emerging field of psychoneuroimmunology, particularly those both the placebo and nocebo effect have demonstrated, the body is not a mere collection of organs but a body, mind, and spirit in which the mind-spirit part of the equation marshals tremendous forces promoting health or disease.

Counseling, health psychology, and *lifestyle modification techniques* are essential modalities for the naturopathic physician. An ND is a holistic physician formally trained in mental, emotional, and family counseling. Various treatment measures include hypnosis and guided imagery, counseling techniques, correcting underlying organic factors, and family systems therapy.

THERAPEUTIC APPROACH

Respect Nature

We are natural organisms, our genomes developed and expressed in the natural world. The patterns and processes inherent in nature are inherent in us. We exist as a part of complex patterns of matter, energy, and spirit. Nature doctors have observed the natural processes of these patterns in health and disease and determined that there is an inherent drive toward health that lives within the patterns and processes of nature.

The drive is not perfect. There are times when unguided, unassisted, or unstopped the drive goes astray, causing preventable harm or even death: the healing intention becomes pathology. The ND is trained to know, respect, and work with this drive and to know when to wait/do nothing, act preventively, assist, amplify, palliate, intervene, manipulate, control or even suppress using the principle of the least force. The challenge of twenty-first century medicine is to support the beneficial effects of this drive and come to a sophisticated application of the least force principle in mainstream health care. This will prevent the last 20 years of life being those of debility from chronic, degenerative disease for the average American and extend healthspan throughout life span.

Because the total organism is involved in the healing attempt, the most effective approach to care must consider the whole person. In addition to physical and laboratory findings, important consideration is given to the patient's mental, emotional, and spiritual attitude; lifestyle; diet; heredity; environment; and family and community life. Careful attention to each person's unique individuality and susceptibility to disease is critical to the proper evaluation and treatment of any health problem.

Naturopathic physicians believe that most disease is the direct result of the ignorance and violation of "natural living laws." These rules are summarized as the consumption of natural, unrefined, organically grown foods; ensuring adequate amounts of exercise and rest; living a moderately paced lifestyle; having constructive and creative thoughts and emotions; avoiding environmental toxins; and maintaining proper elimination. During illness it is also important to control these areas to remove as many unnecessary stresses as possible and to optimize the chances that the organism's healing attempt will be successful. Therefore fundamental to naturopathic practice is patient education and responsibility, lifestyle modification, preventive medicine, and wellness promotion.

The Approach

The therapeutic approach of the naturopathic doctor is therefore basically twofold: to help patients heal themselves and to use the opportunity to guide and educate the patient in developing a more healthful lifestyle. Many supposedly incurable conditions respond very well to naturopathic approaches.

A typical first office visit with an ND takes 1 hour. The goal is to learn as much as possible about the patient using thorough history and review of systems, physical examination, laboratory tests, radiology, and other standard diagnostic procedures; also, the patient's diet, environment, toxic load, exercise, stress, and other aspects of lifestyle are evaluated, and laboratory tests are used to determine physiological function. Once a good understanding of the patient's health and disease status is established (making a diagnosis of a disease is only one part of this process), the ND and patient work together to establish a treatment and health promotion program.

Although every effort is made to treat the whole person and not just his or her disease, the limits of a short description like this necessitate the description of typical naturopathic therapies of specific conditions in a simplified, disease-oriented manner. Following are a few examples of how the person's health can be improved, resulting in alleviation of the disease.

Cervical Dysplasia

The only traditional medical approach to treating cervical dysplasia, a precancerous condition of the cervix, is surgical resection. Nothing is done to treat the underlying causes. The typical naturopathic treatment would include the following:

1. *Education:* about factors that increase the risk of cervical cancer, such as smoking (risk = 3.0), multiple sex partners (risk = 3.4), and the use of oral contraceptives (risk = 3.6) (Clarke et al., 1985).
2. *Prevention:* because 67% of patients with cervical cancer are deficient in one or more nutrients (Orr et al., 1985), and serum β-carotene (critical for the prevention of cancer of cells like those in the cervix) level is only half that of normal women (Dawson et al., 1984), the woman's nutritional status would be optimized (through diet, especially by increasing intake of fruits and vegetables) and with regard to those nutrients known to be deficient (often a result of oral contraceptive use) in women with cervical dysplasia and the deficiencies of which may promote cellular abnormalities: folic acid (Van Niekerk, 1966), β-carotene (Dawson et al., 1984), vitamin C (Romney et al., 1985), vitamin B_6 (Ramaswarmy & Natarajan, 1984), and selenium (Dawson et al., 1984).
3. *Treatment:* the vaginal depletion pack (a traditional mixture of botanical medicines placed against the cervix) would be used to promote sloughing of the abnormal cells.

The advantages of this approach are many: the causes of the cervical dysplasia have been identified and resolved, so the problem should not recur; no surgery is used, thus no scar tissue is formed; and the cost, particularly considering that many women with cervical dysplasia have recurrences when treated with standard surgery, is reasonable. More important, however, is that the woman's health has been improved, and other conditions that could have been caused by the identified nutritional deficiencies have now been prevented.

Migraine Headache

The standard medical treatment is primarily to use drugs to relieve symptoms, a costly and recurrent practice. Nothing is done to address the underlying causes. In contrast, the naturopath recognizes that most migraine headaches are caused by food allergies, and abnormal prostaglandin metabolism caused by nutritional abnormalities results in excessive platelet aggregation. The approach is straightforward:

1. Identify and avoid the allergenic foods because 70% or more of patients have migraines in re-

action to foods to which they are intolerant (Natero et al., 1989).

2. Supplement with magnesium because migraine sufferers have significantly lowered serum and salivary magnesium levels, which are even lower during an attack (Sarchielli et al., 1992). In one study 41% of 32 patients with an acute migraine had low serum magnesium (Baker, 1993). "In another report, magnesium levels in the brain, measured by NMR spectroscopy were significantly lower in patients during an acute migraine than in healthy individuals" (Weaver, 1990) (Gaby, 1998).

3. Reestablish normal prostaglandin balance by decreasing animal fats (high in platelet-aggregating arachadonic acid) and supplementing with essential fatty acids like fish oils (Woodcock et al., 1984).

4. Supplement with riboflavin. "Forty-nine individuals with recurrent migraines were given 400 mg/day of the B-vitamin riboflavin for at least 3 months. The average number of migraine attacks fell by 67% and migraine severity improved by 68%" (Gaby, 1998).

Hypertension

The patients with so-called idiopathic, or essential, hypertension can be very effectively treated if they are willing to make the necessary lifestyle changes.

1. *Diet:* Numerous studies have shown that excessive dietary salt in conjunction with inadequate dietary potassium is a major contributor to hypertension (Fries, 1976; Khaw & Barrett-Connor, 1984; Meneely & Battarbee, 1976), that dietary deficiencies in calcium (Belizan et al., 1983; McCarron et al., 1982), magnesium (Dyckner & Wester, 1983; Resnick et al., 1989), essential fatty acids (Rao et al., 1981; Vergroesen et al., 1978), and vitamin C (Yoshioka et al., 1981) all contribute to increased blood pressure and that increased consumption of sugar (Hodges & Rebello, 1983), caffeine (Lang et al., 1983), and alcohol (Gruchow et al., 1985) are all associated with hypertension.

2. *Lifestyle:* Smoking (Kershbaum et al., 1968), obesity (Havlik et al., 1983), stress (Ford, 1982), and a sedentary lifestyle are all known to contribute to the development of high blood pressure.

3. *Environment:* Exposure to heavy metals such as lead (Pruess, 1992) and cadmium (Glauser et al., 1976) increase blood pressure.

4. *Botanical medicine:* Many herbal medicines are used when necessary for the patient's safety to initially rapidly lower his or her blood pressure until the slower, but more curative, dietary and lifestyle treatments can have their effects. Included are such age-old favorites as garlic *(Allium sativa)* and mistletoe *(Viscum album).*

The causes of high blood pressure are not unknown, but they are generally unheeded.

Lifestyle modification is crucial to the successful implementation of naturopathic techniques—health does not come from a doctor, pills, or surgery but rather from the patients' own efforts to take proper care of themselves. Unfortunately, our society expends considerable resources to induce disease-promoting habits. Although it is relatively easy to tell a patient to stop smoking, get more exercise, and reduce his or her stress, such lifestyle changes are difficult in the context of peer, habit, and commercial pressure. The ND is specifically trained to assist the patient in making the needed changes. This involves many aspects: helping the patient acknowledge the need; setting realistic, progressive goals; identifying and working through barriers; establishing a support group of family and friends or of others with similar problems; identifying the stimuli that reinforce the unhealthy behavior; and giving the patient positive reinforcement for his or her gains.

ACCOUNTABILITY IN NATUROPATHIC MEDICINE

Acceptance of a profession typically is seen to derive from sanctions associated with educational institutions, professional associations and licensing boards.

—ORZACK (1997)

It is extremely important to realize that the establishment of standards and especially credentialling standards is critical for the public to know . . . whatever the discipline is.

—LEVUNDUSKI (1991)

Although naturopathic medicine in the early part of the century was unique, clinically effective, and powerfully vitalistic, it suffered because it had not reached maturity in terms of professional unification, scientific research, and other recognizable standards of public accountability. These goals have finally been achieved during the last two decades (1978-2000).

Naturopathic medicine has responded not only to the need to integrate the best that conventional and natural medicine have to offer but also to issues of public safety, efficacy, and affordability through the following mechanisms:

- Fully accredited naturopathic medical training (regional and professional)
- Standardized science-based naturopathic medical education
- Broad scope licensing laws
- Nationally standardized licensing examinations
- Professional standards of practice and peer review
- Credentialling and quality improvement plans
- Scientific research and efficacy documentation

These are well-accepted mechanisms for public accountability in all forms of licensed health care. Naturopathic medicine's credibility is due in part to these important achievements by a unified profession.

SCOPE OF PRACTICE, LICENSING, AND PROFESSIONAL ORGANIZATIONS

NDs practice as primary care providers. They see patients of all ages, from all walks of life, with every known disease. They make a conventional Western diagnosis using standard diagnostic procedures, such as physical examination, laboratory tests, and radiologic examination. However, they also make a pathophysiological diagnosis using physical and laboratory procedures to assess nutritional status, metabolic function, and toxic load. In addition, a considerable amount of time is spent assessing the patient's mental, emotional, social, and spiritual status.

Therapeutically, NDs use virtually every known natural therapy—dietetics, therapeutic nutrition, botanical medicine (primarily the European, Native American, Chinese, and Ayurvedic), physical therapy, spinal manipulation, lifestyle counseling, exercise therapy, homeopathic medicine, acupuncture, psychological and family counseling, hydrotherapy, and clinical fasting and detoxification. In addition, according to state law, NDs may perform office surgery, administer vaccinations, and prescribe a limited range of drugs. Because NDs consider themselves an integral part of the health care system, they meet public health requirements and work within a referral network of specialists in much the same way as a family practice medical (allopathic) doctor; this network includes the range of conventional and nonconventional providers.

NDs (or NMDs) are licensed in 11 states (Alaska, Arizona, Connecticut, Hawaii, Maine, Montana, New Hampshire, Oregon, Vermont, Utah, and Washington) and have a legal right to practice in another two (Idaho and the District of Columbia). Because no licensing standards exist in these two states and NDs also practice in other states without government approval, individuals with little or no formal education are still able to proclaim themselves NDs to the significant detriment of the public and the profession. The American Association of Naturopathic Physicians, located in Washington, DC, assists consumers in identifying qualified NDs.

The scope of naturopathic practice is stipulated by state law. Legislation typically allows standard diagnostic privileges. Therapeutic scope is more varied, ranging from only natural therapies to vaccinations, limited prescriptive rights, and office surgery. In addition, some states allow the practice of natural childbirth.

In addition to the Council on Naturopathic Medical Education (CNME), two key organizations provide leadership and standardization for the naturopathic profession. The American Association of Naturopathic Physicians (AANP), founded in 1985 by James Sensenig, ND, and others, was established to provide consistent educational and practice standards for the profession and a unified voice for public relations and political activity. Most licensed NDs in the United States are members of the association. The Naturopathic Physicians Licensing Examination (NPLEx) was founded under the auspices of the AANP in 1986 by Ed Hoffman-Smith, PhD, ND, to establish a nationally recognized standardized test for licensing. NPLEx is recognized by all states licensing NDs. All states licensing NDs and all states in the process of attaining licensure have state professional naturopathic associations. The Alliance for State Licensing, a rapidly accelerating state licensure effort, is under way.

INTEGRATION INTO THE MAINSTREAM

The American public has increasingly turned to alternative practitioners in search of healing for a variety of conditions not ameliorated by conventional medical practices (e.g., otitis media, cardiovascular disease, depression, chronic fatigue syndrome, gastrointestinal disorders, chemical sensitivities, recurrent infectious diseases, rheumatoid arthritis, general loss of vitality and wellness, and many other chronic and acute conditions).

Unquestionably, the health care system is undergoing profound change.... Many ... current aspects of health care have resulted from a period of rapid change in the early part of this century. We are returning to a period of rapid change.... What is less certain is exactly where that change will lead. The task ... is to identify and understand the forces of change and describe these forces so that [we] can make [our] decisions more wisely (Bezold, 1986).

Naturopathic medicine has accomplished important steps in integrating into mainstream delivery systems, for example:

Reimbursement—The Every Category of Provider Law: In 1993, during health care reform in Washington state, the "every category of provider law" was passed. This law mandated insurance companies to include access to every category of licensed provider in all types of plans in insurance systems for the treatment of all conditions covered in the Basic Health Plan. Washington State Insurance Commissioner Deborah Senn has vigorously enforced this law in Washington state. She formed the Clinician Working Group on the Integration of Complementary and Alternative Medicine (CWIC), bringing together medical directors, plan representatives, and conventional and CAM providers to identify issues and solutions to integration barriers in insurance systems. This step has been important in increasing consumers' access to the health care providers of their choice, including licensed CAM professionals, as well as providing a solution focus to valid integration challenges. Other reimbursement initiatives in the United States have also been successful. NDs throughout the country are being integrated as primary care providers and specialists in traditional and managed care systems. The Pacific Northwest has emerged as a testing ground or model for integration because of the legislative and regulatory environment in the region.

Health Professional Loan Repayment and Scholarship Program: In 1995 Washington State's Department of Health made naturopathic physicians eligible for student loan repayment in the state's Health Professional Loan Repayment and Scholarship Program. Grants are awarded for student scholarships and student loan reimbursement to health care providers qualified and willing to provide health care in underserved areas or to underserved populations. The first and second naturopathic physician grants for loan repayment were awarded in 1998 and 2000.

King County Natural Medicine Clinic: No conventional model or infrastructure now exists in mainstream medicine for the systematic delivery of care that integrates natural and conventional providers. This integrative model is fundamental to naturopathic medicine. The King County Natural Medicine Clinic in Kent, Washington, is the first publicly funded integrative care clinic in the United States and has been a collaboration between Bastyr University and Community Health Centers of King County (CHCKC) with funding provided by the Seattle King County Department of Public Health. This project forms an unprecedented union between three health forms: conventional medicine, natural medicine, and public health. The clinic has successfully applied a comanagement model by using an interdisciplinary health care team co-led by naturopathic physicians and medical doctors, including nurse practitioners, acupuncturists, and dietitians. The clinic serves the medically underserved. The Centers for Disease Control and Prevention and a team of independent researchers are conducting research to study the provider-to-provider interactions and their effect on health care, patient satisfaction, and cost-effectiveness. There are also several studies under way comparing results from natural and conventional therapies on specific conditions treated using this model.

Comanagement:

Naturopathic medical (co-management) is the practice of medicine by a naturopathic physician (N.D.) in concert with other care givers (N.D., M.D., D.O., L.Ac., D.C., etc.) wherein each care giver operates:
- In communication with others, according to established convention

- Within his licensed scope of practice and acknowledged domain of expertise
- With respect for the other care giver's autonomy, but with recognition of the ultimate responsibility and, therefore, authority of the patient's primary care giver (PCP)
- With respect for the other care giver's expertise, but with recognition of the ultimate responsibility and, therefore, final authority of the informed patient's choices and decisions.

Co-management presents an opportunity to educate other providers to naturopathic medicine as well as a chance to learn from them and expand one's information base and diagnostic and therapeutic potential. Most importantly, however, it greatly increases the therapeutic choices and quality of care to patients, often resulting in more supportive and less invasive therapies (minimizing iatrogenic diseases), while promoting healthier lifestyles and overall reduction in health-care dollars spent (Milliman & Donovan, 1996).

Continuous Quality Improvement

In 1996 the Washington Association of Naturopathic Physicians (WANP) developed a quality assurance program consistent with national accreditation standards. This plan, known as *Continuous Quality Improvement* (CoQI), was completed and adopted by the Washington State Department of Health and was the first naturopathic CoQI Plan approved in the United States. This process is used by all health care professions and enables the profession to define and continuously update its own standards of care. Jennifer Booker, ND, and Bruce Milliman, ND, led this effort.

Residencies
Utah is the first state to require a 1-year residency for naturopathic licensure. Residency opportunities for NDs are growing rapidly through sites established by the naturopathic colleges. Cancer Treatment Centers of America offer a growing number of residencies and staff positions to naturopathic physicians. National College of Naturopathic Medicine and Bastyr University offer a growing number of residencies throughout the United States. All naturopathic colleges also offer residencies on-site.

Hospitals and Hospital Networks
A number of hospitals across the United States are now employing NDs as part of their physician staff in both inpatient and outpatient settings. Following are a few examples of the types of treatment centers:

1. HealthEast Healing Center, a clinic that is part of a larger "hospitals plus provider networks delivery system" employs medical doctors, an ND, an acupuncturist, and body workers, using a "learning organization" model (Alternative Medicine Integration and Coverage, 1997).
2. The Alternative and Complementary Medical Program at St. Elizabeth's Hospital in Massachusetts has a credentialed ND on staff. "The hospital is a teaching center for Tufts University Medical School" (Alternative Medicine Integration and Coverage, 1998).
3. Centura Health (CH), the largest health care system in Colorado, is composed of an association of Catholic and Adventist hospitals. CH owns preferred provider organization Sloans Lake Managed Care. NDs are credentialed along with ND homeopaths and many other CAM providers in this hospital-based network (Alternative Medicine Integration and Coverage, 1998).
4. American Complementary Care Network (ACCN) has recently placed two NDs in key positions—Medical Director of Naturopathic Medicine and Chair of Quality Improvement (Alternative Medicine Integration and Coverage, 1998). Other networks, such as Wisconsin-based CAM Solutions and Seattle-based Alternare, have integrated ND-credentialed medical directors on staff.

When health systems, insurers, and health maintenance organizations (HMOs) decide to cover alternative medicine, NDs are sought out in licensed states. Even in states without naturopathic licensure, health systems and managed care organizations exploring integration have come to understand and value the depth of training of naturopathic physicians (Weeks, 1998).

EDUCATION

The trend of modern medical research and practice in our great colleges and endowed research institutes is almost en-tirely along combative lines, while the individual, progressive physician learns to work more and more along preventive lines.

—LINDLAHR (1914)

The education of the ND is extensive and incorporates much of the diversity that typifies the natural health care movement. The training program has important similarities to conventional medical education (science-based, identical basic sciences, intensive clinical diagnostic sciences), with the primary differences being in the therapeutic sciences, enhanced clinical sciences, clinical theory, and integrative case management. Naturopathic training places the pathology-based training of conventional physicians into the context of the broader naturopathic assessment and management model inclusive of nature, mind, body, and spirit in health care. To be eligible to enroll, prospective students must first successfully complete a conventional premedicine program that typically requires a college degree in a biological science. The naturopathic curriculum then takes an additional 4 years to complete. Residency opportunities are increasing rapidly throughout the United States, at NCNM Bastyr and SCNM. As noted previously, residency is now required for licensure in the state of Utah.

The first 2 years concentrate on the standard human biological sciences, basic diagnostic sciences, and introduction to the various treatment modalities. The conventional basic medical sciences include anatomy, human dissection, histology, physiology, biochemistry, pathology, microbiology, immunology and infectious disease, public health, pharmacology, and biostatistics. The development of diagnostic skills is initiated with courses in physical diagnosis, laboratory diagnosis, and clinical assessment. Natural medicine subjects such as environmental health, pharmacognosy (pharmacology of herbal medicines), botanical medicine, naturopathic philosophy and case management, Chinese medicine, Ayurvedic medicine, homeopathic medicine, spinal manipulation, nutrition, physiotherapy, hydrotherapy, physician well-being, counseling and health psychology, and spirituality and health are also covered.

The second 2 years are oriented toward the clinical sciences of diagnosis and treatment while natural medicine subjects continue. Not only are the standard diagnostic techniques of physical, laboratory, and radiological examination taught, but what makes the diagnostic training unique is its emphasis on preventive diagnosis, such as diet analysis, recognition of the early physical signs of nutritional deficiencies, laboratory methods for assessing physiological dysfunction before it progresses to cellular pathology and end-stage disease, assessment and treatment of lifestyle and spiritual factors, and methods of assessing toxic load and liver detoxification efficacy. The natural therapies, such as nutrition, botanical medicines, homeopathy, acupuncture, natural childbirth, hydrotherapy, fasting, physical therapy, exercise therapy, counseling, and lifestyle modification, are studied extensively. Courses in naturopathic case analysis and management integrate naturopathic philosophy into conventional algorithms using the therapeutic order.

During the last 2 years, students also work in outpatient clinics where they see patients, first as observers and later as primary caregivers under the supervision of licensed NDs. Currently, four schools exist in the United States and one in Canada: Bastyr University (Bastyr), National College of Naturopathic Medicine (NCNM), the Southwest College of Naturopathic Medicine and Health Sciences (Southwest), the University of Bridgeport College of Naturopathic Medicine (UBCNM), and in Canada, the Canadian College of Naturopathic Medicine (CCNM). The oldest institution is NCNM, which was established in 1965, in Portland, Oregon. The largest institution and first to receive accreditation is Bastyr University, established in Seattle, Washington, in 1978. Over the years Bastyr has broadened its mission to also include accredited degree and certificate programs in nutrition, acupuncture and Chinese medicine, midwifery, applied behavioral sciences, health psychology, and spirituality and health. Southwest College, established in 1993, has developed an active research department. The University of Bridgeport, established in 1997, is the most recent addition. Like its counterparts in the United States, CCNM in Toronto, Ontario, has a rapidly increasing enrollment. Naturopathic education is accredited by the U.S. Department of Education recognized Council on Naturopathic Medical Education (CNME). The CNME has granted institutional accreditation to NCNM, accreditation of the Naturopathic Medicine program at Bastyr (Bastyr is also accredited by the Northwest Association of Schools and Colleges), and preaccredited status to Southwest. All states licensing naturopathic physicians recognize the CNME as the official accrediting agency for naturopathic medicine. The offices of the CNME are located in Portland, Oregon.

Research

Science clearly is an essential condition of a right decision.
                                                    —PELLEGRINO (1979)

However, clinical decisions cannot be solely dependent on science, when, with the best of efforts and with billions of public and private dollars spent, medical research has yielded twenty percent and (in some narrow areas up to fifty percent) of medical procedures and practices as scientifically proven and efficacious.

         —OFFICE OF TECHNOLOGY ASSESSMENT (1978)

There is a paucity of theories of medicine. . . . The theory of medicine has lagged seriously behind theories of other sciences . . . any unitary theory of medicine which identifies it exclusively with science is doomed to failure.

                                                    —PELLEGRINO (1979)

The primary intellectual problem facing medicine today is that the information base of medicine is so poor. For a profession with a 2,000 year history which is responsible in the United States for 250 million lives and spends over $600 billion a year, we are astonishingly ignorant. We simply do not know the consequences of a large proportion of medical activities. The . . . task is to change our mind set about what constitutes an acceptable source of knowledge in medicine.

                                                         —EDDY (1993)

The relationship between scientific research and the study of the healing power of nature, a traditionally vitalistic principle, is important. The scientific method is a well-accepted approach to communicating what we learn about medicine's mysteries to others; however, it has been limited in its development by conventional medicine's approach to research. Orthodox research appears to turn on the premise that the universe functions without telos or purpose. Connections are mechanistic. Clinical relevance is directed toward pharmaceutical disease management by means of a single-agent, placebo-controlled, double-blind crossover trial.

What distinguishes naturopathic medicine's clinical research from biomedicine's (a term coined to refer to the currently dominant school of medicine) is not the presence or lack of science. It is a collective confidence in the perception of a vital force or life force. The arguments then follow. What is it? What exactly does it do and how? As Dr. John Bastyr noted,

"We all have an innate ability to understand that there is a moving force in us, that doesn't necessarily need to be understood mechanistically" (interview, August 1989). Future scientific work and naturopathic medical research on this principle is bound by the shared perception (1) that there is a pattern in health and disease; (2) that there is order in the healing process; and (3) that order is based on the life force, which is self-organized, intelligent, and intelligible. Within this paradigm, we can research the life force. Confirming and challenging clinical perceptions and even disproving core assumptions is fundamental to naturopathic medicine's core values. Scientific methods must be challenged to find new approaches to test large quantities and types of clinical data, outcomes, and systems from naturopathic practices. So far, the "Healing Power of Nature's" *(vis medicatrix naturae's)* actuality has not been proved or disproved by the single-agent double-blind study. New models (e.g., outcomes research, field and practice-based research, multifactorial models) provide fertile ground for researching the validity of nonconventional medicine and new opportunities for research on conventional practices.

Until recently, original research at naturopathic institutions has been quite limited. The profession has relied on its clinical traditions and the worldwide published scientific research.

Research in whole practices are only recently gaining interest with the development of methodologies in practice-based and outcomes research. There is a lack of research in whole practices like naturopathy, Oriental medicine, or Ayurveda compared to conventional practice whether in a particular disease or in overall health outcomes. Biomedical research methods which are considered gold-standard by the scientific community have been typically developed to provide reliable data on a single therapeutic intervention for a specific Western disease entity. The requirements of these research methods distort naturopathic practice and may render it apparently less effective than it may actually be. The measures may not take account of residual benefits in a patient's other health problems nor on future health and health care utilization. Compounding the methodological difficulties of research in this medical variant, there are structural obstacles as well. Distinct from the situation in conventional medicine, there is only the beginning of a research infrastructure at the profession's academic centers. Practitioners expert in naturopathic medicine and the individualization of treatment are typically not trained in rigorous comparative trials. Even if the infrastructure and training were in place, sources of funding remain few and small, and most funding agencies make their decisions on the basis of biomedical theories which naturopathy may directly challenge. When research is done on aspects of naturopathic treatment, more studies are done on substances rather than procedures or lifestyle changes. Without the economic incentives which favor the in-depth study of patentable drugs, trials in naturopathic therapeutics, often derived from a long history of human use, are smaller and with fewer replications. Many practices present special methodological or ethical problems for control, randomization, blinding, etc., perhaps making it impossible to perform a study as rigorous as some might wish. Nevertheless, there are numerous studies which yield indications of the effectiveness of individual treatments (Calabrese et al., 1997).

A comprehensive compilation of the scientific documentation of naturopathic philosophy and therapies can be found in *A Textbook of Natural Medicine*, coauthored and edited by Joseph Pizzorno, ND, and Michael Murray, ND. First published in 1985, the *Textbook* was, until 1998, in a looseleaf, two-volume set, published by Bastyr University Publications and updated regularly. The latest edition, published by Churchill Livingstone and released in the fall of 1998, now is made up of more than 200 chapters and references more than 10,000 citations from the peer-reviewed scientific literature.

In the past decade Bastyr University, National College of Naturopathic Medicine, and recently, Southwest College of Naturopathic Medicine have developed active research departments that have resulted in the publication of original research in several peer-reviewed journals, both alternative and mainstream. In October 1994 Bastyr University was awarded a 3-year, $840,000 grant by the U.S. National Institutes of Health Office of Alternative and Complementary Medicine to establish a research center to study alternative therapies for human immunodeficiency virus/acquired immunodeficiency syndrome (HIV/AIDS). Eleven other centers were established in conventional medical schools. The Bastyr group is currently completing a text on alternative therapies in HIV/AIDS for the series *Medical Guides to Complementary and Alternative Medicine*. The profession publishes a peer-reviewed journal, the *Journal of Naturopathic Medicine*, founded in 1990 by Peter D'Adamo, ND, of Norwalk, Connecticut.

THE FUTURE

We could have a significant and immediate impact on costly health care problems if the complementary and alternative medicine disciplines and interventions were widely available.

—DOSSEY & SWYERS (1992)

Naturopathic medicine is enabling patients to regain their health as NDs effectively comanage and integrate care with pertinent providers, to their patients' and the public's benefit. Today's ND, an extensively trained and state-licensed family physician, is equipped with a broad range of conventional and unconventional diagnostic and therapeutic skills. This modern ND considers himself or herself an integral part of the health care system and takes a full share of responsibility for common public health issues.

The scientific tools now exist to assess and appreciate many aspects of naturopathy's approach to health and healing. It is common for conventional medical organizations that in the past have spoken out strongly against naturopathic medicine to now endorse such techniques as lifestyle modification, stress reduction, exercise, consumption of a high-fiber diet rich in whole foods and other dietary measures, supplemental nutrients, toxin reduction, and many others.

These changes in perspective signal the paradigm shift that is occurring in medicine. Emerging knowledge, high health care costs, and unmet health care needs are rapidly forcing this shift in perspective into changes in our current health care system. What was once rejected is now becoming generally accepted as effective. In many instances, it has become recognized that naturopathic alternatives offer benefit over certain orthodox practices. In the future more concepts and practices of naturopathic medicine will undoubtedly be assessed and integrated into mainstream health care.

Historically, emerging bodies of knowledge in health care have formed into schools of thought and professions with standards as the public need for their services increases; naturopathic medicine's reemergence is no accident or anomaly. Naturopathic medicine has followed the developmental stages that health care professions typically undergo while becoming accountable to the public. Access has increased with increasing research and standards.

These models and standards in emerging complementary and alternative medicine fields, including naturopathic medicine, hold answers to health care, delivery, and system issues, which are as singularly significant as the interventions themselves. With accreditation, licensure, reimbursement, ongoing research, and widespread public acceptance, the naturopathic clinical model is reaching professional maturity today.

References

Belizan J, Villar J, Pineda O, et al. 1983. Reduction of blood pressure with calcium supplementation in young adults. JAMA 249:1161-1165

Bensoussan A, Myers S. 1996. Towards a Safer Choice: The Practice of Traditional Chinese Medicine in Australia. Faculty of Health, University of Western Sydney Macarthur, Australia: pp. 20, 82, 109

Bezold C. 1986. Health trends and scenarios: Implications for the health care professions. American Enterprise Institute Studies in Health Policy 449:77-97

Blois M. 1988. Medicine and the nature of vertical reasoning. N Engl J Med 318(13):847-851

Bradley R. 1985. Philosophy of naturopathic medicine—1, in Textbook of Natural Medicine. John Bastyr College Publications, Seattle

Calabrese C, Breed C, Ruhland J. 1997. The effectiveness of naturopathic medicine in disease conditions. The State of the Science in Naturopathic Medicine presentation at the Annual AANP Convention

Clarke E, Hatcher J, McKeown-Essyen G, Liekrish G. 1985. Cervical dysplasia: Association with sexual behavior, smoking, and oral contraceptive use. Am J Obstet Gynecol 151:612-616

Cooper R, Stoflet S. 1996. Trends in the education and practice of alternative medicine clinicians. Health Affairs 15.3:226, 233

Dawson E, Nosovitch J, Hannigan E. 1984. Serum vitamin and selenium changes in cervical dysplasia. Fed Proc 46:612

Dossey L, Swyers J. 1992. Alternative Medicine Expanding Medical Horizons. U.S. Government Printing Office, Washington, DC

Dyckner T, Wester O. 1983. Effect of magnesium on blood pressure. BMJ 286:1847-1849

Eddy D. 1993. Decisions without information, HMO Pract 5(2):58-60

Eddy MB. 1875. Science and health with key to the scriptures

Felter HW, Lloyd JU. 1898. King's American Dispensary

Ford M. 1982. Biofeedback treatment for headaches, Raynaud's disease, essential hypertension, and irritable bowel syndrome: A review of the long term follow-up literature. Biof Self-Reg 7:521-535

Fries E. 1976. Salt, volume and the prevention of hypertension. Circulation 53:589-595

Funk J. 1995. Naturopathic and allopathic healing: A developmental comparison. Townsend Letter for Doctors and Patients October:50-58

Gaby A. 1998. Commentary on migraine. Unpublished

Glauser S, Bello C, Gauser E. 1976. Blood-cadmium levels in normotensive and untreated hypertensive humans. Lancet 1:717-718

Gruchow HW, Sobocinski MS, Barboriak JJ. 1985. Alcohol, nutrient intake, and hypertension in US adults. JAMA 253:1567-1570

Havlik R, Hubert H, Fabsitz R, Feinleib M. 1983. Weight and hypertension. Ann Intern Med 98:855-859

Hodges R, Rebello T. 1983. Carbohydrates and blood pressure. Ann Intern Med 98:838-841

Kershbaum A, Pappajohn D, Bellet S, et al. 1968. Effect of smoking and nicotine on adrenocortical secretion. JAMA 203:113-116

Khaw KT, Barrett-Connor. 1984. Dietary potassium and blood pressure in a population. Am J Clin Nutr 39:963-968

Kirchfield F, Boyle W. 1994. Nature Doctors. Medicina Biological/Buckeye Naturopathic Press: Portland, OR/East Palestine, Ohio: p. 311

Kuts-Cheraux AW. 1953. Naturae Medicina. ANPSA, Des Moines, Iowa

Lang T, Degoulet P, Aime F, et al. 1983. Relationship between coffee drinking and blood pressure: Analysis of 6,321 subjects in the Paris region. Am J Cardiol 52:1238-1242

Levenduski P. 1991. Testimony to U.S. Department of Education, National Advisory Committee on Accreditation and Institutional Eligibility. CNME hearing. Washington, DC

Lindlahr H. 1914a. Nature cure

Lindlahr H. 1914b. Philosophy of Natural Therapeutics. Vol I, II, and III. Dietetics. Maidstone Osteopathic, Maidstone, England

Lust B. 1896. The Naturopathic and Herald of Health

Lust B. 1918. Universal Directory of Naturopathy. Lust Publ, Butler, New Jersey

Lust B. 1945. Program of the 49th Congress of the American Naturopathy Association

McCarron D, Morris C, Cole C. 1982. Dietary calcium in human hypertension. Science 217:267-269

Meneely G, Battarbee. 1976. High sodium-low potassium environment and hypertension. Am J Cardiol 38:768-781

Milliman B, Donovan P. 1996. Naturopathic Medical Co-Management in The Emerging Integrative Care Model. The Best of Naturopathic Medicine Anthology. Southwest College Press. Tucson, AZ

Natero G, et al. 1989. Dietary migraine: Fact or Fiction? Headache 29:315-316

Office of Technology Assessment. 1978. US Department of Commerce National Technical Information Service, Washington, DC

Orr J, Wilson K, Bodiford C, et al. 1985. Nutritional status of patients with untreated cervical cancer, II. Vitamin assessment. Am J Obstet Gynecol 151:632-635

Orzack L. 1997. Professions and world trade diplomacy: national systems and international authority, in Professions, Identity, and Order in Comparative Perspective. Ed. Olgiani, Orzack & Saks, In press

Pellegrino E. 1979. Medicine, science, art: an old controversy revisited. Man Medicine 4:43-52

Pizzo____ Murray MT. 1985-95. A Textbook of Natural M____. John Bastyr College Publications, Seattle

Pizzorno ____ 1995. Using your mind as healer. Delicious! Magazine

____ L. 1997. The roots of herbalism in America. Delicious____ne

Pr___ss HG. 1992. Overview of lead toxicity in early life, effects on intellect loss and hypertension. J Am Coll Nutr ____

____ P, Natarajan R. 1984. Vitamin B_6 status in pa____ with cancer of the uterine cervix. Nutr Cancer ____-180

____ao U, Srikantia S. 1981. Effect of polyunsaturated ____table oils on blood pressure in essential hypertension. Clin Exp Hyperten 3:27-38

____nick LM, Gupta RK, Laragh JH. 1989. Intracellular free magnesium in erythrocytes of essential hypertension: Relationship to blood pressure and serum divalent cations. Proc Natl Acad Sci USA 81:6511-6515

____ney S, Duttagupta C, Basu J, et al. 1985. Plasma vitamin ____nd uterine dysplasia. Am J Obstet Gynecol 151:978-

____ et al. 1992. Serum and salivary magnesium levels in migrain and tension-type headaches: Results in a ____p of adult patients. Cephalgia 12:21-27

____ Zeff J. 1988, 1989. Select Committee on Defini____ Naturopathic Medicine Report: American Asso____on of Naturopathic Physicians: House of Delega____ Portland, OR

____iekerk W. 1966. Cervical cytological abnormalities c____ed by folic acid deficiency. Acta Cytol 10:67-73

____roesen A, Fleischman A, Comberg H, et al. 1978. The influence of increased dietary linoleate on essential hypertension in man. Acta Biol Med Germ Band 37:879-883.

Weeks, J. August, 1998. Personal communication

Werbach M 1996. The American Holistic Health Association ____lete Guide to Alternative Medicine. Werner Books, NY, pp. 118, 123

Whorton J. 1982. Crusaders for Fitness. Princeton Press, Princeton, New Jersey

Woodcock BE, Smith E, Lambert WH, et al. 1984. Beneficial effect of fish oil on blood viscosity in peripheral vascular disease. BMJ 288:592-594

Yoshioka M, Matsushita T, Chuman Y. 1981. Inverse association of serum ascorbic acid level and blood pressure or rate of hypertension in male adults aged 30-39 years.

Int J Vit Nutr Res 54:343-347

Zeff J. 1997. The process of healing: a unifying theory of naturopathic medicine. Journal of Naturopathic Medicine 7(1):122

Zeff J. 1998. J Naturopath Med 8(1):p. 90

Suggested Readings

Beasley JD, Swift JJ. 1989. The Kellogg Report: The Impact of Nutrition, Environment and Lifestyle on the Health of Americans. Annandale-on-Hudson, New York

Benjamin H. 1981. Everybody's Guide to Nature Cure, 7th ed. Thorsons Pub, England

Bilz FE. 1898. The Natural Method of Healing (2 vol). (English Translation) Bilz, Intl News Co, New York

Brown D. 1994. Quarterly Review of Natural Medicine. NPRC, Seattle

Coulter H. 1973. Divided Legacy, vol II. Wehawken Books, Washington, DC

Dejarnette MB. 1939. Technic & Practice of Bloodless Surgery. Private, Nebraska City

Filden JH. 1921. Impaired Health (Its Cause & Cure) 2d ed. Private, Denver

Garlic has to smell bad to do some good. 1992. Fam Prac News 22:31

Graham RL. 1923. Hydro-hygiene. Thompson-Barlow Co, New York

Griggs B. 1981. Green Pharmacy. Jill, Norman, & Hobhouse, London

Hofoss D, Hjort P. The relationship between action and research in health policy. Journal Soc Sci Med Vol 15a:371

Johnson AC. 1946. Principles & Practice of Drugless Therapeutics. Chir Ed Extension Bureau, Los Angeles

Jones D. 1998. Fifth International Symposium on Functional Medicine: Functional Medicine Application to Disorders of Gene Expression, Hawaii

Kellogg JF. 1901, 1902. Rational Hydrotherapy. Battle Creek, Michigan

Kellogg JH. 1923. New Dietetics. Modern Med Publ, Battle Creek, Michigan

Kirschner R, Brinkman R. 1988. American Association of Naturopathic Medicine Conference/Select Committee on Definition of Naturoapathic Medicine, Billings, Montana

Kuhne L: 1918. Neo-naturopathy (New Science of Healing). (Translated by B Lust), Lust Publ, Butler, New Jersey

Lindlahr H. 1914-1919. Philosophy, Practice, and Dietetics of Natural Therapeutics, Vol I-II. Maidstone Osteopathic. Maidstone, England

Lust B. 1918. Universal Directory of Naturopathy. Lust Publ, Butler, New Jersey

MacFadden B. 1904. Building of Vital Power. Phys Cult Publ, New Jersey

McKeown T. 1976. The Role of Medicine: Dream, Mirage, or Nemesis? Nuffield Provincial Hospitals Trust, London, United Kingdom

Murray MT, Pizzorno JE. 1991. Encyclopedia of Natural Medicine. Prima Publishing, Rocklin, California

Murray MT. 1994. Natural Alternatives to Over-the-Counter and Prescription Drugs. William Morrow, New York

Neuberger M. 1932. The doctrine of the healing power of nature throughout the course of time. Trans Linn J. Boyd. J Am Inst Homeo 25:861-884, 1011-1465

Petkov V. 1979. Plants with hypotensive, antiatheromatous and coronary dilating action. A J Chin Med 7:197-236

Pizzorno J. 1996, 1998. Total Wellness. Prima Publishing, p. 14

Richter JT. 1949. Nature—The Healer. Private, Los Angeles

Riley JS. Zone Reflex. Publications of Health Research

Shelton H. 1968. Natural Hygiene, Man's Pristine Way of Life. Published by Dr. Shelton's Health School, San Antonio, Texas, p. 8

Spitler. 1948. Basic Naturopathy. ANA, Des Moines

St. Anthony's Business Report on Alternative and Complementary Medicine. 1997. May, p. 5

St. Anthony's Business Report on Alternative and Complementary Medicine. 1998. July, pp. 6-7

St. Anthony's Business Report on Alternative and Complementary Medicine. 1998. August. pp. 4-5

Starr P. 1983. Social Transformation of American Medicine. Basic Books, New York

Trall RT. 1880. Hydropathic Encyclopedia. 3 vol. SR Wells, New York

Weltmer E. 1913. Practice of Suggestive Therapeutics. Weltmer Inst, Nevada, Missouri

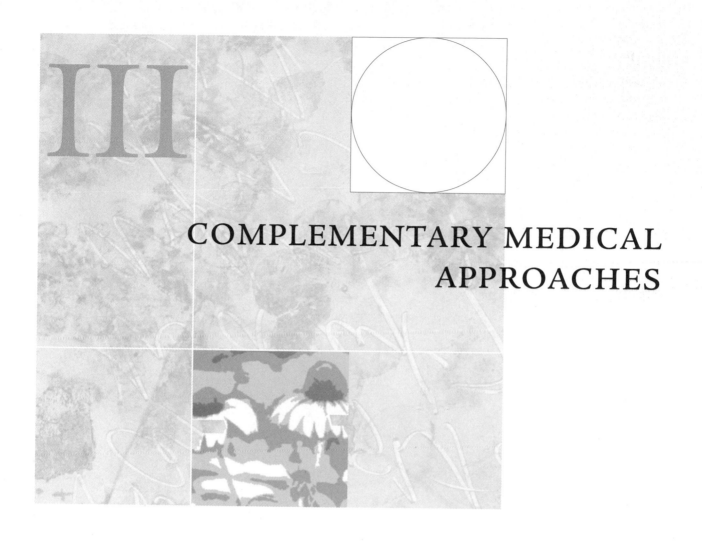

III

COMPLEMENTARY MEDICAL APPROACHES

*A*lthough most forms of complementary and alternative medicine can be seen to draw on a "mind-body" connection, the complementary medical approaches described in this section appear to make use of physiological mechanisms by which mental state may be reflected in direct biological responses. Likewise, although "bioenergy" is invoked in many forms of complementary and alternative medicine, energy medicine itself uses this energetic property as the sole means and primary mode of cure. Ultimately mind and energy may be reflected in the "consciousness" approach of many forms of traditional healing. ◐

193

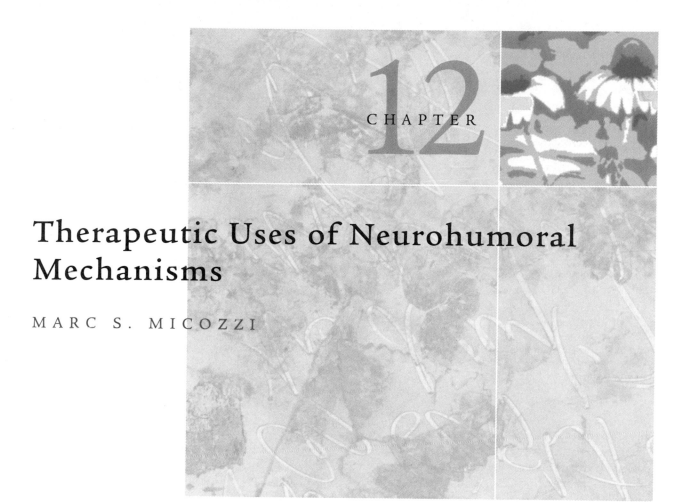

Therapeutic Uses of Neurohumoral Mechanisms

MARC S. MICOZZI

The autonomic nervous system maintains homeostasis by a series of humoral and nervous system interactions that continually occur on a subconscious, involuntary level. The autonomic system sends nervous impulses to all parts of the body as directed by the integration of several complex biofeedback mechanisms.

The information from these biofeedback loops is integrated in the central nervous system, and appropriate neural directives are passed along to the organs of respiration, circulation, digestion, excretion, and reproduction via the autonomic system.

Thus the body is maintained in a state of dynamic equilibrium, continually responsive to stimuli from internally monitored systems and environmental influences.

The functional anatomy of the autonomic nervous system has important implications for therapeutics (Table 12-1). The division of the system into two major parts—the sympathetic and parasympathetic—provides a series of checks and balances to regulate body functions. This division enables an ongoing dialogue between the two parts to maintain dynamic equilibrium. The opposition of two vital forces may be likened to the Asian concept of the yin and the yang (see Chapter 18), whereby the interaction of these opposing forces maintains the balance and harmony of humans and the universe. In addition, each of the two forces may take on some characteristics of the other. Thus the sympathetic and parasympathetic divisions are antagonistic, with a few notable exceptions. Coronary and pulmonary blood vessels are

TABLE 12-1

Autonomic Nervous System

	Sympathetic	Parasympathetic
Synonym	Adrenergic	Cholinergic
Preganglionic fiber	Short	Long
Neurohumoral agent*	Acetylcholine	Acetylcholine
Ganglion location	Paravertebral	End organ
Postganglionic fiber	Long	Short
Neurohumoral agent*	Norepinephrine	Acetylcholine
Extraautonomic sites	Adrenal medulla	Neuromuscular junction
Evolutionary role	Fight-flight/defense-alarm	Relaxation response
		Vegetative functions
Activators	Multiple	Specific
Blockers	Diffuse	Selective
	Nonspecific	Specific
Degradative enzymes	Monoamine oxidase	Cholinesterase
	Methyltransferase	

*These compounds are referred to as *neurohumoral agents* to the extent that they are present both in the general circulation and within nervous tissue. They are neurotransmitters to the extent that they manifest their activity across presynaptic or postsynaptic junctions during transmission of nervous impulses.

dilated by both divisions of the autonomic nervous system, whereas the vessels supplying blood to skeletal muscles may be dilated by the sympathetic system in exercise or by the postganglionic parasympathetic neurotransmitter at rest.

The unique short- and long-term adaptability of the human organism to environmental stimuli is facilitated by the actions of the autonomic system. The so-called fight-flight or defense-alarm responses are promulgated by the sympathetic nervous system, which raises blood oxygenation and pressure, regulates blood flow to the musculoskeletal system for activity and to the skin for thermal regulation, and causes retention of fluids and electrolytes in a state of arousal. These acute physiological responses are adaptive in the short-term and allow long-term survival of the human organism.

The "relaxation response" is mediated by the dynamic opponent of the sympathetic system—the parasympathetic system. This system directs the normative functions of the organism, allowing development of an ongoing state of well-being and physiological equilibrium. The maintenance of vegetative functions has facilitated human development and

cultural evolution. The ability to relax has allowed humans to reserve some portion of physical and mental energy for the pursuit of activities peripheral to primary survival. This ability has given humans their unique cultural attributes, which enable each individual to express the inclination for creativity. The selective responsivity of the autonomic nervous system has enabled humans, both as individuals and as a species, to make the successful adaptation to the environment, which has characterized human evolution.

The anatomical divisions corresponding to the functional autonomy of the sympathetic and parasympathetic nervous system can be traced along the length of the brain and spinal column (Figure 12-1). The autonomic system begins with cranial nerve X, the vagus, a single bundle of parasympathetic nerves that originates from the brainstem and courses throughout the body. Cranial nerves III, VII, and IX also send some parasympathetic fibers to the eyes, nose, and salivary glands. *Vagus* means "wanderer" in Latin, and no other nerve interfaces at so many diverse points along the functional anatomy. Passing down along the spinal cord, the cervical, thoracic, and lumbar divisions send sympathetic nerves through-

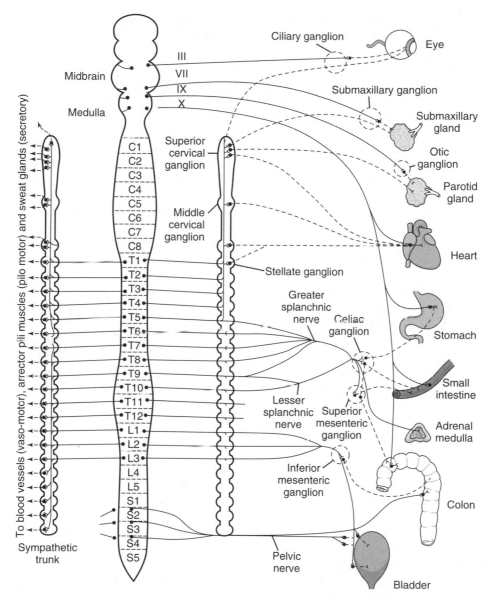

Figure 12-1 Autonomic nervous system and cranial nerves. (From Williams PL: *Gray's anatomy,* Edinburgh, 1995, Churchill Livingstone.)

out the body. Finally, the sacral divisions of the spinal cord send a few parasympathetic nerves to the lower regions of the body.

Each nerve of the autonomic system has two longitudinal divisions as it passes from the central nervous system to the end organs. The initial, or preganglionic, nerve fiber originates in the central nervous system and terminates in a nerve ganglion. Here it synapses with a new continuation—the postganglionic nerve fiber. This postganglionic fiber originates in the ganglion and terminates at a site of action. Autonomic nerve impulses travel in a continuum along the preganglionic fiber, through the synapse, and onto the postganglionic fiber to the site of action. In the sympathetic division, the preganglionic fibers are short and end in nearby ganglia, which occur in chains along the thoracic and lumbar vertebrae. From there, the postganglionic fibers travel to the diverse sites of action. In the parasympathetic system the preganglionic fibers are long and travel into ganglia located near end organs. From there, postganglionic fibers traverse a short distance to the sites of action.

The occurrence of synapses in the ganglia, between the preganglionic and postganglionic fibers, is important to therapy. Local anesthetics effect nerve conduction in the nerve fiber. Otherwise, these nerve impulses may be influenced by activities at the synaptic junction site. The interactions that occur in the synapse are a microcosm of neurophysiology and serve to functionally distinguish the sympathetic from parasympathetic systems. These distinctions are used extensively in therapy. Each of these systems makes use of characteristic neurohumoral agents for the unique transmission of nervous impulses throughout the body. The preganglionic fibers of both divisions use acetylcholine as the neurotransmitter across the synapse. The postganglionic parasympathetic transmitter is also acetylcholine, but the sympathetic transmitter is norepinephrine. The exclusive postganglionic use of acetylcholine as the parasympathetic and norepinephrine as the sympathetic neurotransmitter holds throughout the autonomic nervous system, except in the case of sweating of the palms, soles, and axilla, where the autonomic innervation is adrenergic, but the neurotransmitter is acetylcholine. Because these neurohumoral compounds used in the transmission of impulses across the synaptic junction are distinct chemical entities, there is a tendency for them to accumulate at their sites of release. Such an occurrence would limit effectiveness of the autonomic nervous system in providing sensitive, instantaneous regulation of body systems. Thus the synaptic sites maintain extensive and sophisticated mechanisms for the reuptake and degradation of released neurohumoral transmitters, and the synaptic junctions are kept clear of accumulated active compounds on an ongoing basis.

Specific enzymes degrade norepinephrine in the sympathetic postganglionic synapses, as well as their metabolic products. The concentration of these metabolites may be increased in certain pathological conditions and detected by analytical chemical techniques.

The enzyme responsible for the breakdown of acetylcholine in the postganglionic parasympathetic synapse is acetylcholinesterase. Although acetylcholine itself cannot practically be administered even when its properties are desired, a "functional dose" may be given through inhibition of its breakdown by cholinesterase. Thus anticholinesterases form the basis for parasympathetic nervous stimulation in clinical therapeutics. A phenomenon known as *denervation hypersensitivity* very much depends on this system of reuptake and degradation. When the autonomic innervation to an organ is anatomically interrupted (denervation), the postganglionic synaptic site loses its induced degradative enzymes and the synaptic receptor becomes extremely sensitive (hypersensitivity) to the neurohumoral agent. Thus any amount of the original neurohumoral agent introduced into the site by the circulation, through administration or otherwise, will have a magnified effect because the activity will not be mitigated by action of its appropriate degradative mechanism.

The functional divisions of the autonomic nervous system have great pathophysiological and therapeutic significance. For example, the entire gastrointestinal tract is extensively innervated by nerve fibers from both the sympathetic and parasympathetic divisions. In accordance with the previous discussion of the functional anatomy of this system, the parasympathetic ganglia, where preganglionic synapse with postganglionic fibers, are located near the sites of action in end organs. In the case of the gastrointestinal tract, the parasympathetic ganglia lie in two areas of the esophageal, gastric, intestinal, and colonic walls: Auerbach's myenteric plexus and Meissner's submucous plexus. These ganglia may be congenitally absent, as in Hirschsprung's disease, or destroyed by a number of pathogenic agents. The resultant disease depends on the location of the deficiency or insult along the gastrointestinal tract.

With destruction of the parasympathetic ganglia, there is prolonged, unopposed sympathetic stimulation. The characteristic effect is for the diseased segment to become constricted with impaired motility and loss of peristaltic action. The segment of the gastrointestinal tract proximal to the constriction lesion becomes extensively dilated as a pathological response to the event.

Achalasia of the esophagus is just such a condition, where a local area of constriction leads to proximal dilation of the esophagus. It has been thought that this condition is caused by degenerative disease of the parasympathetic vagus nerve, which innervates this area.

Pyloric stenosis of the gastric outlet is a similar condition. The aforementioned aganglionic mega-colon, or Hirschsprung's disease, is caused by a congenital lack of parasympathetic ganglion cells in the intestinal tract.

Chagas disease, or South American trypanosomiasis, caused by the parasitic organism *Trypanosoma cruzi,* may be associated with both megaesophagus and megacolon caused by the toxic degeneration of the intraluminal nerve plexus caused by *T. cruzi* infection. On the other hand, selective loss of sympathetic activity occurs in Horner's syndrome, with the characteristic triad of ptosis, meiosis, and anhydrosis (lid lag, pupillary constriction, and loss of sweating). This syndrome occurs with injury to the cervical sympathetic trunk and unopposed parasympathetic innervation.

Unfortunately, there are no autonomic therapeutic agents for satisfactory treatment of disorders such as Horner's syndrome or those of the gastrointestinal tract that are irreversible. However, autonomic drugs for the treatment of diseases of the circulatory and respiratory systems are commonplace in medicine. The same neurohumoral mechanisms involved by medical therapeutics may also be used in a nonspecific manner by many of the "mind-body" techniques of alternative and complementary medicine.

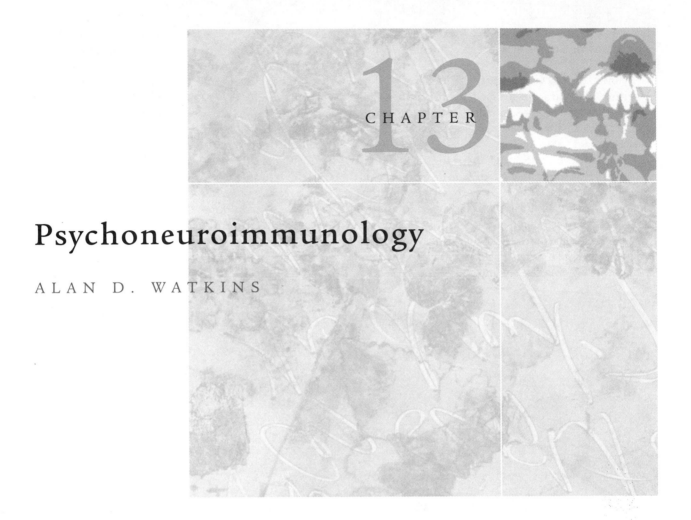

CHAPTER

13

Psychoneuroimmunology

ALAN D. WATKINS

The pursuit of health and the treatment of illness have become major social activities in the Western world. Our society is spending more time and more money on health practices than ever before. For example, the United States now spends more than 12 percent of its gross national product on health care. Within this pursuit of health there is an enormous range of activities, from organ transplantation to meditation. We are changing from a military-industrialized complex to a society dominated by spending on health care and its associated technologies. Fifty years have now passed since the last global war necessitated massive military spending. The fragmentation of the Eastern block and the dissolution of the Cold War also has reduced the need for an enormous financial outlay on military projects. Finally, there has been a steady improvement in general health, wealth, and nutrition during the twentieth century. These changes are reflected in the lower infant mortality rates, increased life expectancies, better nutritional standards, and less poverty-related disease in most Western societies. Because we are no longer preoccupied with basic survival, we have begun to focus more on the issue of improving the quality and quantity of our lives.

Although these fundamental changes in world politics and the world economy have been taking place, there also has been a technologic revolution in science and medicine. At the turn of the twentieth century, doctors had very few drugs at their disposal that could alter the course of disease. Physicians were mostly powerless observers of illness, providing comfort rather than cure. This image presents a sharp contrast to the highly trained specialists of today, who are masters of intervention. Moribund individuals sometimes are literally brought back from the dead, and premature infants with no reasonable hope of independent survival are kept alive to subsequently grow into adults. Lungs unable to breathe are replaced, arteries blocked or fit to burst are bypassed, and cancer cells are sometimes dissolved with toxic chemicals. It is little wonder that many patients perceive modern medicine as omnipotent, and doctors as Godlike figures.

USE OF COMPLEMENTARY MEDICINE

Despite the staggering success of allopathic medicine, record numbers of patients are turning to complementary practitioners in the United States (Office of Technology, 1990), Europe (British Medical Association, 1986; Watt, 1981), Australia (Donnelly et al., 1985), and New Zealand (Clinical Oncology Group, 1987) for a disparate number of ailments. Several surveys have indicated that between 1986 and 1991 the proportion of the population using complementary medicine in the United Kingdom increased by 70 percent (British Medical Association, 1993; Fulder & Munro, 1985) and has tripled in Holland and France (Syndicat National de la Pharmace 1993; Van Dijk, 1993). In 1991, the European over-the-counter market for homeopathy was £590 million, and for herbal remedies, £1.45 billion (Fisher & Ward, 1994). Paradoxically, this boom is occurring at the time when allopathic medicine is able to intervene more powerfully than ever before, looking deep into the very fabric of our bodies with magnetic resonance imaging (MRI) and even genetically engineering the DNA inside the nuclei of our cells.

Why are so many people turning to complementary therapy? Do we feel lost in the technology and uncared for by allopathic medicine? Or are we being misled by the pop medicine we encounter in magazines and newspapers into believing that complementary therapies are as effective as allopathic medicine for all our ills? Recent research suggests that far from being ignorant and ill informed (Charlton, 1992), most individuals visiting complementary therapists are, in fact, well educated and affluent (McGuire, 1988). So why are so many of these individuals deciding that allopathic medicine cannot deliver what they need?

BIOMEDICAL PROWESS

There is no doubt that biomedicine is unequalled for the care of many physical ailments, particularly those related to trauma, emergency medicine, and end-stage disease. However, it is less effective in preventing the development of disease, in altering the course of chronic physical disease, and in addressing the mental, emotional, and spiritual needs of an individual. The biomedical model of illness used by allopathic practitioners largely concerns itself with physical disease—the more advanced, the clearer. Biomedicine finds it very difficult to invest time and resources in prevention, partly because prevention is so difficult to measure. If a disease is prevented by a certain intervention, did that intervention prevent the disease, or did the disease simply not occur as expected?

Allopathic efforts at prevention have focused on screening programs designed to detect early disease, such as cervical smear programs, mammography clinics, and cholesterol and blood pressure checks, rather than on primary prevention. The nonspecific symptoms and signs that are the frequent forerunners to many major diseases are given less attention.

Allopathic medicine also struggles with chronic physical disease. On the basis of the belief that disease, once established, follows an inexorable path of steady deterioration, the allopath seeks to alleviate symptoms for as long as possible, charting the downward progress and deciding when heroic measures are to be called for in a last stand to prevent the patient's demise. In its preoccupation with physical disease, allopathy does not adequately address the mental, emotional, and spiritual needs of its patients. It will address organic mental disease, to which it can give a psychiatric label, but not mental, emotional, or spiritual disease, which is largely viewed as irrelevant or, at best, insoluble and not part of the allopathic practitioner's territory (Charlton, 1993). These limitations of allopathic medicine have led many individuals to seek alternative approaches. This chapter examines the basis of allopathic and complementary medical systems and argues that these approaches are not mutually exclusive on a philosophical, practical, or mechanistic level.

MEANING AND REALITY

A house is made up of a number of bricks. Science comprises a number of facts. The bricks alone do not make the house a reality any more than facts make science a reality. Both must be held together—in the case of the house, by cement and mortar, and in the case of science, by theory and interpretation. Facts usually are elicited to support a theory rather than to be independent of it. In this respect scientific reality is relative. The theories and facts on which health care systems are based change across different cultures. Just as there are differences in architectural interpretation, there are differences in factual interpretation. Thus symptoms and signs are interpreted differently, depending on the underlying culture of each society. Allopathic medicine tends to deny the existence of these multiple realities, perceiving itself as the only true reality and the only reality based on scientific fact. However, the briefest study of the history of Western science and medicine reveals that even the facts that allopathy claims as reality are constantly changing.

EVOLUTION OF SCIENTIFIC MEDICINE

How did allopathic medicine develop its view of a singular reality? In many human societies health care often was provided by a tribal doctor or shaman. These individuals developed powerful intuitive skills and the ability to enter trance states (often drug-induced) to consult with the spirit world. Illness was attributed to the spirits taking away the soul or psyche of the sufferer. The shaman would enter a trance to pursue the soul and to negotiate with the spirits for its return.

Evil spirits were believed to manifest within a subject's body, and the shaman would exorcise the spirit by inducing a trance or convulsions in the possessed individual using drugs, rituals, or rhythm. Thus the earliest forms of therapy involved both attention to the psyche and to the physical body. By the time of the earliest structured civilizations, these two aspects of health care had become separated, with the herbalists becoming the dominant providers of health and the priests and magicians dividing responsibility for spiritualism. Priests were able to consult the gods, and magicians used psychic powers to divine health problems from the study of entrails or the throwing of bones. This early separation of spiritual and physical aspects gave birth to the two schools of thinking, namely, the vitalists and the mechanists.

Vitalists believed illness was the result of psychic or spiritual forces, whereas mechanists believed in more physical explanations. One of the earliest and most influential advocates of the mechanistic school was Hippocrates of Cos. Hippocrates and his followers recognized the natural recuperative powers of the body and did not deny the importance of spiritual energy but still concentrated on treating illness and identifying specific mechanistic causes for ill health. They believed that an imbalance in one of the four humors—blood, phlegm, and black or yellow bile—could produce ill health. The concept that an imbalance of humor could predispose toward illness is remarkably similar to the current view of homeostasis, which dominates much of pathophysiology today.

The homeostatic model suggests that disease occurs, for example, when the balance between inflammatory and antiinflammatory forces is disturbed. This concept is akin to the Chinese notion that ill health is caused by an imbalance in vital energy, or qi. The Greeks used allopathic remedies to treat imbalances in the humors, and mechanistic medicine gradually became synonymous with the administration of allopathic remedies. Another major figure in the development of Western medicine was Galen, the royal physician to Marcus Aurelius, in the second century AD. Galen used all manner of drugs and herbal remedies enthusiastically, often creating bewildering and noxious concoctions. However, Galen recognized the importance of the psyche in physical disease, and his observation that melancholic women were more likely to develop disease of the breast is considered by many to be the earliest Western record of the effects of the psyche on the immune system.

Because many remedies offered by mechanistic allopaths were either toxic or ineffectual, the vitalistic approach resurfaced. This reemergence also was stimulated by the teachings of Jesus and the early Christians. Jesus effected instant cures through the power of faith. Christian healers used the power of a divine force and promoted the manifestation of the spirit within an individual. Such healers relied on inspiration—literally, the spirit inside themselves—for therapeutic guidance. For several centuries the clergy played an active role in healing the sick. By the Middle Ages the teachings of the Christian church (particularly the Vatican) became the dominant force in guiding society. They viewed ecclesiastical intervention in cases of possession, convulsions, and trance states as suspect paganism, bordering on witchcraft, and possibly satanic. As a result the church backed out of its role in healing, and medicine was left to physicians, who were firm followers of the polypharmacy advocated by Galen. Vitalism declined.

THE BIRTH OF REDUCTIONISM

In the mid-sixteenth century polemical changes were occurring throughout society. Copernicus put forth his view that the sun, not the earth, was the center of the universe. Vesalius contested the common practice of fitting the results of medical research (e.g., the discoveries made from cadaver dissection) to fit the theories of the day. This was the birth of scientific thinking. Vitalism was somewhat rehabilitated by Paracelsus, who suggested that there was a mechanistic explanation for miracles, namely, the human imagination. Despite this shift to rational thinking, allopathic treatment lagged behind and was still based largely on Galenic principles of polypharmacy, with little recourse to scientific testing.

Desperate attempts to alter body humors were foisted upon those who could afford to pay for it. For example, eyewitness accounts document the sorry last days of Charles II in the grip of some malady. His surgeon responded by removing 16 ounces of blood from his right arm. Not to be outdone, his physician ordered further blood letting and scarification. Having probably rendered the king anemic, his medical attendants then proceeded to dehydrate him with a potent cocktail of emetics and purgatives. Spanish fly, a blistering agent, was then applied to his shaven scalp, and when this failed to produce therapeutic benefit, someone ordered a red-hot cautery. For the better part of a week, 14 physicians competed in their abuse of the king until finally, one bright spark arranged for the Oriental Bezoar Stone to be transferred from its normal habitat in the stomach of an eastern goat to its final resting place in the body of King Charles. Before he died, Charles apologized to his physicians for taking such a long time to do so.

Fortunately, by the mid-seventeenth century reason began to prevail. Thomas Sydenham, whose name was later associated with an inherited form of chorea, suggested that medical training take place at the bedside rather than in university classrooms. Sydenham also suggested that symptoms be sepa-

rated from the underlying disease, giving birth to the school of nosologists, who began to classify diseases as Linnaeus was classifying plants.

Descartes' assertion that the mind and body were separate entities encouraged the description of physical diseases that did not involve the mind. By the mid-eighteenth century Morgagni suggested that a patient's symptoms could be traced to physical malfunctions in specific organs. Forty years later, Bichat demonstrated that diseased tissues, not organs, were at fault. The great Virchow completed this reductionist trend in 1850 by showing that specific cells within tissue were responsible for disease. Thus in the late nineteenth century the plethora of symptoms and signs presented by the patient could be reduced to a cellular malfunction.

This reductionist approach proved extremely effective in increasing scientific understanding of disease. When the complexity of the body was reduced to simple processes, it became possible to measure these processes. Measurement of bodily functions thus became central to scientific medical thinking. Individual experience, which could not be measured, diminished further, and the intuitive wisdom of healers was dismissed as anecdotal.

Reductionism reinforced the basic separation of the measurable physical body and the unquantifiable psyche. Because changes in the psyche and spirit could not be easily quantified, they were dismissed as irrelevant or nonexistent. Consequently the reality described by science was based largely on a physical reality. Illness was explained in terms of measurable physical malfunction and the role of the spirit was diminished substantially.

By the end of the nineteenth century allopathic practitioners were being taught to elicit a systematic history, search the biochemical and structural integrity of the body for abnormalities, and then reduce all the symptoms and signs of illness to a single diagnostic category.

This biomedical approach produced some early success, particularly in identifying the cause of infectious diseases, which were the major source of ill health in society at the time. However, such advances in scientific thinking had not produced substantial improvement in treatment. The toxic nature of the allopathic remedies of the day spawned the development of less noxious, alternative approaches, such as homeopathy. Thus complementary approaches to health enjoyed a revival, but they often were met with open hostility and derision from the allopathic community (Inglis, 1980).

As scientific thinking and methods became more rigorous, the toxic treatments of the past fell into disuse, more efficacious drugs were discovered and refined, and the gentler, more spiritual complementary therapies were again relegated to the fringe of medical practice. Modern pharmacology fortified the view that psychological factors, such as the placebo response, were irrelevant. The new powerful medicines that had been developed could cure the patient regardless of his or her desires. Allopathic doctors became entrenched even more firmly in their belief that the patient's thoughts, feelings, and emotions were irrelevant to recovery. Promoting an expectation of health using the placebo effect was consequently seen as deceitful, and even unethical.

Although Western society was developing increasing faith in the biomedical model and the power of pharmacological intervention, new scientific discoveries also reinforced the biomedical reductionist view that thoughts, feelings, and emotions were irrelevant to health. For example, the immune system and the endocrine system were being shown to be self-regulatory, independent of the functioning of the mind. The view that health was largely a function of the physical body and unrelated to higher cortical function is the model used in allopathic medicine today. The phenomenal successes of high-tech medicine reinforces this reductionist approach. The biomedical reductionist model appears to be the antithesis of the holistic approach used by most complementary medical practitioners (Rosch & Kearney, 1985).

THERAPEUTIC APPROACHES

Differences between biomedical reductionism and holism are exemplified by their respective approaches to therapy. Biomedicine assumes that all individuals are basically the same; therefore solutions to any one particular diagnosis also will be identical. Treatments are aimed at the antagonism of a single pathological process. By contrast, complementary medicine assumes that all individuals are different; the manifestation of disease depends on the unique characteristics of the individual patient. Therefore a constellation of therapeutic activities is deemed necessary; these may vary daily according to the changing needs of the patient and the changing clinical situation.

These differences also affect research into the efficacy of treatment modalities. Allopathic medicine dissects a therapeutic approach to identify a single mechanism that underpins efficacy. It uses the randomized, placebo-controlled trial (RCT) to aid this dissection and to determine whether a single therapeutic ingredient is active. Complementary medicine places much greater emphasis on the validity of individual therapeutic experience. Research into complementary medicine is made arduous by the difficulty in designing controls for individualized treatments, but with precision and care, such research is possible (Lewith & Aldridge, 1993).

THERAPEUTIC EXCLUSIVITY

Are the therapeutic approaches of allopathy and complementary medicine really mutually exclusive? On a practical level it is possible to integrate complementary medicine into allopathic practice, as has been proven by chiropractic (see Chapter 8). In fact the strong desire to incorporate complementary medicine into allopathic practice is reflected in a 1983 survey that indicated that approximately 80 percent of trainee primary care physicians in the United Kingdom wished to receive training in complementary therapy (Reilly & Taylor, 1983). By 1987 this figure had risen to 92 percent (Reilly, 1993). It was reported in 1986 that approximately 30 percent of primary care physicians in two British counties already had received training in complementary therapy (Anderson & Anderson, 1986; Wharton & Lewith, 1986). So, contrary to the stereotypical image of an unqualified practitioner dispensing untested remedies, a large proportion—in some countries, the majority—of those providing complementary therapies are allopathically qualified (Cassileth et al., 1984).

Thus allopathic and complementary approaches can be used simultaneously in the treatment of disease. Practitioners with training in both allopathic and complementary medicine are well placed to recognize the limitations of both systems. They might be the most suitable practitioners to decide which therapeutic approach, or combination of approaches, best suits the needs of the patient.

Using the skills and knowledge inherent in both systems, he or she is in a position to address the physical, emotional, mental, and spiritual dimensions of health, that is, be truly holistic. In the United Kingdom the realization that allopathy and complementary medical approaches are not mutually exclusive spawned the birth of the British Holistic Medical Association (BHMA) in the early 1980s. One of its founders, Dr. Patrick Pietroni, has written about the paradigm shift that is occurring within allopathic circles (Pietroni, 1990). As allopathic practitioners realize the limits of scientific enquiry, they begin to use other systems that address areas with which science struggles. Thus there is a shift from the reductionist biomedical approach to a holistic approach that incorporates multiple realities and multiple explanations for ill health.

Pietroni also describes models of experimental health centers in the United Kingdom that use this holistic approach. One such health center, situated in the crypt of a London church, incorporates allopathic primary care physicians, osteopaths, psychological counselors, and spiritual healers. The primary care physician has initial contact with the patient and deals with the presenting problem from a biomedical standpoint, involving complementary practitioners within the practice when appropriate. All allopathic and complementary practitioners meet regularly to communicate about individual patients, ensuring that all their physical, mental, emotional, or spiritual needs are being met.

Pietroni's London practice is by no means the only model of holistic practice in the United Kingdom. In Southampton, on the south coast of England, four primary care physicians run the Center for the Study of Complementary Medicine. The physicians at this center are trained in a wide variety of complementary medical techniques. Over the last 15 years they have developed a method of predicting the exact number of consultations a particular problem will require, as well as the likelihood of improvement. Each individual might be treated simultaneously with a number of complementary techniques and allopathic remedies, depending on their individual characteristics and the presentation of the problem.

Many treatments and therapeutic approaches, initially perceived as complementary, have become incorporated into mainstream allopathic practice. For example, at least 25 percent of all prescriptions written in the United States are for drugs that were originally identified from plants by folklore and herbalists (Farnsworth, 1983; Reynolds, 1991). Hypnosis, which was dismissed for many years as a deception, is now widely accepted by psychiatrists and clinical psychol-

ogists as an invaluable therapeutic tool, particularly in the United States. The undoubted success of chiropractic techniques for back pain have ensured that these techniques will complement allopathic approaches permanently.

PHILOSOPHICAL EXCLUSIVITY

Complementary and allopathic therapies also are not mutually exclusive on a philosophical level. Allopathic medicine is often characterized as reductionist and complementary medicine as holistic. It is an oversimplification to suggest that allopathy is entirely reductionist and complementary medicine is entirely holistic. Each type of practice has both elements to varying degrees. Reducing a problem to its component parts does not preclude an analysis of the whole, and it is possible to respond to the patient's needs, as well as the needs of the disease, at the same time. Allopaths often do try to attend to the mental and emotional domain through a referral to a psychiatrist. Complementary practitioners reduce a symptom complex to its component parts in much the same way as an allopath would do. They may even prescribe a complementary technique in the same way that an allopath would prescribe a pill.

It often is argued that complementary medicine cannot be integrated with allopathic medicine because it would then be forced into a reductionist mold. For example, in the classical acupuncture practiced by the Chinese, needles are placed according to the unique characteristics of the individual. In the formula acupuncture practiced in the West, needles are placed at the same points in all patients. This formula has been labeled reductionist and therefore less likely to be effective. However, classical acupuncture must, by definition, also use a formula of sorts, or it would be impossible to know where to place the needles at all.

As highlighted earlier biomedicine tends to see itself as a singular reality, with its validity supported by scientific facts. It views much of the evidence for the efficacy of complementary practices as anecdotal. However, numerous anecdotes can be found in the biomedical literature, called case histories, and the study of these case histories has significantly increased our understanding of basic physiological and pathological processes. For example, in 1986, two types of T lymphocytes were identified in mice and were thought to be crucial to the development of allergic reactions (Mossman et al., 1986). The existence of these subsets in humans was fiercely disputed. However, subsequent case histories demonstrated that such cells did exist in humans (Field et al., 1993). The scientific literature is full of such examples.

In addition, science often studies the isolated extremes of biological malfunction to help explain the mechanisms of normal biological function. Thus individuals with rare genetic deficiencies can tell us a great deal about normal cellular function. This method of gathering information from the investigation of rarities is similar to the gathering of information from the few long-term survivors of malignancy who were treated with a complementary technique. In fact the study of isolated genetic deficiencies has flourished in recent years as a result of genetic engineering, which enables scientists to produce large numbers of animals with a single gene defect. The scientific literature is awash with reports on the effects of such isolated deficiencies and their implications for normal function.

Thus allopathic and complementary medicine can be simultaneously holistic and reductionist, and the philosophical differences are not as broad as some would like to think. Nevertheless, most complementary medical practices may remain unaccepted by allopathic medicine until large-scale RCTs investigating their efficacy have been conducted.

Despite repeated calls for such research by the British Medical Association (British Medical Association, 1993), The Royal College of Physicians (The Royal College of Physicians, 1992), The Royal Society of Medicine (Watt & Wood, 1988), the European Parliament (March 1994), the House of Representatives (Office of Technology, 1990), and the World Health Organization (WHO) (WHO Global Strategy, 1994), few such trials have been performed. Many agencies in control of research funds see complementary therapies as alternative and therefore a threat to orthodoxy. This perception has been fuelled by the antagonistic and divisive opinions of a number of protagonists among both the complementary and allopathic communities. Some allopaths are content to dismiss complementary medicine as ineffectual without any experimental evidence on efficacy from small- or large-scale RCTs; this kind of pejorative attitude is completely unscientific and is usually voiced by individuals who claim to be scientists themselves on the basis of a purported concern for scientific standards.

Investigations of complementary medicine are further hampered by the perception that complementary approaches lack neurophysiological or biochemical explanations. Such explanations could be subjected to scientific testing, thereby helping to bring complementary practices into mainstream medical practice. Scientific explanations occasionally have been found, such as the demonstration that acupuncture relieves pain by stimulating the production of endorphins. As a result acupuncture gained greater acceptance among allopaths, although it still has fallen short of full integration.

MECHANISTIC EXCLUSIVITY

The preceding discussion makes it apparent that complementary and allopathic medicine are not mutually exclusive on a philosophical or a practical level. The only remaining barrier to the integration of complementary and allopathic practices is the question of mechanism of action. If practices such as healing touch, homeopathy, aromatherapy, Ayurveda, curanderismo, or any of the complementary systems are to be integrated, these systems either have to be proven effective by allopathic mechanisms, or allopathy has to accept that they may work by means of mechanisms that are foreign to the present biomedical model. For example, is there a scientific explanation why a homeopathic remedy works when the original compound has been diluted beyond detectable limits? Or should we accept the suggestion that the original compound has in some way left an energetic imprint on water molecules? To determine whether scientific explanations can be found to explain the possible efficacy of complementary practices, it is necessary to examine complementary medical research more closely.

The enormous volume of complementary medical research that has been conducted is astounding. Much of this work has failed to reach allopathic attention because it is rarely published in scientific journals, and journals that do publish such work often are not referenced on the main scientific databases. This partly is because much of this research is not rigorously controlled or of high scientific quality (not unlike a great deal of allopathic research).

The lack of scientific controls in complementary medical research does not necessarily invalidate the research findings; it merely makes them less available to generalization. There are many reasons for this lack of scientific rigor. A nearly complete lack of funding has forced research to be limited to small-scale trials, making it difficult to demonstrate statistically significant results that can be followed up. In addition, controls for many complementary practices are difficult to design. Finally, many allopathic clinicians and scientists are inhibited from investigating this field because they fear that their work will be dismissed by allopathic colleagues as unscientific and irrelevant.

The recent controversy following the investigation of a potential mechanism of action of homeopathic potencies (Davenas et al., 1988) highlights these dangers only too well. Consequently much of the complementary medicine research has been conducted by individuals with little training in clinical trial research and scientific method.

The funding difficulties of complementary medicine have been less acute in Europe, particularly the United Kingdom, where there is a stronger tradition for complementary health practices and research. In the last few years a number of "centers of excellence," based in allopathic teaching hospitals, have evolved. These centers are conducting well-controlled scientific studies on which therapeutic decisions can be made. However, most of this work is still at the stage of determining whether therapeutic efficacy can be established; there has been very little research investigating possible mechanisms of action of complementary therapies. Therefore we will have to look to other areas of scientific research to answer the mechanistic questions.

SUBJECTIVE AND OBJECTIVE BENEFIT

Many of the studies demonstrating the clinical benefit of complementary techniques have reported improvements in what allopaths would call subjective measures of disease activity. These measures are based on the patient's perception of the disease and might be a general feeling of well-being or specific symptoms related to the disease under investigation. Many allopaths dismiss any treatment that has a solely subjective impact. They suggest that such a therapy merely makes the patient feel better, having no real effect on the disease as measured by objective parameters.

This view that only quantifiable objective improvements in disease activity are a valid assessment of therapeutic benefit is inaccurate. Subjective improvements might also be produced by improvements in pathology that are not detectable by currently available tests. Patients may feel better because they *are* better, pathologically.

Furthermore, the subjective assessment of disease activity by the patient and the allopathic doctor usually is what guides clinical practice. For example, if a patient is feeling better, he or she is much more likely to discontinue medication. Similarly, if the patient reports to the doctor that he or she is feeling better, the doctor is equally likely to stop certain medications. Objective benefits might not actually be perceived by the patient. For example, in a study of 82 asthmatic patients, 15 percent of the patients were unable to perceive a 50 percent reduction in their capacity to exhale rapidly (Rubinfeld & Pain, 1976).

It is rather artificial to classify a therapeutic improvement as either entirely objective or subjective because clearly objective measures, such as blood pressure, can be influenced by subjective factors. Thus the subjective well-being of the patient can alter the recorded pressure, and the interpretation of the different sounds heard when measuring a patient's blood pressure also involve a certain degree of subjectivity. In addition, a subjective perception of improved health might result from an objective improvement in the pathological condition (Figure 13-1).

Subjective improvement in symptoms, or an increased sense of well-being, is a valid therapeutic goal, just like objective improvements. Most of the research to date on complementary therapies demonstrates that benefits are predominantly subjective. It is likely that until complementary therapies are able to show consistent objective benefits, they will not be fully integrated into allopathic medicine. However, studies that have reported objective improvements are usually dismissed on the grounds that they are not scientifically robust or because there is no mechanistic explanation for how such objective improvements can be brokered.

One possible explanation for how complementary therapies could produce objective benefit is by first

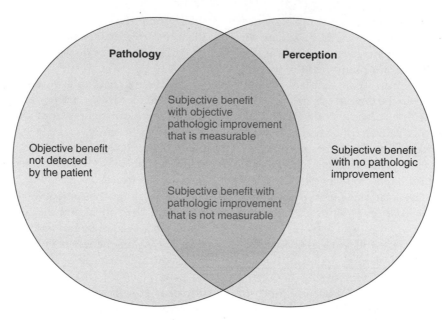

Figure 13-1 Overlap of subjective and objective therapeutic benefit.

producing a subjective benefit. Such subjective, perceptual improvements might promote objective improvements in disease activity. Perception is an evaluative process involving a number of areas of the brain, including the limbic emotional centers. Recent research suggests that higher cortical centers and limbic emotional centers are capable of altering health and disease. The brain communicates with the immune system in a rich flow of hormones, neuropeptides, and cytokines. Thus perception influences pathology and pathology influences perception (Watkins, 1995).

PSYCHONEUROIMMUNOLOGY

An overwhelming amount of evidence suggests that higher cognitive centers and limbic emotional centers are capable of regulating virtually all aspects of the immune system and therefore have a profound effect on health and illness (Ader et al., 1991; Blalock, 1994; Reichlin, 1993). This area of research is referred to as *psycho-* (from the mind, or psyche) *neuro-* (from the brain or neurons) *immunology* (to the immune system) (PNI). Two mind-body pathways of communication have been identified, namely, autonomic and neuroendocrine. The autonomic nervous system innervates the bone marrow, thymus, spleen, and mucosal surfaces where immune cells develop, mature, and encounter foreign proteins (Felten et al., 1992). Some authors have suggested that the development and aging of both the immune and autonomic nervous systems might be related (Ackerman et al., 1989; Bellinger et al., 1988).

The autonomic innervation of immune tissue is extremely complex. There are three different arms to the autonomic innervation of immune tissue, namely, the sympathetic, parasympathetic, and nonadrenergic noncholinergic (NANC). Each neural network communicates with the immune cells directly through the release of chemical messages. These messages range from adrenaline, noradrenaline, and acetylcholine, to small proteins, called *neuropeptides,* that previously were thought to occur only in the brain. These chemical messages may have an inflammatory or antiinflammatory effect on the immune tissue. The situation is further complicated by the finding that a specific neuropeptide can be released from sympathetic, parasympathetic, or NANC nerves and that each type of nerve can store and release both inflammatory and antiinflammatory chemical messages.

The pattern of chemical message released also may vary over time in a specific tissue, depending on the chronicity of the inflammatory process. Furthermore, there is a complicated interaction between the autonomic nerves and the immune cells within each immune compartment, and this relation changes, depending on the immune tissue involved. Thus the nerves may alter the function of the inflammatory cells, and the inflammatory cells may alter the function of the nerves (Watkins, 1995).

In addition to this direct physical communication between nerves and immune tissue, a second indirect chemical communication channel involves hormone production by the hypothalamus and pituitary gland at the base of the brain. These hormones, which normally regulate the function of other glands in the body, are capable of altering the function of virtually every type of immune cell. Immune cells have surface receptors for virtually all of the hormones produced by the brain, including growth hormone, thyroid-stimulating hormone, the sex hormone–releasing hormones, vasopressin, and prolactin, as well as many of the hormones produced by the other endocrine glands in the body (Blalock, 1994; Felten et al., 1992). They also possess receptors for the natural endorphins and enkephalins produced by the brain, which profoundly affect immune system function, some causing suppression, others causing enhancement of the immune system. The release of many of these hormones is intimately related to thoughts and emotions. Each thought and feeling has a chemical consequence within the brain in terms of the chemical messages passing between brain cells and the hormones produced by the emotional centers. For example, after just 5 minutes of stress, an animal's hypothalamus produces the signals that eventually promote increased levels of cortisol (Chover-Gonzalez et al., 1993).

The complex control of the immune system by brain hormones and the autonomic nervous system is complicated further by the demonstration that these two pathways profoundly affect each other as well (Terao et al., 1993). Furthermore, the immune system talks back to the brain by way of the autonomic nervous system and the production of its own chemical signals.

The central nervous system and the immune system function as an integrated whole to maintain a state of healthy balance within the body (Watkins, 1995). The immune system communicates information to the brain that the brain cannot perceive, and the brain informs the immune system about cognitive information that the immune cells are unable to detect. Thus there is now substantial evidence to suggest that thoughts, feelings, emotions, and perceptions do indeed alter immunity (Watkins, 1995). Therefore complementary therapies that alter subjective feelings of well-being might be potentially promoting changes in the pathological condition, by activating these brain-immune pathways (Watkins, 1994).

EVIDENCE FOR PNI MEDIATING THE EFFECTS OF COMPLEMENTARY THERAPIES

Thus the autonomic nervous system and the hormonal system are capable of generating a wide variety of messages that can modulate immune function. Any one of these brain-immune signals might be affected by a complementary therapy. It seems likely that complementary therapies, which rely on a constellation of activities, might affect several brain-immune signals simultaneously. Therefore great care must be taken when designing controls for studies investigating complementary techniques. For example, if acupuncture relieves pain by promoting the local release of endorphins, assessing the analgesic effects of acupuncture by inserting needles into sham acupuncture points may be invalid because sham needles may also stimulate the release of endorphins, thereby producing analgesia in controls and confounding any treatment effect. On the other hand, if acupuncture is effective in asthma by reducing cholinergic tone, then it would be valid to use sham acupuncture points as a control because the release of endorphins would have no significant effect on cholinergic activity and airway caliber.

But what evidence is there that complementary therapies work by way of the brain-immune pathways outlined previously? Few studies have actually investigated the mechanism of action of complementary therapies. Some data do suggest that the activity of the autonomic nervous system may be altered during chiropractic (Beal, 1985; Bouhuys, 1963), hypnosis (DeBeneditts et al., 1994; Neild & Cameron, 1985), conditioning (Hatch et al., 1990), and acupuncture (Han et al., 1980; Jian, 1985). Other studies have suggested that acupuncture (Kasahara et al., 1992) and spinal manipulation (Vernon et al., 1986) might be mediated by endorphin release.

How do these brain-immune pathways relate to the placebo effect? It has been argued that every therapeutic intervention—whether complementary or allopathic—involves a placebo effect. It often is stated that 50 percent of the analgesic effect of painkillers is due to a placebo response. All the same, most allopathic physicians consider it unethical, or even deceitful, to actively encourage a placebo response.

This unwillingness to harness an undoubtedly powerful therapeutic effect is largely because the placebo effect is unpredictable, unreliable, and mediated by nonspecific mechanisms that are dismissed as unmeasurable and irrelevant. However, it is now clear from PNI research that an expectation of recovery can alter subjective feelings of well-being and result in autonomic activation and the production of pituitary hormones. Thus there are specific testable pathways by which expectation (the placebo effect) can alter immunity. It is likely that expectation has different effects in different individuals—producing large shifts in autonomic balance and hormonal output in some

and negligible changes in others. This would explain the unpredictability of the placebo response.

The second factor that has inhibited a greater understanding of the placebo response has been the development of the placebo-controlled trial. The effectiveness of newly developed drugs are established by comparison with identical, but therapeutically inactive, compounds called *placebos*. Placebos are used as if they had no specific effect on the disease in question, rather than a nonspecific effect. Therefore the enormous clinical benefit that could be produced by a placebo response was undermined by the use of inert placebo medications, thereby reinforcing the view that any therapy harnessing placebo effects was at best ineffective and at worst unethical. This view, combined with the view that complementary therapies affect only subjective measures of disease activity, has made it possible for allopathic physicians to

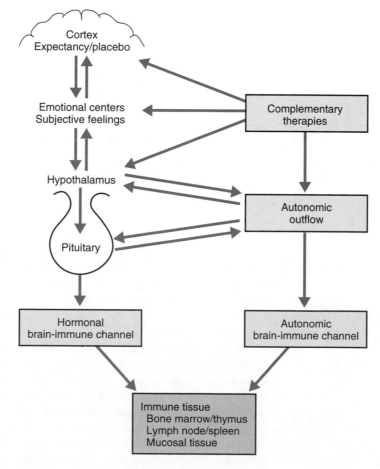

Figure 13-2 Brain-immune pathways of alternative medicine.

argue that complementary practices are of limited benefit.

Such arguments are fallacious. The expectation of recovery that promotes a placebo response is quite separate from a subjective improvement and, incidentally, is also different from hope. It is possible to feel subjectively better, without expecting a full recovery. Similarly, it is possible to expect a recovery without feeling better. Complementary therapies cannot be dismissed as mere placebos; they are producing substantial, subjective, and at times, objective clinical benefit unrelated to the placebo effect.

Thus both expectancy (the placebo response) and subjective feelings of well-being might be produced by the brain-immune pathways identified in PNI research. Complementary therapies may produce clinical benefit by promoting a placebo response, or they may alter subjective feelings of well-being. Alternatively, they may directly activate brain-immune pathways without involving expectancy or subjective feelings (Figure 13-2). For example, hypnosis can alter expectancy or subjective feelings and therefore may be an extremely powerful activator of brain-immune pathways in some individuals. By contrast, acupuncture might directly affect the brain-immune pathways by modulating incoming signals from the immune system to the hypothalamus without involving the higher centers, expectation, or emotions.

Individuals differ in their responsiveness to different activation stimuli—be they expectancy, subjective sensations, or complementary therapies. This would explain why complementary therapies that are supposedly mediated by placebo mechanisms, according to the allopathic argument, can outperform placebos in a double-blind trial (Reilly et al., 1994). It would also explain the need for a constellation of complementary activities to ensure that these pathways were fully activated.

VITAL ENERGY

The importance of energy in health has been recognized for centuries and by many cultures. Many complementary therapies place great emphasis on the concept of energy. Ayurveda suggests an energetic body exists beneath the physical body, not on a biological level but on a quantum level. Traditional Chinese medicine is based on the concept that disruption of vital energy can lead to disease. The therapeutic interventions used in traditional Chinese medicine are designed to unblock or move this energy. In fact encouraging the natural flow of this energy through such practices as tai chi chuan is seen as vital in maintaining health and preventing illness. Acupuncture is claimed to alter the flow of energy around the body through the insertion of needles along the energy meridians.

Such explanations seem, at first glance, to run completely contrary to biomedical explanations because the energy meridians do not conform to allopathic maps of the nervous or vascular systems. But does this energy also flow through the bodies of patients presenting to allopathic practitioners? Allopathic patients do complain about lack of energy, and most allopathic practitioners have difficulty interpreting such statements. The biomedical model does not appear to have any way of incorporating the concept of energy. Lack of energy usually is taken to indicate physical or mental fatigue, but this change in language does not get the allopath off the hook; a cause for fatigue must still be found. Searches for an objective pathological condition, such as anemia, thyroid dysfunction, or occult cancer, usually are fruitless. Unable to find any quantifiable pathological condition but pressed to diagnose the cause of fatigue, allopathic practitioners may assert that there is nothing wrong or allude vaguely to a virus. More recently, chronic fatigue syndrome (myalgic encephalomyelitis) has become a popular diagnosis.

The treatment of such nonspecific diagnoses drains the energy of the allopath. It is difficult to prescribe treatment when there is no firm diagnostic label. Most allopaths end up doing nothing or dispensing some nonspecific advice about fatigue. Brave doctors might suggest some sort of tonic. By contrast, complementary therapies practiced in the West, such as healing touch (see Chapter 9), are specifically directed at dealing with the problems of energy. Despite its own limitations, allopathic biomedicine often dismisses such approaches as scientifically untested and unfounded.

Why does Western biomedicine struggle with the concept of energy? Energy is a complicated and obtuse subject. There are no accepted ways of measuring—and therefore validating—the level of energy within the human body. As a result it is impossible to determine whether energy levels change during an illness and whether they change in response to a treatment, although it is clear that the healthy are more energetic than the ill. Finally, the concept of energy is intimately related to spirituality and religion—intangible concepts.

*A*ctually, allopathic medicine does measure a number of energy systems within the body. For example, the energy produced by the heart is recorded by an electrocardiogram (ECG). The electrical energy of the heart is of particular interest (see Chapter 1).

The heart is a main source of energy within the body. Electrically it is 40 to 60 times more powerful than the brain, emitting 2.5 watts of electrical power. The heart trace seen on the ECG is the averaged electrical signal from all the cardiac muscle cells, and this can be recorded anywhere on the body from the top of the skull to the tip of the toes. What happens to this energy when it reaches the body surface? Does it stop abruptly at the skin? Perhaps more importantly, is the energy altered by the tissue through which it passes?

The height of a heart trace certainly is reduced if there is fluid around the heart (a pericardial effusion) or if there is a large amount of fat in the skin, but does disease in other tissues alter this energy in some subtle way? Perhaps the energy detected by practitioners of healing touch is the heart's electrical energy just above the skin's surface. It has been suggested that if we walk into a room where two people have just been arguing, even if they now are sitting quietly, the atmosphere we can sense is actually the electrical energy emanating from the hearts of the two individuals.

Heart energy is, of course, not the only type of energy in the body. The Hindu concept of chakras also describes other energy centers within the physical body. However, there is no doubt that the heart is the predominant energy source. How is heart energy related to our health? Fascinating answers are being provided by the current detailed analysis of heart energy or heart frequency using modern digital processing computers (Ori et al., 1992; Stein et al., 1994). This hard scientific research has revealed that there are three basic types or patterns of heart energy, and these reflect the ac-

tivity in the autonomic nervous system (McCraty et al., 1995a).

Thus activity or energy in the nervous system is directly related to energy in the heart. Mental stress and negative emotions, such as anger, increase the energy in the sympathetic nervous system (Kamada et al., 1992; Sloan et al., 1994; Williams et al., 1982), and in contrast, positive emotions such as care and compassion increase the energy in the parasympathetic nervous system (McCraty et al., 1995b). Thus the activity of the brain and the vital energy in the body are connected by means of the autonomic nervous system. In addition, because the brain and the immune system work as an integrated unit (*vide infra*), it now becomes possible to see how the brain, the heart, and the immune system are interrelated. Thus energy and matter come together, and this juncture is explained by scientifically testable pathways and mechanisms.

CONCLUSION

It is clear that contemporary biomedicine does not have all the answers; neither does complementary medicine. If we can abstain from linear thinking, we can achieve a breakthrough in understanding. We must put aside the polarized arguments of the allopaths who reduce all individuals to the same, and the complementary advocates who suggest that we are all different. Both systems have something to offer. They are not mutually exclusive on a philosophical, practical, or even mechanistic level. The brain, the heart, the immune system, energy, and matter all work together and so must we. The future of medicine is in our hands. If we open our minds, that future looks very promising indeed.

References

Ackerman KD, Felten SY, Dijkstra CD, et al. 1989. Parallel development of noradrenergic sympathetic innervation and cellular compartmentalisation in the rat spleen. Exp Neurol 103:239-255

Ader R, Felten DL, Cohen N. 1991. Psychoneuroimmunology, 2nd ed. Academic Press, San Diego

Anderson E, Anderson P. 1986. Complementary medicine and the general practitioner (letter). BMJ 293:53

Beal MC. 1985. Viscerosomatic reflexes: a review. J Am Osteopath Assoc 85:786-811

Bellinger DL, Felten SY, Felten DL. 1988. Maintenance of noradrenergic sympathetic innervation in the involuted thymus of the aged Fischer 344 rat. Brain Behav Immunol 2:133-150

Blalock JE. 1994. The immune system: our sixth sense. Immunology 2:8-15

Bouhuys A. 1963. Effects of posture in experimental asthma in man. Am J Med 34:470-476

British Medical Association. 1986. Alternative Therapy: Report of the Board of Science and Education. British Medical Association, London

British Medical Association. 1993. Complementary Medicine: New Approaches to Good Practice. Oxford University Press, Oxford

Cassileth BR, Lusk EJ, Strouse TB, Bodenheimer BJ. 1984. Contemporary unorthodox treatments in cancer medicine: a study of patients, treatments, and practitioners. Ann Intern Med 101:105-112

Charlton BG. 1992. Philosophy of medicine: alternative or science. J R Soc Med 85:436-438

Charlton BG. 1993. The doctor's aim in a pluralistic society: a response to "healing and medicine." J R Soc Med 86:125-126

Chover-Gonzalez AJ, Harbuz MS, Lightman SL. 1993. Effect of adrenalectomy and stress on interleukin-1 beta-mediated activation of hypothalamic corticotropin-releasing factor mRNA. J Neuroimmunol 42:155-160

Clinical Oncology Group. 1987. New Zealand cancer patients and alternative medicine. NZ Med J 100:110-113

Davenas E, Beauvais F, Amara J, et al. 1988. Human basophil degranulation triggered by very dilute antiserum against IgE. Nature 333:816-818

DeBeneditts G, Cigada M, Bianchi A, et al. 1994. Autonomic changes during hypnosis: a heart rate variability power spectrum analysis as a marker of sympatho-vagal balance. Int J Clin Exp Hypnosis XLII(2):140-152

Donnelly WJ, Spykerboer JE, Thong YH. 1985. Are patients who use alternative medicine dissatisfied with orthodox medicine? Med J Aust 142:439-441

European Parliament Committee on the Environment, Public Health and Consumer Protection. 1994. The State of Complementary Medicine Draft Report. Lannoye P, March

Farnsworth NR. 1983. Natural Products and Drug Development. Munksgaard, Copenhagen

Felten SY, Felten DL, Olschowka JA. 1992. Noradrenergic and peptidergic innervation of lymphoid organs. Chem Immunol 52:25-48

Field EH, Noelle RJ, Rouse T, et al. 1993. Evidence for excessive Th2 CD4$^+$ subset activity in vivo. J Immunol 151:48-59

Fisher P, Ward A. 1994. Complementary medicine in Europe. BMJ 309:107-111

Fulder SJ, Munro RE. 1985. Complementary medicine in the United Kingdom: patients, practitioners, and consultations. Lancet 7(2):542-545

Han JS, Tang J, Ren MF, Zhou ZF. 1980. Central neurotransmitters and acupuncture analgesia. Am J Chin Med 8:331-348

Hatch JP, Borcherding S, Norris LK. 1990. Cardiopulmonary adjustments during operant heart rate control. Psychophysiology 27(6):641-647

Inglis B. 1980. Natural Medicine. Fontana/Collins, Glasgow

Jian M. 1985. Influence of adrenergic antagonist and naloxone on the anti-allergic shock effect of electro-acupuncture in mice. Acupunct Electrother Res 10:163-167

Kamada T, Shinji S, Kumashiro M, et al. 1992. Power spectral analysis of heart rate variability in type As and type Bs during mental workload. Psychosom Med 54:462-470

Kasahara T, Wu Y, Sakurai Y, Oguchi K. 1992. Suppressive effects of acupuncture on delayed type hypersensitivity to trinitrochlorobenzene and involvement of opiate receptors. Int J Immunopharmacol 14:661-665

Lewith GT, Aldridge D (eds). 1993. Clinical Research Methodology Within Complementary Medicine. Hodder and Stoughton

L'Homeopathie en 1993. Lyons: Syndicat National de la Pharmacie Homeopathique, 1993. (Quoting COFREMCA and IFOP public opinion surveys)

McCraty R, Atkinson M, Tiller WA, et al. 1995a. The effects of emotions on the short term power spectral analysis of heart rate variability. Am J Cardiol 76:1089-1093

McCraty R, Atkinson M, Tiller WA, Watkins AD. 1995b. The electrophysiological correlates of positive emotions: three patterns of sympathovagal balance in normal subjects. Int J Psychophysiol (in press)

McGuire MB. 1988. Ritual Healing in Suburban America. Rutgers University Press, New Brunswick, New Jersey

Mossman TR, Cherwinski H, Bond MW, et al. 1986. Two types of murine helper T-cell clones. I: definition according to profiles of lymphokine activities and secreted proteins. J Immunol 136:2348-2357

Neild JE, Cameron IR. 1985. Bronchoconstriction in response to suggestion: its prevention by an inhaled anticholinergic agent. BMJ 290:674

Office of Technology Assessment. 1990. Unconventional Cancer Treatments. Washington, DC, Government Printing Office (OTA-H-405)

Ori Z, Monir G, Weiss J, et al. 1992. Heart rate variability. Frequency domain analysis. Cardiol Clin 10(3):499-537

Pietroni P. 1990. The Greening of Medicine. Gollancz Ltd

Reichlin S. 1993. Neuroendocrine-immune interactions. N Engl J Med 329:1246-1253

Reilly DT. 1983. Young doctors' views on alternative medicine. BMJ 287:337-339

Reilly DT, Taylor MA. 1993. Developing integrated medicine: Report of the Research Council for Complementary Medicine Research Fellowship in Complementary
Medicine. 1987-90. RCCM, London

Reilly DT, Taylor MA, Beattie NGM, et al. 1994. Is the evidence for homoeoepathy reproducible? Lancet
344:1601-1606

Reynolds T. 1991. J Natl Cancer Inst 83:594-596

Rosch PJ, Kearney HM. 1985. Holistic medicine and technology: a modern dialectic. Soc Sci Med 21(12):1405-
1409

The Royal College of Physicians. April 1992. Allergy: Conventional and Alternative Concepts. London

Rubinfeld AR, Pain MCF. 1976. Perception of asthma.
Lancet i:882-884

Sloan RP, Shapiro PA, Bagiella E, et al. 1994. Effect of mental stress throughout the day on cardiac autonomic
control. Biol Psychol 37:L89-99

Stein PK, Bosner MS, Kleiger RE, Conger BM. 1994. Heart
rate variability: a measure of cardiac autonomic tone.
Am Heart J 127(5):1376-1381

Terao A, Oikawa M, Saito M. 1993. Cytokine induced
changes in hypothalamic norepinephrine turnover: involvement of corticotrophin-releasing hormone and
prostaglandins. Brain Res 622:257-261

Van Dijk P. 1993. Geneewijzen in Nederland. Ankh-
Hermes, Deventer

Vernon HT, Dhami MSI, Howley TP, Annett R. 1986. Spinal
manipulation and beta-endorphin: a controlled study
of the effects of a spinal manipulation on plasma beta-
endorphin levels in normal males. J Manipulative Physiol Ther 9:115-123

Watkins AD. 1994. The role of alternative therapy in allergic disease. Clin Exp Allergy 24:813-825

Watkins AD. April 1995. Perceptions, emotions and immunity: an integrated homoeostatic network. Q J Med
88:283-294

Watt. 1981.

Watt J, Wood C (eds). 1988. Talking Health: Conventional
and Complementary Approaches. Royal Society of
Medicine, London

Wharton R, Lewith G. 1986. Complementary medicine and
the general practitioner. BMJ 292:1498-1500

WHO Global Strategy for Asthma Management. Feb 1994.
Draft VI. National Heart, Lung, and Blood Institute,
NIH World Health Organization

Williams R, Lane JD, Kuhn CM, et al. 1982. Type A behav-
iour and elevated physiological response to cognitive
tasks. Science 212:483-485

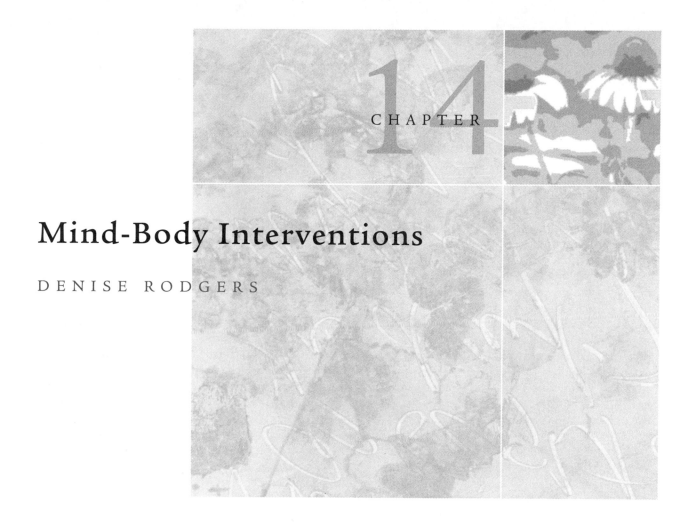

Mind-Body Interventions

DENISE RODGERS

HISTORICAL OVERVIEW

Life and healing are inherently mysterious. The essential stuff of the universe, including the universe of the mind and body, remains essentially unexplained. The void inside every atom is pulsating with information or unseen intelligence. Molecular biologists and geneticists locate this intelligence within DNA, primarily for the sake of convenience. Life unfolds as DNA imparts its coded intelligence into a sequence where energy and information are interchanged for the purpose of building life from matter.

The reality ushered in by quantum physics made it possible to manipulate the invisible intelligence that underlies the visible world. Einstein taught that the physical body, like all material objects, is like an illusion, and trying to manipulate it can be like grasp-

ing the shadow and missing the substance. The unseen world is a real world, and when we are willing to explore the immense creative power that lies within the mind, we can then access the unseen dimensions of the body.

Although mainstream consciousness seems highly aware of the inherent power of the mind, some of the earliest records of certain mind-and-body techniques were found in Babylonia and ancient Sumer well before the rise of experimental science. In the third century BC, Hippocrates was well versed in the art of mental healing. A serpent coiled around a staff, the Hippocratic symbol is used today to portray the medical/healing profession. History reveals that the coiled serpent symbolizes the healing energy possessed by each of us, lying dormant at the base of the spine, with the staff representing life itself. Eastern

215

philosophy posits that when the serpent is unleashed, healing energy spirals up the spine and out the forehead. This energy, said to be mental in nature, can then be used to heal the physical body.

Most ancient and indigenous medical systems make use of the extraordinary interconnectedness of the mind and body. Native American and the Asian Indian cultures are believed to be in contact with natural healing forces through their dreams, visions, and mystical experiences.

The ancient Greeks were also known for their healing temples. These centers existed for more than 800 years and endured until the rise of the Christian era. Patients would travel long distances to experience one of the aesculapian healing temples. The first step in seeking a cure was to create inner cleanliness by taking a purifying bath. Then they were put on a special diet or fast. They would attend one of the great dramas of Euripides or Sophocles, observing the tensions and movements of life. Later they were taken to visit one of the shrines, where healers used imagery to visualize the affected part of the body. During sleep the priests entered the patients' room and touched the diseased parts. Thereafter patients would dream and were said to awaken healed.

Philippus Aureolus Theophrastus Bombast von Hohenhein, known as Paracelsus, was a Swiss, sixteenth-century Renaissance physician. Although considered the father of modern drug therapy and scientific medicine, he nevertheless opposed the idea of separating the mind from the healing processes of the body. Along with his esteemed medical theories, he held that imagination and faith were the cause of healing power. He stated,

Man has a visible and an invisible workshop. The visible one is his body, the invisible one is the imagination of the mind. . . . The spirit is the master, imagination the tool, and the body the plastic material. The power of the imagination is the great factor in medicine. It may produce diseases in man and it may cure them. Ills of the body may be cured by physical remedies or by the power of spirit acting through the soul.

Paracelsus believed that physicians could heal by tapping the power of God. He also believed that dreams gave humans clairvoyance and the ability to diagnose illness from long distances away.

The philosophies of all these cultures had a common belief in a spiritual center that resides within.

They believed in spirit over matter, of mind over body. However, in contrast, modern allopathic medicine has regarded these connections as nonscientific and of secondary importance. Scientific healing, in the form of drug therapy and surgery, has grown to become a dominant Western form of treatment. Since the early 1900s, however, many medical scientists have begun to reinvestigate the role the mind plays in healing. In critical situations physicians have been known to say *"We've done all we can do—it's in God's hands now"* or *"It depends on the patient's will to live."*

Every physician has witnessed miraculous recoveries unexplainable by scientific understanding. Labeling a recovery as a "spontaneous remission" has become common to describe a healing that cannot be explained by medical standards. Physicians have also long recognized the effectiveness of placebos, substances with no known pharmacological action or benefit. In some cases placebos can be as much as 70 percent effective in the treatment of illness, thereby proving the theory that a patient's therapeutic expectation is a contributing factor for healing.

During the past 30 years great strides have been made by the scientific community to explore the mind's capacity to affect the body. This movement has received its impetus from several sources. The rise in incidence of chronic illness over the past few decades combined with the rapidly increasing costs for treatment have set the stage for deeper exploration of mind-body therapies. These therapies show great promise for mobilizing the body's inherent power to heal itself.

Recent studies have begun to further deepen our understanding of the effects of stress on the body. Convincing evidence supports that the immune system, along with other organs and systems in the body, can be and is often influenced by the mind. These research efforts and clinical experiments suggest that the separation between mind and body, long taken for granted in Western philosophy, is difficult to quantify. These challenges are all part of a new approach to medical science. The challenge of proving that the mind—our thoughts and emotions—has a significant impact on the body's health.

For patients this new synthesis has very practical significance. It suggests that by paying attention to and exerting some control over mental and emotional states, these attempts may actually contribute to prevention of or recovery from disease. The conscious participation of the patient in the process of healing not only offers new insight but also raises new questions about the nature and reality of consciousness.

The predominant fundamental tenet of mind-body medicine is the concept of treating the whole person. Another significant tenet is that people can be active participants in their own health care and may be able to prevent disease or shorten its course by taking steps to manage their own mental processes.

Medical researchers are beginning to rediscover what other cultures have historically used in their healing systems, such as meditation, hypnosis, and imagery. Grounded in ancient philosophy, these interventions are capable of stimulating and often facilitating the mind's capacity to affect the body. Experimentation has allowed practitioners the opportunity to offer nontoxic therapies while examining the specific links between mental processes and autonomic, immune, and nervous system functioning.

Evidence grows that states of mind can affect physiology. No one is promising that people can cure themselves of disease by adjusting their mental attitudes; this is not the message of mind-body interventions. However, mind-body approaches can be used to reduce the severity and frequency of biological symptoms and can potentially help strengthen the body's resistance to disease.

This chapter discusses the evidence that supports the mind-body approach, describes some of the more widely used techniques, and summarizes the results of some of the most effective interventions. The approaches discussed in this section not only demonstrate dramatic results in specific areas but also help form the basis for a new perspective for medicine and healing. From this perspective it becomes evident that every interaction between doctor and patient has the potential to affect the mind and, in turn, the body of the patient.

THE ROLE OF CONSCIOUSNESS

The Dismissal of the Mind

Although ancient mystics believed in the power of the human mind, Western science began to question such matters by the mid-1800s. The prevailing philosophy believed by physicians up until that time was that the patient's inner life and social being were vital components of all diagnosis and treatment. Doctors generally believed that medicine should take into account not only biological but also behavioral, moral, psychological, and spiritual factors.

However, these models and methods began to fade by the end of the nineteenth century, and a patient-specific model of treatment gave way to a disease-specific one. During the rise of this era of experimental science, four leading German physiologists (Helmholtz, Ludwig, DuBois-Remond, and Brucke) pledged themselves to account for all bodily processes in purely physiological terms. They determined that any reported relation between mental states and bodily functions was considered biased, subjective, nonmeasurable, and scientifically unreliable (Figure 14-1). More than 15,000 American doctors traveled to Germany to study the fascinating laboratory experimentations being introduced at that time. These innovative breakthroughs were in direct contrast with the style of medicine that had been practiced for centuries. It was believed that proper research could be conducted only in laboratories on isolated constituents—microorganisms, components of blood and urine, tissue, and organs, with the focus on devising universal remedies independent of individual patients. This approach has contemporary medicine in the position of having to learn the scientific basis of something it has known for centuries: that beliefs, thoughts, and feelings affect physiology.

Power of Placebo

The word *placebo* is Latin for "I please." This concept is well illustrated by an anecdote concerning Sir William Osler. One of North America's and England's busiest and most famous doctors, Osler brought new light to the power of placebo near the turn of the nineteenth century. Dr. Osler made a house call to a dying boy, who had been unresponsive to any previous treatments. Osler appeared at the bedside of the boy dressed in magnificent, scarlet academic robes. After a brief examination the doctor sat down at the boy's bedside, peeled a peach, sugared it, and cut it into pieces. He then fed it, bit by bit, with a fork to the entranced patient, telling him that it was a most special fruit and that if he ate it, he would not be sick.

Osler confided to the boy's father that his chances for survival were slim. The doctor continued to visit the boy daily for more than a month, always dressed in his majestic, scarlet robes and offering the boy

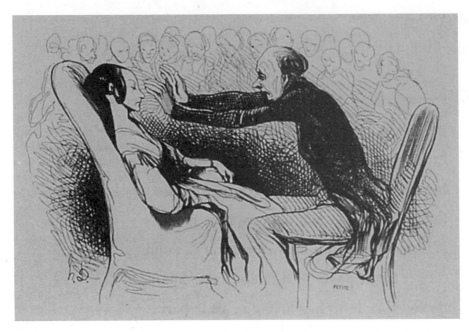

Figure 14-1 Mesmerism and hypnotism were the object of satire and a number of caricatures during the nineteenth century. (Courtesy Bibliothèque Interuniversitaire de Médecine, Paris.)

nourishment with his own two hands. This dramatic presentation inspired magic and belief well beyond laboratory science and helped catalyze the boy's unexpected and complete recovery.

Eloquently summing up the placebo's power, Osler (1953) wrote,

> Faith in the gods or saints cures one, faith in little pills another, hypnotic suggestion a third, faith in a plain common doctor a fourth. . . . The faith with which we work . . . has its limitations [but] such as we find it, faith is the most precious commodity, without which we should be very badly off.

Among the many placebo studies documented are those conduced by Dr. Ronald Katz, chairman of the Department of Anesthesiology at the UCLA School of Medicine. Katz reported a series of observations involving patients who were informed that headaches were a complication of spinal anesthesia. At the last minute the patients were told that the choice of anesthesia had been changed from spinal to general. Despite the change all of the patients experienced the symptoms that went with spinal anesthesia (Katz, 1977).

Similar to Katz's study investigating expectations, Dr. J.W.L. Fielding conducted a similar study at the Department of Surgery at Queen Elizabeth Hospital in Birmingham, England. In compliance with informed consent procedure, 411 patients were told they could expect to lose hair as a result of the chemotherapy being administered. Thirty percent of the patients unknowingly received placebos instead of chemotherapy and suffered hair loss even though the pills they had taken contained no medication (Fielding et al., 1983).

Although it has sometimes confounded as much as clarified, the mechanism of pain has provided fascinating clues to investigators of the mind-body healing response. In one landmark study in 1978, dental patients experiencing the aftereffects of an extracted tooth were given a sugar pill and told it was a powerful painkiller. They reported significant pain relief. Then experimenters added another agent: along with the placebo, a separate group of dental patients were given a chemical known to block the action of the brain's own endorphins. The second group experienced significantly less pain reduction than the first (Levine et al., 1978).

Here was a study that indicated a specific mechanism for placebo—endorphins—without which the magic effect would not have occurred. These studies and many other similar ones led scientists to believe that endorphins mediate much of the mind-body effect, whether that effect is triggered by trauma, placebo, hypnosis, or any other mental agent.

The story does not end there. Two separate studies found that the endorphin-blocker naloxone failed to prevent pain reduction in patients under hypnosis as it had for patients who took a placebo. Yet in another placebo study, pain reduction occurred even with naloxone. One plausible explanation is that other forms of endorphins may stealthily bypass the naloxone blockade. There are likely many mind-body routes, many mechanisms to create similar effects. It may then be that different states of mind affect the body along different pathways or that the same substances have multiple effects. In other words, relief of pain may also stimulate immune function because pain-relieving endorphins are key messenger molecules that also talk to the immune system.

The natural conclusion emerging from placebo research is that expectation or belief affects biology. The emotional responses of individuals to the world around them, stimulating hopes and joys, fears and anguish, has a potential affect on the physical body. This understanding is fundamental to the treatment of illness. It does not mean that conventional medical treatment should be supplanted by psychological or emotional approaches. The most effective and comprehensive strategy of treatment should be expanded to include the awareness of emotional and psychological factors in concert.

Mind and Emotion Everywhere

Former chief of the Brain Biochemistry Section of the National Institute of Mental Health, Candace Pert, PhD, codiscoverer of endorphins, made some startling revelations regarding the existence of neuropeptide receptors throughout the entire body. Pert found that the endocrine system and even the immune system all have these messenger molecules. This means that neuropeptide molecules are involved in a psychosomatic communication network, that the biochemistry of emotion could be mediating the transference of information flowing throughout the body.

Pert maintains that the emotions are the bridge between the mental and the physical, making them prime candidates for a variety of links among thought and healing.

Mind and Immunity

Dr. Robert Ader and Dr. Nicholas Cohen of the University of Rochester showed that the immune system can be trained, or *conditioned,* to respond to a neutral stimulus (placebo). Ader and Cohen found that the administration of an immune-suppressing drug and placebo together "conditioned" the immune system to respond to the placebo alone after the drug was discontinued. They also found that by alternating the administration of real medication and placebos, thus conditioning the body's physiological response to the placebo, the conditioning effects of a drug can be increased. It was also believed that side effects of dependence may be lessened in addition to the reduction of costs (Ader & Cohen, 1991).

Harvard Medical School anesthesiologist Henry Beecher observed that the greater the pain or anxiety, the more effective the placebo. He noted that the usefulness of any given drug is a combination of its chemical ingredients and the confidence of the patient that it will work (Beecher, 1955). This accounts for the effectiveness of the placebos in ameliorating a variety of disorders ranging from angina pectoris and gastrointestinal disorders to asthma, fevers, and the common cold.

Another Harvard-trained physician, Dr. Steven Locke, who specializes in behaviorial medicine and diseases related to disorders of the immune system, studied the power of suggestion using techniques of hypnosis (Locke et al., 1983). Locke has continued to observe a generalized link between hypnotic suggestions and immune reactions and published a bibliography of scientific papers in the field of psychoneuroimmunology titled *Mind and Immunity: Behavioral Immunology.*

It has become increasingly clear that there must be biology behind spontaneous remission, that the anecdotally celebrated power of the mind over the body could be significant. But this research continues to raise more questions about the mechanics of how it works. Why should the anticipation of a physical effect bring about actual physical change? And if anticipation or attitudes have a role in creating physical change, how can that knowledge be used to enhance medical treatment or promote good health? If we can answer those questions, can we determine how the human mind converts ideas and expectations into chemical realities? These are all questions that mind-body practitioners and medical researchers alike must answer.

PSYCHOTHERAPY

The word *psychotherapy* is derived from Greek words meaning "healing of the soul" and means treatment of emotional and mental health, which is obviously closely interwoven with physical health. Psychotherapy encompasses a wide range of specific treatments, including combining medication with discussion, listening to the patient's concerns, and using more active behavioral and emotional approaches. It should also be understood more generally as the matrix of interaction in which all health professionals operate.

An average of "one in every five people in the United States experiences a major psychological disorder every six months—most commonly anxiety, depression, substance abuse, or acute confusion" according to a study by James J. Strain. It is believed that rate is even greater among patients with a chronic illness and among the elderly. Approximately three fifths of patients with psychological problems are seen only by primary care physicians, many of whom are not adequately trained in psychotherapy nor do they have adequate time to spend with each patient discussing these psychological issues. Despite the enormous need for different forms of psychological care, most people who display the greatest need for such care receive less-than-adequate screening and treatment for their psychiatric conditions (Strain, 1993).

Research also indicates that primary care physicians recognize cases of depression in only one fourth to one half of the patients who experience it, and they recognize other types of mental illness less than one fourth of the time. However, these same doctors write most of the prescriptions for antidepressant and antianxiety drugs and may often prescribe them inappropriately. Clearly there is a significant need for better recognition and management of the psychiatric conditions that so often accompany serious illness.

Methods of Psychotherapy

Conventional psychotherapy is conducted primarily by means of psychological methods such as suggestion, persuasion, psychoanalysis, and reeducation. It can be divided into the following six general categories, which can be used individually or in groups.

Psychodynamic therapy. Psychodynamic therapy is derived from psychoanalysis and seeks to understand and resolve emotional conflicts that originate in childhood relationships and repeat themselves in adult life. Sessions usually are devoted to exploring current emotional reactions from past situations. This approach works best if the patient's goal is to make fundamental changes in personality patterns rather than to change one specific behavior.

Behavior therapy. Behavior therapy emphasizes changing specific behavior, such as a phobia, by stopping what has been reinforcing it or by replacing it with a more desirable response. In behavior therapy sessions are usually devoted to analyzing the behavior and devising ways to change it, carrying out specific instructions between sessions. Behavior therapy is more effective with focused problems such as a fear of public speaking.

Cognitive therapy. Cognitive therapy is similar to behavior therapy in changing specific habits; however, it emphasizes the habitual thoughts that underlie those habits. The general strategy is similar to that of behavior therapy, and the two approaches are often used together. Cognitive therapy is effective therapy for treating depression and low self-esteem.

Systems therapy. Systems therapy focuses on relationship patterns, either in couples, between parents and children, or within the whole family. This approach requires that everyone involved attend therapy sessions and often involves experiential practice aimed at changing problem-causing patterns. Systems therapies work well for a troubled marriage or intense conflicts between parent and child, where the problem is in the relationship between them.

Supportive therapy. Supportive therapy concentrates on helping people who are in an intense emotional crisis, such as a deep depression, and may be used in combination with pharmacological support. It focuses on building tools to handle overwhelming day-to-day situations.

Body-oriented therapy. Body-oriented therapy hypothesizes that emotions are encoded in and may be expressed as unexpressed tension and restriction in various parts of the physical body. Various methods of therapy, including breathwork, movement, and manual pressure, are used to help release emotions that are believed to have been held in the muscles and tissues.

• • •

Recent research indicates that psychotherapeutic treatment can hasten recovery from a medical crisis and is in some cases the best treatment for it. According to Strain, brief psychotherapy reduced time spent in hospitals for elderly patients with broken hips by an average of 2 days. These patients returned to the hospital fewer times and spent fewer days in rehabilitation. Other studies show that psychotherapy is most effective when begun soon after a patient is admitted to a hospital. At present, however, most psychological problems associated with physical illnesses remain undiagnosed or are not identified until near the end of a hospital stay.

One of the most common psychological problems medical patients suffer from are "reactive" anxiety and depression—the emotional distress stemming from a patient's reaction to diagnosis. Those with serious or terminal illnesses are particularly vulnerable. In other cases psychiatric symptoms are directly caused by the patient's physical disease. Still other patients experience a shift in their mental or emotional status as a direct result of a specific medication. For instance, some patients taking high levels of steroids may react psychotically, whereas others may experience severe depression.

Role of Group Support and Psychological Counseling

A landmark case was conducted in 1989 by David Spiegel, MD, a professor of psychiatry and behavioral sciences at Stanford School of Medicine, where he studied the benefits of group support on women with metastatic breast cancer. The women who participated in the group psychotherapy lived an average of 18 months longer than those who did not participate, doubling their survival time. The added survival time was longer than any medication or other known medical treatment could be expected to provide for women with advanced breast cancer. The intense social support the women experienced in these sessions appeared to influence the way their bodies coped with

the illness, which suggested that quality of life seemed to affect longevity (Spiegel et al., 1989).

In another well-known study of patients with established coronary artery disease, group support and psychological counseling were combined with diet and exercise. Symptoms such as angina pectoris rapidly diminished or disappeared altogether, and after 1 year the coronary artery obstructions were smaller. This evidence strongly suggested that the nation's most deadly and expensive health care problem could be potentially reversible through a complementary, noninvasive, diet and behavioral modification approach that emphasizes group psychotherapy (Ornish, 1990).

Cost-Effectiveness of Psychotherapy

Psychotherapy has been shown to speed patients' recovery time from illness. Faster recovery leads to reduced costs and fewer return visits to medical practitioners. In one study patients who frequently visited medical clinics were offered short-term psychotherapy, and significant declines were seen in visits to their doctors, days spent in the hospital, emergency department visits, diagnostic procedures, and drug prescriptions. Their overall health care costs were decreased by 10 to 20 percent in the years after brief psychotherapy (Cummings et al., 1988).

A more specific example of cost-effectiveness was demonstrated in a study by Margaret Caudill and colleagues in 1991, in which 10 group sessions of 90 minutes of psychotherapy and relaxation techniques significantly reduced the severity of pain. In a study of clinical use by chronic pain patients, those who participated in the outpatient behavioral medicine program had 36 percent fewer clinic visits than those who did not (Caudill et al., 1991).

A case in point is a 1987 study conducted jointly with Mount Sinai and Northwestern. Psychiatrist George Fulop of Mount Sinai and his colleagues observed that patients hospitalized for medical or surgical reasons had significantly longer hospital stays if they also had concurrent psychiatric problems, especially if they were elderly. In other words, a patient who had a heart attack and who was also depressed tended to remain in the hospital for more days than a similar heart attack patient whose mood was normal. Fulop's study suggested that treating a medical patient's psychological conditions with psychotherapy in adjunct with medication could not only improve psychological well-being but also affect the patient's physical condition (Fulop et al., 1987).

Another well-known study published in 1983 by psychologists Herbert J. Schlesinger and Emily Mumford and their colleagues at the University of Colorado School of Medicine studied patients with four common chronic diseases: asthma, diabetes, coronary heart disease, and high blood pressure. The researchers examined a group of Blue Cross–Blue Shield patients who underwent some form of psychotherapy after having been identified with one of these physical conditions and compared them with a control group who did not receive psychological treatment after similar diagnoses were made (Schlesinger et al., 1983).

Three years after they received their medical diagnoses, patients who had undergone 7 to 20 mental health treatment visits had incurred lower medical charges than those who did not have psychological treatment. The total charges for the first group, including those incurred for psychotherapy and counseling, were more than $300 less than for the other group. In other words, the savings on medical bills offered by psychotherapy more than compensated for its costs. After 21 sessions the savings began to diminish as the cumulative cost of mental health care increased.

Although this study is often cited as "proof" of psychotherapy's financial advantages for the medically ill, the study was not without flaws. For example, it was a retrospective study rather than a prospective study. More scientifically controlled studies are needed in which subjects are selected at random from the beginning of treatment and closely followed after treatment. Another limitation of this particular research approach was that the investigators could not clearly define the type of mental health problems the patients experienced or the specific treatment they received. The information gathered encompassed a large variety of psychiatric interventions.

More rigorous research on specific forms of psychotherapy, including precise diagnoses, will be needed to reach firm conclusions about the economic benefits of psychological treatment for the medically ill. However, there is already sufficient evidence to suggest that this cost/benefit research is important to pursue. For example, one review of 15 studies published between 1965 and 1980 demonstrated that patients who underwent psychotherapy used 13 percent less of other medical services than patients who were not in psychotherapy.

The concept of what constitutes appropriate areas for psychiatric intervention should be expanded. Many people, including health care professionals and academicians, consider psychotherapeutic intervention in physical illness a peripheral concern. Important research questions regarding unexplained mind-body events have long existed but are generally ignored. However, the studies previously cited suggest that psychological intervention could be most beneficial when used early on in the disease process and could potentially affect mortality in certain illnesses.

Although research continues to mount on the effects of psychotherapeutic interventions, further studies are needed to continue researching the interconnectedness of the mind and body and how these methods can potentially offer genuine opportunity to improve health and limit costs simultaneously.

Recent Research on Social Support and Mortality

Thanks to a growing number of large-scale studies, evidence of a link between social support and physical well-being has been prolific. This research shows that having many close social relationships is associated with a lower risk of dying at any age. Research that has looked specifically at sick people shows that once serious illness strikes, social support continues to affect their chances of staying alive. In 1990 epidemiologists Peggy Reynolds and George Kaplan at the University of California at Berkeley studied the number of social contacts that cancer patients had each day. Women with the least amount of social contact were 2.2 times more likely to die of cancer over a 17-year period than were the most socially connected.

Along similar lines, in 1987 internist James Goodwin at the Medical College of Wisconsin and his colleagues published the results of a study on cancer survival in several thousand patients. The married cancer patients did better medically and had lower mortality rates than the unmarried (Goodwin et al., 1987). Similarly, in a study of 1368 patients with coronary artery disease, Redford Williams at Duke University found that having a spouse or other close confidant tripled the chances that a patient would be alive 5 years later.

Naturally, many other potential social factors can account for why one patient survives longer than another. Therefore most studies like this have been careful to eliminate the obvious confounding variables, such as smoking and alcohol use, differences in socioeconomic status, and access to health care. By and large, however, the studies still consistently show that more and better social support from family and friends is associated with lower odds of dying at any given age.

In an overview of research concerning mortality and social relationships, James House observed that the relationship between social isolation and early death is as strong statistically as the relationship between dying and smoking or having high serum cholesterol. Therefore the data suggest that it may be as important to one's health to be socially integrated as it is to stop smoking or to reduce one's cholesterol level. No question, the relationship between social support and health outcome has been greatly underestimated by medical science (House et al., 1988).

MEDITATION

Although the origin of meditation is ancient in its roots, the science of meditation and its physiological effects is in its infancy. Only recently has the concept of meditation been introduced into the realm of modern Western medicine. The Cartesian split between the mind and body in the early seventeenth century resulted in science emphasizing the body and medicine going in the direction of science. The mind and body connection has to do with understanding that the two are not separate (they have always been together!), and they have an interactive influence on each other. Meditation is said to realign the two, consciousness with the physical body, creating a more harmonious interaction.

Similar to the word *medicine,* the word *meditation* suggests something to do with healing. The physicist and author of *Wholeness and Implicate Order,* David Bohm looks at wholeness as a property of the physical, material world. He points out the root in Latin means "to cure" but that its deepest root means "to measure" (Bohm, 1983). But what does medicine or meditation have to do with measure? The ancient Greeks said "Man is the measure of all things." According to Jon Kabat-Zinn, PhD, founder and Director of the Stress Reduction Clinic at the University of

Massachusetts Medical Center, "It has to do with the platonic notion that every shape, every being, every thing has its right inward measure. In other words, a tree has its own quality of wholeness that gives it particular properties. A human being has an individual right inward measure, when everything is balanced and physiologically homeostatic—that's the totality of the individual at that point in time" (Kabat-Zinn, 1993). Kabat-Zinn believes that medicine is the science and art of restoring right inward measure when it is thrown off balance. From the meditative perspective and from the perspective of the new mind-body medicine, health does not have a finite or static destination. Health is a dynamic energy flow that changes over a lifetime, with health and illness coexisting together.

Most meditative practices have come to the West from Asian religious practices, particularly those of India, China, and Japan. Others can be traced to the ancient cultures of the world. Although Western meditators practice a contemplative form of meditation, there are also many active forms of meditation, such as the Chinese martial art, tai chi, the Japanese martial art aikido, and the walking meditations of Zen Buddhism.

Until recently the primary purpose of meditation has been religious or spiritual in nature. However, during the past 20 years it has been explored as a means of reducing stress on both mind and body. Many studies have found that various practices of meditation appear to produce physical and psychological changes.

Meditation is a self-directed practice for the purpose of relaxing and calming the mind and body. Many methods of meditation include focusing on a single thought or word for a specific period of time. Some forms of meditation focus on a physical experience such as the breath or a specific sound or mantra. All forms of meditation have the common objective of stilling the restlessness of the mind so that the focus can be directed inwardly. Meditation, then, is a technique used to calm the mental activity, the endless thoughts, and ways of reacting to our circumstances. As long as these accumulated impressions linger in the inner recesses of the mind, nagging for attention, it remains difficult to experience an inner state of peace, calm, and health. Fast-paced Western society, filled with external stimuli, has conditioned us to push our minds and bodies to the point of exhaustion, often to the detriment of our own well-being. To be still, to experience the peace and contentment that lies within, we must free ourselves from this external materiality. Meditation is the process of calming and releasing the distractions from the mind for the purpose of opening up to and awakening to our true inner natures.

Eastern Techniques and Transcendental Meditation

In the mid-1960s, a popular trend in meditation called *transcendental meditation* (TM) began to emerge. The Vedic philosophy and practice was brought from India to the United States by its founder, Maharishi Mahesh Yogi. The Maharishi had eliminated ancient yogic elements that he considered unnecessary in a contemporary environment. Omitting difficult physical postures and mental exercises, his reformed version became more easily understood and practiced by westerners (see Chapter 20).

TM is relatively simple in application. A student is given a mantra (a word or sound) to repeat silently over and over again while sitting in a comfortable position. The purpose of repeating the sound or word is to prevent distracting thoughts from entering the mind. Students are instructed to be passive and, if thoughts other than the mantra come to mind, to note them and return the attention to the mantra. TM is generally practiced in the morning and in the evening for approximately 20 minutes.

On the Maharishi's first visit to America in 1959, a San Francisco newspaper heralded TM as a "non-medicinal tranquilizer" and praised it as a promising cure for insomnia. TM soon began to ride a crest of popularity with almost half a million Americans learning the technique by 1975, and it was embraced by many celebrities of that day, such as the Beatles. It is believed that today well over 2 million people practice TM.

In 1968 Harvard cardiologist Herbert Benson was asked by Maharishi International University in Fairfield, Iowa, to test TM practitioners on their ability to lower their own blood pressure. Benson initially refused to participate but was later persuaded to do so. Benson's studies and other additional research showed that TM was associated with reduced health care costs, increased longevity, and quality of life (Benson et al., 1977), reduction of chronic pain (Kabat-Zinn et al., 1986), reduced anxiety, reduction of high blood pressure and serum cholesterol levels (Cooper & Aygen, 1978), reduction of substance abuse (Sharma et al., 1991), treatment of posttraumatic stress syndrome in Vietnam veterans (Brooks & Scarano, 1985), blood pressure reduction in African-American persons (Schneider et al., 1992), and lowered blood cortisol levels initially brought on by stress (MacLean et al., 1992).

Western Techniques and Mindfulness Meditations

The term *mindfulness* was coined by Jon Kabat-Zinn, PhD, known for his work using mindfulness meditation to help medical patients with chronic pain and stress-related disorders (Kabat-Zinn, 1993a, b). Like other mind-body therapies, mindfulness meditation can induce deep states of relaxation, at times directly improve physical symptoms, and help patients lead fuller and more satisfying lives. Although Asian forms of meditation involve focusing on a sound, phrase, or prayer to minimize distraction, the practice of mindfulness does the opposite. In mindfulness meditation distractions are not ignored but focused on. This form of meditation practice can be traced originally from the Buddhist tradition and is roughly 2500 years old. The method was developed as a means of cultivating greater awareness and wisdom, with the aim of helping people live each moment of their lives as fully as possible.

Kabat-Zinn points out that mindfulness is about more than feeling relaxed or stress-free. Its true aim is to nurture an inner balance of mind that allows an individual to face life situations with greater clarity, stability, and understanding and to respond more effectively from that sense of clarity (Kabat-Zinn, 1993).

An integral part of mindfulness practice is to accept and welcome the stress, pain, anger, frustration, disappointment, and insecurity when those feelings are present. Kabat-Zinn believes that acknowledgment is paramount. Whether pleasant or unpleasant, admission is the first step toward transforming that reality.

Kabat-Zinn founded the Stress Reduction Clinic at the University of Massachusetts Medical Center in Worcester, where he is an associate professor of medicine. In the 17 years since the clinic was founded, well over 8000 medical patients have gone through his mindfulness meditation programs, almost all referred by their physicians.

Unlike standard medical and psychological approaches, the clinic does not categorize and treat patients differently depending on their illnesses. Their 8-week courses offer the same training program in mindfulness and stress reduction to everyone. They emphasize what is "right" with their patients, rather than what is "wrong" with them, focusing on mobilizing their inner strengths and changing their behaviors in new and innovative ways. Facilitators maintain that their programs are not held out as some kind of magical cure when other approaches failed; rather, they provide a sensible and straightforward way for people to experience and understand the mind-body connection firsthand, using that knowledge to better cope with their illnesses.

In the practice of mindfulness the patient begins by using one-pointed attention to cultivate calmness and stability. When thoughts and feelings arise, it is important that they not be ignored or suppressed, or analyzed or judged by their content; rather, the thoughts are observed intentionally and nonjudgmentally, moment by moment, as events in the field of awareness.

This inclusive noting of thoughts that come and go in the mind can lead to a detachment from them, allowing a deeper perspective about the stresses of life to emerge. By observing the thoughts from this vantage point, one gains a new frame of reference. In this way, valuable insight can be allowed to surface. The key to mindfulness is not the topic focused on but the quality of awareness brought into each moment. Observing the thought processes, without intellectualizing them and without judgment, creates greater clarity. The goal of mindfulness is to become more aware, more in touch with life and its happenings at the time it is happening, in the present.

Acceptance does not mean passivity or resignation. Accepting what each moment offers provides the opportunity to experience life more completely. In this manner any situation can be responded to with greater confidence and clarity.

One way to envision how mindfulness works is to think of the mind as the surface of a lake or ocean. Many people think the goal of meditation is to stop the waves so that the water will be flat, peaceful, and tranquil. The spirit of mindfulness practice is to experience the waves.

RELAXATION

Stress Management

The popular term *stress* was brought into use by Professor Hans Selye, Director of the Institute of Experimental Medicine and Surgery at the University of Montreal. He determined that stress was "the rate of wear and tear on the body." Confusion has continued to this day as to whether stress is the factor that causes the wear and tear, or the resulting damage. Selye termed it "general adaption syndrome" (GAS), which has three phases: an alarm reaction, a stage of resistance, and a stage of exhaustion. A stress cause, or stressor, mobilizes GAS by activating the sympathetic part of the autonomic nervous system. Hormones bring about physiological changes in the body, often referred to as the "fight-or-flight syndrome" (Selye, 1978).

The problem of stress has received wide publicity in the media in recent years. We have also heard the cliché that "stress" is the epidemic of the 1980s and 1990s. Consequently the word *stress* has become a buzzword that has acquired a highly negative connotation. We have also received plenty of advice over the last few years, from all sorts of sources, about the many different approaches to controlling stress. All the alarmist and negative publicity has stimulated further anxiety and concern in many people's minds—a fear of stress, which in itself can lead to further stress. Having become aware of it, everyone now wants to manage their stress and many cater to this growing market. This rapidly growing market consists of various experts, consultants, and therapists. Vitamin regimens, herbal supplements, fitness programs, relaxation techniques, and personal development courses are being offered, all in the name of *stress management*. All sorts of experts, both qualified and self-appointed, are convinced that their particular product or service will banish stress for good.

The fact remains that there are no magic cures and no magic bullets. Stress is essentially a result of an interaction between a negative environment, unhealthful lifestyles, and self-defeating attitudes and beliefs. Therefore, unlike what is believed by stress management consultants, no one particular technique, method, program, or regimen of vitamins or herbs can reduce long-term stress.

Stress is most often seen as the outside pressures and problems that encroach our busy lives: deadlines, excessive work load, noise, traffic, problems with spouse or children, and excessive demands made by others. Stress is the unconscious response to a demand. Stress is not "those things out there," but rather it is what happens inside our mind and body as we react unconsciously to those things or people. Normally we experience some degree of stress in everything we do and everything that happens to us.

In *Magical Child* Joseph Chiltern Pearce states, "Stress is the way intelligence grows." He explains that, under stress, the brain immediately grows massive numbers of new connecting links between the neurons that enable learning. Although the stressed mind/brain grows in ability and the unstressed one lags behind, the overstressed one can collapse into physiological shock. Something is essential to maintain the optimal level of stress, and this of course is relaxation (Pearce, 1992).

When the stress response is minor, we do not notice any symptoms. The greater the stimulation, the more symptoms we notice. Holmes and Rahe's scale of life changes provides a guide to the amount of stress attached to events—such as marriage, relocation, emigration, loss of a job, death of a spouse, or birth of a child. These significant life events can quickly overload our ability to cope (Holmes & Rahe, 1967).

In *The Human Zoo* Desmond Morris posits that modern humans are engaged in the "Stimulus Struggle": "If we abandon it, or tackle it badly, we are in serious trouble." We are trying to maintain the optimal level of stimulation—not the maximum, but that level that is most beneficial, somewhere between understimulation and overstimulation (Morris, 1995).

Stress becomes a problem when it reaches excessive levels, when the demands exceed our ability to respond or to cope effectively. When we are under excessive, prolonged stress and no longer able to cope or adjust, the "stress" becomes "distress." Symptoms are then developed that lead to stress-induced illnesses. The physical body "engine" begins to rev at high speed, totally absorbing restricted, unproductive energy. Over extended periods, this wear and tear begins to take its toll and disease can creep into the body.

We can learn to control our responses to stress by changing the ways that we think. Stress management is developing the ability to assert control over our behaviors. When we become aware of our ability to control attitudes and behaviors, we naturally begin to assert control over our life's situations that seem to be stressful. It is not the stress itself that is harmful, but our reactions to it that create havoc in the body and mind.

The biggest stressor most people experience daily is *change*. Challenges, frustrations, conflicting demands and occasional loss, grief, and suffering are among the many unconscious responses to change. These life events are inevitable and require us to adapt to new situations. If we do not adapt to change by altering our attitudes, our minds and bodies suffer. When changes take place in our environment, career, and personal relationships, it becomes essential to learn how to behave, think, and feel differently to cope with the new situation effectively.

We are all continuously adjusting to changing conditions, rather like an air conditioner that is controlled by a thermostat. As the weather outside changes, the thermostat turns the air conditioner unit on, which begins to bring the interior temperature back to a specified normal level of comfort. The greater the changes outside, the harder the machine has to work to keep up with them. If the external temperature moves into extreme ranges, the machine will be pushed to the limit. If it exceeds its specified limit, it will eventually break down, and the motor will burn out.

So it is with the human machine. Our bodies continuously react to whatever is happening around us or inside of us. We respond physically, mentally, and emotionally to even the most minute changes. This process occurs all of the time, whether we are consciously aware of it or not.

As most are aware, different individuals respond differently to stress. We know people who can remain cool, calm, and collected under the most trying circumstances, and we know others who are unable to cope when faced with even minor situations. The differences are mostly due to the differences in upbringing, past understandings, present experiences, attitudes, belief structures, family values, perceptions, and coping skills developed over years and generations. Furthermore, when different individuals experience distress, the symptoms they develop are also different. This results from the fact that different people seem to channel their excessive stress into different parts of the body. The long-term effects of such different responses include such physical illnesses as ulcers, headaches, chronic backaches, and high blood pressure, which ultimately results in heart disease, cancer, or other chronic disorders.

According to U.S. scientists, stress is now known to be a major contributor, either directly or indirectly, to coronary heart disease, cancer, lung ailments, accidental injuries, cirrhosis of the liver, and suicide.

The Relaxation Response

Harvard-trained physician Herbert Benson investigated the benefits of meditation in the late 1960s. Convinced that the benefits of meditation could potentially lower high blood pressure, Benson continued his research into a variety of psychological and physiological effects that appear common to many mind and body practices. He later identified *the relaxation response,* which elicited a similar response common to meditation, prayer, autogenic training, and some forms of hypnosis (Benson, 1975). He later published his method in a book of the same name.

His research indicated that excessive stress could cause or aggravate hypertension and its related diseases, atherosclerosis, heart attack, and stroke. He then examined the nature of the relaxation response, showing that physiological changes as remarkable as those seen in the fight-or-flight response also occur during true relaxation, including lowering of oxygen consumption, metabolism, heart rate, and blood pressure, as well as increased production of alpha brain waves. A marked decrease in blood lactate was also found. Blood lactate has often been linked with anxiety. Pitts and McLure, of Washington University School of Medicine showed that blood lactate injections increased anxiety attacks in anxiety neurotics.

According to Benson, the following steps elicit the relaxation response:

1. Try to find 10 to 20 minutes in your daily routine; before breakfast is generally a good time.
2. Sit comfortably.
3. For the period you will practice, try to arrange your life so that you will have no distractions. For example, let the answering machine get the phone or ask someone to watch the children.
4. Time yourself by glancing periodically at a clock or watch (but do not set an alarm). Commit yourself to a specific length of practice.

There are several approaches to eliciting the relaxation response; Benson suggests the following:

Step 1: Pick a focus word or short phrase that is firmly rooted in your personal belief system.

For example, a nonreligious individual might choose a neutral word like *one* or *peace* or *love.* A Christian person desiring to use a prayer could pick the opening words of Psalm 23, *The Lord is My Shepherd;* a Jewish person could choose *Shalom.*

Step 2: Sit quietly in a comfortable position.

Step 3: Close your eyes.

Step 4: Relax your muscles.

Step 5: Breathe slowly and naturally, repeating your focus word or phrase silently as you exhale.

Step 6: Throughout, assume a passive attitude. Do not worry about how well you are doing. When other thoughts come to mind, simply say to yourself, "Oh, well," and gently return to the repetition.

Step 7: Continue for 10 to 20 minutes. You may open your eyes to check the time but do not use an alarm. When you finish, sit quietly for a minute or so, at first with your eyes closed and later with your eyes open. Then do not stand for 1 or 2 minutes.

Step 8: Practice the technique once or twice a day.

Benson's subsequent research into the relaxation response covered several efficient techniques of relaxation training, including transcendental meditation, Zen and yoga, autogenic training, progression relaxation, hypnosis, and sentic cycles (Table 14-1). He found that these methods had four common elements: a quiet environment, an object to focus the mind on, a passive attitude, and a comfortable position. Some practices are more effective than others and some are easier to learn and practice than others (Benson, 1993).

Benson's group also found that patients with chronic pain who meditated regularly had a net reduction in general health care costs, suggesting that the effects of relaxation techniques are cost-effective (Caudill et al., 1991).

Exercise for Stress Reduction

Michael Sacks, MD, professor of psychiatry at Cornell University Medical College, found that various forms of exercise can be powerful methods of relaxation effective for dealing with the stress of daily life. Researchers have found in various studies that exercise can decrease anxiety and depression, improve an

TABLE 14-1

Relaxation Response

Technique	Oxygen consumption	Respiratory rate	Heart rate	Alpha waves	Blood pressure	Muscle tension
Transcendental meditation	Decreases	Decreases	Decreases	Increases	Decreases*	Not measured
Zen and yoga	Decreases	Decreases	Decreases	Increases	Decreases*	Not measured
Autogenic training	(Not measured)	Decreases	Decreases	Increases	Inconclusive	Decreases
Progressive relaxation	(Not measured)	(Not measured)	(Not measured)	(Not measured)	Inconclusive	Decreases
Hypnosis with suggested deep relaxation	Decreases	Decreases	Decreases	(Not measured)	Inconclusive	Not measured

*In patients with elevated blood pressure.

individual's self-image, and buffer people from the effects of stress. Not every study has shown the precise benefits researchers were looking for, but taken as a whole, the research strongly supports the common experience that exercise can elevate mood and reduce anxiety and stress (Sacks, 1993).

Although most research has been largely focused on the physical benefits of exercise, virtually any exercise can help people feel more focused and relaxed as long as the activity is enjoyable. Regular exercise does seem to affect one aspect of character in particular: the ability to withstand stress. Exercise and physical fitness can act as a buffer against stress so that stressful events have a less negative impact on psychological and physical health.

HYPNOSIS

Modern hypnosis is said to have begun in the eighteenth century with Franz Anton Mesmer, who used what he called "magnetic healing" to treat a variety of psychological and psychophysiological disorders, such as hysterical blindness, paralysis, headaches, and joint pains. The famous Austrian neuropathologist Sigmund Freud initially found hypnosis to be extremely effective in treating hysteria and then, troubled by the sudden catharsis of powerful emotions by his patients, abandoned its use.

The word *hypnosis* is derived from the Greek word *hypnos,* meaning "sleep." It is believed that hypnotic suggestion has been a part of ancient healing traditions for centuries. The induction of trance states and the use of therapeutic suggestion were a central feature of the early Greek healing temples, and variations of these techniques were practiced throughout the ancient world.

In more recent years hypnosis has experienced a resurgence. Initially this form of therapy became popular with physicians and dentists. Today it is widely used by mental health professionals for the treatment of addictions, pain control, anxiety disorders, and phobias.

During hypnosis a patient enters a state of attentive and focused concentration and becomes relatively unaware of the immediate surroundings. While in this state of deep concentration, people are highly responsive to suggestion. Contrary to popular folklore, however, people cannot be hypnotized against their will or involuntarily. They must be willing to concentrate their thoughts and to follow the suggestions offered. Essentially, all forms of hypnotherapy are actually forms of self-hypnosis.

Hypnosis has three major components: absorption (in the words or images presented by the hypnotherapist), dissociation (from one's ordinary critical faculties), and responsiveness. A hypnotherapist either leads patients through relaxation, mental images, and suggestions or teaches patients to perform the techniques themselves. Many hypnotherapists provide guided audiotapes for their patients so that they can practice the therapy at home. The images presented are specifically tailored to the particular patient's needs and may use one or all of the senses.

Physiologically hypnosis resembles other forms of deep relaxation discussed in this section. It is known to decrease sympathetic nervous system activity, decrease oxygen consumption and carbon dioxide eliminations, and lower blood pressure and heart rate, and it is linked to increasing or decreasing certain kinds of brain wave activity.

Clinical Applications

One of the most dramatic uses of hypnosis is for skin disorders. In the mid-1950s, an anesthesiologist, Arthur Mason, used hypnosis to effectively treat a 16-year-old patient who he thought had warts. Within 10 days the wart fell off and normal skin replaced it (Mason & Black, 1958). Since that time hypnosis has been used to dramatically improve other skin disorders such as ichthyosis.

Depending on the individual's situation, hypnotherapy can be used as a complement to medical care or as a primary treatment. Many people find that hypnotherapy's benefits are enhanced by the use of biofeedback to induce physiological changes. Biofeedback helps patients see that they can indeed control certain bodily functions simply by altering their thoughts, and the added confidence helps them improve more rapidly.

Management of chronic illness. There is little doubt that the regular practice of self-hypnosis is helpful to people with chronic disease. The benefits include reduction of anxiety and fear, decreased requirements for analgesics, increased comfort during medical procedures, and greater stability of functions controlled by the autonomic nervous system, such as blood pressure. Training in self-hypnosis also enhances the patient's sense of control, which is often affected by chronic illness. Hypnotherapy may also have direct clinical effects on certain chronic diseases, such as reducing bleeding in hemophiliac patients, stabilizing blood sugar in diabetic patients, and reducing the severity of asthmatic attacks.

Pain management. Hypnosis can also be quite effective to reduce the fear and anxiety that accompanies pain. Because it is said that anxiety increases pain, hypnotherapy helps a patient gain control over the fear and anxiety, thereby reducing the pain. Many controlled studies have been conducted that demon-

strate that hypnosis is an effective way to reduce migraine attacks in children and teenagers. In one experiment 30 schoolchildren were randomly assigned a placebo or propranol (a blood pressure–lowering agent) or taught self-hypnosis. It was found that only the children who used the self-hypnosis techniques had a significant drop in severity and frequency of headaches (Olness & Gardner, 1988). Another pain study of patients who were chronically ill reported a 113 percent increase in pain tolerance among highly hypnotizable subjects versus a control group who did not receive hypnosis (Debenedittis et al., 1989).

A technique used for surgery in people with little or no tolerance for chemical anesthesia called *spinal anesthesia illusion* was developed by a dentist and psychologist named Philip Ament from Buffalo, New York. In this method a deep state of relaxation is induced by having the patient count mentally or focus on a specific image. The patient is given the suggestion that he or she will feel a growing numbness begin to spread from the navel to the toes as he or she counts to a higher and higher number. Once the patient feels numb, the surgery can proceed. After the surgery the therapist gives the patient suggestions that lead to the gradual return of normal sensations.

Dentistry. Some people have learned to tolerate dental work such as drilling, extraction, and periodontal surgery using hypnosis as the sole anesthesia. Even when an anesthetic is used, hypnotherapy can also be used to reduce fear and anxiety, control bleeding and salivation, and lessen postoperative discomfort. Used with children, it can decrease the chances of developing a dental phobia.

Pregnancy and delivery. It is believed that Lamaze and other popular breathing techniques used during labor and delivery may actually work by inducing a hypnotic state. Women who have used hypnosis before delivery tend to have shorter labors and more comfortable deliveries than other pregnant women. There are even reports of cesarean sections performed with hypnosis as the sole anesthesia.

Anxiety. Hypnosis can be used to establish a new reaction to specific anxiety-causing activities such as stage fright, airplane flight, and other phobias. Typically the hypnotherapist helps the patient undo a conditioned physiological response, such as hyperventilation or nausea. This method can also be used to help calm athletes who are prepared to compete.

Hypnotherapy can be used to quell most any fear whether associated with examinations, public speaking, or social interactions.

BIOFEEDBACK

Biofeedback therapies emerged in the 1960s and 1970s, when advances in psychological and medical research converged with developments in biomedical technology. Improved electronic instruments could convey information to patients about their autonomic nervous systems and their muscles in the form of audio and/or visual signals that patients could understand. The word *biofeedback* became the general term to define the procedures and treatments that make use of these instruments (Green & Green, 1977).

Biofeedback therapy uses special instruments and methods to expand the body's natural internal feedback systems. By watching a monitoring device, patients can learn by trial and error to adjust their thinking and other mental processes to control bodily processes previously thought to be involuntary, such as blood pressure, temperature, gastrointestinal functioning, and brain wave activity. In fact, biofeedback can be used on nearly any bodily process that can be measured accurately.

Biofeedback does not belong to any particular field of health care but is used in many disciplines, including internal medicine, dentistry, physical therapy and rehabilitation, psychology and psychiatry, and pain management. Like all other forms of therapy, biofeedback is more useful for some clinical problems than for others. For example, biofeedback is a useful treatment in Raynaud's disease, a painful and potentially dangerous spasm of the small arteries, and certain types of fecal and urinary incontinence. It has also become an integral part of the treatment of many other disorders, including headaches, anxiety, high blood pressure, teeth clenching, asthma, and muscle disorders.

More recently, researchers have been experimenting with biofeedback treatments for conditions believed to stem from irregular brain wave patterns, such as epilepsy, attention-deficit disorder (ADD), and attention-deficit hyperactivity disorder (ADHD) in children with promising results.

Biofeedback is successful in helping people learn to regulate many physical conditions partly because it puts them in better contact with specific parts of their bodies. For example, biofeedback can help teach people to tighten muscles at the neck of the bladder to better control impaired bladder function. It can help postoperative patients learn to reuse muscles of the legs and arms. It can help teach stroke patients to use alternative muscles to move a limb if the primary ones can no longer do the job. Biofeedback is also helpful in training patients to use artificial limbs after amputation.

In a normal biofeedback session electrodes are attached to the area being monitored. These electrodes feed the information to a small monitoring box that registers the results by a sound tone that varies in pitch or on a visual meter that varies in brightness as the function being monitored decreases or increases. A biofeedback therapist leads the patient in mental exercises to help the patient reach the desired result. Through trial and error, patients gradually train themselves to control the inner mechanism involved. Training for some disorders requires 8 to 10 sessions; however, a single session often can provide symptomatic relief. Patients with long-term or severe disorders may require longer therapy. The aim of the treatment is to teach patients to regulate their own inner mental and bodily processes without the help of a machine.

Five Common Forms of Biofeedback Therapy

Electromyographic biofeedback. Electromyographic (EMG) feedback measures muscular tension. Sensors are attached to the skin to detect electrical activity related to muscle tension in that area. The biofeedback instrument amplifies and converts this activity into useful information, displaying the various degrees of muscle tension. This form of biofeedback therapy is most often used for tension headaches, physical rehabilitation, chronic muscle pain, incontinence, and general relaxation purposes.

Thermal biofeedback therapy. Thermal biofeedback therapy is used to measure skin temperature, as an index of blood flow changes from the constriction and dilation of blood vessels. Low skin temperature usually means decreased blood flow in that area. A temperature-sensitive probe is taped to the skin, often on a finger. The instrument converts information into feedback that can be seen and heard and can be used to reduce or increase blood flow to the hands and feet. Thermal biofeedback is often used for Raynaud's disease, migraine headaches, hypertension, and anxiety disorders, and to promote general relaxation.

Electrodermal activity therapy. Electrodermal activity therapy is used to measure changes in sweat activity too minimal to feel. Two sensors are attached to the palm side of the fingers or hand to measure sweat activity. They produce a tiny electrical current that measures skin conductance on the basis of the amount of moisture present. Increased sweat can mean arousal of part of the autonomic nervous system. Electrodermal activity therapy can be used to measure the sweat output stemming from stressful thoughts or rapid deep breathing. It is most often used for anxiety and hyperhidrosis.

Finger pulse therapy. Finger pulse therapy measures pulse rate and force. With this method a sensor is attached to a finger and helps measure heart activity as a sign of arousal of part of the autonomic nervous system. It is most often used for hypertension, anxiety, and some cardiac arrhythmias.

Breathing biofeedback therapy. Breathing biofeedback therapy measures breath rate, volume, rhythm, and location. Sensors are placed around the chest and abdomen to measure air flow from the mouth and nose. The feedback is usually visual, and patients learn to take deeper, slower, lower, and more regular breaths using abdominal muscles. This simple form of biofeedback is most often used for asthma and other respiratory conditions, hyperventilation, and anxiety.

• • •

The general goal of biofeedback therapy is to lower body tension and change faulty biological patterns to reduce symptoms. Many people can and do reach goals of relaxation without the use of biofeedback. Although biofeedback may not be necessary, it can potentially add something useful to any treatment.

A major reason why many patients like biofeedback training is that, like behavioral approaches in general, it puts the patient in charge, giving him or her a sense of mastery and self-reliance over the illnesses. It is believed that such an attitude can play a critical role in shortening recovery time, reducing incidence, and lowering health care costs.

Research Considerations

Biofeedback-assisted relaxation training has been shown to be associated with a decrease in medical care costs, a decrease in the number of claims and costs to insurers in claims payments, reductions of medication and physician use, reduction in hospital stays and rehospitalization, reduction of mortality and morbidity, and enhanced quality of life (Basmajian, 1989).

Efforts are being made to further increase the cost-effectiveness of biofeedback therapy through the use of group instruction, reduced therapist contact, and home-based training. No studies have yet been conducted that discuss cost/benefit ratios for non-relaxation-based biofeedback therapies, such as neuromuscular education and seizure reduction training.

Research on exactly how biofeedback works is inconclusive. Some studies link its benefits directly to physiological changes that the patient learns to make voluntarily. Other experiments find benefits even for patients who do not make the desired changes in the physiological measures. Biofeedback may help some patients increase their sense of control, heighten their optimism, and lessen feelings of hopelessness triggered by chronic health problems (Hatch et al., 1987). However, the proper question is not whether the therapy works or even how it works, but if some form of biofeedback as adjunct therapy would add something useful to an already existing therapy.

IMAGERY

Since human societies began analyzing human experiences, philosophers have tried to define and explain the interior processes of the mind—all of those experiences that are invisible to another person because they do not have physical referents. Philosophers have speculated at length on the nature of mental imagery, and scientists have found the phenomenon difficult to verify or measure. Behavioral psychologists of the 1920s went so far as to say that mental images simply did not exist.

Since 1960 psychologists have done a great deal of work exploring and categorizing mental imagery and inner processes. Contemporary psychologists distinguish several types of imagery. Probably the most common kind of imagery that people experience is memory. If a person tries to remember a friend, the bed in his or her room, or what the seats of his or her car feel like, that person immediately perceives an image in his or her mind, the *mind's eye*. People refer to this experience as forming a mental picture. Some people feel that they do not "see" the scene but that they simply have a strong sense of the scene and "know" what it looks like.

Imagery is both a mental process and a wide variety of procedures used in therapy to encourage changes in attitudes, behaviors, or physiological reactions. As a mental process, it is often defined as "any thought representing a sensory quality" (Horowitz, 1983). In addition to the visual, it includes all the senses—aural, tactile, olfactory, proprioceptive, and kinesthetic. *Imagery* is often used synonymously with *visualization*. However, the latter refers only to "seeing" something in the "mind's eye," whereas imagery can use one sense or combination of senses to produce an image.

Creating images with the mind is also a way of communicating with the deeper-than-conscious aspects of the mind. This is obvious when considering the dream state, which communicates mainly in images, which are then interpreted to make a story. This communicative quality of imagery is very important because feelings and behaviors are primarily motivated by subconscious and unconscious aspects of ourselves.

Imagery can be taught either individually or in groups, and the therapist often uses it to affect a particular result, such as quitting any addictive behavior or bolstering the immune system to attack cancer cells. Because it often involves directed concentration, it can also be thought of as a form of guided meditation.

Many practices discussed in this chapter use a component of imagery. Psychotherapy, hypnosis, and biofeedback all use various elements of this process. Virtually any therapy that relies on the imagination to stimulate, communicate, solve problems, or evoke a heightened awareness or sensitivity could be described as a form of imagery.

Numerous studies indicate that mental imagery can bring about significant physiological and biochemical changes. These findings, which have encouraged the development of imagery as a health care tool, have found it to have the capacity to dramatically affect the following: oxygen supply in tissues (Olness & Conroy, 1988), cardiovascular changes (Barber, 1969), vascular or thermal changes (Green & Green, 1977), the pupil and cochlear reflex (Luria, 1968), heart rate and galvanic skin response (Jordan & Lenington, 1979), and salivation (Barber et al., 1984; White, 1978).

Clinical Applications

Communication with the unconscious has previously been the domain of hypnosis, which basically consists of two components: first, the use of a technique to induce a state of consciousness where there is a freer access to the deeper part of the mind, and second, a method of communicating with that deeper part of the mind. Often this communication will involve making suggestions to the inner depths of the mind, suggesting items or behaviors that the individual desires for his or her betterment. Several different techniques are used to induce the necessary state of consciousness, some of them quite similar to more commonly known relaxation techniques and to meditation techniques (Jordan & Lenington, 1979).

Self-directed imagery. More and more attention is currently being paid to the ability of individuals to use these principles for their own healing purposes. Through the practice of effective deep relaxation techniques, individuals can bring themselves to a state of consciousness where they have increased access to deeper parts of their minds. Then, using imagery, they can "reprogram" new healthy images (Achterberg, 1985).

Self-directed imagery is another powerful way in which individuals can have more control over their own healing processes. Imagery can be used to contribute to the healing of physical problems and has been used extensively in the area of pain control. In one method the individual allows an image for his or her pain to emerge. For example, an individual may come up with an image that characterizes the area of pain and then creates a second image to counteract the pain image. Once the images are formed, the individual would then use a relaxation or meditation technique to open access to the levels where his or her self-healing power resides and imagine the healing image. This process could be repeated as often as necessary, allowing changes in the healing image that might either spontaneously appear or be appropriate if the image associated with the pain were to change.

Self-directed imagery can also be used to stimulate personal growth and change by repeatedly entering a relaxed or meditative state and strongly imaging a new desired behavior. Similarly, by repeatedly imaging oneself as having already achieved a desired goal, the deeper mind gradually accepts this new image and works to bring it into reality.

Carl O. Simonton, MD, and his wife Stephanie brought the use of meditation and imagery for cancer self-help to popular attention. They emphasized several aspects characteristic of a powerful healing image: (1) that the image be created by the healee himself or herself, that it involve as many sense modalities as possible, and (2) that it have as much dynamism and energy behind it as possible. The image must be vital because that vitality is what stimulates the image to take root (Simonton et al., 1978).

Recent studies suggest a direct impact between imagery and its corresponding effects on the body. These findings include the following.

1. Correlations between various types of leukocytes and components of cancer patients' images of their disease, treatment, and immune system (Achterberg & Lawlis, 1984)
2. Enhanced natural killer cell function after a relaxation and imagery training procedure with geriatric patients (Kiecolt-Glaser et al., 1985) and in adult cancer patients with metastatic disease (Gruber et al., 1988)
3. Specificity of imagery training was suggested by a study on training patients in cell-specific imagery of either T lymphocytes or neutrophils

The effects of training, which were assessed after 6 weeks, were statistically associated with the type of imagery procedure used (Achterberg et al., 1989).

MENTAL HEALING

The idea that consciousness can affect the physical body has a time-honored and respected historical base. The observation that "there is a measure of consciousness throughout the body" is scattered about the 2000-year-old Hippocratic writings. The ancient Persians expounded on this concept considerably. They insisted that a person's mind can intervene not just in his or her own body but also in that of another individual located far away. It was later postulated by the great Muslim physician Abu Ali ibn Sina (Avicenna in Latinized form, AD 980-1037) that it was the faculty of imagination that man uses to make himself ill or restores health.

The attitudes of the ancient Greeks and Persians toward the interaction between minds and bodies gave rise to two very different types of healing: local and nonlocal. The Greeks believed that the action of the mind on the body was a local event in the here and now. The Persians, however, viewed the mind-body relationship as nonlocal. They held that the mind was not localized or confined to the body but extended beyond the body. This implied that the mind was capable of affecting any physical body, local or nonlocal.

Implications of Nonlocality

Modern physicists have long recognized the concept of nonlocality. These developments rest largely on an idea in physics called Bell's theorem, introduced in 1964 by the Irish physicist John Stewart Bell, and subsequent experiments. Bell showed that if distant objects have once been in contact, a change thereafter in one causes an immediate change in the other, even if they are separated to the opposite ends of the universe. Thus it is important to realize that nonlocality is not just a theoretical idea in physics, but its proof rests on actual experiments.

The idea prevalent in contemporary science is that the mind and consciousness are entirely local phenomenon, localized to the brain/body and confined to the present moment. From this perspective nonlocal healing cannot occur in principle because the mind is bound by the "here and now." Research studies conducted in distant mental influence challenge these modern-day assumptions. Dozens of experiments, specifically conducted over the past 20 years, suggest that the mind can bring about changes in nonlocal physical bodies, even when shielded from all sensory and electromagnetic influences. This suggests that mind and consciousness may not be located at fixed points in space (Braud, 1992; Braud & Schlitz, 1991; Jahn & Dunne, 1987).

Some physicists believe that nonlocality applies not just to the domain of electrons and other subatomic particles but also to our familiar world consisting of dense matter. A growing number of physicists think that nonlocality may apply to the mind. Physicist Nick Herbert, in his book *Quantum Reality*, states "Bell's theorem requires our quantum knowledge to be non-local, instantly linked to everything it has previously touched" (Herbert, 1987).

For the Western model of medicine, the implications of a nonlocal concept are profound. Among them are the following:

1. Nonlocal models of the mind could be helpful in understanding the actual dynamics of the healing process. They may help to understand why in some instances a cure suddenly appears unexpectedly or when a healing appears to be influenced by events occurring nonlocally.

2. Nonlocal manifestations of consciousness may complicate traditional experimental designs and require innovative research methods because they suggest that the mental state of the healer may influence the experiment's outcome, even under "blind" conditions (Solfvin, 1984).

These assumptions give rise to the idea that consciousness could prevail after the death of the body/brain, suggesting that there is some aspect of the psyche that is not bound to points in space or time. This idea in turn leads toward a nonlocal model of consciousness, which allows for the possibility of distant healing exchange.

This nonlocal model of consciousness implies that at some level of the psyche there are no fundamental separations between individual minds. Nobel physicist Erwin Schroedinger suggested that at some level and in some sense there may be unity and oneness of all minds (Schroedinger, 1969). In the nonlocal model distance is not fundamental but is completely overcome. In other words, because of the unification of consciousness, the healer and the patient are not separated by physical distance.

For 30 years psychologist Lawrence LeShan investigated the local and nonlocal effects of prayer and healing. He taught these techniques to more than 400 people and ultimately became a healer himself. He maintained that healing changes were observed to have taken place 15 to 20 percent of the time but never could be predicted in advance of any specific healing (LeShan, 1966).

LeShan found that mental-spiritual healing methods are of two main types:

Type I (nonlocal): The healer enters a prayerful, altered state of consciousness in which he or she views himself or herself and the patient as a single entity. There is no physical contact or any attempt to offer anything of a physical nature to the person in need, only the desire to connect and unite. These healers emphasize the importance of empathy, love, and caring in this process. When the healing takes place, it does so in the context of unity, compassion, and love. This type of healing is considered a natural process and merely speeds up the normal healing processes.

Type II (local): The healer does touch the patient and may imagine some "flow of energy" through his or her hands to the patient's area receiving the healing. Feelings of heat are common in both the healer and patient. In this mode, unlike type I, the healer holds the intention for healing.

Research about the origins of consciousness and how it relates to the physical brain are practically nonexistent. Although hypotheses purporting to explain consciousness do exist, there is no agreement among researchers as to its nature, local or nonlocal.

SPIRITUALITY AND HEALING

Throughout the ages, ancient mystical traditions have valued the spiritual qualities of humans over the physical, emphasizing the transcendence of one over the other. In the background of most mystical traditions is the idea that the body is somehow at odds with the spirit. A war wages, and one must battle the war to achieve an enlightened status. Still other theologians postulate that the greatest spiritual achievement of all may lie in the realization that the spiritual and the physical are but one and that perhaps the ultimate spiritual goal is to transcend nothing but to realize the integration and oneness of our being.

A new quality of spiritual awakening has been emerging worldwide over the past 25 years. This innovative approach encourages people to develop faith in their own capacity to create their own reality in partnership with the God-force within. In many cultures, both Eastern and Western, prayer-based spiritual healing is an integral part of modern religious practices.

The premise of creating our own reality is, in essence, a spiritual one. This concept is sometimes contrary to many fundamental religious positions that embrace God as an external being because spirituality emphasizes a "God-within" reality. Transcending the boundaries and limitations of specific religions, a spiritual practice honors the relationship between the individual and the God-force as a partnership.

When people consider the possibility that they create their own realities, the question that invariably arises is "Through what source? What is the source of this power of creation that runs through my being?" The answer to this question is not found externally, but internally. This internal seeking to understand our own nature is the study of divinity in action, incarnated into each person.

The blending of spirituality with the tenets of alternative and complementary therapies provides individuals with a means of understanding how they contribute to the creation of their illness and to their healing. This consideration is not made from a place of self-blame and not as the result of the will of God but rather as a result of attempting to understand a spiritual purpose for suffering in a physical body. The relationship that is cultivated ultimately transcends the human value system of punishment versus reward and grows into a relationship based on principles of cocreation and coresponsibility. Therefore the journey of healing, as well as the journey of life, is thereby freed of the burden of feeling victimized by fate, circumstances, or God, free to have faith and hope not only in God but in themselves as well.

Power of Prayer

The use of prayer in healing may have begun in human prehistory and continues to this day as an underlying tenet in almost all religions. The records of many of the great religious traditions, including the mystical traditions of Christianity, Taoism, Hinduism, Buddhism, and Islam, give the very strong impression that enlightenment comes when one begins to explore the dynamic qualities of interrelation and interconnection between the self and the source of all beings.

The word *prayer* comes from the Latin *precarious,* "obtained by begging," and *precari,* "to entreat"—to ask earnestly, beseech, implore. This suggests two of the most common forms of prayer—petition, asking something for one's self, and intercession, asking something for others.

Prayer is a genuinely nonlocal event, not confined to a specific place in space or to a specific moment in time. Prayer reaches outside the here and now; it operates at a distance and outside the present moment. Because prayer is initiated by a mental action, this implies that there is some aspect of our psyche that also is genuinely nonlocal. Nonlocality implies infinitude in space and time because a limited nonlocality is a contradiction in terms. In the West this infinite aspect of the psyche has been referred to as the *soul.* Empirical evidence for the power of prayer, then, may be seen as indirect evidence for the soul.

Scientific attempts to assess the effects of prayer and spiritual practices on health began in the nineteenth century with Sir Francis Galton's treatise "Statistical Inquiries into the Efficacy of Prayer" (Galton, 1872). Galton assessed the longevity of people frequently prayed for, such as clergy, monarchs, and heads of state. He concluded that there was no demonstrable effect of prayer on longevity. By current scientific standards, Galton's study was flawed. He was, however, successful in promoting the idea that prayer is subject to empirical scrutiny. Galton did acknowledge that praying could make a person feel better. In the end he maintained that although his attempts to prove the efficacy of prayer had failed, he could see no good reason to abandon prayer.

Those who practice healing with prayer claim uniformly that the effects are not diminished with distance; therefore it falls within the nonlocal perspective discussed in this chapter under Mental Healing. Claims about the effectiveness of prayer do not rely on anecdote or single case studies; numerous controlled studies have validated the nonlocal nature of prayer. Moreover, much of this evidence suggests that praying individuals—or people involved in compassionate imagery or mental intent, whether or not it is called *prayer,* can purposefully affect the physiology of distant people without the "receiver's" awareness.

Anecdotal accounts of the power of prayer are legendary, and countless books on these subjects are available; however, most literature contains little of scientific value. Although the validated evidence continues to build concerning the efficacy of prayer, Larry Dossey, MD, maintains that some serious questions arise in the wake of these experiments (Dossey, 1993). The evidence clearly shows that mental activity can be used to influence people nonlocally, at a distance, without their knowledge. Scores of experiments on prayer also show that it can be used to great effect without the subjects' awareness. The question then is whether it is ethical to use these techniques if recipients are unaware that they are being used. This question becomes even more compelling as we consider the possibility that prayer, or any other form of mind-to-mind communication, may be used at a distance to harm people without their knowledge. Institutional review committees, whose job it is to oversee the design of experiments involving humans and to ensure their safety, have rarely had to consider these types of ethical questions.

References

Achterberg J. 1985. Imagery in Healing: Shamanism and Modern Medicine. Shambhala, Boston.

Achterberg J, Lawlis GF. 1984. Imagery and Disease: Diagnostic Tools. Institute for Personality and Ability Testing, Champaign, Illinois.

Achterberg J, Lawlis GF, Rider MS. 1989. The effects of music-mediated imagery on neutrophils and lymphocytes. Biofeedback Self-Regulation 114:247-257.

Ader R, Cohen N. 1991. Psychoneuroimmunology. 2nd ed. Academic Press, San Diego.

Barber TX. 1969. A Scientific Approach. Van Nostrand, New York.

Barber TX. 1984. Changing 'unchangeable' bodily processes by hypnotic suggestions: a new look at hypnosis, imaging and the mind/body problem. Advances 1(2):7-40.

Barber TX, Chauncey HM, Winer RA. 1964. The effect of hypnotic and nonhypnotic suggestion on parotid gland response to gustatory stimuli. Psychosom Med 26:374-380.

Basmajian JV. (ed). 1989 Biofeedback: Principles and Practice for Clinicians. Williams & Wilkins, Baltimore.

Beecher HK. 1955. The powerful placebo. Journal of American Medical Association 159:1602-1606.

Benson H. 1975. The Relaxation Response. Morrow, New York.

Benson H, Kotch JB, Crassweller KD. 1977. Relaxation response: bridge between psychiatry and medicine. Med Clin North Am 61:929-938.

Benson HR. 1993. The Relaxation Response. Mind & Body Medicine. Goleman and Gurin (eds). Consumer Reports Books, New York.

Bohm D. 1983. Wholeness and Implicate Order. Rutledge, London.

Braud WG. 1992. Human interconnectedness: research indications. ReVision 14:140-148.

Braud WG, Schlitz M. 1991. Consciousness interactions with remote biological systems: anomalous intentionality effects. Subtle Energies 2.

Brooks JS, Scarano T. 1985. Transcendental meditation in the treatment of post-Vietnam adjustment. Journal of Counseling and Development 65:212-215.

Caudill M, et al. 1991. Decreased clinic use by chronic pain patients: response to behavioral medicine intervention. Journal of Chronic Pain 7:305-310.

Cooper M, Aygen M. 1978. Effects of meditation on blood cholesterol and blood pressure. Journal of the Israel Medical Association 95:1-2.

Cummings NA, Bragman JI. 1988. Triaging the "somatizer" out of the medical system into psychological system. In Stern and Stern (eds). Psychotherapy and the Somatizing Patient. Hayward Press, New York.

Debenedittis C, Panerai AA, Villamira MA. 1989. Effect of hypnotic analgesia and hypnotizability on experimental ischemic pain. Int J Clin Experimental Hypnosis 37:55-69.

Dossey L. 1993. Healing Words: The Power of Prayer and the Practice of Medicine. Harper, San Francisco.

Fielding JWL, et al. 1983. An interim report of a prospective, randomized, controlled study of adjuvant chemotherapy in operable gastric cancer: British stomach cancer group. World Journal of Surgery 7:390–399.

Fulop G, Strain JJ, Vita J, et al. 1987. Impact of psychiatric comorbidity on length of stay for medical/surgical patients: a preliminary report. Am J Psychiatry 144:878-882.

Galton F. 1872. Statistical inquiries into the efficacy of prayer. Fortnightly Review 12:11225.

Goodwin JS, Hunt WC, et al. 1987. The effect of marital status on stage, treatment and survival of cancer patients. Journal of American Medical Association 258:3125-3130.

Green E, Green A. 1977. Beyond Biofeedback. Delta, New York.

Gruber BL, Hall NR, Hersh SP, Dubois P. 1988. Immune system and psychological changes in metastatic cancer patients using relaxation and guided imagery: a pilot study. Scandinavian Journal of Behavior Therapy 17:25-46.

Hatch JP, Fisher JG, Rugh JD. 1987. Biofeedback: Studies in Clinical Efficacy. Plenum, New York.

Herbert N. 1987. Quantum Reality. Anchor/Doubleday, Garden City, New York.

Holmes TH, Rahe RH. 1967. The Social Readjustment Rating Scale. Journal of Psychosomatic Research 11:213-218.

Horowitz M. 1983. Image Formation. Jason Aronson, Inc., New York.

House J, Landis KR, Umberson D. 1988. Social relationships and health. Science 241:540–545.

Jahn RG, Dunn BJ. 1987. Precognitive remote perception. In Margins of Reality: The Role of Consciousness in the Physical World. Harcourt Brace, New York, pp. 149–191.

Jordan CS, Lenington KT. 1979. Psychological correlates of eidetic imagery and induced anxiety. Journal of Mental Imagery 3:31-42.

Kabat-Zinn J. 1993a. Meditation in Healing and the Mind. Flowers BS, Grubin D, Meryman-Bruner E (eds). Bantam Doubleday, New York.

Kabat-Zinn J. 1993b. Mindfulness Meditation in Mind Body Medicine. Goleman D, and Gurin J (eds). Consumer Reports Books, New York.

Kabat-Zinn J. 1993c. Wherever You Go, There You Are: Mindfulness Meditation In Everyday Life. Hyperion, New York.

Kabat-Zinn J, Lipworth L, et al. 1986. Four-year follow-up of a meditation-based program for the self-regulation of chronic pain. Journal of Behavioral Medicine 8: 163-190.

Katz R. 1977. Informed consent—Is it bad medicine? The Western Journal of Medicine 126:426-428.

Kiecolt-Glaser JK, Glaser R, Williger D, et al. 1985. Psychosocial enhancement of immunocompetence in a geriatric population. Health Psychology 4:25-41.

LeShan L. 1966. The Medium, the Mystic, and the Physicist. Viking, New York.

Levine JD, Gordon NC, Fields HL. 1978. The mechanism of placebo analgesia. Lancet 2:654-657.

Locke S, Hornig-Rohan M. 1983. Mind and Immunity: Behavioral Immunology. Institute for the Advancement of Health, New York.

Luria AR. 1968. The Mind of a Mnemonist. Basic Books, New York.

MacLean CRK, Walton KG, et al. 1992. Altered cortisol response to stress after four months' practice of the transcendental meditation program. Presented at the 18th Annual Meeting of the Society for Neuroscience, Anaheim, California, October 30, 1992.

Mason AA, Black S. 1958. Allergic skin responses abolished under treatment of asthma and hay fever by hypnosis. Lancet 1:877-880.

Morris, D. 1995. The Human Zoo. Oxford University Press, Oxford.

Olness K, Gardner GG. 1988. Hypnosis and Hypnotherapy with Children. (2nd ed.) W.B. Saunders, Orlando.

Ornish D. 1990. Can lifestyle changes reverse coronary artery disease? Lancet 336:129.

Osler W. 1953. Aequanimitas. 3rd ed. Blakiston Company, New York.

Pearce JC. 1992. The Magical Child. Penguin, New York.

Sacks M. 1993. Exercise for Stress Control. In Mind & Body Medicine. In Goleman and Gurin (eds). Consumer Reports Books, New York.

Schlesinger HJ, Mumford E, Glass GV. 1983. Mental health treatment and medical care utilization . . . following onset of a chronic disease. American Journal of Public Health 73:422-429.

Schneider RH, Alexander CN, et al. 1992. In search of an optimal behavioral treatment for hypertension: a review and focus on transcendental meditation. In Johnson EH (ed). Hypertension. Hemisphere, Washington, D.C.

Schroedinger E. 1969. What is Life? And Mind and Matter. Cambridge University Press: London.

Selye H. 1978. The Stress of Life. McGraw-Hill, New York.

Sharma HM. Triguna BD, Chopra D. 1991. Maharishi Ayur-Veda: modern insights into ancient meditation. Journal of American Medical Association 265: 2633-2634, 2637.

Simonton OC, Simonton S, Creighton J. 1978. Getting Well Again. Tarcher, Los Angeles.

Solfvin J. 1984. Mental Healing. In Krippner S. (ed.) Advances in Parapsychological Research. Vol. 4. McFarland and Company, Jefferson, North Carolina.

Spiegel D, et al. 1989. Effect of psychosocial treatment on survival of patients with metastatic breast cancer. Lancet 2 (8668):888-891.

Strain JJ. 1993. Psychotherapy and medical conditions. In Goleman D, and Gurin J (eds). Mind/Body Medicine. Consumer Reports Books, New York.

White KD. 1978. Salivation: the significance of imagery in its voluntary control. Psychophysiology 15(3):196-203.

Suggested Readings

Barber TX. 1978. Hypnosis, suggestion and psychosomatic phenomena. American Journal Clinical Hypnosis 21: 12-27.

Gentry WD, Julius S (eds). Personality, Elevated Blood Pressure and Essential Hypertension.

Goleman DJ. 1977. The varieties of the meditative experience. Irvington Association 258:3125-3130.

Moyers B. 1993. Healing and the Mind. In Flowers BS, Grubin D, Meryman-Brunner E (eds). Bantam Doubleday, New York.

Schneider CJ. 1987. Cost-effectiveness of biofeedback and behavioral medicine treatment: a review of the literature. Biofeedback Self Regulation 12(2):71-92.

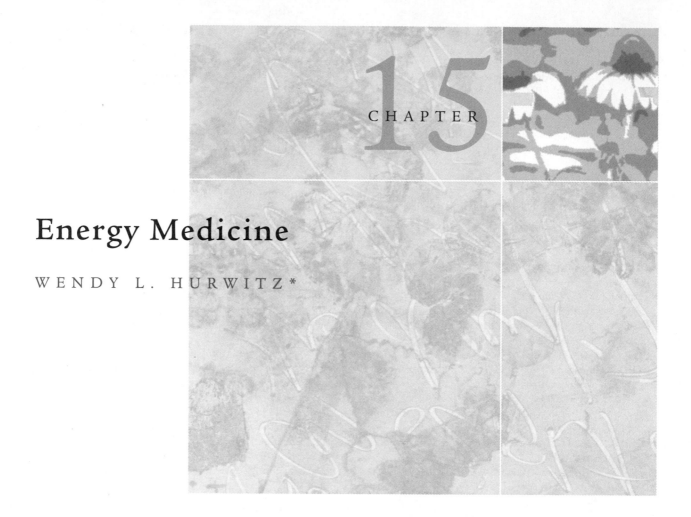

Energy Medicine

WENDY L. HURWITZ*

Energy medicine is based on the belief that in addition to a system of physical and biochemical processes, the human being is made up of a complex system of energy. This energy, denoted by different words in different cultures, is defined in China as *chi* or *Qi* (pronounced "chee"), in India as *prana* (pronounced "prah-nah"), and in Japan as *ki* (pronounced "kee") (Table 15-1). In English *Qi* defies exact description but is most commonly defined as vital life force. In his book, *Encounters with Qi,* Dr. David Eisenberg, Director of the Center for Alternative Medicine Research at Harvard Medical School, refers to energy as "that which differentiates life from death, animate from inanimate. To live is to have Qi in every part of your body. To die is to be a body without Qi" (Eisenberg & Wright, 1987).

Energy permeates and flows through all living things, continually circulating within and throughout the body in a proscribed pattern, just as blood flows through the body. Unlike blood, however, energy does not stop at the surface of the skin but extends beyond the body, thereby creating an individual's energy field (NIH, 1994). When energy flows freely and in a balanced manner, the body can maintain good health. When the normal flow of energy is disrupted, or becomes blocked, stagnated, or weakened, an energetic imbalance occurs. This energetic imbalance, which presents as an excess or deficit of energy, predisposes the body to disease.

Scientists have yet to characterize energy or vital life force. Hypotheses about what constitutes ener-

---

*Chapter copyright owned by Wendy Hurwitz, MD.

238

TABLE 15-1

Cultural Terms to Denote Energy

Term	Source
Ankh	Ancient Egypt
Arunquiltha	Australian aborigine
Bioenergy	United States, United Kingdom
Biomagnetism	United States, United Kingdom
Gana	South America
Ki	Japan
Life force	General usage
Mana	Polynesia
Manitou	Algonquia
M'gbe	Hiru pygmy
Mulungu	Ghana
Mumia	Paracelsus
Ntoro	Ashanti
Ntu	Bantu
Oki	Huron
Orenda	Iroquois
Pneuma	Ancient Greece
Prana	India
Qi (chi)	China
Ruach	Ancient Hebrew
Sila	Inuit
Subtle energy	United States, United Kingdom
Tane	Hawaii
T(ix)	Mayan
Ton	Dakota
Wakan	Lakota

Adapted from National Institutes of Health. 1994. Alternative Medicine: Expanding Medical Horizons—A Report to the National Institutes of Health on Alternative Medical Systems and Practices in the United States. US Government Printing Office, Washington, DC.

getic matter include explanations from electromagnetic theory, quantum physics, and subatomic "subtle" energy. While some debate exists regarding the underlying reasoning, theorists generally agree that:

Matter is no longer considered inert. The basic components of matter are particles that are constantly emitting and absorbing energy, changing position, yet at the same time maintaining equilibrium. There is an underlying dynamism associated with material objects, although it may not always be visible to the naked eye. At the basis of life are subatomic particles, continually in motion and continually emitting or taking in energy. Living beings, by virtue of their molecular makeup, participate in this energy (Wager, 1996).

ENERGY ANATOMY

The pattern of the flow of energy through an individual's energy field has an anatomy that includes chakras, meridians, and etheric levels.

Chakras

The term *chakra* (pronounced "shah-krah") is derived from the Sanskrit word for "wheel." Sometimes referred to as "wheels of energy" or energy centers, chakras function as power plants for the body that input energy from the environment and output energy to the environment. Chakras supply energy to different regions of the body, their organs, neural ganglia, and endocrine glands. There are seven major chakras: crown, brow, throat, heart, solar plexus, sacral, and coccygeal (Figure 15-1). In addition, there are multiple minor chakras located throughout the body.

Meridians

Meridians are pathways of energetic flow that are distributed symmetrically throughout the body, similar to the body's organization of blood flow. Meridians create a network which conducts the flow of energy through the body, extending externally to the skin and sensory organs and internally to the viscera and major organs. There are 12 major meridians corresponding to the following organs: lungs, heart, pericardium, liver, spleen, kidney, bladder, stomach, gallbladder, large intestine, small intestine, and "triple warmer." There are eight collateral meridians (also known as "extra" meridians) and multiple minor meridians. Acupuncture points are found along these pathways (Figure 15-2).

Etheric Levels

As one moves farther away from the skin's surface, the human energy field is divided into layers. Each of these layers is three-dimensional and envelops the body like a sheath or shell. Four to seven layers have been described (Brennan, 1988; Kunz, 1995). The three layers closest to the physical body are the physical, emotional, and mental layers (Figure 15-3).

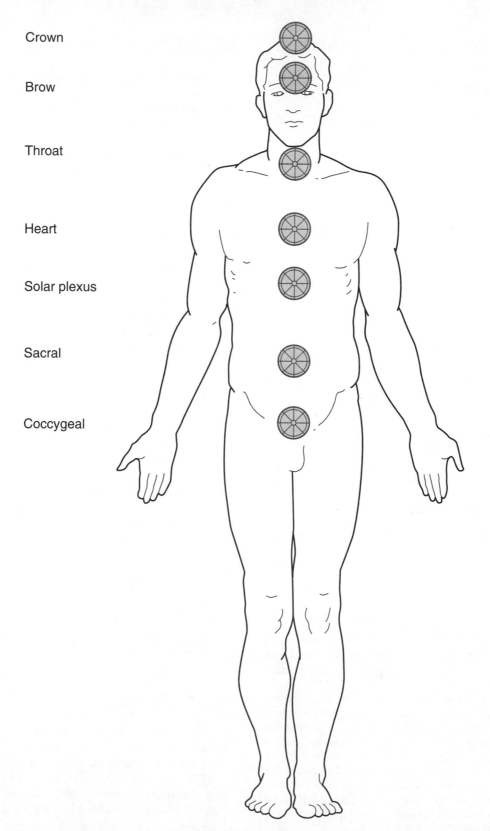

Crown

Brow

Throat

Heart

Solar plexus

Sacral

Coccygeal

Figure 15-1 The major chakras. (Adapted from Brennan BA. 1988. Hands of Light: A Guide to Healing Through the Human Energy Field. Bantam Books, New York.)

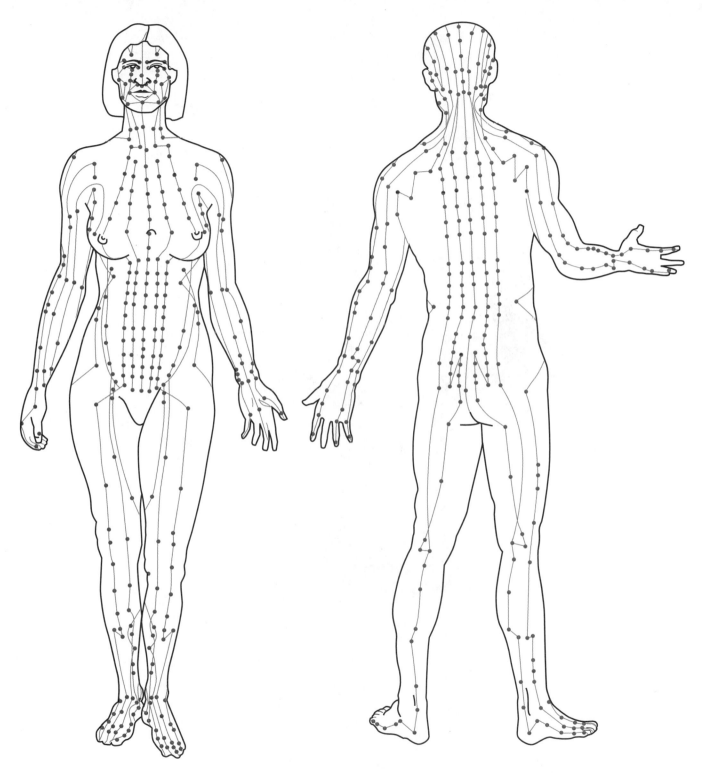

Figure 15-2 The major meridians. **A,** Anterior view. **B,** Posterior view. (From Beinfield H, Korngold E. 1991. *Between Heaven and Earth: A Guide to Chinese Medicine.* Random House, New York.)

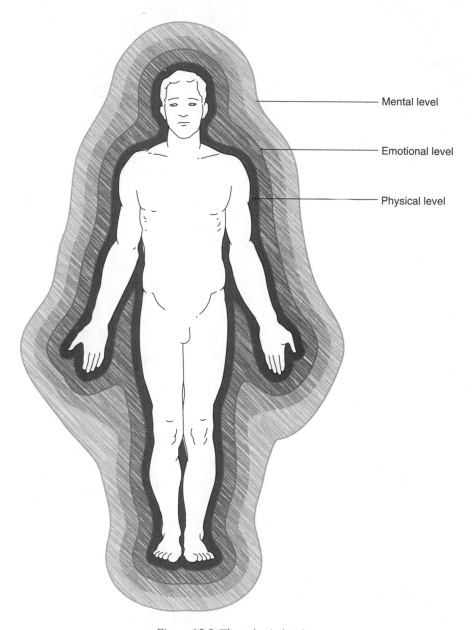

Mental level

Emotional level

Physical level

Figure 15-3 The etheric levels.

The Physical Level

Also known as the physical field, vital field, etheric level, or etheric body, this layer contains the energy most closely associated with physical sensation, the body's vitality, and the autonomic functioning of cells, tissues, and organs. Energy from this layer is closest to the surface of the skin.

The Emotional Level

Also known as the emotional field or emotional body, this layer contains the energy associated with feelings from positive emotions such as happiness and affection or from negative emotions such as anxiety and despair. Energy from this layer surrounds and interpenetrates energy from the physical level. Because emotional and physical energies are interconnected, emotions can have a profound effect on how the body functions.

The Mental Level

Also known as the mental field or mental body, this layer contains the energy associated with thought, conceptualization, rationalization, and interpretation of events. Energy from this layer surrounds and interfaces with the emotional level, intensifying the relationship between thoughts and feelings.

THE ROLE OF ENERGY

The role of energy is to perform two vital functions:

1. In proper balance, energy improves vitality and nourishes the body's cells, rendering them robust and healthy.
2. Energy provides the template upon which the pattern of cellular regeneration is based.

All cells regenerate over time. But how do they know in what form or pattern to regenerate? An individual's energy field acts as a "blueprint," helping to direct the pattern in which cells are "laid down."

When energy flows freely through and about the body in a balanced symmetrical manner, good health can be maintained. When energy flow becomes restricted, disordered, imbalanced, or asymmetrical, ill health can follow. In the short term, an imbalance in the energy field can decrease one's vitality, limit one's resilience, and impair the functioning of cells, tissues, and organs. In the long term, an energetic imbalance may damage one's blueprint, disrupting the body's pattern of cellular regeneration, predisposing the individual to chronic pain, chronic disease, and illness such as cancer.

DISRUPTIONS TO ENERGY FLOW

When the free flow of energy through and about the body is disrupted, the result is a compromised energy field which leads to compromised health. Disruptions to energy flow can be caused by physical trauma, stored emotions, habitual patterns of negative emotion, or habitual patterns of negative thought.

Physical Trauma

When individuals sustain a wound, such as a laceration (including surgical incision or excision), bruise, fracture, or burn, they not only injure their physical cells but also damage their energy fields. Repairing this field through energetic intervention has been found to accelerate healing and reduce a patient's predisposition to chronic pain or atrophy.

Stored Emotions

Unexpressed or buried feelings, and emotions from unaddressed issues, unresolved conflicts, or emotional traumas become stored in the body in pockets called *energy cysts*. These cysts impede the free flow of energy to vital organs or regions of the body, impairing the body's ability to heal and predisposing one to chronic illness. Expressing stored emotions, addressing relevant issues, and resolving underlying conflicts can improve or restore energy flow. Energetic intervention has been found to facilitate the expression of emotions, the addressing of issues, and the resolution of conflicts.

Habitual Patterns of Negative Emotion

Habitual patterns of negative emotion (e.g., fear, anxiety, anger, resentment, depression, and guilt) restrict the amount of energy available to nourish cells, tissues, and organs, decreasing vitality and disrupting autonomic functioning. In contrast, habitual positive emotions (e.g., happiness, joy, hope, appreciation, affection, and contentment) can enhance energy flow. Energetic intervention has been found to facilitate the expression and release of negative emotions, support the shift toward positive emotions, and induce a sense of peace and well-being.

Habitual Patterns of Negative Thought

Repetitive patterns of negative thought, negative attitudes, self-defeating beliefs, and stress can disrupt the free flow of energy to vital regions of the body, lowering resilience and predisposing one to chronic disease. Resolution of negative thought patterns and replacement with realistic beliefs can enhance and restore energy flow. Energetic intervention has been found to reduce stress, improve perspective and mental clarity, facilitate the integration of positive thought, and induce relaxation.

HISTORY

The act of healing by using the hands to direct energy has been evident throughout recorded history. From the earliest cultures, hieroglyphics, cuneiform writings, and pictographs contain evidence of the use of hands to facilitate healing. Cave paintings in the Pyrenees, estimated to date as far back as 15,000 years ago, depict the laying on of hands to help the sick, as do rock carvings from Ancient Egypt, Third Dynasty (2700 BC). Writings from the Ebers Papyrus (Egypt, 1552 BC) reveal therapeutic use of the hands to heal the infirm. Aristophanes in Ancient Greece (450-385 BC) wrote of energy healing, and manuscripts of ancient Greeks (400 BC) detail the use of the laying on of hands in Aesculapian temples to alleviate illness. Hippocrates (Greece, 460-377 BC) referred to energy as "the force which flows from many people's hands" (NIH, 1994). His writings relate:

It has often appeared while I have been soothing my patients, that there was a singular property in my hand to pull and draw away from the affected parts, aches and impurities by laying my hands upon the place and by extending my fingers toward it.

—HIPPOCRATES (MacManaway and Turcan, 1983)

The earliest Eastern reference, *The Yellow Emperor of Internal Medicine* (Huang Ti Nei Ching Su Wen), dated 2500 to 5000 years ago, and Tibetan sutras (holy writings), dated 2500 years ago, make reference to the therapeutic use of hands to heal. For many centuries historical records from China and India contain energetic healing practices including external chi-gong and pranic healing, traditions passed from Master to student. In the Western Hemisphere earliest reports of Native Americans contain evidence of the use of hands to "cast out infirmity."

Judeo-Christian writings reveal many references to the laying on of hands. In early Christian history healing was considered as much a part of the ministry as was preaching or administering the sacraments. Roman emperors Vespasian (69-79 AD) and Hadrian (117-138 AD) and monarchs such as King Olaf II of Norway (995-1030 AD) and King Philip I of France (1052-1108 AD) were reported to minister to the sick by energetic healing; hence, the laying on of hands came to be known as the "King's Touch" or "Royal Touch." Such healings were based on the belief in the power of God and the King as a designated healer who had special dispensation from God. Later, scholars, including Paracelsus (Germany, fifteenth century), theorized that the act of healing from laying on of hands did not result from connection to a higher source of power but instead emanated from the magnetic nature of energies. In the late 1700s Franz Mesmer (France, 1778) claimed that remarkable therapeutic success in energetic healing was possible without the need of the patient's faith in God or in the healer himself. Mesmer theorized that a subtle life-energy of a magnetic nature was exchanged between healer and patient during the laying on of hands, with the palms as the most active points of energetic flow.

Touching with the intent to heal was used in Europe until the 1600s when, with the rise of the Puritan culture, touch became equated with sex and sin. The strong puritanical ethic in Europe and America discouraged all "unnecessary" touch, and the rise of Western scientific medicine that followed in the eighteenth and nineteenth centuries replaced energetic practices.

In the mid-1800s the hands-on healing practice of Reiki, based on Tibetan sutras, was developed in Japan by Mikao Usui; it was brought to the United States in the 1930s. Renewed interest in touch as a therapeutic intervention commenced in the 1950s. In the early 1960s Bernard Grad, a Canadian biochemist, together with noted healer Oskar Estebany, began extensive research on the practice of laying on of hands by conducting double-blind studies on wounded mice. Results showed that mice treated with the laying on of hands healed at an accelerated rate compared to controls.

In 1971 and 1973 controlled studies on humans conducted by Dolores Krieger, PhD, RN, Professor of Nursing at New York University, showed that patients' hemoglobin levels significantly improved following treatment with the laying on of hands. Krieger and Dora Kunz, a renowned healer, collaborated in 1972 to develop Therapeutic Touch, a technique based on the laying on of hands with the intent to help or heal, independent of religious or spiritual belief. Other energetic modalities followed. In 1974 Rosalyn Bruyere developed Natural Healing; in 1978 Barbara Ann Brennan created Healing Science, and in the 1980s Janet Mentgen developed Healing Touch utilizing techniques from Krieger and Kunz, Bruyere, Brennan, and others. In 1994 the North American Nursing Diagnosis Association (NANDA) added "Energy Field Disturbance" to its classification of nursing diagnoses.

ENERGY-BASED THERAPIES

Energy-based therapeutic modalities involve the use of the practitioner's hands to repattern the patient's energy field in areas of energetic disruption. Energetic intervention can correct imbalances in energy flow, restore symmetry, and re-establish the free flow of energy. Energy-based therapeutic techniques are predicated on the following assumptions:

1. Energy moves through and around the human body.
2. Every individual is surrounded by an energy field.
3. This energy field is dynamic; it moves and flows.
4. This energy field can be perceived, and the ability to perceive energy is a learnable skill.
5. Disorder or imbalance of one's energy field is associated with disease.
6. Orderly repatterning of one's energy field restores balance, creating an improved environment in which healing can occur.
7. One's energy field exists within a universal energy field.
8. The patient and the practitioner are not separate but are interconnected and integral with the universal energy field.

Therapeutic Touch, Healing Touch, and Reiki are energy-based therapeutic modalities that are to be used in addition to, not in lieu of, traditional medical therapies. Each has been used successfully in hospital, hospice, and outpatient settings. Each technique has been found to:

- Accelerate healing
- Reduce pain
- Alleviate physical symptoms
- Reduce stress and anxiety
- Facilitate expression of stored emotions
- Facilitate the shift from negative to positive emotion
- Facilitate the replacement of negative thought with realistic beliefs
- Induce relaxation
- Induce a sense of peace and well-being

THERAPEUTIC TOUCH

History

Therapeutic Touch is a "consciously directed process of energy exchange during which the practitioner uses the hands as a focus to facilitate healing" (NHPA, 1992). The technique was developed in 1972 by Dolores Krieger, PhD, RN, Professor of Nursing at New York University, and Dora Kunz, a noted healer who worked closely with many physicians and scientists. Observing the art of healing by laying on of hands, Kunz hypothesized that the ability to assist healing was a talent not bestowed to certain special individuals but accessible to everyone, a capacity innate in all human beings, a "natural potential" that one could actualize under the appropriate circumstances. Together, Krieger and Kunz studied healers to determine the factors involved in facilitating patient healing. The result of their work was the development of an energy-based healing modality that could be taught to others. Krieger coined the name "Therapeutic Touch" to differentiate the technique from other types of touch and massage. Krieger did extensive research on Therapeutic Touch, published results in peer-reviewed journals, taught numerous courses to health care professionals, and in 1977 established Nurse Healers-Professional Associates, an organization for Therapeutic Touch practitioners.

Since its development, Therapeutic Touch has continued to be extensively researched, its techniques further refined, and its effects documented. One small uncontrolled study drew conclusions beyond its results and asserted that energy did not exist and that use of Therapeutic Touch was unjustified (Rosa, 1998).

Therapeutic Touch is included in the nursing curricula of many colleges and universities, recognized by the American Nurses Association (ANA, 1998), American Holistic Nurses Association (AHNA, 1998), and the National League for Nursing (NLN, 1998).

Nursing Interventions Classification (NIC) includes Therapeutic Touch as a direct care nursing treatment (McCloskey & Bulechek, 1992). Utilized in hospital, hospice, and outpatient settings, Therapeutic Touch has also been successfully taught to patients and their families for use in the home.

Typical Therapeutic Session

In a typical therapeutic session, the patient is lying down or sitting comfortably, fully clothed but with shoes removed and arms and legs uncrossed, so as not to obstruct the free flow of energy. The practitioner may stand or sit. In treating the patient, the practitioner uses four steps: centering, assessing, decongesting the energy field, and balancing the energy field.

The practitioner always begins a treatment session by centering. This is accomplished by the practitioner's consciously focusing his or her attention inward to release any tensions or distractions; the practitioner is then able to turn his or her full attention to helping the patient, with intent for the patient's highest good. Centering results in an enhanced state of concentration and awareness, free of any physical or mental tension. For this reason, Therapeutic Touch has been described as a "healing meditation." Studies have shown that centering and intent are an integral and significant part of the Therapeutic Touch process; sham procedures, in which hand gesturing was done without centering or intent, show a significant reduction in effectiveness (Quinn, 1984).

Once centered, the practitioner assesses the patient and takes a history, picking up cues from the patient's vocal inflection, posture, and gait. The practitioner then assesses the patient's energy field. Placing his or her hands, palms down, 1 to 6 inches above the skin surface, the practitioner scans the patient, generally beginning at the head and moving downward along the body to the feet. While scanning, the practitioner notes any focal differences in temperature, pressure, pulsation, or sensation, as well as any differences in symmetry.

When the assessment is complete, the practitioner mobilizes any perceived areas of energetic congestion (in which flow is blocked and energy cannot flow freely). He or she then liberates the congested energy by moving the hands in a sweeping or "unruffling" motion down the length of the body, parallel to the skin surface, or outward from the body, perpendicu-

lar to the body surface. Practitioners describe this action as that of pushing a pressure front; sweeping is continued until the sense of pressure or congestion is alleviated. Following this procedure the practitioner often shakes, wipes, or washes his or her hands.

After decongesting the patient's energy field, the practitioner, acting as a conduit for universal life energy, uses his or her hands to transfer energy to the patient. By transferring energy to the patient as needed, the practitioner helps to repattern the patient's energies and create symmetry in the patient's energy field (Quinn & Strelkauskas, 1993).

When the practitioner perceives that the patient's energy field is "balanced" (without any energetic excess, deficit, or disorder), he or she will end the treatment. Treatment usually takes 10 to 20 minutes; following treatment, it is recommended that the patient rest quietly. More than one practitioner can treat a patient at the same time. Frequency and duration of treatments are individualized, dependent on the patient's status. In general, acute conditions are treated once a day on consecutive days until symptoms are relieved; chronic conditions are treated once a week until symptoms are improved (Denison, 1998). Treatments can take place in the hospital, hospice, nursing home, or outpatient setting. Inpatient Therapeutic Touch is considered part of routine nursing care and can be requested in health care facilities that provide the technique. Costs of outpatient sessions vary by region but tend to parallel that of a massage.

Effects

Following treatment with Therapeutic Touch, patients report a reduction in pain, a profound state of relaxation, and a sense of well-being. Studies have shown that Therapeutic Touch elicits a profound generalized relaxation response in the patient (Krieger, 1979). EEG studies reveal that patients receiving Therapeutic Touch go into a low amplitude alpha state, consistent with calmness, and remain in this state throughout the treatment process (Krieger et al., 1979). Other signs of this relaxation response include: a deepening of the patient's voice level, slowing and deepening of the patient's respirations, audible sigh or breath with the feeling of relaxation, and flushing of the skin, associated with dilatation of the patient's peripheral blood vessels (Krieger, 1979).

Studies have shown that patients experience a significant increase in hemoglobin levels (Krieger, 1975), a decrease in diastolic blood pressure (Quinn, 1989), as well as a significant reduction in suppressor T-cells (in recently bereaved patients) (Quinn & Strelkauskas, 1993). Improvement in patient affect, with dramatic increase in positive emotions (e.g., joy and contentment) and dramatic decrease in negative emotions (e.g., anxiety, guilt, hostility, and depression) has also been documented following treatment with Therapeutic Touch (Quinn & Strelkauskas, 1993).

Therapeutic Touch is purported to work through a combination of these mechanisms:

1. Its induction of the Relaxation Response, a state of being that reduces stress and is reported to facilitate healing (Benson, 1993).
2. A process of resonance with the practitioner. As demonstrated by controlled studies (Quinn, 1984), for Therapeutic Touch to be effective, the practitioner must be centered with intent for the patient's highest good. This centering leads to a state of internal calm or "quietude" (Krieger, 1979). Since being in the presence of calm can make one calm, interaction with the centered practitioner may help the patient achieve a state of inner calm, reducing anxiety and improving mood.
3. Repatterning of the patient's energy field through a process of energy transfer from the practitioner acting as a conduit for universal life energy, able to supply and modulate energy where needed, thereby creating balance in the patient's energy field, facilitating healing.

Uses

Since Therapeutic Touch reduces anxiety and stress, relieves tension, and improves mood, it has been found to be of benefit in stress-related disorders and in facilitating mental, as well as physical, health. Therapeutic Touch has been used successfully to:

- Reduce and eliminate preoccupational thoughts and obsessive behaviors (Hill & Oliver, 1993)
- Decrease irritability in premature babies (Krieger, 1979)
- Decrease irritability of colicky babies (Krieger, 1993; Macrae, 1996)
- Decrease anxiety and stress of hospitalized children (Kramer, 1990)

- Decrease anxiety and stress of hospitalized cardiovascular patients (Heidt, 1981, 1991; Quinn, 1984, 1989)
- Decrease agitation of hospitalized patients (Krieger, 1979)
- Decrease anxiety of institutionalized elderly patients (Simington & Laing, 1993)
- Soothe women in childbirth (Macrae, 1996)
- Give comfort to the terminally ill (Kunz, 1997; Sayre-Adams & Wright, 1995)

Studies have shown Therapeutic Touch to be effective in the treatment of the following:

- Wounds, with accelerated rate of healing (Wirth et al., 1993)
- Headaches, with pain reduction sustained 4 hours after treatment (Keller & Bzdek, 1986)
- Arthritis, with improvement after the first treatment session and progressive improvement with subsequent sessions (Eckes Peck, 1997)

In addition, Therapeutic Touch has been reported anecdotally to be useful in:

- Reducing distress and agitation of Alzheimer's patients, increasing their awareness and independence (Wager, 1996)
- Improving sleep (Kramer, 1990)
- Relieving acute and chronic pain (Sayre-Adams & Wright, 1995)
- Treating muscle tension (Krieger, 1979)
- Enhancing tissue granulation in open wounds (Denison, 1998)
- Accelerating the healing of burns (Krieger, 1979), fractures (Kramer, 1990), bruises (Denison, 1998), and diabetic skin ulcers (Wager, 1996)
- Reducing edema (Krieger, 1979)
- Reducing fever (Kramer, 1990)
- Facilitating the healing of infections (Sayre-Adams & Wright, 1995)
- Reducing allergies (Krieger, 1979)
- Improving asthma, with quelling of an asthmatic attack within 2 to 4 minutes (Krieger, 1979)
- Alleviating gastrointestinal upset (Krieger, 1979)
- Decreasing peri-procedural reactions, when used before procedures such as spinal taps, or during preinduction of anesthesia (Krieger, 1979, 1993)
- Providing supportive care during radiation therapy and chemotherapy (Krieger, 1979), re-

ducing and alleviating untoward effects (Wager, 1996)

- Improving the thriving of premature babies, with reduced respiratory problems, improved neurological status, and improved weight gain (Krieger, 1979; Wager, 1996)
- Reducing the symptoms of chronic fatigue syndrome and premenstrual syndrome (Krieger, 1997)
- Alleviating the symptoms of AIDS (Newshan, 1989), including peripheral neuropathy (Wager, 1996)

Precautions and Contraindications

In Therapeutic Touch, precautions are indicated for the following patient populations:

- Neonates, infants, and children (as with medication, children require smaller doses than adults)
- Pregnant women (the practitioner has to respect two energy fields—that of the mother and that of the fetus)
- Patients with cardiovascular disease
- Patients with neurological disorders (e.g., epilepsy, traumatic brain injury, and Alzheimer's disease)
- Patients with psychiatric disorders
- The elderly and/or debilitated

For these patients Therapeutic Touch is to be delivered in gentler doses of shorter duration. If precautions are not followed, sensitive patients may temporarily experience light-headedness, dizziness, irritability, or agitation. There are no reported contraindications for Therapeutic Touch.

Training and Certification

Courses in Therapeutic Touch are generally given as part of the nursing curricula in colleges and universities or as seminars in hospitals and other health care settings nationally and internationally. The NH-PA recommends that training in Therapeutic Touch be divided into three levels: Beginner, Intermediate, and Advanced. Each level consists of 6 to 12 hours of training and involves didactic and experiential components. Instruction at the Beginner level includes history, theory, scientific foundation, and basic training in the tech-

nique of Therapeutic Touch, indications for its use, precautions, and contraindications. Following completion of Beginner's level courses, a student is qualified to practice on family or friends only. NH-PA recommends that a student practice, under the supervision of a mentor, a minimum of twice a week for 6 to 12 months before progressing to the Intermediate level (NH-PA, 1992).

The Intermediate level expands the student's knowledge of energetic theory, meditative skills, ability to modulate energy, and current research. Upon completion of Intermediate level training, practitioners are qualified to treat patients. The NH-PA recommends that practitioners spend 3 years to gain experience before participating in Advanced level training. Advanced level training expands the practitioner's knowledge and further refines his or her skills. There is no formal certification or appellation for those who have completed training (NH-PA, 1994).

To become a qualified teacher of Therapeutic Touch, the NH-PA recommends completion of a minimum of two Advanced courses, at least 5 years' experience as a practitioner, and continued practice of Therapeutic Touch. There is no formal certification or appellation for qualified teachers; however, the NH-PA utilizes a peer-review process to select membership in the NH-PA Therapeutic Touch Teachers Co-operative (NH-PA, 1997). A list of academic programs and health care facilities in the United States and abroad that include Therapeutic Touch as part of their curricula is compiled by the Nurse Healers-Professional Associates, Inc., Philadelphia, and is published in Dolores Krieger's *Therapeutic Touch: Inner Workbook, 1997.*

Practitioner Availability and Resources for Referral

Therapeutic Touch is taught as part of the nursing curricula in more than 100 colleges and universities in the United States and Canada and in more than 75 countries throughout the world. Utilized in hospital, hospice, nursing homes, and outpatient settings, Therapeutic Touch is practiced by nurses as well as physicians, physical therapists, massage therapists, and other health care professionals. It has also been successfully taught to patients and their families. As a result, there are no estimates for the number of practitioners available nationally or internationally.

A list of more than 100 health care facilities in the United States and abroad that currently provide Therapeutic Touch is available from Nurse Healers-Professional Associates. For information or referral, contact:

Nurse Healers-Professional Associates, Inc.
3760 South Highland Drive, Suite 429
Salt Lake City, UT 84106
Telephone: (801) 273-3399; Telefax: (801) 273-3352
E-mail: uh-pai@therapeutic-touch.org

The Therapeutic Touch Network
P.O. Box 85551
875 Eglinton Avenue West
Toronto, Ontario, Canada M6C4A8
Telephone: (416) 65-TOUCH

British Association of Therapeutic Touch
33 Grange Thorpe Drive
Burnage, Manchester UK M192LR

HEALING TOUCH

History

Healing Touch was developed in the 1980s by Janet Mentgen, BSN, RN, in Colorado. Mentgen combined a number of her own energy-based techniques with those from a variety of sources including (Hover-Kramer et al., 1996; Mentgen & Trapp Bulbrook, 1996a, b):
- Dolores Krieger, PhD, RN, Professor of Nursing, New York University and Dora Kunz, noted healer, developers of therapeutic touch
- Barbara Ann Brennan, MS, former NASA research scientist, Founder and Director of Barbara Brennan School of Healing, East Hampton, NY, developer of Healing Science
- Reverend Rosalyn Bruyere, research assistant on the human energy field at UCLA, Founder and Director of Healing Light Center Church, Glendale, CA, developer of Natural Healing
- Valerie Hunt, EdD, principal investigator on the human energy field at UCLA, chairman and president of Bioenergy Fields Foundation, Malibu, CA
- W. Brugh Joy, MD, physician and author
- Reverend Rudy Noel, student of Rosalyn Bruyere, developer of a mind-clearing technique

- Reverend John Scudder, developer of the Scudder relaxation technique
- Native American (Hopi Indian) tradition
- Rod Campbell, Australian sheepherder and healer

In 1989 the name Healing Touch was coined by Mentgen; Sharon Scandrett-Hibdon, PhD, RN; Dorothea Hover-Kramer, EdD, RN; and Myra Till-Tovey, BSN, RN, in order to distinguish this integrated technique from Therapeutic Touch. In that same year Mentgen developed The Healing Touch Program, a course of instruction initially offered through the American Holistic Nurses Association (AHNA). In 1996 Healing Touch International, a professional corporation that administers certification in Healing Touch, was established by Mentgen. Healing Touch is offered as part of continuing education in nursing and is endorsed by the AHNA (AHNA, 1998).

Typical Therapeutic Session

In a typical therapeutic session, the patient is in a prone position, wearing loose, comfortable clothing, with shoes and jewelry removed. Arms and legs are uncrossed so as to permit the free flow of energy. The practitioner uses four steps in his or her treatment of the patient: centering, assessment, selection and employment of modalities, and reassessment.

The practitioner begins a treatment session by centering and setting the intention for the patient's highest good. As in Therapeutic Touch, this involves practitioners' conscious effort to free themselves of inner tensions or distractions to enter a calm, focused state of being and to turn their full attention to the patient's needs. The practitioner then takes a patient history, and assesses the patient's energetic status by one or more of the following means: (1) placing the hands lightly on the patient, or 1 to 6 inches over the patient, to detect temperature, pressure or vibrational differences, or asymmetry; (2) using a resonant tone from a chime or bell to detect vibrational imbalances; or (3) using a pendulum to detect imbalances in energetic spin.

After the assessment is completed, the practitioner selects from more than 20 techniques those most appropriate for the patient's condition. These modalities include:
- Therapeutic Touch (the Krieger-Kunz method)
- Magnetic unruffle

- Etheric unruffle
- Scudder relaxation technique
- Mind clearing
- Spiral meditation
- Magnetic pain drain
- Hopi Indian technique
- Lymphatic drain technique
- Wound sealing
- Leak sealing technique
- Spinal cleansing
- Back and neck techniques
- Headache techniques
- Chakra spread
- Chakra connection
- Full body connection
- Double hand chakra balance
- Vertebral spiral technique
- "Ultrasound" technique
- "Laser" technique
- "Chelation" technique
- Pyramid technique

Each of these techniques involves the use of the practitioner's hands placed gently on or over the patient's body. Depending on the individual needs of the patient, treatment typically takes 20 to 40 minutes. At the end of a treatment session, the practitioner reassesses the patient's energy field and recommends follow-up treatment as indicated (Hover-Kramer et al., 1996; Mentgen & Trapp Bulbrook, 1996a, b).

Following treatment, patients report feeling alleviation of pain, reduction of stress and anxiety, and an enhanced sense of well-being. Since therapy induces relaxation, patients are encouraged to rest following a session. Cost of outpatient treatment varies regionally but typically parallels that of a massage.

Uses

The use of Healing Touch is reported to have been successful in the treatment of a number of physical and psychological conditions. Anecdotal reports include (Hover-Kramer et al., 1996; Mentgen & Trapp Bulbrook, 1996 a, b; Turner, 1997; Wetzel, 1993):

- Accelerated healing of wounds, burns, and fractures
- Accelerated healing of infections
- Facilitation of lymph drainage
- Facilitation of elimination of toxins from addictive or chemotherapeutic agents

- Decreased anxiety, reducing need for preoperative medication
- Reduced peri-procedural untoward effects when used before and after surgery, chemotherapy, radiation therapy, diagnostic testing, or dialysis
- Easing of labor
- Reduction of acute and chronic pain
- Reduction of symptoms in migraine headaches, sinusitis, neck and back problems, arthritis, and gout
- Reduction of symptoms in premenstrual syndrome
- Improvement in autoimmune disease
- Improvement in chronic conditions such as diabetes, hypertension, and chronic fatigue
- Improvement in cancer
- Decreased irritability and improved weight gain in neonates
- Improved rehabilitation
- Enhanced relaxation and improved sleep
- Calming of the agitated, anxious, or distressed
- Facilitation of expression of suppressed emotions or repressed memory
- Facilitation of the release of negative emotions
- Facilitation of grief management
- Supportive help for bipolar mood swings
- Calming of addictive cravings and easing of physical discomfort from withdrawal
- Soothing of the dying

Precautions and Contraindications

There are no established precautions for Healing Touch. In general, practitioners follow precautions similar to those in Therapeutic Touch, delivering gentler doses of shorter duration to the following patient populations:

- Neonates, infants, and children (as with medications, children need smaller doses than adults)
- Pregnant women (the practitioner has to respect two energy fields—that of the mother and that of the fetus)
- Patients with serious illness, including cardiovascular disease
- The elderly and/or debilitated

At this time Healing Touch uses the literature from Therapeutic Touch as its clinical research base.

Since Healing Touch incorporates multiple modalities, research on each of its component techniques may be indicated. Controlled studies and/or wider observation over time may help establish clinical efficacy and safety. At the time of this writing, Healing Touch International reports that a number of research projects are under way; information may be obtained from Healing Touch International as it becomes available. There are no reported contraindications to Healing Touch.

Training and Certification

Healing Touch International requires that a practitioner successfully complete three levels of training to become eligible for certification; each level includes didactic and experiential components as well as recommended reading. Level I consists of 15 to 20 hours of continuing education. Instruction is given in energetic theory, centering and assessment techniques, Therapeutic Touch, and several other treatment modalities. Level II is divided into two parts (Levels IIA and IIB); each consists of 15 to 20 hours of continuing education. These courses increase the number of techniques available to the practitioner and provide instruction in advanced energetic theory and interviewing and assessment skills.

Level III is divided into two parts (Levels IIIA and IIIB); each consists of 30 hours of continuing education. Level IIIA focuses on integration and advancement of skills, a relationship with a mentor, and development of a practice. A practitioner must wait at least 1 year after completion of Level IIIA before taking Level IIIB. To become eligible for Level IIIB, a practitioner must provide documentation of more than 100 treatment sessions as well as successful completion of a mentor relationship. After completion of Level IIIB, a practitioner may apply for certification from Healing Touch International. If approved, a practitioner is designated a Certified Healing Touch Practitioner (CHTP). Practitioner certification must be renewed every 5 years (HTI, 1996a).

Completion of a fourth level of training is required to become a Certified Healing Touch Instructor (CHTI). Level IV consists of didactic and experiential requirements and includes practice teaching as an assistant instructor and lead instructor in Level I Healing Touch program courses. Healing Touch International recommends that instruc-

tors meet annually to advance their skills. Instructor certification must be renewed every 5 years (HTI, 1996b).

Practitioner Availability and Resources for Referral

Healing Touch has been taught in the United States, Canada, Great Britain, the Netherlands, South Africa, Australia, and New Zealand. Healing Touch International, Inc., reports that throughout the world there are approximately 500 CHTPs (413 are in the United States) and 100 CHTIs (79 are in the United States).

For information or referral to a Certified Healing Touch Practitioner, contact:

Healing Touch International, Inc.
12477 West Cedar Drive, Suite 202
Lakewood, Colorado 80228
Telephone: (303) 989-7982; Telefax: (303) 980-8683
E-mail: HTIheal@aol.com

REIKI

History

The word *Reiki* (pronounced "ray-kee") is derived from a combination of the Japanese characters *rei,* meaning "boundless and universal," and *ki,* meaning "energy" or "vital life force." In Japanese the word is used to denote universal life energy as well as to describe the ancient method of healing based on this energy (Figure 15-4).

Reiki was developed in Japan in the mid-1800s by Dr. Mikao Usui, a theologian minister, President of Doshisha University, Kyoto. Usui is said to have been challenged by his students to explain how noted spiritual leaders such as Jesus and Buddha were able to heal the sick. Traveling extensively in search of an answer, Usui found references in the Tibetan sutras (holy writings) describing the use of universal life energy for healing through the laying on of hands. Through meditation and prayer, Usui discovered a means for accessing this energy. He translated his findings into a series of sacred ceremonial procedures known as "attunements," "alignments," or "initiations." During these procedures the practitioner's en-

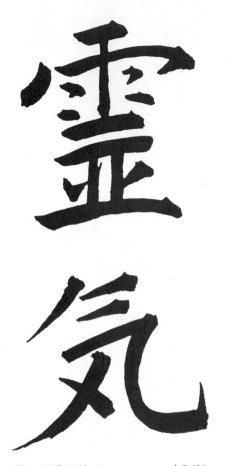

Figure 15-4 The Japanese word *Reiki*.

ergy field becomes aligned so that he or she is able to access the flow of universal life energy and transfer this energy to others through the hands.

Reiki is an oral tradition, passed from Master to practitioner. Usui passed the practice and teaching of Reiki to Dr. Chujiro Hayashi, who passed it on to Hawayo Takata, a Hawaiian woman who introduced Reiki to the United States in the late 1930s (Brown, 1992). Since then, a number of organizations for Reiki practitioners have been founded; these societies vary in their interpretations of history, philosophy, and methodology. The organization that follows most closely the Usui tradition is The Reiki Alliance, led by Takata's granddaughter, Phyllis Lei Furumoto. Reiki has been utilized in hospital, hospice, and outpatient settings, nationally and internationally.

Typical Therapeutic Session

A typical Reiki session lasts 60 to 90 minutes and treats the entire body; however, there can be treatments of shorter duration or treatments focused on specific areas only. The patient is usually in a prone position, although treatment can take place with the patient in a sitting position. To ensure the free flow of energy, the patient does not cross his or her arms or legs, as this may obstruct energetic flow. The patient typically wears loose comfortable clothing, with shoes, eyeglasses, and sometimes belts or jewelry removed.

Similar to Therapeutic Touch and Healing Touch, in Reiki the practitioner begins a therapeutic session by centering, with intent for the patient's highest good. Although a patient history may be taken, Reiki differs from Therapeutic Touch and Healing Touch in that often no initial physical or energetic assessment is made. Once the patient is in a comfortable position, the Reiki practitioner uses Japanese symbols ("kanji") and a sequence of hand positions to transfer energy to the patient. With fingers gently held together and palms down, the practitioner's hands are placed lightly on the patient beginning at the head, then moving down the body. During these hand placements, universal life energy is said to flow through the practitioner and transfer from the practitioner's hands to the patient, to balance the patient's energy where needed. Each hand position is held for approximately 5 minutes, or longer if the practitioner senses continued need and flow. Unlike Therapeutic Touch and Healing Touch, Reiki is traditionally practiced "hands-on," although "hands-over" (hands held 1 to 2 inches above the skin) can be used in specific situations, such as treating a patient with a burn or an infectious disease. "Hands-over" can also be used if the patient is uncomfortable with being touched. More than one practitioner can treat the patient at the same time; these sessions are called team treatments (Baginski & Sharaman, 1988; Morris, 1996).

During a session the patient may feel the transfer of energy as a change in temperature (warm/cold), change in pressure (heavy/light), vibration (tingling, pulsing), or "magnetic" sensation. Following a session patients generally report feeling a reduction in stress and anxiety, and an overall feeling of relaxation, inner calm, peace, and "balance." Patients also report feeling a reduction in pain. It should be noted that, in certain circumstances, pain may be temporarily intensified (see Precautions and Contraindications). After a session, it is recommended that a patient drink water to facilitate the energetic shift. Practitioners typically wash their hands and cleanse the room when treatment is completed.

Reiki is felt to work best when performed on consecutive days. Depending on the nature of the problem, the traditional approach is to provide treatment on 3 or 4 consecutive days, with subsequent treatment as indicated. Cost of a typical session varies from region to region but usually will parallel that of a massage.

Uses

Reiki is purported to work by creating energetic balance within the body, where needed, thereby helping the body to heal itself. In addition to pain reduction and stress reduction, with concomitant enhancement of relaxation, Reiki has been reported to be useful in a number of physical and psychological conditions. Anecdotal reports include (Baginski & Sharaman, 1988; Mitchell, 1997; Morris, 1996):

- Accelerated healing of insect bites, burns, sprains, and fractures
- Use during dental surgery, precluding the necessity for novocaine
- Accelerated healing of infections such as colds, flus, strep throat, pneumonia, and cellulitis
- Accelerated healing of inflammatory conditions such as bursitis and arthritis
- Pain reduction, including alleviation of headaches
- Improvement in chronic diseases such as emphysema and amyotrophic lateral sclerosis (ALS)
- Improvement in asthma, hypertension, and diabetes, with reduction of medication
- Improvement in chronic conditions such as scoliosis, endometriosis, psoriasis, and chronic fatigue syndrome
- Improvement in ovarian cysts and benign and malignant tumors
- Enhancement of the efficacy of radiation therapy and chemotherapy, supporting the toward effects and reducing the untoward effects
- Improvement in depression, schizophrenia, post-traumatic stress disorder, and alcoholism

Precautions and Contraindications

Following Reiki treatment, some patients may experience a temporary increase in symptoms, fever, discharge, or pain as the body undergoes the energetic shift. Reiki practitioners attribute this transient intensification to the patient's experiencing all of the stages of healing at an accelerated rate. Reiki is reported to be safe and effective for use during pregnancy, labor, and delivery.

Reiki is contraindicated for use in:
- Fractures that require setting, until *after* they have been set
- Skin wounds that require stitching, until *after* they have been stitched
- Severed limbs or digits (or anything requiring re-anastomosis), until *after* reattachment is completed

Reiki practitioners report that this is because Reiki accelerates the natural course of healing of the bone, blood vessel, and skin edges, and they will then not reoppose and reknit properly.

Training and Certification

There are three levels of Reiki training. Completion of the first level renders one a first-degree Reiki practitioner, qualified to treat self, family, and friends only. Completion of the second degree qualifies a Reiki practitioner to treat patients. After completing the third degree, a practitioner becomes a Reiki Master and is qualified to teach other practitioners as well as treat patients.

In the first level of Reiki training, students learn the uses of Reiki, its history, spiritual precepts, and hand positions for healing. Students undergo four "attunements" or "initiations," ceremonial procedures that are said to open, balance, and align their energy field, allowing them to access the flow of universal life energy and transfer it to others through their hands. According to Reiki tradition, the ability to access and transfer energy is predicated on these sacred "attunements." First-degree training takes approximately four 3-hour sessions to complete. General guidelines advise that students wait at least 3 months after completing the first degree before beginning the second, a time in which to gather experience.

The second level of training increases the practitioner's capability by augmenting the amount of energy he or she is able to access or transfer. At this level the practitioner undergoes another "attunement" and learns three Japanese characters or "kanji." The nature of these symbols and the techniques for their use are considered sacred knowledge and, in keeping with tradition, are not to be published. Second-degree training is generally completed in two 3-hour sessions. Second-degree practitioners must gather experience for at least 1 year before beginning third-level training.

The third level consists of one-on-one training with a Reiki Master for at least 1 year. During this apprenticeship practitioners receive another "attunement," learn an additional sacred symbol, receive instruction to train and attune first- and second-degree practitioners, and become initiated as Masters. Following this training, practitioners must teach at the first- and second-degree level for at least 3 years before becoming qualified to teach at the third-degree level or to "initiate" another Master (Mitchell, 1997).

Practitioner Availability and Resources for Referral

The number of second-degree Reiki practitioners is not known, nor is the total number of Masters. The Reiki Alliance, an international organization of Reiki Masters who practice and teach the Usui System of Reiki Healing, reports membership of 282 Masters in the United States, 69 in Canada, and 900 worldwide. For information or a referral to a Reiki practitioner, contact:

The Reiki Alliance
P. O. Box 41
Cataldo, Idaho 83810
Telephone: (208) 783 3535; Telefax: (208) 783-4848
E-mail: reikialliance@compuserve.com

Stichting The Reiki Alliance
Postbus 75523, 1070 AM
Amsterdam, Netherlands
Telephone: 31-294-290022; Telefax: 31-294-290931
E-mail: 100125.466@compuserve.com

SUMMARY

Energy medicine is based on the belief that in addition to a system of physical and biochemical processes, the human being is made up of a complex system of energy. This energy does not stop at the surface of the skin but extends beyond the body, thereby creating an individual's energy field. The pattern of energy flow through this energy field has an anatomy that includes chakras, meridians, and etheric levels. The role of energy is to perform two vital functions: (1) in proper balance, energy improves vitality and nourishes the body's cells, rendering them robust and healthy; and (2) energy provides the template upon which the pattern of cellular regeneration is based.

When energy flows freely through and about the body in a balanced symmetrical manner, good health can be maintained. When energy flow becomes restricted, disordered, imbalanced, or asymmetrical, ill health can follow. Physical trauma, stored emotions, habitual patterns of negative emotion, and habitual patterns of negative thought disrupt the free flow of energy, causing energetic imbalance. In the short term energetic imbalance can decrease vitality, limit resilience, and impair the functioning of cells, tissues, and organs. In the long term, energetic imbalance may damage one's "blueprint," disrupting the body's pattern of cellular regeneration, impairing the body's ability to heal, and predisposing one to chronic pain and chronic disease.

Energy-based therapeutic modalities involve repatterning of the patient's energy field, correcting imbalances, and restoring energy flow. Therapeutic Touch, Healing Touch, and Reiki are energetic techniques that have been used successfully in hospital, hospice, and outpatient settings. Each has been found to accelerate healing, alleviate symptoms, reduce pain, reduce stress and anxiety, induce relaxation, and provide a sense of peace and well-being. Shown to be effective tools in preventive health measures and disease intervention, energy-based therapeutic modalities are to be used in addition to, not in lieu of, traditional medical therapies.

According to NIH reports, the United States falls behind other countries in the recognition of energy healing. In the United Kingdom, for example, energy medicine is approved for use at 1500 government hospitals, more than 8500 registered healers are licensed to practice, and physicians receive postgraduate education credits for study.

It is important for health care providers to consider the role of energy medicine in the treatment of patients. Recognition and assessment of a patient's energy field is a significant complement to physical examination and laboratory analysis. When used in combination with traditional medicine, energy medicine is a powerful tool. Energetic intervention can reduce pain and stress, alleviate symptoms, and create an improved environment in which accelerated healing can occur.

Bibliography

American Holistic Nurses Association. 1998. McKivergin M, Executive Director. Flagstaff, Arizona. Personal communication.

American Nurses Association. 1998. Foer S, Spokesperson. Washington, DC. Personal communication.

Baginski BJ, Sharaman S. 1988. Reiki: Universal Life Energy. Life Rhythm, Mendocino, California

Beinfield H, Korngold E. 1991. Between Heaven and Earth: A Guide to Chinese Medicine. Random House, New York.

Benson H. 1993. The Relaxation Response. In Goleman D and Gurin J (eds): Mind/Body Medicine. Consumer Reports Books, Yonkers, New York.

Brennan BA. 1988. Hands of Light: A Guide to Healing Through the Human Energy Field. Bantam Books, New York.

Brennan BA. 1993. Light Emerging: The Journey of Personal Healing. Bantam Books, New York.

Brown F. 1992. Living Reiki: Takata's Teachings. Life Rhythm, Mendocino, California.

Bruyere RL. 1994. Wheels of Light: Chakras, Auras, and the Healing Energy of the Body. Simon and Schuster, New York.

Clark PE, Clark MJ. 1984. Therapeutic Touch: is there a scientific basis for the practice? Nursing Review 33(1): 37-41.

Denison B. 1998. Chairperson of Programs and Education, Nurse Healers—Professional Associates and Coordinator, Complementary Healing Services, Via Christi Regional Medical Center, Wichita, Kansas. Personal communication.

Easter A. 1997. The state of research on the effects of Therapeutic Touch. Journal of Holistic Nursing 15(2):158-175.

Eckes Peck SD. 1997. The effectiveness of Therapeutic Touch for decreasing pain in elders with degenerative arthritis. Journal of Holistic Nursing 15(2):176-198.

Eisenberg D, Wright TL. 1987. Encounters with Qi: Exploring Chinese Medicine. Penguin Books, New York.

Gagne D. Toye RC. 1994. The effects of Therapeutic Touch and relaxation therapy in reducing anxiety. Archives of Psychiatric Nursing 8(3):184-189.

Healing Touch International. 1996a. Healing Touch Certificate Program: Practitioner Certification Process. Healing Touch International, Inc., Lakewood, Colorado.

Healing Touch International. 1996b. Healing Touch Certificate Program: Instructor Certification Process. Healing Touch International, Inc., Lakewood, Colorado.

Heidt P. 1981. Effect of Therapeutic Touch on anxiety level of hospitalized patients. Nursing Research 30(1):32-37.

Heidt PR. 1991. Helping patients to rest: clinical studies in Therapeutic Touch. Holistic Nursing Practice 5(4):57-66.

Hill L, Oliver N. 1993. Therapeutic Touch and theory-based mental-health nursing. Journal of Psychosocial Nursing 31(2):19-27.

Hover-Kramer D, Mentgen J, Scandrett-Hibdon S. 1996. Healing Touch: A Resource for Health Care Professionals. Delmar, Albany, New York.

Hunt VV. 1995. Infinite Mind: The Science of Human Vibrations. Malibu Publishing, Malibu, California.

Joy WB. 1979. Joy's Way: A Map for the Transformational Journey—An Introduction to the Potentials for Healing with Body Energies. G.P. Putnam's Sons, New York.

Jurgens A, Meehan TC, Wilson HL. 1987. Therapeutic Touch as a nursing intervention. Holistic Nursing Practice 2(1):1-13.

Kaptchuk TJ. 1983. The Web That Has No Weaver: Understanding Chinese Medicine. Congdon and Weed, Inc., Chicago.

Keller E, Bzdek VM. 1986. Effects of Therapeutic Touch on tension headache pain. Nursing Research 35(2): 101-106.

Kramer NA. 1990. Comparison of Therapeutic Touch and casual touch in stress reduction of hospitalized children. Pediatric Nursing 16(5):483-485.

Krieger D. 1975. Therapeutic Touch: the imprimatur of nursing. American Journal of Nursing 75(5):784-787.

Krieger D. 1979. The Therapeutic Touch: How to Use Your Hands to Help or to Heal. Simon and Schuster, New York.

Krieger D. 1993. Accepting Your Power to Heal: The Personal Practice of Therapeutic Touch. Bear and Company, Inc., Santa Fe, New Mexico.

Krieger D. 1997. Therapeutic Touch: Inner Workbook—Ventures in Transpersonal Healing. Bear and Company, Inc., Santa Fe, New Mexico.

Krieger D, Peper E, Ancoli S. 1979. Therapeutic Touch: searching for evidence of physiological change. American Journal of Nursing 79(4):660-662.

Kunz D. 1995. Spiritual Healing: Doctors Examine Therapeutic Touch and Other Holistic Treatments. Theosophical Publishing House, Wheaton, Illinois.

Kunz D. 1997. Co-developer of Therapeutic Touch. Rye, New York. Personal communication.

Lyons AS, Petrucelli RJ. 1978. Medicine: An Illustrated History. Harry N. Abrams, Inc., New York.

Mackey RB. 1995. Complementary modalities (part 1): discover the healing power of Therapeutic Touch. American Journal of Nursing 95(4):26-32.

MacManaway B, Turcan J. 1983. Healing. Thorsons, Wellingborough, England.

Macrae J. 1979. Therapeutic Touch in practice. American Journal of Nursing 79(4):664-665.

Macrae J. 1996. Therapeutic Touch: A Practical Guide. Alfred A. Knopf, New York.

McCloskey JC, Bulechek GM (eds). 1992. Nursing Interventions Classification (NIC). Mosby-Year Book, Inc., Philadelphia.

Mentgen J, Trapp Bulbrook MJ. 1996a. Healing Touch: Level I Notebook. North Carolina Center for Healing Touch, Carrboro, North Carolina.

Mentgen, J, Trapp Bulbrook MJ. 1996b. Healing Touch: Level II Notebook. North Carolina Center for Healing Touch, Carrboro, North Carolina.

Mitchell PD. 1985a. The Usui System of Natural Healing. The Reiki Alliance, Cataldo, Idaho.

Mitchell PD. 1985b. The Usui System of Reiki Healing. The Reiki Alliance, Cataldo, Idaho.

Mitchell S. 1997. Executive Director, The Reiki Alliance, Cataldo, Idaho. Personal communication.

Morris JJ. 1996. Reiki: Hands That Heal. The Center Bookstore, Encino, California.

Morris JJ. 1997. Director, Reiki Center of Los Angeles and Author: Reiki Hands That Heal. Los Angeles, and Pittsfield, Massachusetts. Personal communication.

National Institutes of Health. 1994. Alternative Medicine: Expanding Medical Horizons—A Report to the National Institutes of Health on Alternative Medical Systems and Practices in the United States. US Government Printing Office, Washington, DC.

National League for Nursing. 1998. Crawford L, Director of Professional Development. New York. Personal communication.

Newshan G. 1989. Therapeutic Touch for symptom control in persons with AIDS. Holistic Nursing Practice 3(4):45-51.

North American Nursing Diagnosis Association. 1996. Nursing Diagnoses: Definitions and Classifications 1997-98. NANDA, Philadelphia.

Nurse Healers-Professional Associates. 1991. Therapeutic Touch Policy and Procedure for Health Professionals. Nurse Healers-Professional Associates, Inc., Philadelphia.

Nurse Healers-Professional Associates. 1992. Guidelines for Teaching Therapeutic Touch by the Krieger/Kunz Method: Beginner's Level. Nurse Healers-Professional Associates, Inc., Philadelphia.

Nurse Healers-Professional Associates. 1994. Guidelines for Teaching Therapeutic Touch by the Krieger/Kunz Method: Intermediate Level. Nurse Healers-Professional Associates, Inc., Philadelphia.

Nurse Healers-Professional Associates. 1997. Guidelines for Qualified Teachers of Therapeutic Touch. Nurse Healers-Professional Associates, Inc., Philadelphia.

Olson M, et al. 1992. Therapeutic Touch and post-hurricane Hugo stress. Journal of Holistic Nursing 10(2):120-136.

Potter-Hughes P, Meize-Grochowski R, Duncan-Harris CN. 1996. Therapeutic Touch with adolescent psychiatric patients. Journal of Holistic Nursing 14(1):6-23.

Poznanski-Hutchison C. 1998. Research Coordinator, Healing Touch International, Boulder, Colorado. Personal communication.

Quinn JF. 1984. Therapeutic Touch as energy exchange: testing the theory. Advances in Nursing Science 6(2):42-49.

Quinn JF. 1989. Therapeutic Touch as energy exchange: replication and extension. Nursing Science Quarterly 2(2):79-87.

Quinn JF, Strelkauskas AJ. 1993. Psychoimmunologic effects of Therapeutic Touch on practitioners and recently bereaved recipients: a pilot study. Advances in Nursing Science 15(4):13-26.

Randolph GL. 1984. Therapeutic and physical touch: physiological response to stressful stimuli. Nursing Research 33(1):33-36.

Rosa L, et al. 1998. A Close Look at Therapeutic Touch. Journal of the American Medical Association 279(13):1005-1010.

Sayre-Adams J, Wright S. 1995. The Theory and Practice of Therapeutic Touch. Churchill Livingstone, New York.

Simington J, Laing G. 1993. Effects of Therapeutic Touch on anxiety in the institutionalized elderly. Clinical Nursing Research 2(4):438-450.

Slater VE. 1996. Healing Touch. In Micozzi MS (ed): Fundamentals of Complementary and Alternative Medicine. Churchill Livingstone, New York.

Sui, CK. 1990. Pranic Healing. Samuel Weiser, Inc. York Beach, Maine.

Turner J. 1997. Healing Touch Program Director, Lakewood, Colorado. Personal communication.

Vieth I. 1972. Huang Ti Nei Ching Su Wên: The Yellow Emperor's Classic of Internal Medicine, chapters 1–34 translated from the Chinese with an introductory study. University of California Press, Los Angeles.

Wager S. 1996. A Doctor's Guide to Therapeutic Touch: Enhancing the Body's Energy to Promote Healing. The Berkley Publishing Group, New York.

Wetzel WS. 1993. Healing Touch as a nursing intervention: wound infection following cesarean birth—an anecdotal case study. Journal of Holistic Nursing 11(3):277-285.

Wirth DP, et al. 1993. Full thickness dermal wounds treated with non-contact Therapeutic Touch: a replication and extension. Complementary Therapies in Medicine 1(3):127-132.

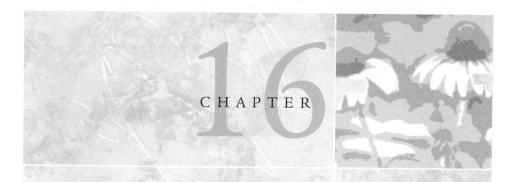

CHAPTER
16

Expressive and Creative Arts Therapies

RICHARD A. LIPPIN

The new image of humanity emerging in our century is that of the divine artist in everyone.

—JUDITH CORNELL

The capacity for the arts to enhance health has been known since antiquity. We are currently experiencing a resurgence of interest in this topic based on several megatrends in medicine. Among these megatrends are a shift from reductionism to holism and a shift from paternalism to consumerism. Other fundamental factors contributing to the serious study of the relation of the creative and the healing arts are major scientific advances in neuroscience and the concurrent growth of so-called mind-body medicine and the resurgence of interest in the application of physics, including energy concepts, to human health. Passive exposure to the arts alone, including music, dance,

painting, sculpture, poetry, and drama, has proven health-giving properties, and interestingly, passive exposure to live or original arts can be differentiated from exposure to electronic or printed reproductions. The central theme of this chapter, however, is the relationship of so-called expressive or active creative arts therapies to human health and well-being, where patients actively engage in one or more of the creative arts. This creative process enhances or augments the life force through classical biophysiological responses such as movement, relaxation, and emotional catharsis, as well as through self-discovery and awareness, increases in self-esteem, pleasure, hope and optimism, and the achievement of transcendence, which enhances our spiritual selves. Perhaps most important, the creation of beauty itself is a profound and powerful source of health and well-being.

HISTORY

Contemporary physician Michael Samuels has written that art, prayer, and healing all come from the same source. Other scholars have said that every child, every adult, and every culture gives form to its feelings and ideas through art. Even before objective language was used in science with conceptual thought, it is believed that early preliterate humans naturally embodied feelings, attitudes, and thoughts in symbols. Thus some believe that the metaphorical use of language preceded the literal and scientific. Don Blacking hypothesizes that singing and dancing preceded the development of verbal interchange. Eighteenth century Italian philosopher Giambattista Vico has suggested that human beings danced before they walked and that poetry came before prose. This is echoed by social theorist Jean-Jacques Rousseau, who believed that musical sounds accompanied or preceded speech as we know it.

I believe that the most basic roots of the impact of the arts on health can be traced to the dawn of *Homo sapiens* himself (or herself) and man's unique awareness of himself. This existential jolt of separateness or aloneness and awareness of mortality has been a driver of artistic expression ever since. The early cave drawings in Southern France may have served many purposes for early humans. Through them, for example, humans communicated and hence connected with fellow human beings, mastered and taught others about a vast and potentially hostile environment by rendering it, recorded their accomplishments and existence, and simply enjoyed the pleasure of beautiful images, rhythmic sound, and elegant movement. All of these were individual and cultural survival mechanisms and health giving in the broadest sense.

The ancient Greeks recognized the connection between healing and the arts by their building of aesculapia or temples of medicine, constructed in places of natural beauty, where, among other interventions, arts played a prominent role in the healing process. According to Aristotle, Pythagoras began the daily practice of singing and playing as the means by which the soul achieved catharsis. Homer told of his hero Ulysses being treated for hemorrhage with both bandages and incantation. Anathaneum reported a cure for sciatica in which flutists were hired to play music in the Pythagorean mode for the affected area. In other non-Western traditions, as early as the Han dynasty, Chinese scholars began to realize that music could affect the human body, not only psychologically but physiologically, and during the Tsin dynasty (265-420 BC) music was known and used as a means of cultivating pleasant personality and positive mood.

During the Renaissance music as one art form pervaded medieval medical practice and theory. Music prescribed was not only for good digestion and for bodily preparation before surgery but also as a stimulus to wound healing, a mood changer, and a critical accompaniment to bloodletting. Specifically composed medical music (the shivaree) graced the wedding chamber to ensure erotic coupling at the astrologically auspicious moment.

Although in the modern era highly creative individuals in the arts and health continued to make individual contributions, the roots of the modern application of the arts to medical science belong to the professional creative arts therapy movement. Stimulated by the growth of modern mental health science after World War II, art therapists, music therapists, dance or movement therapists, poetry therapists, and drama therapists have provided meaningful therapeutic opportunities for people of all ages in a wide variety of settings, but with a particular emphasis on mental health settings.

The creative arts therapists have established a solid professional base through education, training, professional publications (including journals), credentialing mechanisms, and scientific research. There are currently more than 5000 music therapists, 10,200 dance therapists, 2250 art therapists, and several hundred drama and poetry therapists in the United States. The arts therapy movement now includes more than 140 undergraduate and postgraduate degree programs. At least 10 professional associations are in existence in various creative arts therapies and several first-rate professional journals are being published.

The growth of the application of the arts in medicine owes a debt to this creative professional community. It is noteworthy that two hearings were held in 1991 and 1992 under the jurisdiction of the U.S. Senate's Select Committee on Aging dealing with the healing power of music, the visual arts, and dance in the aging population. These hearings led to changes in the Older Americans' Act that enhanced insurance coverage for the creative arts therapies and provided increased professional credibility and acceptance of these interventions.

Also, one would be remiss not to cite the recent hospital arts movement. This successful and growing movement emphasizes improving the environmental quality of health care institutions through the architectural design, interior design, and placement of fine art in strategic health care setting locations and performances in a variety of hospital arts settings such as lobbies, waiting rooms, patient rooms, and high-tech intervention venues. These individuals and organizations generally do not state that they are engaging in therapy per se but have a general belief in the salutary effect of aesthetic environments on patients, visitors, family members, staff, and the overall health care institution community. Among the leading organizations in this important new field are the Society for the Arts in Healthcare, the Foundation for Hospital Arts, Art that Heals, Arts as a Healing Force, the British Healthcare Arts Centre, and the Center for Health Design and Aesthetics. Collaboration with the professional architectural and interior design community provides exciting opportunities. Some of these professionals have recently begun incorporating not only performance but also specific sounds into the holistic health care environment. In one case, Annette Ridenour, President of Aesthetics, Inc., works with a composer who writes music that integrates with the architecture, the color, and the intention of the selected space. Patients and staff often participate in the production of such art and performances. As noted previously, these activities are not categorized as therapeutic per se, but leaders in the field are encouraging at least some outcome measurement studies. Economics, of course, may demand this.

In recent years there has been a growing interest in the application of the arts to all specialties of medicine in addition to the previous emphasis on the application of the arts in psychiatry. In part, this trend has to do with the recognition of the problems associated with the excesses of pharmacological and surgical intervention. In 1985 I published an article calling for the formation of a new medical specialty known as *Arts Medicine,* which sought to explore the many synergistic relationships between the healing and the creative arts. It was stated that the arts could be explored for their etiological, diagnostic, educational, therapeutic, and environmental impact on health. Also, in recent years creative arts and expressive arts therapists are increasingly expanding their emphasis on applying their work in mental health settings to other medical specialties, most notably pe-

diatrics, gerontology, oncology, cardiology, physical medicine and rehabilitation (physiatry), and thanatology (death and dying). For several reasons there appears to be differential capacity to apply these interventions to pediatric populations, geriatric populations, and to other "special" populations that are explored later in this chapter.

Definitions

Arts: For this chapter we are limiting our definition to music, dance, visual arts, poetry, and drama. (A case can be made that all human activities, such as avocational cooking and gardening or work for pay, can be engaged in artistically when aesthetics becomes an ontology or way of being.)

Creativity: Mihali Csikszentmihaly defines creativity as "the ability to produce something that changes the existing patterns and thoughts in a domain."

Creative Arts Therapy: The National Coalition of Arts Therapies Associations (NCATA) states that creative arts therapies include art therapy, dance/movement therapy, drama therapy, music therapy, psychodrama, and poetry therapy. These therapies use arts modalities and creative processes during intentional intervention in therapeutic, rehabilitative, community, or educational settings to foster health, communication and expression, promotion of the integration of physical, emotional, cognitive, and social functioning, enhancing self-awareness and facilitating change.

Arts Medicine: The International Arts Medicine Association states that arts medicine studies the relationship of human health to the arts. Arts and artistic activities are explored for their etiological, diagnostic, educational, therapeutic, and environmental potential.

Expressive Therapies: Natalie Rogers, a leader in this field, states that expressive therapies are the use of the expressive arts in a supportive setting to facilitate awareness, growth, and healing. Various art modes interrelate simultaneously in what Rogers calls the *creative connection.*

Imagery and Visualization: Imagery is both a mental process and a wide variety of procedures used in therapy to encourage changes in attitudes,

Continued

Continued

behavior, or physiological reactions. As a mental process, it can be defined as "any thought representing a sensory quality which might include the visual, oral, tactile, olfactory, proprioceptive and kinesthetic." Whereas *visualization* refers to "seeing something in the mind's eye" only, procedures for imagery fall into at least three major categories: evaluation or diagnostic imagery, mental rehearsal, and therapeutic intervention.

Recently some leaders in the creative arts therapies field and others have been introducing newer terms such as *musicmedicine, medical art therapy,* and *medical dance therapy,* reflecting the increasing use of the creative arts therapies in medical settings other than mental health settings. Of particular note is the pioneering work of Drs. Ralph Spintge and Roland Droh, who founded the International Society for Music in Medicine after studying music's anxiolytic and analgesic properties in thousands of surgical patients in a hospital wired throughout for music in Ludenscheid, Germany. ∾

THEORETICAL CONSIDERATIONS AND MECHANISMS OF ACTION

Before we embark on a discussion of the various types, current practices, and research in expressive or creative arts therapies, an elaboration on some general theoretical considerations and some possible mechanisms of action seems appropriate. Expressive arts therapies are often categorized as mind-body therapies or embracing the holistic model of medicine. Fueled by advances in neuroscience, mind-body or holistic medicine recognizes that the entire universe and everything in it, including one's perceptions of it through the human brain, affect human physiology and medical outcomes ranging from accidents to dysfunction and disease to wellness and peak performance.

One fundamental shift that is gaining credibility is support for a transformation from our current pathology-based health care system to a health care system that embraces a fundamental view of humans as good and empowered to seek and achieve increas-ingly higher levels of health or wellness. The arts play an essential role in realizing the preceding health care model, because the arts promote the salutary effects of freedom, self-esteem, growth, pleasure, communication, love, a sense of community, and the connectedness to a universal life force.

Another fundamental concept associated with the expressive arts therapies is that human beings can deterministically choose to perceive the innate and abundant beauty of themselves and the universe and can incorporate this beauty into their lives on a conscious decision basis. Therefore the role of the health professional or healer is to recognize, validate, nurture, support, and facilitate the expression of the innate goodness and beauty of the patient and the universe. Therefore, in this model, physicians and other health professionals do not direct behavior or provide interventions; instead, they allow or provide permission to enjoy the beauty and bounty of human existence. Thus they do not extinguish negative behaviors as much as they encourage innate positive ones. Finally, I believe that all human beings have an innate desire to counter both individual and collective destructiveness and decay (entropy)—in short, to choose life over death. Engaging in the arts is thus life-affirming and life-enhancing. Neurosurgeon Dr. Michael Salcman has stated "at the heart of both the arts and the sciences is a desire to leave the world marginally better than one finds it. Thus the will to create and heal is the moral force and guiding principal of the medical profession." Finally, a fundamental theoretical consideration is the growing call for what could be referred to as the *democratization of the arts.* Judith Cornell states that the new image of humanity emerging in our century is that of the divine artist in everyone. Thus everyone can engage in the arts without fearing shame, ridicule, derision, or embarrassment. I have referred to some of these concepts as the emergence of a new paradigm of medical optimism. This paradigm is essentially one that is based on a love of life, self-determination, and responsibility, in contradistinction to our current predominant medical paradigm of pathology and paternalism, which is based on a fear of death, dependency, and victimhood. A proven and potential biological mechanism of action for arts interventions includes muscular movement, which is a central feature of expression in all the arts. Furthermore, engaging in the arts can induce relaxation and pleasure. The arts can also lead to self-knowledge, self-discovery, mood change, and emotional catharsis (e.g., weeping, laughing, sexual activity). Finally, the arts can elicit and augment spiritual and transcendental states and their associated psychological and physiological benefits.

Musculoskeletal Movement

Artistic creation involves musculoskeletal movement, which is a reaffirmation and augmentation of life force itself, because movement is central to the living state. To some degree, all expressive arts involve muscular movement. Although the most obvious is dance, movement is also involved in the making of music, singing, painting, sculpting, drama, and even the act of writing. Musculoskeletal movement involved in the creation of art may have special relevance to pediatric and geriatric populations and those categorized as having disorders of movement regardless of the specific cause.

In addition to the basic musculoskeletal and cardiopulmonary benefits of movement, from a psychiatric perspective, movement "frees up" and allows the discharge of suppressed emotions and trapped energy from psychic and somatic blocks. Such an energy release facilitates new levels of perception that may lead to integration of body, mind, and spirit. Dance therapists have stated that movement is our primary realm of expression on which all other means depend. For example, the movement impulse can be transformed into words, tones, lines, and color. Our inner experience is externalized through movement to some material apart from ourselves.

From a musculoskeletal or exercise perspective, it is said that the demands of ballet exceed those of professional football. For example, in dance, the deceleration of the "rigid" body is of the order of 40g. At the professional level virtually all forms of art require an extraordinary level of sensorimotor control, precision, speed, endurance, and strength. For example, in one study forearm blood flow changes in pianists increased an average of 232 percent over basal state blood flow rates, and cardiac index increased 62 percent at the highest stages of piano playing. Heart rates of up to 60 percent and blood pressure up to 34 percent above basal can be achieved, demonstrating that not only is forearm activity significant in piano playing but it is truly a total body experience. One of the theories also associated with longevity of orchestral conductors is the amount of musculoskeletal

movement or aerobic exercise in which conductors routinely engage as they practice their art.

In singing, so-called classic (opera quality) and "belting" (e.g., Ethel Merman) singing techniques have been analyzed by electromyography, measuring both intrinsic and extrinsic muscles associated with the act of singing.

Many studies have demonstrated the antidepressant effect of musculoskeletal movement in exercise. Exercise has been proven to be time and cost-effective compared with psychotherapy and drug treatment for depression and is potentially useful as a preventive measure for future depressive episodes. Hence exercise, including movement in the arts, may become a primary treatment of choice. Also, exercise is probably safer than a lifelong commitment to pharmacotherapy.

Relaxation Response

Herbert Benson's classic description of the relaxation response did not specifically reference the arts per se. His emphasis was on mental focusing devices and a passive attitude toward distracting thoughts. However, other authors believe that the arts, either passively experienced or actively pursued, can elicit the relaxation response. Steven Halpern has documented music's impact on the relaxation response through what he calls his "antifrenetic alternative" music, which he contrasts with other forms of New Age music. In Western culture a passive relaxation response can be supplemented with what some have called *active meditation,* in which engaging in the arts produces a timeless experience associated with deep relaxation and neurophysiological changes. Psychiatrist and music therapist John Diamond, for example, refers to the arts as the "royal yoga" or the supreme meditation.

In the music area, for example, there are three explanations for how music promotes a relaxation response. Biochemical theory states that music is the sensory stimulus that is processed through the sense of hearing. Sound vibrations are transformed into neurological impulses that activate biochemical changes either through the sympathetic or parasympathetic nervous system. Entrainment theory suggests that oscillations produced by music are received by the human energy field, and various physiological systems entrain with or match the hertz or oscillation frequency of the music. Metaphysical theory suggests that music is divine in nature and puts us in touch with or augments our spiritual selves, thus inducing a highly relaxed state.

Emotional Catharsis

Among the art's healing capacities is its ability to stimulate or augment emotion and the biological and behavioral concomitants of emotions. These range from simple mood alteration to full-blown emotional catharsis. In addition to a body of serious psychiatric literature on the complex topic of emotional catharsis, in 1985 I listed among stress-releasing techniques the so-called weep response (crying), the mirth response (laughing), and the sexual response (orgasm).

It is becoming increasingly clear that the arts can both stimulate and augment weeping, laughing, and sexual behaviors. The physiology of all three of these important human behaviors and their benefit is being increasingly studied and validated by the scientific community.

Music, poetry, and photographs can be used to stimulate conscious memories or may subconsciously precipitate sad and wistful mood changes leading to weeping. Laughing can be stimulated through all of the arts, but especially through the joy of dancing, music, theater and clowning, and popular singing such as barbershop quartets.

The capacity for stimulating healthy sexuality through tasteful art is well known, especially as it relates to the stimulatory effect of depictions of sexuality and beauty of the human form in visual arts and the enhanced libido associated with dancing.

Self-Discovery

Knowledge of oneself has been defined as a cornerstone of health in most cultures. Some authors believe it is the single most important goal of any psychotherapeutic intervention. This can be characterized as a lifelong intrapsychic discovery or "self-diagnostic process" for everyone. It is theorized that only through self-knowledge can rational, hence healthy, choices be made.

Carl Rogers, developer of person-centered psychotherapy, incorporates the belief that each individual has worth, dignity, and the capacity for expres-

sion and self-direction. Rogers' philosophy is based on a trust in the inherent impulse all human beings have toward growth and his very deep faith in the innate capacity of each person to reach toward his or her full potential. This is a major theoretical foundation for the value of expressive arts therapy. I have referred to this concept as the *doctrine of original beauty,* which states that each of us is born with beauty within us that we desire to make manifest and share during our lifetime. Furthermore, Sigmund Freud believed that love and work are central to health. I would add the word *creative* or *meaningful* before the word *work* in Freud's conceptualization.

Noted sociologist Jean Houston describes "entelechy" or the discovery and dynamic unfolding of our essence of who we are and who we are meant to be, our essence, if you will. It has long been known that the arts can play a key role in the self-discovery process. Engaging in the creative arts can provide a safe, direct path to both the personal unconscious and/or the universal collective unconscious as described by Carl Jung. It also provides a path to spiritual discovery. For example, the more one regularly creates, the more one will notice an image often repeated in various ways. That is described as the true self made visible. Lockhart states that not only specific organs but also physiological processes have the capacity to stimulate the production of psychic images meaningfully related to the type of physical disturbance and its location. This may come about by means of electrical and/or chemical messages from the diseased part of the body to the brain, which are interpreted in our minds as images. We may comprehend that the human being can and does convey through wordless communications and in his or her own idiom (the arts) both somatic and psychological conditions. Somatically, pictures, for instance, may point to events in the past relevant to anamnesis (recall), early diagnosis, and prognosis. Psychologically we may see what goes on and has been going on deep in the mind (e.g., in past traumas how drawings can help express hopes, fears, and forebodings). Furthermore, drawings can serve as bridges between the health provider and the patient, the family and the surrounding world. Indeed, their meaning and what it implies could guide the healing profession to assist especially the critically ill patient in living as near to his or her essential being as possible whether in recovery, in the midst of illness, or on being close to death. Finally we may ask how it could be that spontaneous drawings, for instance, as dreams do, reflect the total situation of a human person. D'Arcy Hayman has stated that the expressive arts give voice to the self, the highest form of individuality. Natalie Rogers, one of the founders of expressive arts therapies, says we express our inner feelings by creating outer forms. She states that expressive art refers to using the emotional, intuitive aspects of ourselves in various media. To use the arts expressively means going into our inner realms to discover feelings and to express them through visual art, movement, sound, writing, or drama. In the therapeutic model based on humanistic principles the term *expressive therapy* has been reserved for nonverbal and/or metaphoric expressions. Humanistic expressive arts therapy differs from analytical or the medical model of arts therapies in which the arts are used to diagnose, analyze, and "treat" people. Most of us have already discovered some aspect of expressive art as being helpful in our daily lives. One may doodle as one speaks on the telephone and find it soothing. One might write or keep a personal journal and find that as he or she writes, feelings and ideas change, perhaps as one writes down one's dreams and looks for patterns and symbols. One might paint or sculpt as a hobby and realize that the intensity of the experience transports him or her out of the everyday problems, or perhaps one sings while driving or going for long walks. These activities exemplify self-expression through movement, sound, writing, and art to alter one's state of being. They are ways to release one's feelings, clear one's mind, raise one's spirits, and bring oneself into higher states of consciousness. The process is indeed therapeutic, says Rogers. When using the arts for self-healing, or therapeutic purposes, the expressive arts therapist is not concerned about the beauty of the visual art, the grammar and/or the style of writing, or the harmonic flow of the song. The expressive arts therapist uses the arts to let go, to express, and to release. One can also gain insight by studying the symbolic and metaphorical messages. Art speaks back to us if we take the time to let in those messages. In regard to music, Therese Marie West states that music bypasses the intellectual defenses and goes to the nexus that connects the body, mind, emotion, and spirit. People are often afraid to experience themselves fully because of the possible pain they may discover. Music is a nonverbal form in which to explore all aspects of oneself on a multisensory level. The expressive arts thus lead us into the unconscious as

they allow us to express previously unknown facets of ourselves. This brings to light new information and awareness.

Creativity

Because it is believed to be increasingly strategic in the business world and is supported by scientific discovery, much has been written recently on the topic of creativity. Little, however, is known about the fundamental biology and health impact of creativity. Noted psychologist Abraham Maslow believed that creativity is a fundamental characteristic inherent in human beings at birth. Carl Rogers, founder of person-centered psychotherapy, stated that from the very nature of the inner condition of creativity it is clear that it cannot be forced but must be permitted to emerge. A limited amount of early childhood research has shown that exposure to and/or involvement in the arts has a potential trophic or growth influence on the brain and on the body.

In expressive arts therapies, although the expressive product itself may have value and can provide important feedback cybernetically to the individual, it is the process of creation that can be profoundly transformative. Norman Cousins described an encounter with the cellist Pablo Casals in which Cousins observed Casals at age 90 literally transformed from a frail and slow 90-year-old to a vibrant thoroughly engaged musician while playing the cello, demonstrating extraordinary intellectual and physiological performance. Cousins attributed this to Casals being thoroughly engaged in his own creativity and his desire to accomplish a specific purpose, not just a physical exercise of playing the cello. Creativity expert Mihaly Csikszentmihalyi references the term *flow* and describes creative individuals as having the personality traits of independence, self-confidence, unconventionality, alertness, ambition, commitment to work, willingness to confront hostility, inquisitiveness, a high degree of self-organization, and the ability to work effectively for long periods without sleep. Their cognitive style, the way they think, rather than their native intelligence, seems to set creative individuals apart from their peers. Intrinsic factors (a passion for pursuing a particular activity for the sake of the activity itself) rather than extrinsic factors, such as fame, fortune, status, or prizes, seem to motivate creative individuals.

Although some believe there is a correlation of creativity to mental illness or emotional pain, most experts would argue that it is unlikely that mental illness could be routinely advantageous to the creative process because the concentration required for creative endeavors is likely to be hampered by symptoms of the illness that would make "flow" difficult to achieve. A high rate of psychosis and neurosis among artists and performing artists does not mean that emotional turmoil is the source of creativity. Instead, most people who have mental illness, including major mood disorders, show little evidence of creativity.

Neurobiology of the Creative Process

The therapeutic benefits of activities that involve the experience of creativity provide powerful evidence for a biologically adaptive function that may be independent of any specific kinesthetic, visual, or musical art form. University of Tennessee ethologist Neil Greenberg believes that important insights into the nature of creativity can be obtained by looking into its biological causes and consequences. He has drawn on his work into the neuroendocrine aspects of behavior to develop a model of creativity as a highly evolved mechanism for coping with stress. In his view creativity is part of the ensemble of neurobehavioral mechanisms that enable organisms to respond to real or perceived needs of varying urgency. In other words, creativity is a key mechanism for coping with possible challenges to the dynamic balance within itself and between itself and its environment. The fullest expression of creativity involves contributions from systems that mediate affect, motivation, and cognition and that are orchestrated in large measure by the neural and endocrine mechanisms of the stress response. The needs these mechanisms address range from coping with life-threatening emergencies through the resolution of cognitive dissonance.

The well-studied selective effects of the stress response on different forms of learning and on pathologies associated with creativity such as depression and temporal lobe epilepsy provide a framework for examining the roles of ancient and recently evolved brain mechanisms in creativity.

Creativity is energized and focused by neural mechanisms yoked to hormonal responses that evolved to cope with stress and that are woven throughout the nervous system. Specific patterns of neuroendocrine responses evoked are determined by the duration and intensity of a stressor and apparent prospects for its control. Furthermore, the way the stress response is activated can determine whether creative work will be impaired or enhanced. Specific neural mechanisms involved in creativity that are believed to be affected by elements of the stress response include heightened reactivity, long-term potentiation, perceptual restructuring, and selective memory.

The study of creativity has been handicapped by its traditional focus on one element or another of the dynamic ensemble of processes that underlie it. Furthermore, the concept is torn between two points of view: (1) that creativity is only rarely expressed, and then only in gifted individuals, and (2) that it is so ubiquitous as to barely deserve special comment. Drawing on the work of Margaret Boden and working with University of Tennessee computer scientist Bruce MacLennan, a University of Tennessee computer scientist specializing in neural connectionism, Greenberg is working to bridge the gap and build a framework for understanding when and why creativity is manifest.

Tinnin has written about neurophysiology and the aesthetic response. He puts forth a theory of the aesthetic response that makes it so resistant to verbal analysis. He states that there is a mimetic response to art that is not available for verbal reflection not only because it is automatic and unintended but also because its nonverbal, cerebral initiative is actively denied by consciousness, which reflexly owns all mental initiative. Human perception of nonverbal communication, including art, is an active unconscious process in which the receiver creates the perception by active mimicry. The viewer's response to a picture, for example, begins with an active, nonverbal experience that is largely outside of consciousness and involves kinesthetic and visceral mimicry preceding verbal interpretation. The viewer circumscribes the lines and volumes with movement of the scanning eyes while mimetic movement of other body parts follows the contours of the figure. The listener's response to music is played out with movement by the head, shoulders, and other body parts. Observers of sculpture unknowingly imitate the implied movement of the sculpture. This kinesthetic imitation is automatic and unintended, and it predicts the person's pleasure in the art. Thus is it the sensation produced by mimetic motor activity combined with an emotional pattern of visceral arousal that constitutes the aesthetic experience? Any inhibition of either kinesthetic or autonomic mimicry determines the pleasure of the response to the artistic stimuli. This resistance is universal and is a necessary consequence of the ego's requisite maintenance of mental unity. Arieti defined creativity as the "magic synthesis" of primary process and secondary process thinking into what he called *tertiary process,* thus building on Freud's topographical model of the mind as consisting of conscious and unconscious portions, each with very different systems of logic. In addition to Arieti's "magic synthesis," other theorists have put forth proposals to account for creativity in terms of the conscious/unconscious dichotomy, including sexual sublimation, regression in the service of the ego, freedom from neurosis, schizophrenic thinking, and a race against the human awareness of mortality. I have put forth a potential neurophysiological definition of creativity that states that creativity is that noble and elegant neurophysiological activity that takes place within the human central nervous system when a maximal state of biochemical and bioelectric fluidity exists among all components of a human brain in its relation to a human body and the cosmos.

Pleasure and Play

There has been increasing societal acceptance in modern Western culture that pleasure is not a sin, which I believe relates to a growing fundamental shift in our view of humans as essentially good rather than evil. The role of physicians as finger waggers, admonishing patients not to succumb to their bestial instincts, is changing. Rather, physicians can trust their patients or even encourage them to engage in responsible pleasures that do not harm others or society, and a new role of the physician is to give permission, even encouragement, to enjoy the beauties and bounties of life (including the arts) without guilt. I refer to this trend as the reemergence of the paradigm of medical optimism, requiring the imperative for the inclusion of pleasure and creativity into life as a prescription for total health.

On an intuitive and anecdotal basis, the capacity for the arts to induce pleasure is well known. When journalist Bill Moyers asked me what differentiated the arts from other alternative medical interventions, I answered that among the most prominent and important capacities for the arts is the capacity to induce the state of pleasure. Although explanation of the neurophysiology of human pleasure is still in its infancy, this topic is being studied more carefully. Using research findings in the fields of medicine, biology, and psychology, Drs. Robert Ornstein and David Sobel in their book *Healthy Pleasures* have been pioneers in articulating the crucial role of pleasure in health. Dr. Sobel has defined pleasure as having a central role in human evolution in that pleasure can serve as a guide to survival behaviors. Creativity expert Mihaly Csikszentmihalyi states that eight main elements were reported repeatedly to describe how it feels when an experience is pleasurable. Among these are (1) there are clear goals every step of the way—the musician knows what note to play next; (2) there is immediate feedback to one's actions—the artist sees what color he has placed on the canvas; (3) there is a fine balance and congruence between challenge and skills; (4) action and awareness are merged; (5) abstractions are excluded from consciousness, that is, there is total engagement—the musician becomes the music, the dancer becomes the dance; (6) there is no worry of failure, and self-consciousness disappears; (7) the sense of time becomes distorted (in a positive sense), and thus dancers and figure skaters may report that a quick turn that in real time seems to take only seconds seems to stretch out for 10 times as long; (8) the activity becomes "autotelic," that is, something that becomes an end in itself. Although the arts can provide the product or even money and/or status gains, most people engaging in the arts do so because of the sheer pleasure of engaging in these activities.

Related to pleasure is the concept of play. Because stress is proven to be linked with ill health, engaging playfully in music, art, dance, poetry, and drama can move a person from puritanical emphasis on "doing something productive" into becoming a receptive being. In this state there is increased activation of the parasympathetic nervous system, which is one of the reasons why play could be so essential to health. We may seek creative experience because it is pleasurable, but pleasure, like creativity itself, exists not for its own sake but because it serves the needs of organisms to thrive and reproduce. Pleasure is nevertheless an ardently sought emotion. In 1971 Michel Cabanac derived the equation *pleasant = useful* from his extensive review of responses of people to external thermal stimuli when they possess differing internal thermal states. *Pleasure,* Robert Wright reminds us, is *not* the end purpose of life—contrary to some traditional views such as that of J.S. Mill, *pleasure is a device for steering the organism in the right direction.* Our seeking of pleasure, Wright believes, is "sponsored by [our] genes, whose primary goal . . . is to make us prolific, not lastingly happy." Pleasure is addictive; "we are designed to feel that the next great goal will bring bliss, and the bliss is designed to evaporate shortly after we get there."

The adaptive function of pleasure is also emphasized by Nesse and Berridge (1997) in their interpretation of our vulnerability to addiction. It is an emotional experience, and emotions after all "are coordinated states, shaped by natural selection, that adjust physiological and behavioral responses to take advantage of opportunities and to cope with threats that have recurred over the course of evolution. . . . Thus, the characteristics and regulation of basic emotions match the requirements of specific situations that have often influenced fitness. Emotions influence motivation, learning and decisions and, therefore, influence behavior and, ultimately, fitness."

Optimism and Hope

Hope is currently viewed as a significant determinant of health and health outcomes. Again, however, we are in the early stages of understanding the physiology of these feelings. In his book on optimism, psychologist Martin Seligman explores the limited research on optimism's impact on the immune system. The relationship of hope and optimism to health is linked also to the concept of meaning in life (Frankl). Palomore studied social factors such as work satisfaction and predictors of longevity, and Wong described the need for personal meaning in successful aging. Engaging in the arts can provide a person with a sense of hope and meaning by actively expressing the self, producing a beautiful product, and sharing it with loved ones or the public. Perhaps the most important function of the arts from a medical standpoint, however, is its revitalization function, in which the creative process itself reaffirms and augments the desire of humans to consciously and deterministically choose life over death in this critical and tenuous period in the history of human culture.

Spirituality and Transcendental States

The arts are playing an increasing role in the Western world's spiritual renewal. Addressing the National Coalition of Arts Therapies Associations (NCATA) in Washington, DC, in November of 1990, renowned psychoanalyst Rollo May described art therapists as "harbingers or sparks of a new world—a new religion based on man's endless search for beauty and the joy of human beings helping other human beings." The excesses of materialism and alienation, rebellion and shock seen in modern art (the so-called culture of transgression) is yielding to a postmodern emphasis and rebirth of arts that connect us to our spiritual selves with an emphasis on enduring values, including beauty and harmony within ourselves and within the universe. For many, engaging in the arts is fundamentally a spiritual path or transformational process, a way of being, a shift from scientism and materialism to the treatment of the soul. Michael Samuels and colleagues believe that the arts free the body's own internal healing mechanisms, uniting body, mind, and spirit as art is produced; no interpretation or therapy is necessary. The creative process itself is the healer. In music Reverend Cynthia Snodgrass states that "we need to reclaim our sound traditions. From the Genesis passages of creation to the collapsing walls of Jericho to the healing of King David, with the melodies of the harp, we must revive those testimonies from the Hebrew scriptures that stand as witness to music's power."

Deep within us Samuels believes we have a memory of the beautiful place where our spirit was given breath by traveling inward and that only through art we can experience this spiritual essence, this loving and healing force. Thus art is the voice of the spirit and is the energy of healing. Today, the artist and the healer feel the rebirth of these ancient traditions. At the source they and we are all connected. In the place of birth is the universal land, a land of awesome power and beauty. From it comes painting of stars, of swirls of light, of radiance, from that universal realm comes early movement and the softest sounds like "ohm," "amen," or "mama." Closer to the surface we find radiant colors, still abstract, and in the next world we see the birth of archetypal symbols and dream figures and finally, upward we are in "body land" and the so-called material world. Because art acts at the level of the spirit, energy is involved. Music therapist Shawn McNiff says whenever illness is associated with the loss of soul, the arts emerge spontaneously as remedies, soul medicine, if you will. Creation is interactive, and all the players are instruments of the soul's instinctual process of ministering to the self. Art historian and psychiatrist Hans Prinz has believed that patients' art was a natural antidote to schizophrenic disintegration and alienation. Louise Montello, a music therapist, writes about the loss of self or the loss of one's connection to the so-called divine child, which she believes is the root of much chronic illness. "Once the self, however, is awakened through the arts which is some sort of playful and/or prayerful activity, the healing process is awakened from within. Once there is self established, then the soul can be consciously cared for." Thomas Moore, in his famous book *Care of the Soul*, says "art is not about the expression of talent or the making of pretty things—it is about the preservation and containment of soul." Art captures the eternal in the everyday, and it is the eternal that seeds the soul. In Montello's description of working with emotionally disturbed ("soul-starved") children, she states that these children hunger for beauty, love, and goodness that art can provide. McNiff states that art as a medicine is in a postheroic phase in art's history. Individual heroics are replaced by the individuation of expression within a group that supports each member's natural and spontaneous emanations. Connection exists between our life force, our inner core or soul, the essence of all things. Therefore, as we journey inward to discover our essence or wholeness, we discover our relatedness to the outer world. The shamanic community of the creator is in our genes, is waiting to be released. This collective involvement is yet another shamanic element that survives to manifest itself in every aspect of the current application of art as medicine. Painters influence and stimulate one another with their images like musicians improvising with related sounds. Participants become what the romantic poets call "agencies of the flying sparks." Soul moves about through charges and counter-charges. In this world pathology and health are not limited to patients, they are in all of us. Tribal societies knew how to make use of those who were possessed by emotional upheavals. In contemporary Western society we do not. By trying to fix them, improve them, eliminate them, drug them, and cure

them, we are demonstrating that we have not grasped how they can help us. McNiff says that the best medicine one can offer to a troubled person is a sense of purpose, the feeling that what he or she is going through may contribute to the vitality of the community and that the process is reciprocal. During the biblical age of prophets, harp players would perform special pieces of music to produce a mental state in which extrasensory powers were thought to be activated and it is said of Elisha—"and it came to pass when the minstrel played that the hand of the Lord came upon him." David played for King Saul to help him recover from depression and paranoia. In this spiritual renaissance, especially among so-called Evangelicals, the arts are playing an increasing role in church and synagogue services throughout the world. Thus making a joyful noise unto the Lord becomes increasingly manifest in such phrases as "God respects you when you work. He loves you when you sing." Many believe the basic purpose of the creative or expressive arts therapies is to access the deepest centers of the spirit and bring back the abducted soul from the excesses of a modern excessively materialistic and increasingly uncivil society.

CURRENT PRACTICE AND GOALS

Dance and movement therapists' goals are numerous and vary according to the population served. For the emotionally disturbed, goals are to uncover and express feelings, gain insight, and develop therapeutic bonds and attachments; for the physically disabled, the goals are to increase movement and self-mastery and esteem, have fun, and heighten creativity; for the elderly, to maintain a healthy body, enhance vitality, develop relationships, and express fear and grief; and, for the mentally retarded, to motiv increase bodily awareness, and deve An underlying goal in dance and is that visible movement c chosocial potential and f by altering mood, re memories, organi ing isolation movemen such ne and joints to reduce body tension and body armoring. Other known clinical effects are the reduction of chronic pain, depression, and suicidal ideation.

Music therapy goals include physical and emotional stimulation for those in chronic pain and those with impaired movement. Music can invoke a wide range of emotional responses. It has both sedative and stimulant qualities. Music is also a unique form of communication. Music can be used with patients who are nonverbal or who have difficulty communicating, such as in autism, where there can be a facilitation of social interaction. Music can be used to express a wide range of emotions, from anger and frustration to affection and tenderness. Selecting music from an individual's past may evoke memories of times, places, events, and persons. Such memories can contribute additional information to the treatment of the individual.

Art therapy can be effectively used as a therapy and especially as a diagnostic tool. Patients may focus on parts of their bodies that unconsciously concern them, which they have been unable to verbalize. Patients may draw images about their disease processes and explore all the medical and psychological manifestations of their disorder.

Poetry therapy uses poetry for the purposes of healing and personal growth. The participant's own creative writings are viewed as avenues toward self-discovery. Poems used as a method of a life review and reminiscence have been particularly effective in assisting the elderly. A life review involves the person writing his or her own autobiography using photo albums, letters, memoirs, and interviewing techniques to gather and integrate a person's life experiences into a meaningful whole. Telling one's own "story" through poems, songs, journals, and so forth produces vital narrative material for the therapeutic process. Among the special goals of poetry therapy are to increase the patient's spontaneity and capacity for playing with words and ideas; to strengthen communication, particularly listening and speaking and writing skills; and to help the patient experience the life-giving and nourishing qualities of beautiful writing. Poems serve as catalysts to evoke feelings within and can help focus on the other person's reaction to the words. Poetry enables individuals to express experiences they may be unable to say in any other way, may be the first step in speaking about shame-subjects. The single most powerful representation through

metaphor. When patients externalize feelings into poetry, the product is a tangible, literally black and white, testament to feelings and thoughts previously without literal form. The externalization gives the participant a feeling of mastery and allows individuals to view their own feelings from a different perspective. Patients often are comforted by a poem, which they can literally carry on their persons as they do with biblical and other quotes. Poetry may have layers of meaning with an ability to conceal and reveal, thus providing both psychological closeness and distance when necessary. Reading poetry aloud together, like prayer, can build cohesion, can boost ego, and can enable individuals and groups to respond to the rhythm and beauty of the poem together.

Practices that use the techniques of imagery include biofeedback, systematic desensitization, counterconditioning, echosynthesis, neurolinguistic programming, Gestalt therapy, rational-emotive therapy, meditation, relaxation techniques, and hypnosis. Procedures for imagery fall into at least three major categories: (1) evaluation or diagnostic imagery, (2) mental rehearsal, and (3) therapeutic interventions. Techniques used in evaluation or diagnostic imagery involve asking the patient to describe his or her condition in sensory terms. Mental rehearsal is an imagery technique used before medical techniques, usually in an attempt to relieve anxiety, pain, and side effects that are exacerbated by a heightened emotional reaction. Surgery or a difficult treatment is rehearsed before the event so that the patient is prepared and is rid of any unrealistic fantasies.

Imagery as a therapeutic intervention is based on the concept that images have either a direct or indirect effect on human physiology and health outcomes. Patients are taught how to use their own flow of images about the healing process or alternatively are guided through a series of images that are intended to soothe and/or distract them to reduce sympathetic nervous system arousal or generally enhance relaxation.

Whether imagery is merely an antidote to feelings of helplessness or whether the image itself has the capacity to induce the desired physiological effect is still unclear. Existing research suggests that both conclusions are justified, depending on the particular situation being studied. Among the research accomplishments in imagery, there is a great deal of emphasis on immunology. Findings include correlations between various types of leukocytes and components of cancer patients' images of their disease, treatment, and immune system:

Enhanced natural killer cell function after relaxation and imagery training procedure with geriatric patients and in adult cancer patients with metastatic disease.

Altered neutrophil adherence or margination and white blood cell count after an imagery procedure.

Increased secretory immunoglobulin A (IgA) following training in location activity and morphology of IgA after 6 weeks of daily imaging.

The specificity of imagery training was suggested by a study on training patients in cell-specific imagery of either T lymphocytes or neutrophils. Effects of training were statistically associated with the type of imagery procedure used.

MEDICAL ART THERAPY

In 1993 a special issue of *Art Therapy* was published on the topic of art and medicine noting the term *medical art therapy* and stating that there are distinct differences between art therapy conducted in the psychiatric milieu and art therapy conducted in a medical setting because of the environmental realities and goals of each. Appleton cites the need for crisis intervention in medical art therapy as differentiated from short- or long-term psychotherapy settings. Also, the physical conditions of patients affected determine how often therapy can be presented and used. Healing is not just defined by improved blood chemistries, x-ray films, or the eradication of a tumor. Healing is the process of being made whole, physically, psychologically, and spiritually. Healing can take place even as the body weakens and dies. Thus the greatest impact of engaging in the art of expressive therapies could be the potential of these processes to synthesize and integrate patient issues such as pain, loss, and death, and the art therapies assist patients in doing this through art making and the creative process. Medical art therapy is defined as the use of art, expression, and imagery with individuals who are physically ill, experiencing trauma to the body, or undergoing aggressive medical treatment such as surgery or chemotherapy. In some cases in which the patient is fragile and susceptible to infection, the therapist must be cognizant of maintaining a sterile environ-

ment through the appropriate use of art therapy media and tools. At other times the patient may be unable to participate actively without physical adjustments such as arranging for the therapist to be at the bedside or creation of special devices to assist the patient in the creative act. Other art therapists have discussed necessary adaptations in art experiences for patients with dementia and for pediatric patients who have experienced serious burns. Art therapy with pediatric cancer patients may be offered in the hospital waiting room, where children await chemotherapy and radiation treatments or checkups. Family, including siblings, may be present and may become part of the art therapy, but confidentiality is not easily maintained in this type of open environment where patients come and go at will and where art therapy essentially takes place in a quasipublic arena such as a waiting area or at a bedside.

RESEARCH

Advances in neuroscience, psychoneuroimmunology, and psychoneurocardiology, have provided necessary tools to engage in solid scientific research on creative and expressive arts therapies. The impact of music in particular on human physiology has been well studied and demonstrates great promise. For instance, music's capacity as an analgesic or anxiolytic agent is well documented as is the impact of music on mood. Music has been studied with burn patients, the terminally ill, and patients with cerebral palsy, stroke, and Parkinson's disease. The impact of music on the immune system has also been studied, including the impact on patients with acquired immunodeficiency syndrome (AIDS) and on patients with other immune disorders. Furthermore, music has been studied extensively among the elderly as a means to improve quality-of-life measures. Other studies have demonstrated the effect of music on physiological measures such as galvanic skin response, vasoconstriction, muscle tension, respiratory rate, heart rate variability, pulse rate, and blood pressure. Music has been used to relieve anxiety and depression in coronary care units and to promote recovery from heart attacks. It has also been shown that listening to different types of music can lower levels of the stress hormones cortisol, adrenaline, and noradrenaline and increase levels of atriol and natriurectic peptide, a potent antihypertensive hormone produced by the atria of the heart. Neurophysiology researchers have postulated that music affects brain function in at least two ways: (1) it acts as a nonverbal medium that can move through the auditory cortex directly to the limbic system (an important part of the emotional response system), and (2) it may stimulate the release of endorphins, thereby allowing these polypeptides to act on specific brain receptors. This theory is supported by direct recording of neuronal discharge rates while listening to music. However, because music can alter mood and emotional states, it is also likely that the immune and hormonal changes seen after subjects listen to music are mediated by the autonomic nervous system. The Institute of Heart and Math previously investigated the effects of music on autonomic activity with powered spectral density analysis of heart rate variability and of immunity, measuring levels of secretory IgA from saliva samples. This work demonstrated a relationship between increased autonomic activity and increased salivary IgA. The term *designer music* was introduced by the music industry to describe a new genre of music designed to affect the listener in specific ways. This term has also been used in the scientific literature to specify this type of music. Research and clinical studies have shown that so-called designer music produces a significant effect on listeners' physiological and psychological status. After U.S. Senate hearings in 1991 on the impact of music on the elderly, the Older Americans Act Amendments of 1992 listed music therapy as both a supportive and preventive medical service. Furthermore, among the initial grants of the National Institutes of Health Office of Alternative Medicine was one to investigate the effects of specific music therapy interactions on empirical measurements in persons with brain injuries. In the visual or "plastic" art therapy field, research has occurred on psychiatry and burn patients; on patients with eating disorders, chemical addictions, deafness, aphasia, and autism; and as a prognosticator in childhood cancer, in childhood bereavement cases, and in sexually abused adolescents. The visual arts, because they produce a permanent visual "record," lend themselves to high-quality research in art as a diagnostic tool. Dance therapy research has demonstrated clinical efficacy in ameliorating depression; decreasing bodily tension; expressing anger; reducing chronic pain; and enhancing circulatory, respiratory, and musculoskeletal function.

Although music and the other arts have been used successfully as treatment modalities for mood and other psychiatric disorders and medical conditions, there remains uncertainty as to how such effects are mediated within the brain. There is speculation that benefits are achieved through music's ability to directly modify the neuronal substrates (neurological locii) of affective states, which then have widespread effects on the autonomic, hormonal, and immunological mechanisms of the body. In dance, studies could be done to quantify specific components of dance, including exercise, social contact, bonding, spontaneous versus instructional dance, male-female relationships versus male-male or female-female dancing versus group dancing, touch versus no touch dancing, with and without music, and so on. Manfred Clynes postulates so-called essentic forms, which he describes as "biologically given expressive dynamic forms for a specific emotion" and theorizes that the neurobiological process of recognition of pure emotion essentic forms may release specific substances in the brain, which then act to transmit and activate those specific emotional experiences. The so-called iso principle, first described in 1948, seeks to match the musical mood of the patient, which helps him or her gain insight into internal thoughts and memories. These concepts require further research.

Entrainment, as noted earlier, is an aspect of sound that is closely related to rhythm and the way these rhythms affect human beings. Powerful rhythmic vibrations of one object will cause the less-powerful vibrations of another object to quote "lock in step" and oscillate at the same frequency. The music potential (rider) lies with the fact that the hypothalamus has strong connections to the limbic system. Thus the connection between music and health is very likely to have a mechanism involving a "neural" hypothalamic frontal limbic loop and a neuroendocrine hypothalamic-immunological loop.

New research is beginning to explain the physiology of hope and positive expectations. In one series of studies, patients entering the hospital for open-heart surgery or surgical repair of a detached retina were evaluated before and after surgery. Those who expressed greater optimism regarding surgical results, confidence in the ability to cope with the surgical outcome, and trust in their surgeon recovered more quickly. Among patients undergoing heart surgery, death rates were lower. Hopeful expectations in another study may also predict who has cancer of the cervix. The more optimistic the woman, the less likely she was to have cervical cancer.

A study of patients with advanced breast and skin cancer revealed that a joyful attitude and optimistic style were the strongest psychological predictors of how long patients would remain cancer free before the disease returned. Webster says optimism is "an inclination to anticipate the best possible outcome—a tendency to seek out, remember and expect a pleasurable experience." Optimists have a high level of so-called locus of control and feel challenged, not threatened, by the current environment and the future. Also related to optimism is the capacity for love. Bernie Siegel has stated that if he teaches AIDS patients to love themselves and others fully there is an automatic increase in the immune globulins and killer T cells. Green and Shilenberg defined love as a positive energy and presented data from several sources including psychology, sociology, medicine, epidemiology, and healing to explain the healing-promoting effects of love and the psychophysiological, psychophysical, and psychosocial behavioral processes involved with this phenomenon. In the aesthetic paradigm, where the arts are used, unlike the athletic or militaristic paradigm, the fundamental goal of the artist is to communicate, share, or even love compared with the athlete or soldier whose fundamental purpose is to compete or even destroy.

Another interesting article titled "Putting Stress into Words" published in the *Journal of Health Promotion* by Francis Pennebaker of Southern Methodist University in Dallas indicated that individuals who wrote about upsetting personal events evidenced significant changes in psychometric surveys and selected serum chemistry measurements compared with those who wrote about nontraumatic topics. This has implications for creative writing and poetry.

In summary, generally, research issues in creative or expressive arts therapies for the future could include the following: (1) What is the impact of aesthetic stimuli, including color, form, sound, rhythm, movement, words, or even beauty itself on human physiology? (2) Specifically, how does the human brain perceive, process, integrate, and/or react to aesthetic stimuli? (3) What is the neurophysiological nature of creativity and its relationship to human health? (4) What are the biopsychosocial characteristics of living, performing, and visual artists as they re-late to a more complete understanding of the limits of human capacities? (5) How can the study of highly successful elderly artists and performers contribute to understanding the role of the arts in the aging process? (6) How can the arts be effectively used to enhance early brain development and early childhood education? (7) How can the arts contribute to the development of individual and cultural self-esteem in that self-esteem is increasingly viewed as central to the development of mental health and cultural well-being? (8) How can the arts be used to improve diagnostic and prognostic capabilities in medicine? (9) Which already-developed models are most promising for the successful integration of the arts to improve the environmental quality of health care settings? and (10) What specific steps must be taken to ensure inclusion of arts medicine topics in formal art or medical curricula?

SPECIAL POPULATIONS

Although the expressive arts therapies can be applied to most patients in most medical settings, they are of special value to the following special patient subgroups:

Pediatrics: Children are by definition more freely expressive and in the early years less verbal than other medical populations. Children also can engage in creative play more easily.

Geriatrics: The geriatric population is especially vulnerable to the excesses of pharmacological and surgical interventions. The arts can serve as an alternative and/or supplement. Also, musculoskeletal movement associated with expressive arts in this population can be a fundamental therapeutic goal. Finally, disorders of the central nervous system, especially those associated with memory loss (e.g., Alzheimer's disease) seem to be differentially benefitted by creative or expressive arts therapies.

AIDS patients: Since the AIDS epidemic became manifest in the early 1980s, the expressive arts have played a key role in assisting patients, their loved ones, and their families in dealing with this devastating disease. Much art has been produced by and for patients with AIDS. This in part is due to the differential effect that this disease has had on the artistic workforce sector. The famous AIDS quilt project is an example of this phenomenon.

Health professionals: Health professionals have always been subject to differential physical and psychological stresses inherent in their profession. Increased incidences of serious forms of psychopathology, sociopathy, and burnout are seen in these populations. Also disabled or ill health professionals can cause significant harm to patients in their charge. In recent years a massive transition in the enterprise of health care has added additional transition and career stresses to health professionals. On the positive side, same studies have demonstrated that physicians in particular possess differential creative skills. It is for these reasons that health professionals are encouraged to engage in the arts, especially as a stress-reduction technique or for stress prevention. Also, when physicians engage in the arts, they share and demonstrate their common humanity with their patients. Contemporary physician/poet John Graham-Pole says "such self-revealing [writing poetry] opens my vulnerability to others, helps me lick my wounds without leaving a scar, washes me clean, releases my tensions, redresses my balance, captures painful and delicious sense, validates me as a sentient human being."

Chronic diseases and chronic pain: Engaging in the arts by individuals with these disorders provides hope, pleasure, beauty, and quality of life to individuals who are coping with chronic disease and chronic pain syndromes.

The dying: Faced with the realization of imminent mortality, dying patients often seek to resolve lifelong psychosocial and, of great importance, spiritual issues. This can be greatly facilitated and enhanced through artistic expression. Dying patients often express lifelong conflicts and desires through artistic expression. Also, the creation of artistic products allows the dying patient to leave something of value to loved ones, friends, and society-at-large. Finally, the product of self-generated art often puts beauty, joy, and meaning into the last days of the dying patient's life. Dying patients often are depressed and may be in pain. The arts can assist with these conditions as well.

CONCLUSION

As the excesses of the predominant scientific and theoretical paradigms in medicine yield to the new and emerging paradigms, the application of the arts will play an increasing role in health in the broadest sense of the term. We are entering into an era where art is viewed as a major positive force able to unlock each human being's potential for goodness and individual growth reflected in a healthier society composed of remoralized, revitalized, healthier human beings.

The arts will continue to unfold as a major cost-effective contribution to individual, institutional, and societal health. Researchers, educators, and practitioners and those who pay for and regulate these endeavors will increasingly appreciate the role that the arts can play in producing healthy individuals, healthy families, healthy communities, healthy schools, healthy workplaces, and a healthy planet.

Acknowledgments

I wish to acknowledge the following individuals and organizations for their assistance in the preparation of this chapter: Natalie Rogers, Author of Creative Connection,® Neil Greenberg, University of Tennessee; Susan Kleinman, Chair of NCATA; Alicia Seeger, Administrator of NAPT; Eric Miller of Expressive Therapies Concepts and the entire creative arts therapy community on whose shoulders the modern arts-medicine movement stands; my physician colleagues within the arts-medicine movement, including John Graham-Pole, John Diamond, Sheila Katz, Michael Samuels, Patch Adams, Michael Salcman, Eric Avery, Joel Elkes, Ralph Spintge, Yoshihito Tokuda, and Itzhak Siev-Ner, also, David Hinkamp from the ACOEM Section on Arts-Medicine and Naj Wikoff from the Koop Institute. From the hospital arts movement, Janice Palmer and John Feight. My colleagues in IAMA; Allegheny University Arts in Therapy Program Directors Ronald Hayes, Paul Nolan, and Sherry Goodill; Marjorie Smink of the College of Physicians of Philadelphia, Section on Arts-Medicine; the leaders of the Office of Alternative Medicine (NIH OAM), Joe Jacobs, Alan Trachtenberg, and Wayne Jonas. I wish to thank Karen Barton, Robert Hand, and Roberta Dougert for assistance in the preparation of this manuscript.

Appreciation to my wife, Lynn Lippin, for her patience with me and her love and, most of all, to my colleague, trusted advisor, and close friend, Marc Micozzi, for providing this opportunity.

Suggested Readings

Achterberg J. 1985. Imagery and Healing: Shamanism and Modern Medicine. New Science Library. Boston

Ackerman D. 1990. A Natural History of the Senses. Random House. New York. pp. 175-285

Anonymous. 1992. Alternative Medicine: Expanding Medical Horizons. A Report to the National Institutes of Health on Alternative Medical Systems and Practices in the United States. Prepared under the auspices of the Workshop on Alternative Medicine, Chantilly, Virginia, September 14-16, 1992. pp. 25-30

Anonymous. 1993. AIDS and the arts. Newsweek. January 18, pp. 16-23

Arieti D. 1976. Creativity: The Magic Synthesis. Basic. New York. pp. 16-20

Benson H, Beary JF, Carol MP. 1974. The relaxation response. Psychiatry. 37:37-46

Benson H, Stuart EM. 1992. The Wellness Book. Birch Lane Press. New York. pp. 33-65, 121

Bertman SL. 1991. Facing Death: Images, Insights, and Interventions: A Handbook for Educators, Healthcare Professionals, and Counselors. Hemisphere Publishing Corporation. New York. pp. 1-9, 169-200

Bonny H. 1978. Music listening for intensive coronary care units: A pilot project. In: Music Rx. A Tape Set with Accompanying Booklet. Institute for Consciousness and Music. Port Townsend, Washington

Cabanac M. 1971. Physiological role of pleasure. Science 173:1103-1107

Campbell D. 1991. Music: Physician for Times to Come. Quest Books. Wheaton, Illinois

Campbell DG. 1989. The Roar of Silence: The Healing Powers of Breath, Tone, and Music. Theosophical Publishing House. Wheaton, Illinois

Clynes M (ed). 1982. Music, Mind, and Brain: The Neurophysiology of Music. Plenum Press. New York

Cousins N. 1979. Anatomy of an Illness as Perceived by the Patient. WW Norton. New York. pp. 72-87

Csikszentmihalyi M. 1990. Flow: The Physiology of Optimal Experience. Harper & Row. New York

Csikszentmihalyi M. 1996. Creativity: Flow and the Psychology of Discovery and Invention. HarperCollins Publishers. New York. pp. 58-76, 110-113

Davis W, Thaut M. 1989. The influence of preferred relaxing music on measures of state anxiety, relaxation, and physiological responses. J Music Ther 26:168-187

Estill J. 1988. Belting and classic voice quality: some physiological differences. Medical Problems of Performing Artists 3(1):37-43

Fox J. 1992. The healing pulse of poetry: the life-giving power of your own words. The Quest (Autumn): 65-70

Goodill SW, Morningstar DM. 1993. The role of dance/movement therapy with medically involved children. Int J Arts Med 2(2):24-27

Gorelick K. 1989. Poetry on the final common pathways of the psychotherapies: private self, social self, self-in-the-world. J Poetry Ther 3(1)

Graham-Pole J. 1997. Why I write poetry. Int J Arts Med 5(1):34-39

Greenberg N. 1997. Creativity: The adaptationist view. University of Tennessee University Studies Colloquy on Creativity working paper. Published on the Worldwide Web at http://utk-biogw.bio.utk.edu/Neils.nsf/

Hanna JL. 1995. The power of dance: health and healing. J Alternative Complementary Med 1(4):323-331

Hanser S. 1989. Music therapy with depressed older adults. In Spingte R, Droh R (eds). Music Medicine. [proceedings] International Society for Music in Medicine. IV. International MUSICMEDICINE Symposium. Rancho Mirage, California, October 25-29, 1989, pp. 3-5, 10-11, 149-150, 195-196

Harvey A, Rapp L. 1988. Music soothes the troubled soul... Ad Nurse March/April:19-22

Hayman D. 1969. The Arts and Man: A World View of the Role and Function of the Arts in Society. Prentice Hall. Englewood Cliffs, New Jersey

Higgins JM. 1997. Escape from the Maze: 9 Steps to Personal Creativity. The New Management Publishing Company. New York

Houston J. 1982. The Possible Human: A Course in Enhancing Your Physical, Mental, and Creative Abilities. J. P. Tarcher. Los Angeles

Johnson DR. 1988. Introduction to the special issue—creative arts therapists as contemporary shamans: reality or romance? The Arts in Psychotherapy 15:269-270

Laws K. 1986. Physics and the potential for dance injury. Medical Problems of Performing Artists 1(3):73-79

Laws K. 1988. The physics and forces of partnered lifts in dance. Medical Problems of Performing Artists 3(3):88-93

Leedy JJ. 1985. Poetry as Healer: Mending the Troubled Mind. Vanguard. New York, pp. 200-212

Lerner A, Mahlendorf UR (eds.). 1991. Life Guidance Through Literature. American Library Association. Chicago

Lippin R. 1985. Arts medicine: a call for a new medical specialty. Philadelphia Medicine. 81:14-15

Lippin R. 1991. A message from the president of IAMA. Int J Arts Med 1(1):4-7

Malchiodi California. 1993. Introduction to special issue: art and medicine. Art Therapy 10(2):66-69

Malchiodi California. 1993. Medical art therapy: contributions to the field of arts medicine. Int J Arts Med II(2):28-31

Malchiodi California. 1994. Commentary on "Art for Recovery": using art to humanize the medical milieu. Int J Arts Med 3(1):24-25

McCraty R, Barrios-Choplin B, Atkinson M, Tomasino D. 1998. The effects of different types of music on mood, tension, and mental clarity. Alternative Therapies 4(1):75-84

McNiff S. 1981. The Arts and Psychotherapy. Charles C Thomas. Springfield, Illinois

McNiff S. 1992. Art as Medicine: Creating a Therapy of the Imagination. Shambhala. Boston. pp. 1, 14-17, 22, 25

Montello L. 1992. Arts medicine. Int J Arts Med 1(2):33-34

Montello L. 1994. Arts medicine editorial. Int J Arts Med 3(2):34-35

Moore N. 1998. Alternatives. Alternative Therapies. 4(1): 37-40

Nemetz LD. 1995. Dance/movement therapy: speaking the language of self. Int J Arts Med 4(2):26-31

Ornstein R, Sobel D. 1989. Healthy Pleasures. Addison-Wesley. Menlo Park, California

Palmer J, Nash F. 1991. The hospital arts movement. Int J Arts Med 1(1):34-38

Palomore EB. 1995. Physical, mental and social factors in predicting longevity. American Psychological Association. Sum. Vol. 9(2 Pt. 1):103-108

Panksepp J, Bekkedal MYV. 1996. The affective cerebral consequence of music: happy vs sad effects on the EEG and clinical implications. Int J Arts Med 5(1):18-27

Parr SM. 1988. The effects of graduated exercise at the piano on the pianist's cardiac output, forearm blood flow, heart rate, and blood pressure. Medical Problems of Performing Artists 3(3):100-104

Pennebaker JR, Francis ME. 1992. Putting stress into words: the impact of writing on physiological, absentee, and self-reported emotional well-being measures. Am J Health Promot 6(4):280-287

Pratt RR. 1985. The history of music and medicine. In Pratt RR (ed). The Third International Symposium on Music in Medicine, Education, and Therapy for the Handicapped. University Press of America. Lanham, MD. pp. 237-268

Pratt RR. 1992. Healing and art. Int J Arts Med 1(2):3

Pratt RR. 1992. The new interface between music and medicine. In: Spingte R, Droh R, eds. Music Medicine. MMB Music. St. Louis 2:6-18

Pratt RR, Tokuda Y (eds.). 1997. Arts Medicine. [proceedings] First U. S./Japan Arts Medicine Leadership Conference. Tokyo, 8–9 October 1993. MMB Music, Inc. St. Louis

Reiter S. 1984. Enhancing the quality of life for the frail elderly: Rx: the poetic prescription. Journal of Long-Term Home Health Care 13(2)

Rogers CR. 1951. Client-centered Therapy: Its Current Practices, Implications, and Theory. Houghton Mifflin. New York

Rogers CR. 1961. On Becoming a Person. Houghton Mifflin. Boston

Rogers CR. 1980. A Way of Being. Houghton Mifflin. Boston

Rogers N. 1993. The Creative Connection: Expressive Arts as Healing. Science & Behavior Books. Palo Alto, California. pp. 1-9, 50-64, 86-90

Salcman M. 1992. Presidential address: The education of a neurosurgeon: The two cultures revisited. Neurosurgery 31(4):686-696

Samuels M. 1991. Art as a Healing Force. Published on the occasion of the exhibition *Art as Healing Force,* organized by the Bolinas Museum. March 1-April 21

Sataloff RT, Brandfonbrener AG, Lederman RJ (eds.). 1991. Textbook of Performing Arts Medicine. Raven Press. New York. pp. 30-31

Schindler AG. 1996. Contemplating Creativity. In: Encyclopedia Britannica. 1997 Medical and Health Annual. Chicago. pp. 44-61

Seligman M. 1990. Learned Optimism. Knopf. New York. pp. 168-177

Siegel B. 1987. Images in Disease and Healing. In: Siegel. Love, Medicine, and Miracles. Harper & Row. New York. pp. 50-51, 157-160

Sobel R. 1989. Healthy Pleasures. Addison-Wesley. Philadelphia. pp. 168-169, 277-282

Spencer MJ. 1996. Live Arts Experiences: Their Impact on Health and Wellness: A Work in Progress. Hospital Audience. New York. pp. 49-72

Spingte R. 1982. Psychophysiological surgery preparation with and without anxiolytic music. In: Droh R, Spingte R (eds.). Angst, Schmerz, Musik in der Anasthesie. Editiones Roche. Basel. pp. 77-88

Spingte R, Droh R (eds.). 1989. Music Medicine. [proceedings] International Society for Music in Medicine. IV. International MUSICMEDICINE Symposium. Rancho Mirage, California, October 25-29, 1989, pp. 3-5, 10-11, 149-150, 195-196.

Standley J. 1989. Meta-analysis of research in music and medical treatment effect size as a basis for comparison across multiple dependent and independent variables. In: Spingte R, Droh R (eds.). Music Medicine. [proceedings] International Society for Music in Medicine. IV. International MUSICMEDICINE Symposium. Rancho Mirage, CA, October 25-29 pp. 364-378

Stoll B. 1991. Art Therapy: From Isolation to International Visibility. Int J Arts Med 1(1):27-32

Storr A. 1992. Music and the Mind. Ballantine Books. New York. pp. 12-13

Tinnin L. 1990. Biologic processes in nonverbal communication and their role in the making and interpretation of art. Am J Art Ther 29:9-13

Tinnin L. 1991. Creativity and mental unity. Perspect Biol Med 34:347-354

Tinnin LW. 1992. The Neurophysiological Process of Mimicry as a Model for the Aesthetic Response. Presented at the MedArt International World Congress on Arts and Medicine, New York, February 1992

Turner SS. 1989. Expression Through Dance for the Well-Elderly. In Spingte R, Droh R (eds). Music Medicine. [proceedings] International Society for Music in Medicine. IV. International MUSICMEDICINE Symposium. Rancho Mirage, California, October 25-29, 1989, pp. 3-5, 10-11, 149-150, 195-196

Wikström B-M, Theorell T, Sandström S. 1992. Psychophysiological effects of stimulation with pictures of works of art in old age. International Journal of Psychosomatics 39(1-4):68-75

Wong PTP. 1989. Personal meaning and successful aging. Canadian Psychology 30:3

Zhuo D. 1992. The tradition of music therapy in the People's Republic of China. Int J Arts Med 1(2):4-6

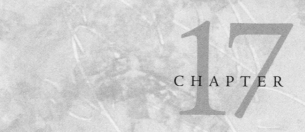

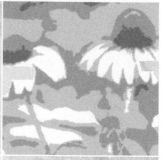

Humor as Context and Therapy

PATCH ADAMS, WILLIAM F. FRY,
LEE GLICKSTEIN, ANNETTE GOODHEART,
CHRISTIAN HAGESETH III, RUTH HAMILTON,
ALLEN KLEIN, VERA M. ROBINSON,
PATTY WOOTEN

The arrival of a good clown exercises a more beneficial influence upon the health of a town than of twenty asses laden with drugs.

—THOMAS SYDENHAM, MD,
SEVENTEENTH-CENTURY PHYSICIAN

*B*efore tackling what humor therapy might be, I would like to introduce where I think it fits into complementary medicine in a discussion on wellness or preventive medicine. Allopathic medicine has generally ignored this field. What could be more complementary to any system of disease care than a sound emphasis on being well? As the economic crisis in medicine worsens, it seems both prudent and inevitable that we focus much greater attention on living healthful lives. The complementary therapies have all had a greater emphasis on wellness partly (see Chapter 1) because they fit into their more holistic approaches. Often, in spending more time with patients, the intimacy that happens leads toward a compassionate desire to help the patient feel better. The primary care health provider clearly sees the difference in the way healthy people on a wellness program respond to illness from the way people respond to illness who do not do wellness care for their health. We also see less frequent illness in people on wellness programs.

WELLNESS—RECOGNIZING WHOLE POTENTIAL

Exercise and recreation are as necessary as reading. I will say rather more necessary because health is worth more than learning.

—THOMAS JEFFERSON

The practice of family medicine can be an exercise in frustration. Current medical education focuses on disease care: a patient comes to the doctor sick, does the prescribed treatment, and returns to the world. Why he or she got sick in the first place is glossed over with a few quick questions, partly because in the short dialogue between doctor and patient, there is no time to address the patient's lifestyle. I have chosen to spend long hours with patients for these past 25 years to try to understand the processes that lead to illness. In medical school, health was defined as the absence of disease, so those not complaining of symptoms were healthy. Yet, so few adults I have spoken with speak of life as a wondrous zestful journey, and most illnesses seen by a family doctor have a huge lifestyle component, frustrating the physician because they could have been prevented with self-care.

Health

Health is obviously so much more than a disease-free interlude. To be healthy is to have a body toned to its maximum performance potential, a clear mind exploding with wonder and curiosity, and a spirit happy and at peace with the world. Most adults, however, exist in a gray area between health and sickness, a zone where people say, "I'm fine," when asked how they feel. This "fine" can be chock full of disease as diverse and inhibiting as (1) the chronic fatigue or "blah" experienced by those labile fluctuations in blood sugar as a result of a high-sugar diet, (2) the foot problems that come from wearing shoes geared for fashion, not fitness, and (3) the distraction and anger that linger on after poor communication with a spouse or friend. In fact, our lifestyle is assaulting us now and anticipating future expression in disease in hundreds of silent ways.

Because wellness is the summation of all factors leading us to being healthier, this chapter can only touch, ever so briefly, on some of those of paramount importance, ideally stimulating a thirst in each person to discover individual parameters. In the wellness model, patients become responsible for their own health because health results from an active participation that only the self can give. The health professional's role then shifts from that of mechanic fixing the breakdowns to a gardener nurturing growth.

So much of illness, from minor to profound, has a powerful stress component. It is the intention of the wellness movement to offer many insights and paths to eliminate unhealthy stress and make good use of positive stress. It is time to lighten up and live life in deepest appreciation of all its gifts.

Wellness is a great investment with many repercussions. A long-term investment in good health opens the door to a lifetime of quality living for the investor. The physical body becomes the vehicle for indulging in every activity one desires, never limited because of being out of shape. However, the benefits of wellness extend far beyond the self. Family life can become a rich, creative, and happy experience on the train of communication and cooperation. The workplace can become a fun place, as a well-dressed attitude and personality help make all employees a team and every task a delight. Separating self, family, and work is arbitrary and possibly even dangerous, because the health of one so obviously has an impact on all the others. People who are at maximum health will be happier and more loving in all their relationships and hence prepared to give their best work performance. An individual striving to be healthy, full of caring and curiosity, brings loving management and creativity to the workplace. A body in tone and at proper weight is ready for the tasks at hand. If any of these areas are ignored in one's pursuit of health, the others will suffer. Studies have shown that emphasizing a human-centered, healthy workplace and providing space and time to exercise and be more personal cuts absenteeism and turnover and increases honesty and productivity.

Unfortunately one of life's ironies is that wisdom mostly comes with age. By the time we realize that a habit has profoundly hurt us, we feel helpless to change the habit, even justifying it as intrinsic to our nature. Luckily the design of a great organism is such that it can recover remarkably well; in fact, it begins to repair itself as soon as we alter the unhealthy habit. Wellness is not some kind of end product; it is a process, a journey, where each day presents its unique face, and we must choose from many choices which paths to follow. We cannot rest on the health of our past, because it must be renewed each day.

Life is a cascade of choices, and we are so much an expression of both the short- and long-term choices we make. To manage the number of choices we have to make daily, we fall into habits, and a routine substitutes for a choice. These habits can be a double-edged sword: Although it is true we do not have to concern ourselves any longer with an immediate choice, once entrenched, a habit is incredibly hard to break. When the habit is an unhealthy one and we want to break it, the task is arduous. Wellness seems like an emerging system to help people restructure or balance habits, so how we live becomes healthy, not as a task of effort but simply as a collection of positive, intentional habits. As medical practitioners focus on the causes and prevention of illness, they are finding that many major diseases could have been prevented or dramatically postponed through lifestyle changes. Most of this information has been reiterated throughout medical literature from Hippocrates to the present.

Nutrition

Take nutrition, for example. Simplified, we are a sack of water with chemicals in solution. How these chemicals interact determines what we are to be, but in many of the interactions, chemicals are used up or altered and must be replenished. Nutrition consists of the proper consumption and assimilation of foods containing those necessary chemicals. Because few foods contain all or most of the needed nutrients, we have to get them in a variety of foods. As people have moved further from food sources and food companies have changed the foods grown to have longer shelf life, our diets have changed dramatically. For the last 100 years or so, synthetic chemicals, refined foods, sugar, and salt have replaced many of the natural foods our ancestors ate.

Refined simple sugars so dominate our lives that they are ubiquitous, present even in table salt. In the United States 100 years ago, we consumed 3 pounds of sugar per person per year; we now consume 140 to 180 pounds. Many believe this has had a profound effect on our health. Certainly it plays a major role in one of the most devastating diseases—obesity. The federal government has stepped in to encourage some nutrition changes: (1) dramatic cutbacks in sugar and salt consumption, (2) increase in foods containing fiber, and (3) vast decrease in milk products and other animal fat products. I would expand on this to say eat mostly whole grains, fresh fruit, and vegetables and, if eating meats, eat mostly fish and poultry.

Exercise

If nutrition is the fuel, then exercise is the toner for the body. Modern civilization has changed few things in our lives as severely as the amount of exercise we get. We have never been as sedentary as we are today, and this, combined with dietary changes, has made much of our adult population overweight and flabby. There is a popular quip that says, "If you do not use it, you lose it." The interplay of muscles, bones, tendons, ligaments, and joints demands consistent stimulation to stay in tone. Being in shape does not mean simply being slender but having all the muscles trained. There are four kinds of exercise to consider. The body's internal toner in heart-lung (aerobic) exercise that strengthens the heart, exercises the bellows to supply oxygen to the body and rid it of carbon dioxide, and tones the muscles used in exercise, all giving the body endurance. Joint flexibility exercises, like stretching or yoga-style exercises, keep the body limber and relaxed. Strength exercises are important to tone those muscles not covered in the heart-lung exercises. Balancing exercises like dance, gymnastics, or circus skills add yet another dimension to maximum performance. Being in shape has obvious rewards as far as being physically able to do whatever you want to do, and regular exercise also has other benefits. It has been shown to lower blood pressure, to have a positive effect on mental health, to diminish stress, and to aid digestion. I believe that regular exercise does such good for the body that it appears to slow the aging process.

Emotional Life

Just as we must exercise our bodies to be fit, so must we exercise our minds to keep awake and alert. The greatest instruments for the mind's stimulation are wonder and curiosity. Boredom is a major disease, eroding the health of many adults who over time narrow their spheres of interest. Wonder and curiosity are the tools that all children carry with them in their interactions with the world. In fact, that wonder and curiosity are what make kids seem so alive. For adults, somewhere along the line, sunsets become routine and life's pace too hectic. But wonder and curiosity can be recaptured. There are no stimulants that begin to awaken a person like a new interest captivating one's life or consuming ongoing exploration. The next time a person is excited about something, instead of turning it off, jump right into it and share in their interest. Carry your wonder and curiosity into your older years and you take your youth with you. Often, having such a vibrant interest is a major impetus and motivation for staying healthy, so the exploration goes unimpeded.

It goes without saying that love is the most important wellness factor in sustaining a healthy, happy life. Love, that passionate abstract, has captured the arts from the beginning as they attempt to define and elucidate it. As a healing force, love can be defined as that unconditional surrender to the overwhelming wonderful feeling experienced in giving to or receiving from an object. We most commonly express it toward family, friends, God, self, lovers, pets, nature, or hobbies. By surrender I mean to lose oneself in awe, trust, respect, fun, and tenderness for the object of surrender. In striving for maximum wellness, one could pursue love in all the parameters just mentioned. It appears that the more one submits to unconditional love toward one object, the easier it is to do so for others. The unconditional aspect is so important because without it love is often lost to expectations, doubts, and fears.

If love is the foundation for happiness, then fun, play, and laughter are the vehicles for its expression. The great physician Sir William Osler said that laughter is the "music of life." Humor and laughter are the subject of this chapter.

Faith

Faith is the cornerstone of our inner strength. Faith is a personal, passionate, immutable belief in something of inexhaustible power and mystery. Whenever we have to face any kind of devastating change without some kind of solid belief, we become prey to confusion, fear, and panic. Often these present crises present questions that have no answers; the discomfort arising from this uncertainty is healed in the domain of our beliefs. Faith has no physical characteristics, no external requirements; it is not a commodity. To acquire a belief, one simply needs to have an interest and a willingness to submit to its mystery. Although there are many great religious traditions that promote a common interpretation of belief, I think the truth is that each person has to find an individual, meaningful faith. Faith is not summarized by a label but expressed by an inner experience of strength that lives in each, day by day.

Nature

Whereas faith is intangible, requiring sweet surrender, nature is a physical, sensual thing. Our relationship with nature has had great historical significance as part of our healthy life. It is little surprise that most symbols in early religions were from nature. Our moods are often described in terms of nature: a synonym for "happy" is "sunny." The first warm bright day after winter heightens spirits like few days of the year. Love has a metaphorical connection to the moon. Most early celebrations grew out of ties with and reliance on the seasons. We have such strong needs to connect with nature that billions of dollars are spent to bring nature into our homes in the form of pets and house plants. Medical literature is currently peppered with the therapeutic significance of putting pets in the lives of the elderly and mentally ill

Flowers are a major communication of love at sick beds, deaths, marriages, and special occasions. The few weeks we take during a year to relax on vacation are mostly spent with a natural setting in mind: the beach or the mountains, for instance. Let's face it—nature is the mother of wonder. If we are to be fully well, we need a daily communion with nature, both in the spectacular sunset and in the tenacious blade of grass as it pushes up through the sidewalk.

Creativity

Our imagination, hands, and senses are the tools for the next major wellness factor—creativity. Life is experienced as a rich journey if we believe we have a creative hand in its passage. Creativity is not just expressed through hobbies and arts but can touch every aspect of our life: our work, family, and even how we wait in line. The importance seems to be in the enjoyment of the process rather than in the quality of the final product. Creativity works like our muscles: the more it is exercised, the greater its tone. Explore the next idea, activity, or interest in your life that catches your eye. Whenever exploring, do not settle for one point of view; set it aside and insist on other perspectives. Explore the spontaneous. The key here is to be open and susceptible. Do not catalogue your hobbies and interests as indulgences; respect them as major medicines. Our interests often decline with age, and this can be deadly. Try to see each day as a building block to the next. Be sure to take advantage

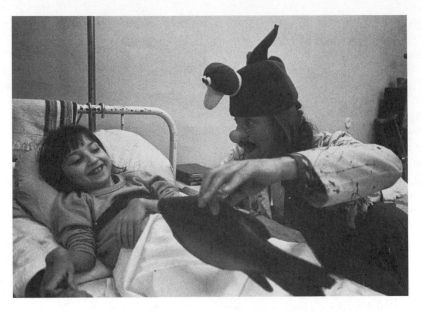

Copyright Patch Adams.

of all the human creativity in existence, because the arts give such a sense of well-being.

Service

As soon as people recognize how fortunate they are to be well, there arises the urge to give thanks. The healthy expression of that thanks is in service. Unless individuals believe they live a life of service, in whatever form suits them, I believe that they will have a hard time feeling life is ultimately fulfilling. John Donne wrote, "No man is an island," acknowledging that we are all connected in some way. It is through helping others that we find this deepest interdependence. It is important that this service be done out of thanks in the joy of giving, because service can easily slide into a debit and credit mentality. Service can take many forms, from simply being a loving friend or parent to stopping to help someone in need. These are very personal forms of service. I suggest that there is also an important wellness connection to our community and our planet.

Synergy

To these components of wellness could be added passion, hope, relaxation, wisdom, and peace. In the wellness lifestyle each of these components suggests a context in which men and women could live their lives so that they can feel healthy and that dramatically softens the experience when they do get sick. I think it safe to say that these components of wellness, regularly practiced, are healthy to individuals and families. When these two are healthier, it helps make the community and society healthier.

All of these wellness components act uniquely in each person within a specific culture, and they all act together in a person at the same time without a measurement of relative value.

Most of these wellness components are dramatically affected by the others; for example, humor is different in a jolly, friendly person than in an angry, lonely one. If one were to use these in a therapeutic way, it would make sense to have the medical environment exude these qualities to create a context of love, wonder, curiosity, and humor. This atmosphere would have a positive health effect on patients, staff, and visitors, whether in an office or in a hospital.

The examination of these wellness qualities, until the modern day, has not been by science; rather, it has been made by art, philosophy, and religions. However, some of the most exciting research in medicine today is finding the connections in biochemistry and physiology between the mind and its thoughts on the health of the body. This new field is evolving and is now popularly called *mind-body medicine* or *psychoneuroimmunology* (see Chapters 13 and 14).

HUMOR

This chapter looks at one component of wellness—humor. Many of the wellness components are difficult to measure (e.g., love, passion, faith) with some scientific precision or standard. Humor is believed to be different because it has a handle to measure it—laughter. Laughter has wide variation within genders, ages, and cultures, making actual studies point to a direction rather than establish a fact. This is one area of study in which anecdotal experience may have to count as science. I do not think one who uses humor in therapy does so because he or she found that laboratory studies showed value. Humor therapy is not a static regimen of memorized jokes and numbers of chuckles per hour. Humor therapy comes out when therapists decide to let their humorous parts join the interaction with a patient. This can be in many forms, such as laughter, theater, verbal, and physical play. With humor, the one who practices (whether laugher, funny person, clown, or comic) the craft—the laboratory—is the patient, audience, or friend. All of one's past experience in that laboratory is brought to the spontaneous act with the patient, and if it is effective, smiling and laughter occur. This positive feedback is the determining feature in reproducing the gesture, statement, or behavior that elicited the laughter. When a patient says "my doctor has a good bedside manner," he or she is not speaking about expertise but of qualities of interaction. A friendly, playful sense of humor is at the core of a good bedside manner. The patient's appreciation perpetuates the behavior. Friendship is the safest context for humor to work in, so when humor has missed its mark, instead of offense, forgiveness is felt.

A merry heart doeth good like a medicine.

—PROVERBS 17:22

History

There is little history of the use of laughter therapy. A lot of it is being made now. However, there is a large body of comments on humor and laughter from philosophy, religion, and the arts.

Arthur Koestler summarizes a fraction of these comments in his book *The Act of Creation:*

Among the theories of laughter that have been proposed since the days of Aristotle, the "theory of degradation" appears as the most persistent. For Aristotle himself laughter was closely related to ugliness and debasement; for Cicero "the province of the ridiculous . . . lies in certain baseness and deformity"; for Descartes laughter is a manifestation of joy "mixed with surprise or hate or sometimes with both"; in Francis Bacon's list of laughable objects, the first place is taken by "deformity" (Koestler, 1964).

The essence of the "theory of degradation" is defined in Hobbes's *Leviathan:*

The passion of laughter is nothing else but sudden glory arising from a sudden conception of some eminency in ourselves by comparison with the infirmity of others, or with our own formerly.

Bain, one of the founders of modern psychology, followed on the whole the same theory:

Not in physical effects alone, but in everything where a man can achieve a stroke of superiority, in surpassing or discomforting a rival, is the disposition of laughter apparent.

For Bergson laughter is the corrective punishment inflicted by society upon the unsocial individual: "In laughter we always find an unavowed intention to humiliate and consequently to correct our neighbor." Max Beerbohm found "two elements in the public's humour: delight in suffering, contempt for the unfamiliar." McDougall believed that "laughter has been evolved in the human race as an antidote to sympathy, a protective reaction shielding us from the depressive influence of the shortcomings of our fellow men."

The first to make the suggestion that laughter is a discharge mechanism for "nervous energy" seems to have been Herbert Spencer. His essay on the "Physiology of Laughter" (1860) starts with the proposition: "Nervous energy always *tends* to beget muscular motion; and when it rises to a certain intensity always does beget it. . . . Emotions and sensations tend to generate bodily movements, and . . . the movements are violent in proportion as the emotions or sensations are intense." Hence, he concludes, "when consciousness is unawares transferred from great things to small" the "liberated nerve force" will expand itself along the channels of least resistance, which are the muscular movements of laughter.

One wonders where in their descriptions appears something useful in helping patients or caregivers in the delivery of care. For this we turn to research done in the twentieth century.

Research

According to Ruxton (1988) humor can help establish rapport and verbalize emotionally charged interpersonal events. Using humor, patients may find it easier to bring embarrassing or frightening parts of their history, and with nurses using funny anecdotes and being more vulnerable with a patient, it appears to strengthen the staff-patient bond. Coser (1959) looked closely at a hospital's social structure and found that humor helped relieve tension, reassure, transfer information, and draw people together. Norman Cousins (1979, 1989) put humor back on the therapeutic map when he laughed himself well from a profound painful, chronic illness, dramatically reducing the pain of his ankylosing spondylitis. He spent the rest of his life working at the University of California School of Medicine investigating the positive emotions and their relationship to health. Dr. William Fry studied humor for 30 years and believes it is an exercise for the body. Mirthful laughter exercises the diaphragm and cardiovascular systems, initially causing an increased heart rate and blood pressure but after a short while a much longer lasting decrease in heart rate and blood pressure, a relaxation response. Paskind (1932) showed that skeletal muscle tone was diminished during mirthful laughter in muscles not actually participating in the laughter. Lloyd (1938) showed an expiratory predominance with mirthful laughter manifesting in a decrease in residual air in the lungs and increased oxygenation of the blood. From work done by Schachter and Wheeler (1962) and Levi (1965) there appears to be an elevation of catecholamines with mirthful laughter. Lee Berk will describe later the body's immune response to laughter.

Freud (1964) suggests that the psychotherapeutic use of humor causes a release of stress, tension, and anxiety. Psychotherapists use humor to facilitate insight (through metaphor, joke, or story) and offer a sense of detachment or perspective. Humor can build a tighter relationship between therapist and patient. Humor can be offered as a tool for coping with life's troubles. Mahrer and Gervaize (1974) looked at their review of the research literature on laughter in psychotherapy and found that strong laughter is a valuable indication of the presence of strong feelings and is seen by most therapeutic approaches as a desirable event. Strong laughter seems to correlate with increased self-esteem and heightened experiencing.

Although no research has conclusively shown a release of endorphins with mirthful laughter, the anecdotal literature about laughter's pain-killing properties is massive. Cousins (1979) opened this door. The Clemson nurses program did a study with elderly residents in a long-term care facility. The residents were divided into two groups. One group watched a comedy video nightly for 6 weeks; the other watched a serious drama. The nurses checked the need for analgesics. There were fewer requests for pain killers from the comedy group. Texas Tech Medical School did another test. Research participants were shown comedy or serious material for just 20 minutes. Relaxation therapy was given to another group. The researchers then determined the participants' pain thresholds using inflated blood pressure cuffs. The comedy group had the greatest pain tolerance of these groups.

I would like to relate a powerful story of a time when humor quite clearly was a pain killer.

Context

I have been doing street clowning almost daily for 30 years, increasingly all over the world. In my 25 years of being a physician I have always practiced in a humorous context. With a group called Gesundheit Institute, we are building the first hospital to fully incorporate humor. Although disconcerting at first, in the many lectures to lay and medical audiences I have given for the last 8 years about our work, when asked which ward they would choose—a serious, solemn one or a fun, silly one—more than 85 percent have chosen the fun one. Few people need more than their personal experience to be completely convinced that humor is necessary for their personal health and the health of their relationships.

The primary practice of medicine is a delicate balance between science and art. Ideally this relationship is one of friendship in which, although radically different in approach, there is a mutual appreciation for the value of all parties involved and a thankfulness and a necessity that they can work together in harmony. Science and art play different roles in the healing interaction. Medical science works at tackling the disease (the organ or systems afflicted) using a well mapped out series of thought processes, tests, and treatments. The "art of medicine" is concerned with how the disease affects the patient, the family, and their society—the larger repercussions of the disease.

These concepts are beautifully discussed in the recent books *The Illness Narratives* by Arthur Kleinman, MD, and *The Nature of Suffering* by Eric Cassell, MD. The art of medicine comes from the intuition and inherent magic found in compassion, love, humor, wonder, and curiosity. For these reasons one is hard put to break down the components or mechanics of what is working in the art of medicine. Simply put, science serves reductionism, and art serves holism. For this reason, when I do clowning, I am free to explore all of these healing abstractions. I use all of these in a multitude of combinations, not because they are well mapped out but because they can more freely arise within the clown persona.

I am both a professional clown and a physician. Each discipline took about the same number of years to master. The difficulties in becoming each were also similar. In one I had to master information and the ability to synthesize information to make responsible decisions, and in the other I had to master the art of spontaneity and freedom of behavior. I could never say which parts of my clown persona did the trick in a healing interaction, and I bet the patient could not either. I can only say that my character brings a blatant expression of love, innocence, fun, joy, and friendliness to which people readily respond.

I believe humor and love are at the core of good bedside manner, burnout prevention, and malpractice prevention, and for these alone, humor deserves a central place in a medical practice, but let us not deny its value in just raw fun. Despite my long, deep experiences with humor, I still can be brought to tears of joy over its power.

This was all brought home to me in November 1991 in a children's burn unit in a hospital in Tallinn, the capital of Estonia.

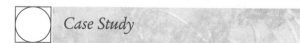

Case Study

For 4 years I have taken a group of clowns to the former Soviet Union to promote good relations between our countries, to spread good cheer, and to provide a 2-week seminar in clowning for both beginners and professionals. We clown in hospitals, orphanages, prisons, and schools, and we perform a tremendous amount in the street. Everywhere we go, patients, staff, and clowns are tremendously uplifted; at times it even seemed to help their medical problems.

Estonia was the footnote to a trip that normally just visits Moscow and St. Petersburg. I added it this year so that we could explore a new country. We arrived 25 clowns strong at the burn hospital, where right off I noticed a woman crying outside a closed door. My medical training told me that this was a mother crying so agonizingly over a severely ill child. I knew that to touch her pain I should not clown with her—but with her child. Against strong protestations from the smiling staff, I went inside the room.

I walked in on three women (one physician and two assistants) who had just begun to change dressings and perform debridement on a 5-year-old boy, Raido, with at least 60 percent third-degree burns solid from ears to knees on both sides of his body. He was in his third week of recovery. I was first struck by the medical supply and pharmaceutical shortages so devastating in the Soviet Union in the winter of 1991. There were no masks or gloves and no strong painkillers. But the work had to be done. With the utmost in loving tenderness on the staff's part and commanding bravery on the boy's, I watched the bandages come off his wound, revealing a bloody exudative, meaty field, slowly healing from the edges with no evidence of grafts. The silence was punctuated by Raido's screams with each tug of the bandages. At first I felt the horror of a parent for his suffering. From this came a gushing empathy moving the clown to act instinctively;

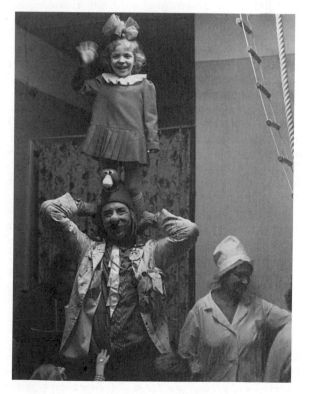

Copyright Patch Adams.

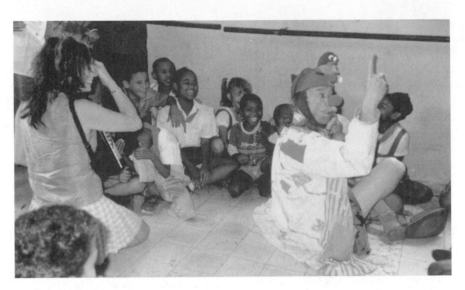

Copyright Patch Adams.

to love, comfort, care for, and bring forth laughter. Without fear.

I watched only for the first third of removal because I was not sure how to proceed. Raido's neck involvement prevented him from looking up at me. When they took a short break I went over, (dressed in full clown regalia) bent over him and smiled. Spontaneously he looked surprised and delighted and said in Estonian, "You look beautiful." My heart was captured. I immediately went around to the head of his stretcher and spent the next hour stroking his face and hair, smiling and laughing and talking with him. We played. He stopped screaming entirely. I was only 1 foot from his small unburned face, and I fell in love with him (having a 4-year-old son myself). I had never seen humor's power so raw. I kept telling him he was beautiful and strong and that he was going to live.

It is clear that the child is the one who changed himself from being sad to being cheerful. I was my clown self. His response "you're beautiful" came as a surprise. My character is not "beautiful." It was his willingness to let me inside that made me be of value to him. Another child could have been spooked and cried. Unlike an operation, the impact of humor on the patient wholly has to do with the patient.

I cannot say what I did that was, in this case, the catalyst for a pain-free experience. Was it the sparkle in my eye, the duck hat on my head, the soothing stroking of his head, the words of love and encouragement—or was it simply skilled diversion?

He asked me to come back to his room—so I wheeled his mummified body (bandages already bloody) back to his bed. There for 1 hour I entertained him with clown silliness, still peering into his sky blue eyes and stroking his face. I don't know who benefited more, because my whole body shook, thrilled for being there. I left most of my toys with Raido—even dressed up his dad like a clown while Raido laughed heartily. It was hard to leave him; I felt like he had given me so much. ∾

Humor as Therapy

So what is humor therapy? In its broadest sense it is whatever one does to put mirth into a patient encounter or hospital setting. This is a brand new field, and many are exploring how to add humor to the medical setting.

Ruth Hamilton has been using humor carts at Duke University Medical Center since 1989. Peggy Bushey is a nurse who has used the same carts in the intensive care unit at Medical Hospital of Vermont for several years. These carts have comic videos and cassettes, funny and cartoon books, props, makeup, costumes, and a host of volunteers called in on consultation for patients or staff who request it. Patients have given wonderful feedback on the painkilling and relaxing results of cart use. There is a suggestion that they improve communication, help visitors to hospitals to relax, and even increase motivation in rehabilitation programs. Greater staff relaxation may also be a factor.

Other hospitals, like Dekalb near Atlanta, have created lively rooms—like an expanded cart with all the same things and a place to use them. Of course, carts and rooms do not make humor; here the volunteer becomes the key.

Eleven years ago, Michael Christensen of the Big Apple Circus started taking clowns into children's hospitals to make regular, three-times-a-week rounds to the children. What started out as a whim for him has become a full-time passion. He now has 45 clowns in six hospitals in New York City. Clowns who have worked for him have since set up similar programs in France, Germany, and Holland. The wonderful, positive feedback by staff, patients, and family keeps this program alive.

Others, like Annette Goodheart, insist they do laughing therapy not humor therapy. There are laughter meditations and workshops on laughter and play. For many the decision has simply been how to bring more laughter, play, and levity to the medical setting. I suggest a broader view for humor therapy. In our society that harbors alienation, depression, anxiety, and boredom one could decide to be indiscriminately humorous and joyous to try to add these elements to every human encounter. I believe it would help our general societal health.

Humor therapy could include a loud bow-tie, singing on the ward, word play, cartoons put up around the hospital, and even inviting comedians to come into the hospital. One note of caution, some believe humor can be harmful in some situations, especially in psychotherapy. I would certainly suggest humor that is not racist or sexist. I suggest first becoming quite close to your patients and have them be sure of your tenderness and sincerity so that if a funny situation or joke hurts, someone can simply apologize. It behooves the medical history taker to make an exploration into the patient's sense of humor and act on it. Because humor in therapy is so new to medicine, I thought I would let a dozen of the leading voices in humor today make a few statements about their place in the use of humor. I encourage people considering putting more humor in their practice to contact the resources for much greater depth.

HUMOR THERAPY IN PRACTICE

Big Apple Circus Clown Care Unit

The Big Apple Circus Clown Care Unit (CCU) is a community outreach program of the Big Apple Circus, a not-for-profit performing arts organization presenting the finest classic circus in America. The

CCU transforms the performance of classic circus arts to aid in the care and healing of hospitalized children and teens, their parents, and caregivers.

As classic circus defines a specific body of knowledge, so too does classic clowning. The classic clown types, White, Auguste, and Eccentric, appeared as horsemen, acrobats, jugglers, dancers, musicians, and of course, actors and actresses. Using all of these skills, they had a singular focus—to make people laugh. To this end, they used parody. They parodied all circus acts, rules, structures, and authority as symbolized in one circus figure, the black-booted, top-hatted, red-coated, riding-cropped ring master.

For the Big Apple Circus CCU the hospital room replaces the circus ring; the doctor replaces the ring master; and all of the rules, charts, formulas, procedures, machines, straight-laced, white-washed corridors of the hospital become the source of endless parody. The focus is still to bring laughter to their hearts.

Using juggling, mime, music, and magic, 35 specially trained "doctors of delight" bring the joy and excitement of classic circus to the bedsides of hospitalized children 2 and 3 days each week, 50 weeks per year. The Big Apple CCU makes "clown rounds," a parody of medical rounds in which the healing power of laughter is the chief medical treatment. Using sophisticated medical-clown techniques (including red nose transplants, rubber chicken soup, and kitty cat scans), professional CCU performers work one-on-one with hospitalized children, their parents, and caregivers to ease the stress of serious illness by reintroducing laughter and fun as natural parts of life.

In the Beginning

The CCU was created in 1986 by Michael Christensen, Director of Clowning at the Big Apple Circus, in cooperation with the medical staff at Babies & Children's Hospital of New York at Columbia-Presbyterian Medical Center. The first CCU clowns, "Dr. Stubs" and "Disorderly Gordon," learned that they could reduce children's fears about their hospital experiences by using medical instruments as props (e.g., blowing bubbles through a stethoscope) or performing silly medical procedures that echo real medical procedures (e.g., chocolate milk transfusions). The "red-nose transplant," for example, was created specifically to ease the fears of heart transplant patients at Babies & Children's Hospital.

At every CCU host-hospital the medical staff has recognized the healing effect of the CCU—how joy and delight relieve the stress of pediatric patients and their worried parents; how music, magic, and mayhem in the halls make patients easier to treat and enhance the effectiveness of the medical staff; how a happy child appears to get better faster. Dr. Driscoll, Chairman of Pediatrics at Babies and Children's Hospital of New York, stated in a recent news article, "When a child begins to laugh, it means he's probably beginning to feel better. I see the clowns as healers. When someone gets around to studying it, I wouldn't be at all surprised to see a connection between programs like the CCU and shorter hospital stays."

In addition to numerous news articles and television features, Michael Christensen and the CCU have received wide public recognition for their innovative work in the field of health and humor including the prestigious *Raoul Wallenberg Humanitarian Award,* the *Red Skelton Award,* and the Northeast Clown Convention's annual *Gold Nose Award.*

Resident Hospital Programs

The Big Apple Circus currently operates CCU programs in seven prominent metropolitan hospitals: Babies & Children's Hospital of New York at Columbia-Presbyterian Medical Center, Harlem Hospital Center, The Hospital for Special Surgery, Memorial Sloan-Kettering Cancer Center, Mount Sinai Medical Center, New York University Medical Center, and Schneider Children's Hospital of Long Island Jewish Medical Center. Each CCU clown team works under the direct supervision of the hospital's Chief of Pediatrics.

In addition, the CCU is resident each summer at Queens Hospital Center and Paul Newman's Hole in the Wall Gang Camp for children with cancer and chronic blood diseases.

Working in close partnership with the medical staff at each hospital, the CCU tailors its activities to meet the special needs of each facility. The supervising clown consults daily with nurses, child life staff, and chief residents on the status of individual children. The clown team visits children in all areas of the hospital, including at their bedsides in wards, in intensive care units, and in clinic and acute care waiting rooms. The CCU clowns also visit specialty clinics such as the bone marrow transplant unit at Memorial Sloan-Kettering Cancer Center and the HIV/AIDS clinic at Harlem Hospital.

All CCU clowns are professional performers who have been auditioned and selected for their professionalism, artistry, and sensitivity. They undergo a rigorous CCU training program to prepare them for working safely and appropriately in the hospital environment. The CCU continually improves its level of quality through rehearsals, continuing education, and procedural and artistic reviews.

The CCU has plans to expand to preeminent children's hospitals in major cities throughout the country. Affiliate programs begun by Big Apple Circus CCU-trained performers currently operate in Paris, France; Sao Paulo, Brazil; and Wiesbaden, Germany.

If you would like further information about the CCU, please contact us:

Big Apple Circus Clown Care Unit
35 West 35th Street, 9th Floor
New York, New York 10001
(212) 268-2500

THE GROWING WORLD OF HUMOR

When I first started my humor studies in 1953, there was a vast dearth of scientific investigation of the subject. Literary analyses of humor and comedy abounded, there was ample hypothesizing and theorizing, particularly around the question of what is the crucial element of humor that precipitates the mirthful reaction. And there were a few psychological and anthropological studies that carried out examinations of humor preferences, humor values, interactive uses of humor, communication, and humor. That is as close as we got to science. Mind you, it was not a complete wasteland, but it looked like an Edward Hopper canvas; it certainly was not Times Square at midnight on New Year's Eve.

I had entered the field through the gate of humor and communications, as a member of ethnologist Gregory Bateson's research team. The research team had been originally assembled by Gregory to explore the roles of the "paradoxes of logical type" in communication (Fry, 1971). As a psychiatrist, I was the team member with training most closely related to the so-called hard sciences, with university classes in a large variety of chemistries, physics, embryology, bacteriology, laboratory technology, physiology, and biochemistry. The scientific method had been portrayed to me as the criterion for research purity and rigor. I did and still do hold the scientific method in high respect. During my psychiatric residency I had exercised my understanding of scientific discipline by designing, conducting, and reporting in the literature a postdoctoral psychophysiological study of schizophrenia.

In the 1950s a certain excitement had been stirred in the humor studies field by psychologist D. E. Berlyne, a very talented and innovative scholar. Up to the time of his contributions, humor theory was strongly dominated by the views Freud had adopted from philosopher Herbert Spencer's "discharge of energy" postulate (Bainy, 1993). This dominance directed most views of humor to observing it primarily as a cathartic phenomenon, a sudden diminution of repressed psychic energy involving a release from inhibition. Berlyne's contribution shifted emphasis to the state of arousal, which he proposed to be the dominant element of the humor response—"laughter . . . is restricted to situations in which a spell or moment of aversely high arousal is followed by sudden and pronounced arousal reduction" (Berlyne, 1972). Needless to say, this attempt to supplant Freud's doctrine aroused much controversy and energy. Some of the energy was channeled into research procedures aimed at proving or disproving one or the other of the main themes and their various corollaries. As these experiments proceeded and were reported in the scientific literature, I became increasingly distressed by what I perceived as defective protocols, in that much of the test ratings were based on what were in my perception subjective and vaguely defined and arbitrary criteria; in many instances test results were measured by degrees of humor identified as "much," "moderate," or "slight"—or by some similar system. I believed that conclusions based on these studies were flawed by deficiencies of objectivity. I agonized over this scientific design issue for many months, even several years into the 1960s.

I finally came to the conclusion that the best readily available source of objectivity in humor experimentation would be the physiological phenomena that both the Freudians and the Berlynians agreed accompany the perception of humor and the experiencing of reactive mirth. A National Institutes of Mental Health Small Grant in 1963-1964 made it possible for me to develop an answer to the question of whether it is possible to observe experimentally the somewhat ephemeral physiology of mirth in such artificial and

rigid environments as those that often develop in scientific pursuits (when the fun of science is lost sight of or is ignored). The outcome of my feasibility exploration was "certainly yes" and, after wasting months during the Vietnam War buildup time futilely trying to obtain financial support from government scientific agencies (when armaments had so much greater priority than laughter) I got to work on designing and carrying out a series of basic science studies of the physiology of mirth and laughter. That research program continued during the following approximately 15 years. I am (I hope not immodestly) proud that I and my colleagues in those studies were able to perform contributive research in most of the human body's major physiology system areas (Fry, 1994). We have been able to demonstrate significant impacts of mirth and mirthful laughter in the cardiovascular, respiratory, muscular, immune, endocrine, and central nervous systems. With that basic science information being established and disseminated, many other professional persons subsequently have found it possible and desirable to extend their speculations and practice outside spheres of scholarly study into many directions, much of it having to do with health issues, both prevention of disease and with uses of humor as adjunctive to traditional treatment procedures.

During the years in which I was absorbed in that research adventure (the 1960s, 1970s, and early 1980s), several other themes and ventures were forming, developing, building, expanding, and arousing the interest and participation of more and more persons throughout North America, in the United Kingdom, and to a certain extent in Europe, especially in France, the Netherlands, and Belgium. This process was a vital component of a truly revolutionary movement throughout the world. The worldwide movement has been designated by several different titles, depending on the specific location or years being designated. Broader titles identify this movement as a modern renaissance, a new style of life, the Deconstruction era; more specific titles designate the Hippy Revolution, the Free Speech Movement, an overturning of old values. The period for awhile was named The Age of Aquarius. There are other, less enthusiastic, designations that characterize the new era as being a time of Satan's dominance over humankind or an ascendancy of evil and libertine practices. Whatever the values ascribed, there is little argument over the presence of new beliefs and values and social practices, over the revolutions of social customs, garb, artistic expression, communication, lifestyles, music, interpersonal interactions of many varieties, and religious practices. There can be no doubt that this revolution built on the shoulders of earlier times, as is the way of the world. However, this was a watershed era, a parametric cultural shift.

Tons of paper and miles of words have been exchanged during the past three decades regarding this parametric revolution. Discussion of the underlying implications, dealing with issues of the past and future of humanity, is far beyond the scope of this contribution. Suffice it to say that a vast proportion of the revolutionary changes has had to do with what can be called the "pragmatics" of human life and human behavior. Changes brought during these turbulent years have been more in the everyday ways of humans, less so in consideration of the many and deep implications of the turbulence and its innovative consequences. To be sure, these implications have received some attention, but to large extent in the more traditional manner of analysis and consideration. The changes of lifestyle and performance have been huge and have been little inhibited by the paucity of reflective attention turned toward them. There has been much change in daily ways of life, not only in so-called developed cultures; the revolution has been universal over the globe—with varied intensities and varied specifics of behavior.

Returning to the issues of humor in health care, it is apparent that a part of the revolution has been a process of reshaping the pragmatics of health care, making it possible to consider many new features of health care, including interrelationships between health care and humor, wherein humor takes adjunctive roles such as cited previously. Underlying the pragmatics that predominate with this mutation is new emphasis on the principle of one's personal responsibility for one's own health care (Cousins, 1979). More so than many other products of the revolutionary era, this issue of health care responsibility received more and more attention during the 1970s and 1980s. With this expanding orientation and under the title of holistic medicine, implementation of adjunctive roles in healing and health care for humor, and many other alternative and complementary nontraditional medical practices, became not only possible but realized. Many uses of the opportunity for using humor and mirthful laughter have been in-

stituted and operated successfully. Physician Patch Adams is one of the luminous pioneers in this humor movement. The movement is spread throughout areas of the world where humans attempt to improve the quality of their lives, both in health and at times of disease.

The nature of many humor–health care innovations is such that adjunctive use of humor, mirth, and laughter is having increasingly interesting application. Facilities have been established in hospitals, convalescent homes, day-care centers, long-term care units, and rehabilitation centers in which sources of humor are made available. This availability is usually intended primarily for the patient or resident, but this practice has also brought forth recognition that benefits of humor can be experienced by others in the broader health care environment: staff members, patients' family members, volunteers, community contacts—all have been demonstrated to have benefited by having humor "tonics" available at times when beset by the various "negative emotions" so common in such circumstances. Patient benefits are demonstrated to come doubly, both from direct impact and from the energizing and positive effects on those who are participating with the patient in his or her struggle for return to or maintenance of health. It has been indicative of this double value that much of the encouragement for humor facility establishment in health care institutions has come from nursing staffs, who it must be admitted experience the greater degree of patient-provider interaction, both in terms of quantity and intensity.

This health care facilities use of humor as adjunctive to other, more traditional, medical procedures and practices does not stand alone in the new orientation about humor in health care. A rising enthusiasm for humor in wider use, beyond institutional use and beyond the age-old popularity of humor as an important source of entertainment and amusement, is fueling spread of humor forms among populations throughout the world (Berger, 1993). This enthusiasm has broken down many of the customary prejudices against humor, which have previously characterized humor as frivolous, unimportant, or vulgar and reprehensible. People have shaken the sense of guilt or shame or flippancy that earlier restricted their access to their natural, genetically inculcated sense of humor (Morreall, 1983). Individuals in their inner lives, in their relationships with family members, in the workplace, in their public activities increasingly avail themselves of this element of their biological inheritance for enriching their existence and for making unexpected discoveries about the complexities of life (Blumenfeld & Alpern, 1994; Klein, 1989). Workshops, seminars, lectures, and discussion groups throughout the world explore new and beneficial values of humor and laughter for leading healthful lives, for helping patients recover from illness, and for helping patients maintain higher quality of life during illness. Humor has even been admitted into the quiet privacy of psychotherapy and counseling (Fry & Salameh, 1993).

Humor continues to be a major source of entertainment, a major component of the array of pleasures to be enjoyed in this world. All evidence indicates sturdy continuation of that status. Now humor and laughter, with new knowledge and new attitudes about their values and benefits, increasingly spread their magic into areas of human experience that had previously not been visualized as appropriate places for their presence.

LAUGHING SPIRIT LISTENING CIRCLES

The potential for healing laughter bubbles deep within us like natural hot springs. It just *is*. For me, humor therapy is about providing the safe space that *allows* us to erupt in our uniquely unpredictable, often socially unacceptable way, fluidly carrying warm chuckles, hot guffaws, and tender tears to the places within and without that serve our body, our soul, and our community.

The laughter that is the *best* medicine is that which lies *beneath* seriousness and respects gravity, sadness, fear, frustration, and anger. It is not the surface, over-the-counter, diluted gigglery we call "lightening up."

Robust tears are no less potent than lusty laughter, and when "lightening up" is even slightly more valued over "getting heavy," therapy is dead and community is crippled.

I practice humor therapy in a form I call *Laughing Spirit Listening Circles*. Each participant in a group of 6 to 10 gets equal time to receive absolute positive, silent attention, first for 3 minutes, then for 5 minutes. The guidelines are "dare to be boring."

You do not even have to speak. When you do, just tell the truth without trying to be funny. Stay in connection with individuals when you speak. *Receive* your support, rather than trying to *give*. The first time around is often serious, even grave, as people feel the safety and respect and build the integrity of the community. By the second time around, laughter and tears often flow, sometimes interchangeably.

THREE MYTHS ABOUT LAUGHTER THAT KEEP US FROM LAUGHING

The *first major myth* about laughter that prevents us from laughing as much as we need to is that we must have a reason to laugh. The people who respond to my opening laughter with great seriousness at my workshops may feel that there is no reason for me to be laughing, or if there is, they missed it. Not only must we have a reason to laugh, but the reason must be so good that when someone challenges us with "Why are you laughing? What's so funny?" when we explain it, they too will laugh. If they do not laugh, very often we are presented with a puzzled face and a remark, such as, "That was it? Boy, do you have a weird sense of humor!"

Many of us unconsciously censor our laughter because at some level we think our reason for laughing is not good enough. It is important to note here that the reality is that laughter is unreasonable, illogical, and irrational. I propose that we do not need a reason to laugh. When we see a 6-month-old baby laughing, we do not demand "What's so funny?" but rather delight in the response and often join in. We can do so with adults. Insisting on a reason to laugh is an excellent way of stopping someone, or ourselves, from laughing. This is important to remember when we are in situations in which laughter is inappropriate. We may want to ask ourselves, "Why am I laughing right now?" so that we can stop—for instance, if you get the giggles when pulled over by a policeman for speeding or some other infraction of the law.

The *second major myth* about laughter is that we laugh because we are happy, when the reality is we are happy because we laugh. I ask my groups how many feel better after they have laughed, and there is always a unanimous show of hands. At this point I remark that if laughter came out of happiness, we would not feel better after laughing—we would have already felt better before laughing.

I think that laughter has been assigned the job of indicating happiness because we have been so desperate for some outward sign of this vague, undefined, but treasured state. Actually most people (I am certainly one of them) do not know what happiness is. We know that the Declaration of Independence mandates us to pursue it, but judging by our national behavior, we are somewhat confused about where happiness lies. If we feel better after we laugh, then laughter must come from a source other than happiness.

Those of us who have laughed until we have cried know that in the middle of the process, we cannot tell which is which. We do not laugh because we are happy and cry because we are sad—we laugh or cry because we have tension, stress, or pain. Laughter and tears rebalance the chemicals our bodies create when these distressed states are present, so we feel better after we have laughed or cried.

The *third major myth* is that a sense of humor is the same thing as laughter. I suggest that even though the two terms are used interchangeably, they are very different processes. The reality is that you do not need a sense of humor to laugh. Again, when we see a 6-month-old baby laughing, we do not remark, "Doesn't that baby have a wonderful sense of humor!" A sense of humor is learned; laughter is innate. A sense of humor is an intellectual process, whereas laughter spontaneously engages every major system in the body.

There is absolutely no agreement on what a sense of humor is or what makes something funny. Senses of humor vary according to culture, age, ethnic, or economic background, race, sex, and so on. I remarked to one of my groups that women in the ladies' room laugh at different things than men in the men's room. A man raised his hand and said, "Men don't laugh in the men's room." I didn't realize this, having spent very little time in the men's room. (Later on, a man came up to me and said he knew why men didn't laugh in the men's room. . . . It is hard to laugh and aim at the same time!)

A sense of humor does not guarantee laughter in the person to whom we give that designation. Many people with great senses of humor do not laugh.

Groucho Marx was known to have laughed only once, publicly or privately. Very often people who make other people laugh do so because they can control when the laughter will occur. The emphasis on humor diverts us from the broad scope of laughter that is available, making laughter a specialty that is then possible only occasionally.

A DEFINITION OF HUMOR

A clear understanding of what constitutes humor and what does not is a necessary starting point to prevent the inevitable misunderstandings that arise when the subject is considered.

1. Humor is not the equivalent of laughter. Humor may or may not stimulate laughter, sometimes merely a quiet smile or even an inner glow of delight. Laughter may accompany humor, but it also accompanies aggression, surprise, and sometimes even grief.

2. Joking comprises a minor percentage of humor experience. Only about 4 percent of the adult population admits to remembering and telling jokes well; whereas more than 90 percent consider that they "have a pretty dog-gone good sense of humor." Humor is conveyed between persons much more nonverbally such as in the eye twinkle and the smile.

3. Humor is not a form of therapy per se. It is a perspective and appropriate behaviors integrated in the overall conduct of our lives.

4. Humor does not cure cancer, baldness, or major depression. Humor is a marvelous adjunct to the overall conduct of one's psychological life, especially when confronting illness, tragedy, or death.

5. Although the observational evidence is intriguing, humor as yet has not been demonstrated conclusively to release endorphins. (Endorphins: Small children without parents who live in the house all the time.)

Humor is a mature psychological response to stress in which the stressful issue is maintained in conscious, without distortion, and is responded to with amusement when double meanings, ironies, or some other inconsistency is noted. Humor does not increase the discomfort of the individual nor those in his company.

Until recently (1970s) humor was looked down on in the conduct of medicine as being unprofessional or uncaring or even as beneath the standard of care. Such an attitude was in response to immature psychological defenses masquerading as humor (e.g., passive aggression, schizoid fantasy, projection).

Applying humor with kindness, compassion, and empathy is the key. For the most part, humor in medical practice should take the form of gentle amusement, twinkling eye contact, and only in the rarest situations, jokes.

The following is a short listing of specific guides to the conduct of humor (Hageseth, 1988).

Five mature ego mechanisms of defense (after Vaillant): altruism, humor, anticipation, suppression, and sublimation.

Three pathways to a humor experience (Hageseth):
- Nonverbal interactive—smiling, eye twinkle, etc.
- Stimulation of forbidden subjects
- Jokes and other forms of verbal humor

Four elements to successful communication of humor: relationship, rapport, setting, and timing

THE LAUGH MOBILE PROGRAM

Carolina Health and Humor Association is an educational service organization dedicated to promoting humor in health care and for personal growth. As founder and executive director, I started the Duke Humor Project with the department of Duke Oncology Recreation Therapy in 1986. At Duke University Medical Center in Durham, North Carolina, oncology patients may come for as long as 6 weeks for various cancer treatments. One difficulty with recreational programming is that patients must feel well enough to attend a group craft or entertainment program. Often the patient is too ill to leave the room during the intensive treatments. The Laugh Mobile was created to bring humorous media bedside to these patients. Volunteers from Carolina Health and Humor Association use the Laugh Mobile to deliver bedside laughs and to initiate a humor intervention. A humor intervention may be described as a plan to promote joy and laughter in the treatment program for patient care.

The Duke Humor Project continues to bring joy bedside to cancer patients at Duke Medical Center. The Laugh Mobile delivers humorous media bedside to patients and family twice weekly. Humor volunteers engage in yo-yo demonstrations, guitar playing, and practical jokes. For example, the patient may want to set up a whoopee cushion under the covers of his or her bed and then invite the doctor to have a seat and take a load off. Water guns are also dispensed to allow the patient a way to fight back. It is all in the interest of building fun-loving relationships, and the staff is highly receptive to any humor statements from the patient, and especially practical jokes.

One of the evolving aspects of the Duke Humor Project and the Laugh Mobile Program is the referral procedure used for targeting the patients. The professional oncology recreation staff attends grand rounds and gathers information about the patients that may be most receptive to humor. Background information is reported in a notebook that goes with the Laugh Mobile. This reports pertinent information on the patient and suggestions for the best approach. For example, the staff may relate that the patient is hard of hearing or that the patient may enjoy learning to juggle scarves. The humor volunteer comes in and sees each patient on referral. A comment by the volunteer reports back to the staff about how the humor intervention worked. This gives the hospital staff an opportunity to follow-up between Laugh Mobile visits.

As a designer of humor programs like the Laugh Mobile Program, I see humor and intentional laughter programs expanding to reach patients in all stages of recovery. I believe that to be effective, I must continue to volunteer with the cancer patients and the Laugh Mobile Program weekly. I am now opening new avenues for spreading the humor programming by the design of programs for bone marrow transplant and for cardiac care patients. Each illness seems to have its own set of humorous episodes and strategies. It is my challenge to explore with the patient the areas that need more humor and to suggest funny coping strategies. Perhaps my greatest challenge is to continually seek new ways for the humor impaired to laugh and to invite the medical staff to enjoy more playfulness. I am confident that community-based groups like Carolina Ha Ha, which offers both trained volunteers and professional program implementation, will continue to plant the seeds of comic caring and loving laughter.

IT MAY BE SERIOUS BUT IT NEEDN'T BE SOLEMN

These healing hot springs of holistic "laughtears" are what I'm after in humor therapy.

I try to be playful but others won't respond.

If I ever needed humor it is now.

I want to smile and laugh, but that upsets my family.

—HOSPICE PATIENTS' COMMENTS
(*AMERICAN JOURNAL OF HOSPICE CARE,* 1990)

A couple of years ago my father-in-law was very ill. Once, when he came home from the hospital, it was his and my mother-in-law's wedding anniversary. I suggested that they invite a few friends over for dinner and I would cook a turkey.

Jimmy managed to get out of bed to join us. He enjoyed the meal but the strain of feeding himself and the presence of guests were obviously tiring him. Noticing this and knowing that he could not hear very well, my mother-in-law wrote a note and passed it to me to give to him. I read it and got hysterical. She remembered what she just wrote and laughed out loud too.

The note said, "Happy Anniversary dear. Do you want to go to bed?"

Jimmy read what his wife had written, looked up across the table, and with a twinkle in his eye and a smile on his face slowly said to her, "I would love to dear, but we have company."

It was only a brief moment of levity in his difficult last days, but it was a moment that was long remembered after he was gone.

Looking for humor in the not-so-funny world of serious illness may seem like a disrespectful thing to those who are suffering. However, situational humor, which inevitably arises during stressful times, is very appropriate. Because of humor's ability to give a new perspective to any situation, it is an important coping tool for everyone involved in the dying process, including the physician.

Laughter is a powerful tool in powerless situations. It can give hope and an upper hand to patients, who are experiencing both physical and mental loss, as well as to physicians who cannot change that loss or stop the demise of the patient.

The safest way for a physician to find that laughter is to first establish a rapport with the patient. Then look for humor by listening to what the patient jokes about. Above all, do not go into a patient's room with a battery of jokes. First, jokes can be offensive, and second, when you enter a patient's room, you have no knowledge whether they will be receptive to your kidding around. Keep in mind that humor is a wonderful bonding tool, but it can also backfire and create alienation.

My friend, Patty Wooten (AKA Nancy Nurse), once told me a story about the time she was bathing a patient who had a rather large surgical scar down her front. The patient said, "Nurse, look at my scar. It looks just like Market Street in San Francisco." Puzzled by this remark, Patty questioned, "What do you mean, 'Market Street in San Francisco?'" "Well," replied the patient, "it goes from Twin Peaks to the waterfront." (Indeed, Market Street in San Francisco does run from Twin Peaks to the waterfront!)

Patty and the patient laughed uproariously together. Then, months later, Patty was bathing another woman who had a similar scar and told her this joke. The patient got highly insulted.

In the first case humor came from a woman who was comfortable enough to laugh at what she had experienced; the second patient was not.

The best way to find humor when working with the seriously ill is to listen to what they are saying. The patient is the one who will often give you the laugh lines.

One example comes from a friend of mine who had AIDS for 8 years. One day I walked into Rick's house and found a Star of David, a Crucifix, and a picture of Buddha on the wall.

"Rick," I said, "you are a Quaker, why do you have these opposing religious items around?" Rick, who never missed a moment for some levity, replied, "Well, you never know who's right. I'm covering all bases!"

Rick was someone with whom I could joke about his illness because he would be the first one to poke fun at his difficulties. Your patients are the ones who will let you know if it is O.K. to kid around with them, supply you with laughs, and help you see death as less of a grave matter.

HUMOR IN HEALTH CARE

We think of humor as just fun and play—not serious. Yet, it is one of the most healthy, healing phenomena human beings have. It is a cognitive, emotional, and physical response to stress. It gives us balance and a perspective and provides a comic relief and survival from all the seriousness of living.

Within the health care arena, which is probably one of the most stressful and craziest areas in which we live, humor is a major coping mechanism for patients and staff and a powerful tool for healing. It is the perfect mind-body connection! The humor, verbal or nonverbal, stimulates the feeling of mirth and the laughter, which researchers have found produces a healthy biochemical response in the body.

As an indirect form of communication, humor facilitates all the relationships and manages all the delicate situations that occur. It conveys messages and helps us get in touch with our feelings. And, when we laugh, we release those associated feelings.

Humor reduces all the social conflicts inherent in health care, and facilitates change and survival in the system. As a major relief mechanism, it reduces anxiety, provides a healthy outlet for anger and frustration, and is a healthy denial of all the heaviness of crises, tragedy, and death.

Humor is also a major source of coping for the caregiver and for the prevention of burnout. The health professional who can accept and value his or her need for laughter and comedy can then be comfortable using and encouraging humor with clients.

Humor as a communication should be an integral part of the total healing caring process. Humor conveys our concern, understanding, warmth, and caring. As one patient said, when staff laughed and joked with him, he knew they cared!

For the health professional the key to the therapeutic use of humor is being sensitive to whose needs are being met and being sensitive to the right time, the right place, and the right amount, like a judicious dose of good medicine. And always, it must be used in the context of caring, a laughing with and not a laughing at.

HUMOR—ANTIDOTE FOR STRESS

Humor is a perceptual quality that enables us to experience joy even when faced with adversity. Health professionals work in stress-filled environments that place demands on their physical, emotional, and spiritual well-being (Maslach, 1982). Most caregivers are compassionate and sensitive individuals working with people who are suffering. This too can be a source of stress. Caregivers can experience what is known as *compassion fatigue*—feeling that they have very little left to give (Ritz, 1995). Finding humor in our work and our life can be one way to replenish ourselves from compassion fatigue (Ritz, 1995; Robinson, 1991; Wooten, 1995). This can be an effective self-care tool.

In his book *Stress without Distress,* Selye (1974) clarified that a person's interpretation of stress is not dependent solely on an external event but also depends on their perception of the event and the meaning they give it; how you look at a situation determines whether you will respond to it as threatening or challenging (Kobassa, 1983). In this context, humor can be an empowerment tool because it gives us a different perspective on our problems and, with an attitude of detachment, we feel a sense of self-protection and control in our environment (Klein, 1989; McGhee, 1994). As comedian Bill Cosby is fond of saying, "If you can laugh at it, you can survive it."

There is a type of humor called *gallows humor* (McGhee, 1994; Robinson, 1991) that is unique to people who deal with tragedy and suffering. Those outside of the caregiving professions often do not understand our sometimes desperate need to laugh and may not appreciate this type of humor. The term *gallows humor* supposedly came into being when two brothers were being executed by hanging. Both were standing on the gallows and one brother was already hanged when the other brother said, "Look at my brother there, making a spectacle of himself. Pretty soon we'll be a pair of spectacles."

This laughing bravado, in the face of death, is what caregivers also use to maintain their sanity amidst the horror. It is well documented that there is more laughter in the intensive care unit (ICU), emergency room, and operating room than in other places in the hospital setting. Much of the humor is sexual, obscene, or jokes directly about the tragedy and suffering (Ritz, 1995; Rosenburg, 1991; Wooten, 1995). This appears to be a psychological game one plays with oneself and others, hoping to communicate: "See, I'm doing okay amidst all this horror. Really. See? I'm laughing!"

An ICU nurse shared with me a sign that the staff had placed in the visitor waiting area to explain what might be overheard and misunderstood (Box 17-1).

We attempt to maintain balance by offsetting tragedy in our lives with comedy. Another true story of this cathartic activity was shared by Wayne Johnston, an emergency room nurse:

You saw me laugh after your father died. . . . To you I must have appeared calloused and uncaring. . . . Please understand, much of the stress health care workers suffer comes about because we do care. Sooner or later we will all laugh at the wrong time. I hope your father would understand, my laugh meant no disrespect, it was a grab at balance. I knew there was another patient who needed my full care and attention . . . my laugh was no less cleansing for me than your tears were for you (Johnston, 1985).

Laughter can provide a cathartic release, a purifying of emotions, and a release of emotional tension. Laughter, crying, raging, and trembling are all cathartic activities that can unblock energy flow (Goodheart, 1996).

An ability to laugh at our situation or problem gives us a feeling of superiority and power. We are less likely to succumb to feelings of depression had helplessness if we are able to laugh at what is troubling us. Humor gives us a sense of perspective on our problems. Laughter provides an opportunity for the release of uncomfortable emotions, which, if held inside, may create biochemical changes that are harmful to the body.

As the famous American humorist Mark Twain once said:

Humor is the great thing, the saving thing. Afterall, the moment it arises, all our hardnesses yield, our irritations and resentments slip away, and a sunny spirit takes their place (Klein, 1989).

References

Bainey, M. *Why do we laugh and cry?* Sunlight Publications, West Ryde, Australia, 1993.

Berger, A.A. *An anatomy of humor.* Transaction Publishers, New Brunswick, NJ, 1993.

Berlyne, D.E. Humor and its kin. In Goldstein J.H. & McGhee P.E. (eds.). *The psychology of humor.* Academic Press, New York, 1972.

Blumenfeld, E., & Alpern L. *Humor at work.* Peachtree Publishers, Atlanta, 1994.

Cassell, E. *The nature of suffering.* Oxford University Press, New York, 1991.

Coser, R.L. Some social functions of laughter: A study of humor in a hospital setting. *Human Relations* 12:171-182, 1959.

Cousins, N. *Anatomy of an illness as perceived by the patient.* W.W. Norton, New York, 1979.

Fry, W.F. Laughter. Is it the best medicine? *Stanford M.D.* (Stanford Medical Alumni Association) 10(1):16-20, 1971.

Fry, W.F. The biology of humor. *Humor: International Journal of Humor Research* 7(2):111-126, 1994.

Fry, W.F., & Salameh W. *Advances in humor and psychotherapy.* Professional Resources Press, Sarasota, Florida, 1993.

Goodheart, A. *Laughter therapy.* Stress Less Press, Santa Barbara, California, 1994.

Hageseth, C.M. *A laughing place.* Berwick Publishing, Ft. Collins, CO., 1988.

Johnston, W. To the ones left behind. *American Journal of Nursing* 85(8):936, 1985.

BOX 17-1

Laughter in the Intensive Care Unit

If you are waiting . . .
You may possibly see us laughing; or even take note of some jest;
Know that we are giving your loved one our care at its very best!
There are times when tension is highest;
There are times when our systems are stressed;
We've discovered humor, a factor in keeping our sanity blessed.
So, if you're a patient in waiting, or a relative or friend of one seeing,
Don't hold our smiling against us, it's a way that we keep from screaming.

Sincerely,
The ICU Staff (anon)

Klein, A. *Healing power of humor.* J.P. Tarcher, Los Angeles, 1989.

Kleinman, A. *The illness narratives.* Basic Books, New York, 1988.

Kobassa, S.C. Personality and social resources in stress resistance. *Journal of Personality and Social Psychology* 45:839, 1983.

Koestler, A. *The act of creation.* New York, Macmillan, 1964.

Levi, L. The urinary output of adrenaline and noradrenaline during pleasant and unpleasant states. *Psychosomatic Medicine* 27:80-85, 1965.

Lloyd, E.L. The respiratory rate in laughter. *Journal of General Psychology* 10:179-189, 1938.

Mahrer, A., & Gervaize, P. An integrative review of strong laughter in psychotherapy: What it is and how it works. *Psychotherapy* 21:510-516, 1974.

Maslach, C. *Burnout—The cost of caring.* Prentice Hall, Upper Saddle River, New Jersey, 1982.

McGhee P. *How to develop your sense of humor.* Kendall-Hunt, Dubuque, Iowa, 1994.

Morreall, J. *Taking laughter seriously.* State University of New York Press, Albany, New York, 1983.

Ritz, S. Survivor humor and disaster nursing. In Buxman, K. *Humor and nursing.* A.D. Von Publishers, New York, 1995.

Paskind, H.A. Effect of laughter on muscle tone. *Archives of Neurology and Psychiatry* 23:623-628, 1932.

Robinson, V. *Humor and the health professions,* 2nd ed. C.B. Slack, Thorofare, New Jersey, 1991.

Rosenburg, L. Clinical articles: a qualitative investigation of the use of humor by emergency personnel as a strategy for coping with stress. *Journal of Emergency Nursing* 17(4), 1991.

Ruxton, S.P. Humor deserves our attention. *Holistic Nursing Practice* 2(3):54-62, 1988.

Schachter, S., & Wheeler, L. Epinephrine, chlorpromazine, and amusement. *Journal of Abnormal and Social Psychology,* 1962.

Selye, H. *Stress without distress.* Lippincott & Crowell, New York, 1974.

Wooten, P. Interview with Sandy Ritz. *Journal of Nursing Jocularity* 5(1):46-47, 1995.

Suggested Readings

Ader, R., Felten, D.L., & Cohen, N (eds.). *Psychoneuroimmunology,* 2nd ed. Academic Press, San Diego, 1991.

Arieti, S. New views on the psychology of wit and the comic. *Psychiatry* 13:43-82, 1950.

Averill, J.R. Autonomic response patterns during sadness and mirth. *Psychophysiology* 5(4):399-414, 1969.

Baron, R.A., & Ball, R.L. The aggression-inhibition influence of nonhostile humor. *Journal of Experimental Social Psychology* 10:23-33, 1974.

Barra, J.M. High kicks in the ICU. *RN* 49:45-46, 1986.

Baudelaire, C. The essence of laughter. In *Essays.* Meridian Books, New York, 1956.

Bergson, H. *Laughter: An essay on the meaning of the comic.* Macmillan, New York, 1911.

Berk, L.S., et al. Modulation of human natural killer cells by catecholamines. *Clinical Research* 32(1):1984.

Berk, L.S., et al. Eustress of mirthful laughter modifies natural killer cell activity. *Clinical Research* 37(1), 1989.

Berk, L.S., et al. Neuroendocrine and stress hormone changes during mirthful laughter. *The American Journal of Medical Sciences* 296(7):390-396, 1989.

Berkowitz, L. Aggressive humor as a stimulus to aggressive responses. *Journal of Personality and Social Psychology* 16:710-717, 1970.

Beyondananda, S. *When you see a sacred cow . . . milk it for all it's worth.* Aslan Publishing, Lower Lake, California, 1993.

Bhargava, K.P. An overview of endorphins' probable role in health and disease. In Dhawan, B.N. (ed.). *Current status of centrally acting peptides.* Pergamon Press, Oxford, 1982.

Blair, W. What's funny about doctors. *Perspectives in Biology and Medicine* 21(1):89-98, 1977.

Bloch, S., & McGrath, G. Humor in group psychotherapy. *British Journal of Medical Psychology* 56:88-97, 1983.

Blumenfeld, E., & Alpern, L. *The smile connection.* Prentice Hall, Englewood Cliffs, New Jersey, 1986.

Bokun, B. *Humour therapy.* Vita Books, London, 1986.

Boston, R. *An anatomy of laughter.* Collins, London, 1974.

Brill, A.A. The mechanism of wit and humor in normal and psychopathic states. *Psychiatric Quarterly* 14:731-749, 1940.

Brody, M.W. The meaning of laughter. *Psychoanalytic Quarterly* 19:192-201, 1950.

Burton, R. *The anatomy of melancholy.* Tudor Publishing, New York, 1927.

Buxman, K. Humor in therapy for the mentally ill. *Journal of Psychological Nursing* 29(12):15-18, 1991.

Byrne, D.E. The relationship between humor and the expression of hostility. *Journal of Abnormal and Social Psychology* 53:84-89, 1956.

Byrne, D.E., Terril, S., & McReynolds, P. Incongruence as a predictor of response to humor. *Journal of Abnormal and Social Psychology* 62:435-438, 1961.

Cassell, E. *The healer's art.* MIT Press, Boston, 1986.

Cassell, J. The function of humor in the counseling process. *Rehabilitation Counseling* 17:240-245, 1974.

Chapman, A.J. An experimental study of socially facilitated humorous laughter. *Psychological Reports* 35:727-734, 1974.

Chapman, A.J., & Foot, H.C. (eds.). *It's a funny thing, humor.* International Conference on Humor and Laughter. Pergamon Press, Oxford, 1976.

Dana, B., & Laurence, P. *The laughter prescription.* Ballantine, New York, 1982.

Dearbom, G.V.N. The nature of the smile and the laugh. *Science*, 1900.

Dillon, K.M., et al. Positive emotional states and enhancement of the immune system. *International Journal of Psychiatry in Medicine* 15(1):13-18, 1985-1986.

Domis, J., & Fierman, E. Humor and anxiety. *Journal of Abnormal and Social Psychology* 53:59-62, 1956.

Elliot-Binns, C.P. Laughter and medicine. *Journal of the Royal College of General Practitioners* 37(277):364-365, 1985.

Erdman, L. Laughter therapy for patients with cancer. *Oncology Nursing Forum* 18(8):1359-1363, 1991.

Euck, J.J., Forter, E., & Whitley, A. (eds.). *The comic in theory and practice*. Appleton-Century-Crofts, New York, 1960.

Fairbanks, D. *Laugh and live*. Britton Publishing, New York, 1917.

Feibleman, J. *In praise of comedy*. Horizon Press, New York, 1970.

Flugel, J.C. Humor and laughter. In Lindsay, G. (ed.). *Handbook of social psychology*. Addison-Wesley, Cambridge, Massachusetts, 1954.

Freud, S. *Jokes and their relationship to the unconscious*. W.W. Norton, New York, 1964.

Fry, W.F., Jr. *Sweet madness: A study of humor*. Pacific Books, Palo Alto, California, 1963.

Fry, W.F., Jr. *Make 'em laugh*. Science and Behavior Books, Palo Alto, California, 1975.

Fry, W.F., Jr. Humor and the cardiovascular system. Paper presented at the 2nd International Conference on Humor and Laughter. Los Angeles, August, 1979.

Professional Resource Press, Sarasota, Florida, 1993.

Fry, W.F., Jr., & Rader, C. The respiratory components of mirthful laughter. *Journal of Biological Psychology* 19:39-50, 1977.

Fry, W.F., Jr., & Stoft, P.E. Mirth and oxygen saturation levels of peripheral blood. *Psychotherapy and psychosomatics* 19:76-84, 1971.

Gaberson, K.B. The effect of humorous distraction on preoperative anxiety. *AORN Journal* 54(6):1258-1264, 1991.

Greenwald, H. Humor in psychotherapy. *Journal of Contemporary Psychotherapy* 7:113-116, 1975.

Grotjahn, M. *Beyond laughter*. McGraw-Hill, New York, 1956.

Haller, B., & Zarai, R. *Rire c'est la sante*. Editions Soleil, Geneva, 1986.

Harlow, H.F. The anatomy of humor. *Impact of Science on Society*, 1969.

Hassett, J., & Schwartz, G.E. Why can't people take humor seriously? *New York Times Magazine* February, 1977.

The healing power of laughter and play: Uses of humor in the healing arts. Twelve tapes. P.O. Box 94305. Portola Valley, California: IAHB, 1983.

Herth, K.A. Laughter: a nursing Rx. *American Journal of Nursing* 84(8):991-992, 1984.

Heuscher, J. The role of humor and folklore themes of psychotherapy. *American Journal of Psychiatry* 137:1546-1549, 1980.

Holden, R. *Laughter is the best medicine*. Thorsons, London, 1993.

Holland, N. *Laughing: The psychology of humor*. Cornell University Press, New York, 1982.

Joubert, L. *Treatise on laughter*. University of Alabama Press, Birmingham, Alabama, 1970.

Kaplan, H., & Boyd, I. The social functions of humor on an open psychiatric ward. *Psychiatric Quarterly* 39:502-515, 1965.

Keller, D. *Humor as therapy*. Med-Psych Publications, Wauwatosa, Wisconsin, 1984.

Klein, A. *The healing power of humor*. Jeremy Tarcher, Los Angeles, 1989.

Kubie, L.S. The destructive potential of humor in psychotherapy. *American Journal of Psychiatry* 127:861-886, 1971.

Lefcourt, H., & Martin, R. *Humor and life stress*. Springer-Verlag, New York, 1986.

Leiber, D.B. Laughter and humor in critical care. *Dimensions in Critical Care* 5(3):162-170, 1986.

Levine, J. Humor as a form of therapy. In Chapman, A.J., Foot, H.C. (eds.). *It's a funny thing, humor*. Pergamon Press, Oxford, 1976.

McConnell, J. Confessions of a scientific humorist. In *Impact of Science on Society*, 1969.

McGhee, P., & Goldstein, J.H. (eds.). *Handbook of humor research, vol. 1, basic issues and vol. 2, applied studies*. Springer-Verlag, New York, 1983.

McHale, M. Getting the joke: Interpreting humor in group therapy. *Journal of Psychological Nursing* 27(9):24-28, 1989.

Metcalf, C.W., & Felible, R. *Lighten up*. Addison-Wesley Publishing, Reading, Massachusetts, 1992.

Mind, H. The use and abuse of humor in psychotherapy. In Chapman, A.J., & Foot, H.C. (eds.). *Humor and laughter: Theory, research and application*. John Wiley & Sons, New York, 1976.

Mindess, H., et al. (eds.). *The antioch humor test*. Avon, New York, 1985.

Mindess, H. Laughter and humor in medical practice. *Behavioral Medicine*, 1979.

Mindess, H., *Laughter and liberation*. Nash, Los Angeles, 1971.

Moody, R.A., Jr. *Laugh after laugh: The healing power of humor*. Headwaters, Press, Jacksonville, Florida, 1978.

Nussbaum, K., & Michaux, W.W. Response to humor in depression: A predictor and evaluator of patient change. *Psychiatric Quarterly* 37:527-539, 1963.

O'Connell, W.E. The adaptive functions of wit and humor. *Journal of Abnormal and Social Psychology* 61:263-270, 1960.

O'Connell, W.E. Humor and death. *Psychological Reports* 22:391-402, 1968.

Pasquali, E.A. Learning to laugh: Humor as therapy. *Journal of Psychological Nursing* 28(3), 1990.

Pirandello, L. *On humor.* University of North Carolina Press, Chapel Hill, North Carolina, 1974.

Poland, W.S. The place of humor in psychotherapy. *American Journal of Psychiatry* 28:635-637, 1971.

Potter, S. *The sense of humor.* Penguin Books, Middlesex, England, 1954.

Powell, B.S. Laughter and healing: The use of humor in hospitals treating children. *Association for the Care of Children in Hospitals Journal,* Biv., 10-16, 1974.

Robinson, V. *Humor and health.* In Goldstein, J.H., & McGhee, P. (eds.). *Handbook of humor research.* Springer-Verlag, New York, 1983.

Robinson, V.M. Humor is a serious business. *Dimensions in Critical Care,* 5(3):132-133, 1986.

Rosenheim, E. Humor in psychotherapy: An interactive experience. *American Journal of Psychotherapy* 28:584-591, 1974.

Samra, C. *The joyful chant: The healing power of humor.* Harper & Row, San Francisco, 1986.

Schaller, C.T. *Rire pour gai-rire.* Editions Vivez Soleil, Geneva, 1994.

Spenser, H. The physiology of laughter. *Macmillan's Magazine,* 1860.

Vaillant, G. *Empirical studies in ego mechanisms of defense.* American Psychiatric Press, Washington, D.C., 1986.

Vaillant, G. *The wisdom of the ego.* Harvard University Press, Cambridge, 1993.

Vergeer, G., & MacRae, A. Therapeutic use of humor in occupational therapy. *American Journal of Occupational Therapy* 47(8), 1993.

Williams, H. Humor and healing: Therapeutic effects in geriatrics. *Gerontion* 1(3):14-17, 1986.

Wooten, P. (ed.). *Heart, humor, and healing.* Commune-A-Key Publishing, Mt. Shasta, California, 1994.

Zillman, D., et al. Does humor facilitate coping with physical discomfort. *Motivation and Emotion* 17(1), 1993.

Health and Humor Resources:
Individuals, Organizations, and Publications

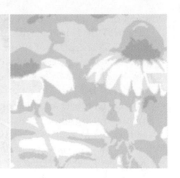

Alan Agins, PhD, Asst. Professor of Nursing, University of Virginia, School of Nursing, McLeod Hall, Charlottesville, VA 22903-3395, (804) 924-1647

Steve Allen, Jr., MD, 8 LeGrand Ct., Ithica, NY 19850, (607) 277-1795, physician lecturer on humor

Al's Magic Shop, 1012 Vermont Avenue, Washington, DC 20005, (202) 789-2800

Dale Anderson, MD, 2982 West Owasso Blvd., Roseville, MN 55113, (612) 484-5162, physician doing humor programs

Lee Berk, 11645 Wiley St., Loma Linda, CA 92354, (909) 796-4112, research into biochemistry and physiology of laughter, esp. neuroimmunology

Steve Bhaerman, "Swami Beyondananda," P.O. Box 110, Burnet, TX 78611, (512) 756-2791, lectures, workshops, books, tapes

Michael Christensen, Clown Care Unit, Big Apple Circus, 35 W. 35th St., New York, NY 10001, (212) 268-2500, clowns who visit pediatric wards

Clown Hall of Fame, Museum & Gifts, 212 E. Walworth, Delavan, WI 53115, (414) 728-9075

Eric de Bont, Bont's Adventures In Clown Arts, Pardoestheater, postbus 419, 6800 AK Arnheim, The Netherlands, center for learning clown arts

Mouton DeGruyter, W. DeGruyter Inc., 200 Saw Mill River Rd., Hawthorne, NY 10532, publishes humor

Glenn C. Ellenbogen, Wry-Bred Press, Inc., 10 Waterside Plaza, New York, NY 10010, (212) 689-5476, 1985 published directory of humor magazines and organizations in America and Canada

Fellowship of Merry Christians, Cal Samra, P.O. Box 895, Portage, MI 49081, network of Christian humorists publishes *The Joyful Noiseletter*

Laura Fernandez, Die Clown Doktoren, Klaren Thaler Str. 3, 65197 Wiesbaden, Germany, 0611-9490981, clown created hospital clown units in Germany

William Fry, 156 Grove Street, Nevada City, CA 95959, (916) 265-5125, physician researcher on humor

Cathy Gibbons, Fun Technicians, P.O. Box 160, Syracuse, NY 13215, (315) 492-4523, fax 469-1392, *Laughmaker's Magazine*

Leslie Gibson, RN, The Comedy Connection, 323 Jeffords St., Clearwater, FL 34617, (813) 462-7842, lectures and creates hospital humor carts

Lee Glickstein, Center for the Laughing Spirit, 288 Juanita Way, San Francisco, CA 94127, (415) 731-6640

Art Gliner, Humor Communications, 8902 Maine Avenue, Silver Spring, MD 20910, (301) 588-3561, lectures/workshops

Annette Goodheart, P.O. Box 40297, Santa Barbara, CA 93103, (605) 966-4725, laughter therapist, lectures & workshops

Joel Goodman, The Humor Project, 179 Spring Street, Box L, Saratoga Springs, NY 12866, qrtrly newsletter *Laughing Matters*, lectures, workshops, annual humor conference

Christian Hageseth, MD, 1113 Stoneyhill Dr., Ft. Collins, CO 80525, psychotherapist doing humor programs

Ruth Hamilton, Carolina Health and Humor Assn., 5223 Revere Rd., Durham, NC 27713, (919) 544-2370, newsletter workshops

International Humor Institute, 32362 Saddle Mt. Road, Westlake Village, CA 91361, (818) 879-9085

International Laughter Society, 16000 Glen Una Dr., Los Gatos, CA 95030, (408) 354-3456

Steve Kissel, 1227 Manchester Avenue, Norfolk, VA 23508-1122, (804) 423-3867

Alan Klein, The Whole Mirth Catalog, 1034 Page Street, San Francisco, CA 94117, catalog of books and toys

Karen Lee, The Laughter Prescription, 7720 El Camino Real B-225, Carlsbad, CA 92009, (800), RxHUMOR

Paul McGhee, The Laughter Remedy, 380 Claremont Avenue, Montclair, NJ 07042, (201) 783-8383, researcher/lecturer

C.W. Metcalf, The Humor Option, 2801 S. Remington, Suite 2, Ft. Collins, CO 80525, (303) 226-0610, workshops and presentations on humor

Jeff Moore, Orthopedic Coordinator, Physical Medicine/Saint Paul Medical Center, 5909 Harry Hines Blvd., Dallas, TX 75235, (214) 879-3848, entertains patients

Jim Pelley, Laughter Works, P.O. Box 1076, Fair Oaks, CA 95628, (916) 863-1593, workshops, newsletter

Dr. Karen Peterson, 1320 S. Dixie Hwy., Coral Gables, FL 33146, (305) 662-2654

Caroline Simonds, Le Rire Medecin, 75 Avenue Parmenitier, 7509 Paris, France, 42-58-39-91, French version of clown care units

Dhyan Sutorius, MD, Secretariat of the Center In Favor of Laughter, Jupiter, 1008, NL-1115 TX, Duivendrecht, Holland, 31-0-20-690028

Christian tal Schaller, 15 Francois Jacquier CH1235 Chene-Bourg, Geneva, Switzerland

Tumor Humor, Uniquest, P.O. Box 97391, Raleigh, NC 27624

Lex Van Someren, Batstangveien 81, 3200 Sandefjord Norway, 034-59644, "The Mystic Clown," teacher of workshops

Joan White, Joygerms, P.O. Box 219, Syracuse, NY 13206, (315) 472-2779, spreader of good cheer, resources

Patty Wooten, RN, "Nancy Nurse", P.O. Box 4040, Davis, CA 95617, (916) 758-3826, author of *Humor, Heart & Healing*

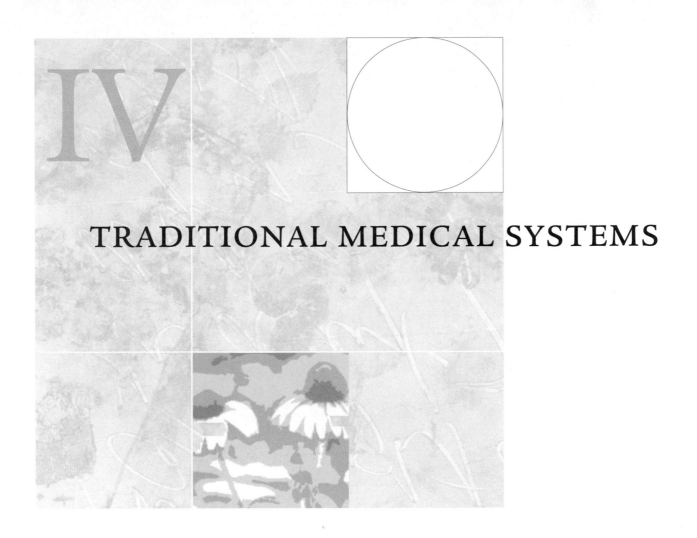

TRADITIONAL MEDICAL SYSTEMS

This section provides a survey of the fundamentals of global health traditions that form integrated systems of thought and practice, following from an explanation of their relevant world views. Although this book aims to present a unified body of the theories and practices of alternatives, many world healing traditions are marked by a significant degree of heterogeneity, consistent with their historical evolution and their underlying philosophies. ∽

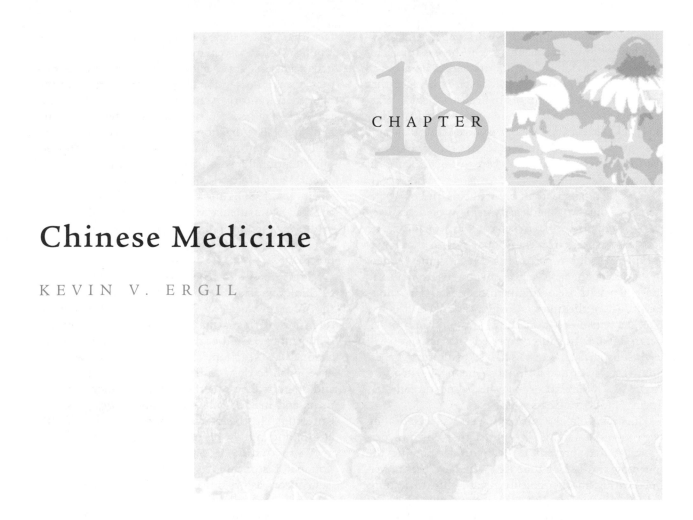

Chinese Medicine

KEVIN V. ERGIL

CHINA'S TRADITIONAL MEDICINE IN CULTURAL PERSPECTIVE

Certain considerations are important to understanding ethnomedical systems in general and Chinese medicine in particular. Medicine is a human endeavor and as such is shaped by the considerations of the human beings using and practicing it. These considerations sometimes have very little to do with curing disease in the most simple and efficient way and a great deal to do with economics, politics, and culture. Ideology, belief, and even simple ignorance have influenced the practice of medicine more than rationality. A medical historian or a physician might perceive medicine to be a steady march from ignorance to the light, but these are typically revisionist histories.

Medicine is a human enterprise embedded in and intersected by myriad other human projects. Even the choice of how to conduct a medical procedure or what kind of health care to choose may have more to do with habit or economics than with rationality or efficacy. For instance, American gynecologists position their patients for maximum visual exposure during routine examinations, whereas physicians in the United Kingdom allow the patient to lie on her side, assuming a more relaxed posture during the examination (Payer, 1988). An example closer to our subject is the case of a Chinese patient choosing traditional herbal medicine to manage painful and debilitating kidney stones. Although the treatment was ultimately efficacious, the patient's choice was not motivated by a desire for efficacy. Undergoing surgery would have meant that the patient would have been classified as an invalid on the work papers and therefore barred from advancement. Or, there is the example of a hospital in California that closes its doors to the practice of acupuncture despite the fact that acupuncturists in the state are licensed medical practitioners and their services are routinely requested by hospital patients. In each instance, considerations that are not directly linked to the rational and effective delivery of medical care influence medical choices.

Our own perspectives on medicine and our experience of our own medical systems provide us with ideas of what is normal or typical for medicine. We respond to aspects of a traditional system that correspond with our expectations. We imagine Chinese herbal medicine as a gentle therapy using nontoxic ingredients. Its use of highly toxic substances or drastic purgative therapies is easily overlooked. It is unlikely, for instance, that the traditional form of Tibetan therapeutic cautery applied with a hot iron will elicit substantial interest as a form of alternative therapy. Naturalistic and rational elements of systems intrigue us. Unfamiliar or magical diagnostic and therapeutic modes cause us concern.

It is easy to make intellectual errors when dealing with medical systems. We forget that our own perspectives may prevent us from understanding the meaning and use of practices that have been developed within another culture. That failure to account for our own needs and biases also can lead to the overenthusiastic acceptance of ideas whose genesis and application we really do not understand.

If we want to avoid these errors, we must think about medical systems as being embedded in their respective cultures. Each system's structure and elements are vital to their practice in a particular cultural context. Culture, in this sense, does not imply an all-embracing system of meaning subscribed to by all members of a community, country, or ethnicity. Culture is a complex network of signification, elements of which might resonate only in a very local sense, whereas other aspects have almost global relevance. This does not mean that the medical ideas and practices of one society cannot or will not be successfully appropriated by another, but rather that aspects of a system that are meaningful to one group of people might not be meaningful at all to another.

For example, the concept of neurasthenia *(sheng jin shuai ruo)* is an important syndrome in traditional Chinese medicine and Chinese psychiatry, despite the fact that this diagnosis has fallen into disrepute among Western psychiatrists and is no longer classified as a disease entity in diagnostic manuals. Neurasthenia was an exceptionally popular diagnosis in the nineteenth century during periods of extensive medical exchange between the United States and China and Japan. The diagnosis has continued to be clinically important in China because it fits well into certain traditional medical models and responds well to cultural and political concerns about mental illness (Kleinman, 1986). Americans and Europeans who encounter neurasthenia within the corpus of Chinese medicine sometimes find it an unusual or obscure concept despite its relevance for Chinese medical practice.

Sometimes, on encountering a new idea, we like to think about it in familiar terms. One example is the use of the word *energy* to express the idea of qi. An extension of this is the frequent translation of the therapeutic method of draining evil influences from channels as "sedation." Neither energy nor sedation have much to do with the concepts that underlie qi and draining; however, these terms are more familiar to us and make Chinese medicine more accessible. Unfortunately, this practice can obscure the breadth of meaning in these terms (Wiseman & Boss, 1990).

We try to make sense of the world from our position in it, historically as well as culturally. We tend to view history as progressing, as if by design, to a specific end. Events of the past, viewed from the perspective of the present, offer tempting opportunities for reinterpretation in relation to current experience. For example, in the context of current perspectives on disease causation, Wu You Ke's statements that "miscellaneous qi" could cause epidemic disease, and his concept of "one disease, one qi" (Wiseman, 1993) have led contemporary sources in China to suggest that coming before the invention of the microscope, such an insight is quite remarkable (Wiseman et al., 1995). The implication that Wu You Ke's observation represented a precursor of germ theory is attractive to Chinese practitioners who are trying to find a place for traditional practices in an increasingly biomedicalized world. In fact, the concept of miscellaneous or pestilential qi has been used extensively in adapting traditional theory to the management of human immunodeficiency virus (HIV) infection. However, as Wiseman points out, it never was explored in relation to the causation of disease by microscopic organisms, nor was it ever conceived as a basis for such an exploration. Its relation to the concept is a retrospective interpretation.

The preceding points are generally relevant to almost any system or collection of medical practices. Some additional points are crucial to understanding the progression of medical thought in China. Although we tend to think that Chinese medicine has been practiced without any significant change for millennia, this is simply not true. Chinese medicine has undergone significant change and development over the centuries. Ideas that once were important are now almost invisible, and ideas that were left by the wayside for centuries found favor in later times. Recent ideas have been relatively significant in the organization of the system. Changes in technology, for instance, have broadened the clinical use of acupuncture and increased its safety. Ideas, substances, and medical practices have come to China from all over the world, some of which have become significant parts of traditional Chinese medicine and some of which remain only as observations in ancient texts.

Within China itself, many competing ideas have existed side-by-side. Old theories have been rejected or discovered anew and accorded even more importance than they had at their conception. Some ideas found more fertile ground in other Asian countries, as is the case with transmission of acupuncture and Chinese herbal medicine to Japan, where particular aspects of the Chinese tradition were emphasized and adapted.

Historian and anthropologist Paul Unschuld critiques the perspective of Chinese medicine as a homogenous monolithic structure.

Proponents of this view depict "Chinese Medicine" as an identifiable, coherent system, the contents of which they attempt to characterize. Such an approach is both ahistorical and selective. It focuses on but one of the many distinctly conceptualized systems of therapy in Chinese history, that is the medicine of systematic correspondence, and it neglects both the changing interpretations of basic paradigms offered by Chinese authors through the ages and the synchronic plurality of differing opinions and ideas that existed for twenty centuries concerning even fundamental aspects of this therapy system such as pulse-diagnosis (Unschuld, 1985).

This is a particularly important point, because it is extremely tempting to encounter medical systems with the expectation that they be possessed of an internal logic that reconciles all of their aspects. Although many aspects of Chinese medicine can be applied with complete consistency, other aspects or concepts seem to be quite contradictory. This trait leads us to what has been probably the most important aspect of Chinese medicine throughout its history: it is a medical tradition that never threw anything away. Certain medical practices might have been relegated to the attic, but they were available if necessary. A striking example of this is the work of Zhang Zhong Jing, whose system of diagnosis and therapy did not attract much attention during his lifetime but became highly influential centuries after his death. Later, authors believed his theory to be incomplete and broadened its perspective, but his theories and these new theories that emerged in response to them are still important to the contemporary clinician. In the West an incomplete theory is rejected and disappears. In the history of Chinese medicine, theories, practices, and concepts may fade, but they do not entirely disappear. A new theory can exist beside the one that it sought to correct. The clinician can choose to apply the perspective that he believes is most applicable. In this way conflicting concepts of cause, systems of diagnosis, and treatment have continued to exist side-by-side.

Unschuld considers this one of the basic characteristics distinguishing traditional Chinese thought from modern Western science (Unschuld, 1985). It also is the aspect of Chinese medicine that is most challenging to Western students. The extent to which deductive reasoning and its necessary condition of "either this or that but not both" are pervasive in our society have made it difficult to approach a medical tradition that dispenses with what we view as a necessary precondition of valid human knowledge. Even European or American advocates of Chinese medical traditions sometimes err and insist that only certain theoretical perspectives or therapeutic methods are correct or authentic.

Years earlier, Lin Yutang wrote that systematic metaphysics or epistemology were alien to traditional Chinese thought.

The temperament for systematic philosophy simply wasn't there, and will not be there so long as the Chinese remain Chinese. They have too much sense for that. The sea of human life forever laps upon the shores of Chinese thought, and the arrogance and absurdities of the logician, the assumption that "I am exclusively right and you are exclusively wrong," are not Chinese faults, whatever other faults they may have (Lin, 1942).

Of course, the history of Chinese medical thought includes plenty of individuals who thought that they were exclusively right, but the breadth of traditional Chinese medical thought was sustained by an intellectual climate that retained all possible ideas for use and exploration. A given philosopher or clinician might reject an idea, but the idea itself would remain available for future use.

For example, during the Ming dynasty, Wu You Ke (circa 1644) was the leading exponent of the "offensive precipitation sect" (*gong xia pai*) of physicians whose tenets included a distinctive set of ideas concerning the management of epidemic disease and a wholehearted rejection of many established ideas in Chinese medicine (Wong & Wu, 1985). He was subsequently viewed alternatively as a contributor to Chinese medical thought; a proponent of a divergent and uninformed theory; and finally (as noted previously) as the intellectual antecedent of Koch, the discoverer of the tuberculosis bacillus. At no point were his ideas discarded.

Interestingly enough, in modern China, where the sheer volume of information and the nation's health care needs makes it necessary to teach a standard curriculum to thousands of students each year, this tolerance for varying clinical perspectives continues. There are for instance herbal physicians known as Minor Bupleurum Decoction (*Xiao Chai Hu Tang*) doctors because their prescriptions are organized around one formula from the *Treatise on Cold Damage (Shang Han Lun)*, an early text on diagnosis and herbal therapy written during the Han dynasty (206 BCE-220 CE). Also some herbal physicians reject traditional formulas entirely and use contemporary perspectives on the Chinese pharmacopeia to organize their prescriptions.

There are acupuncturists whose clinical focus might be dedicated almost entirely to six acupuncture points and who use computed tomography scans to plan clinical interventions. At the same time two floors down in the same hospital, physicians base their selection of acupuncture points on obscure and complex aspects of traditional calendrics and systems such as the "Magic Turtle."

Once it is understood that Chinese medicine is a large and various tradition with many manifestations and philosophies, it is possible to begin its exploration.

HISTORY

Chinese medicine has an extensive history. As is the case with most medical traditions, this history can be approached from several perspectives. There is the ancient mythology of Chinese medicine, which attributes the birth of medicine to the legendary emperors Fu Xi, Shen Nong, and Huang Di. There is the history that can be deduced from the careful study of available ancient texts and records, which indicate, for example, that there is no reference to acupuncture as a therapeutic method in any Chinese text before 90 BCE (Unschuld, 1985) and that the oldest existing text to discuss medical practices that faintly resemble current Chinese medicine date from the end of the third century BCE (Unschuld, 1985). Finally, there are the more extravagant interpretations of archaeological evidence and textual materials that seek to establish the ancient character of certain Chinese medical practices. An example would be the frequent assertion that the stone "needles" excavated at different times in various parts of China were remnants of ancient acupuncture (Chuang, 1982; Wang, 1986). This assertion is based on references to the ancient surgical application of sharp stones in texts from later periods and morphological similarities between the excavated stones and later metal needles.

Legendary Origins

The origins of Chinese medicine are mythically linked to three legendary emperors: Fu Xi, or the Ox Tamer (ca 2953 BCE), taught people how to domesticate animals and divined the *Ba Gua*, eight symbols that became the basis for the *Yi Jing*, or *Book of Changes*. Shen Nong, or the Divine Husbandman, also is known as the Fire Emperor. Shen Nong is said to have lived from 2838 to 2698 BCE and is considered the founder of agriculture in China. He taught the Chinese people how to cultivate plants and raise livestock. He also is considered the originator of herbal medicine in China, having learned the therapeutic properties of herbs and substances by tasting them. Later authors would attribute their work to him to indicate the antiquity and importance of their text. The *Divine Husbandman's Classic of the Materia Medica (Shen Nong Ben Cao Jing)* is a case in point. The text probably was written in 220 CE and reconstructed in 500 CE by Tao Hong Jing. Given that all historical evidence points to the ancient character of herbal medicine in China, it is appropriate that Shen Nong is considered its originator (Figure 18-1).

Huang Di, the Yellow Emperor (2698-2598), is known as the originator of the traditional medicine of China. He also is seen as the "Father of the Chinese Nation." He is credited with teaching the Chinese how to make wooden houses, silk cloth, boats, carts, the bow and arrow, ceramics, and the art of writing. Legend has it that he gained his knowledge from visiting the immortals. Most important to our discussion is his work *Yellow Emperor's Inner Classic (Huang Di Nei Jing)*, in which the traditional medicine of China is first expressed in a form that is familiar to us today. The text is divided into two books. *Simple Questions (Su Wen)* is concerned with medical theory, such as the principles of yin and yang, the five phases, and the effects of seasons. The *Spiritual Axis (Ling Shu)* deals predominantly with acupuncture and moxibustion. The texts are written as a series of dialogues between the Emperor and his ministers. Qi Bo, the most famous among the ministers, is said to have tested the actions of drugs, cured people's sickness, and written books on medicine and therapeutics.

QI BO EXPLAINS THE ORDERLY LIFE OF TIMES PAST

The first book of *Simple Questions* begins with the Yellow Emperor asking Qi Bo why peoples' life spans are now so short when in the past they lived close to a hundred years. Qi Bo explains that in the past people maintained an or-derly life. "In ancient times those people who understood Dao patterned themselves upon the yin and the yang and they lived in harmony with the arts of divination" (Veith, 1972).

Today it is generally agreed that the Yellow Emperor's Inner Classic was first compiled around 200 BCE. Both in terms of legend and practice, it remains a text that is critical to Chinese medicine.

Ancient Medicine 2205 to 206 BCE

Little is actually known about the practice of medicine in China before 200 BCE. The Shang dynasty (1766-1121 BCE) is the first dynasty of which there exists clear archaeological evidence. It appears likely that before the Shang, nomadic cultures were scattered across Northern China. Interaction among these groups eventually led to the development of the Shang. This dynasty leaves us the first traces of some sort of therapeutic activity. In addition to developing the first Chinese scripts, the Shang had clearly defined social relations. There was a king and nobility and, perhaps most importantly, the people were no longer nomadic. The Shang response to illness is documented by archaeological finds and writings from the succeeding Zhou dynasty (1122-221 BCE). During this period ideas developed that would be central to Chinese culture, specifically a relationship between the living and the dead that developed into a ritualized veneration of ancestors. Ancestors could be consulted concerning a variety of issues, including the cause of illness, through the use of oracle bones. Tortoise shells and the scapula of oxen were heated and rapidly cooled, causing them to crack. The resulting patterns would be used for guidance in resolving questions. Often the question posed to the ancestors would be inscribed on the bone itself. Bones could be used for more than one divination. One tomb has yielded more than 100,000 oracle bones, displaying questions such as "Swelling of the abdomen. Is there a curse? Does the deceased Chin-wu desire something of the king?" (Unschuld, 1985). The ancestors were appropriately placated according to the response. Natural causes of illness also were encountered, but these appear to have been addressed through the intervention of ancestors as well.

The Zhou dynasty resulted from a political conflict with a group of Chinese-speaking descendants of the same neolithic peoples who had settled to form

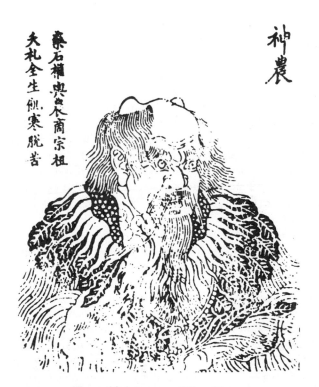

Figure 18-1 Image of Shen Nong.

the Shang. The defeat of the Shang established one of China's longest dynasties, as well as a pattern of governance that would characterize Chinese society—a central government working in relation to smaller principalities.

The Zhou continued the practices of the Shang rulers, consulting tortoise shell oracles with the aid of *wu,* or shamans. The *wu* acted as intermediaries between the living and the dead, played important ritual roles in court activities and the weather, and were called on to combat the demons who caused illness. During this period the shamanic activity of chasing evil spirits away from towns and homes with spears might have been transferred to the human body, and the practice of acupuncture emerged. Later accounts (eighth century CE) describe the needling techniques used by the physician Bian Qu (fifth century BCE) to drive out demons. However, we have no clear evidence of this.

The Warring States period, toward the close of the Zhou, was marked by political strife and social upheaval. This era saw the emergence of two philosophers, Kong Fu Zi (Confucius) and Lao Zi, whose ideas about social and natural order were to have a lasting impact on Chinese culture. A similar trend occurred within medicine: the human body no longer was seen as subject only to the whims of spirits and demons, but as a part of nature, and subject to discernible natural relationships. Those ideas were elaborated on during the Han dynasty.

The Flowering of Chinese Medicine 206 BCE to 907 CE

In 206 BCE the empire was reunited under the Han. The Han (206 BCE-219 CE) created a stable aristocratic social order, expanded geographically and economically and spread Chinese political influence throughout Vietnam and Korea. The Chinese people today refer to themselves as the Han. This dynasty was a period of great development for the Chinese, including the integration of the Confucian doctrine, elements of yin and yang, and the five-phase theory into the political picture. Textual evidence reveals the emergence of a medicine that is similar to the Chinese medicine we know today.

The earliest texts available were recovered from three tombs dating to 168 BCE that were excavated at Ma Wang Dui in Hunan province (Unschuld, 1985).

These texts discuss magical and demonologic concepts, as well as some ideas about yin and yang in relation to the body. The texts present an early concept of channels in the body, but in a less developed fashion than the later *Yellow Emperor's Inner Classic.* Ma Wang Dui texts mention moxibustion and the use of heated stones, but they do not speak about acupuncture or specific points on the body, implying that the idea of acupuncture had not yet emerged at this time.

A biography written by a contemporary in 90 BCE describes Chun Yu Yi, the first known physician to record personal observations of clinical cases. Interestingly he also was tried for malpractice because of his use of the apparently unfamiliar method of acupuncture to change the flow of qi (Unschuld, 1985).

The *Divine Husbandman's Classic of Materia Medica (Shen Nong Ben Cao)* appears during this era as well. This text is the first known formal presentation of individual medicinal substances, the first in a long line of such texts.

The *Classic of Difficult Issues (Nan Jing)* was compiled sometime during the first or second century CE, although its authorship is attributed to the legendary physician Bian Qu. This text has had and continues to have a marked influence on the practice of Chinese medicine and, to an even greater extent, on the practice of Chinese medicine in Japan. It marks a drastic shift in medical thinking, systematically organizing the theory and practice of therapeutic acupuncture in terms of body structure, illness, diagnosis, and treatment. It is almost entirely devoid of magical elements. The author(s) of the *Classic of Difficult Issues* reconciled the contradictions of the *Inner Classic,* in addition to providing many new observations. It is thought to have been written as an independent text but met with so much resistance as a result of its radical organization that it became known as a commentary on the *Inner Classic.*

The *Treatise on Cold Damage (Shang Han Lun)* and the *Survey of Important Elements from the Golden Cabinet and Jade Container (Jin Gui Yao Lue)* were written in the second century CE by Zhang Zhong Jing also known as Zhang Ji (142-220 CE). Chinese medical texts of this period were primarily philosophical, but like the authors of the *Classic of Difficult Issues,* Zhang studied disease from a clinical standpoint, emphasizing the physical signs, symptoms, and course of disease; the method of treatment; and the action of the substances used. He was interested especially in fevers because most of his village was wiped out by fever epidemics (possibly typhoid). Although the texts were published during the Han dynasty, they remained relatively obscure until the Sung dynasty (after 960 CE) when medical thinkers realized that the concepts of diagnosis and therapy presented reflected their own concerns. These texts enormously influenced the practice of herbal medicine in Japan (see p. 328). We examine an herbal formula derived from the Treatise on Cold Damage later in this chapter.

Hua Tou (110-207 CE), acupuncturist, herbalist, and surgeon, is an almost legendary figure in Chinese medicine. He is reported to have used acupuncture and herbs, and his adaptation of animal postures is one of the early forms of Qigong. He is said to have used the anesthetic properties of plants to render a patient insensible to pain, enabling him to successfully practice surgery.

Despite Hua Tou's reputation his surgical innovations seem to have departed with him. Chinese medical history reveals the practice of a variety of minor surgical interventions for growths, hemorrhoids, and wound healing, but none of the significant abdominal surgeries attributed to Hua Tou. The surgical castration used to produce eunuchs for the imperial court was medically significant, and there is textual evidence of Chinese exposure to the surgical practices developed in India for the treatment of cataracts, but these did not form surgical traditions per se.

Huang Pu Mi (215-286 CE) wrote the *Systematic Classic of Acupuncture (Zhen Jiu Jia Yi Jing),* which exercised substantial influence over the acupuncture traditions of China, Korea, and Japan. This text presented and reorganized material from the *Inner Classic* and earlier texts.

It is important to realize that the histories of individual physicians and the texts that have come down to us reflect the medicine of the literate elite of China more than the medical traditions of that nation as a whole. About 80 percent of the total population consisted of farmers, peasants, and farming villages. These people lived at a level of bare subsistence and worked extremely hard to stay there, entirely dependent on the soil and the weather. They were not exposed to formal education and typically were illiterate. Very little is known of what these people knew or thought at any particular time. Their traditions were regionally oriented, full of folk superstition, his-

torical legend, and aspirations dominated by the hope of survival.

Some authors, especially compilers of materia medica texts, would explore the nonliterate traditions of the Chinese people, but the first systematic publication of this material did not occur until late in the Qing dynasty (Unschuld, 1985). Folk herbal and medical traditions were most systematically explored under the guidance of the postrevolutionary government of China. Texts such as *The Barefoot Doctor's Manual* reflect the inclusion of this type of material.

In 220 CE, after approximately 30 years of strife and religious rebellion by Daoist sects, the Han dynasty fell. After the Han there was another long period of division in China, although not as violent or as divisive as the Warring States period after the Zhou dynasty. In 589 CE the Sui dynasty reunified China and soon was succeeded by the Tang dynasty, considered by many to be the height of China's cultural development. The Tang dynasty spread China's influence as far as Mongolia, Vietnam, Central Asia, Korea, and Japan. During this period both Buddhism and Daoism strongly influenced medical thought.

Sun Si Miao (581-682), a famous physician of the period, was a prolific author and a productive scholar who was well versed in both Daoist and Buddhist practice. His *Thousand Ducat Prescriptions (Qian Jin Yao Fang),* a text on eye disorders, and *The Classic of Spells,* a guide to magic in medicine, are some of the texts he wrote. The *Thousand Ducat Prescriptions* contains a section titled "On the absolute sincerity of great physicians" that established him as China's first medical ethicist. He addresses the need for diligent scholarship, compassion toward the patient, and high moral standards in the physician, which remain pertinent and seem to speak directly to issues in medicine today.

SUN SI MIAO EXPLAINS THE INCURABLE NATURE OF PHYSICIANS

Finally, it is inappropriate to emphasize one's reputation, to belittle the rest of the physicians and to praise only one's own virtue. Indeed, in actual life someone who has accidentally healed a disease, then stalks around with his head raised, shows conceit and announces that no one in the entire world could measure up to him. In this respect all physicians are evidently incurable (Unschuld, 1979).

Academic Medicine and Systematic Therapeutics 960 CE-1368 CE

By the time of the Sung dynasty the practice of medicine had become more specialized, and efforts were made to systematically integrate past insights. The number of texts published in this dynasty may have exceeded the number written during all of the previous dynasties put together. In 1027 Wang Wei Yi designed and oversaw the casting of two bronze figures designed to illustrate the location of acupuncture points. One of these was used in the imperial medical college. The bronzes were pierced at the location of the acupuncture points, covered with wax, and filled with water. When a student found the hole under the wax with a needle, water would drip out, indicating it to be the correct spot.

During the Sung dynasty there was a huge advance in herbal therapeutics and the publication, under imperial decree, of several complete herbal texts that contained illustrations. It was during this time that tastes and properties were assigned to herbs according to their yin or yang nature, and functions were assigned that were a result of the herb's nature and its ability to treat specific symptoms. Efforts were made to systematize herbal therapeutics. The writings of Zhang Zhong Jing received great interest because of his systematic application of traditional theoretical principles to the use of herbal medicine. The revival of the *Treatise on Cold Damage* influenced medicine for the next several hundred years because it precipitated warm-induced disease theory *(wen bing xue)* during the Ming dynasty.

During the Sung dynasty the education of physicians became more formal. The Imperial College, which had provided for the training of the emperor's physicians, was expanded. In 1076 an Imperial Medical College was founded with an enrollment of 300 students. There were regional schools as well.

The Jin and the Yuan dynasties saw the continuation of specialized medical thought and independent inquiry. Much of what we recognize as Chinese medicine today—and what we shall discuss in the section on fundamental concepts—stems from the Sung, Jin, and Yuan dynasties. Physicians of this period developed ideas involving the elaboration of therapeutic approaches on the basis of early theory. They espoused the application of five-phase theory in relation to seasonal influences, supplementing the body,

purging the body to eliminate evil influences, and supplementing the yin.

Medicine in the Ming and Qing Dynasties 1368-1911

Physicians continued to pursue lines of inquiry pursued in preceding dynasties, such as the far-reaching naturalistic explorations of Li Shi Zhen (1518-1593). His *Grand Materia Medica (Ben Cao Gang Mu)* included discussions of 1892 substances and, among its topics, described the use of kelp and deer thyroid to treat goiter.

The exploration of more precise linkages between factors in disease causation and therapeutics continued, and a number of medical sects emerged. During a virulent epidemic that struck from 1641 to 1644, Wu You Ke (Xing) (1592-1672) used an unorthodox method that was highly successful. His text, *Discussion of Warm Epidemics (Wen Yi Lun)*, explored the theoretical basis for his treatment.

Some authors consider the Ming dynasty to be the peak of the cultural expression of acupuncture and moxibustion in China (Qiu, 1993). This period saw the production of numerous texts on the subject. One of the most influential acupuncture texts, *The Great Compendium of Acupuncture and Moxibustion (Zhen Jiu Da Cheng)*, was written by Yang Ji Zhou toward the end of the dynasty.

Intellectual trends of the Ming continued into the Qing dynasty. *The Discussion of Warm Disease (Wen Re Lun)* by Ye Tian Shi complemented Zhang Zhong Jing's method of diagnosing and treating diseases caused by cold with an equally systematic method of diagnosing and treating those caused by heat.

Political, economic, and social trends during the Qing dynasty exacerbated the isolation of the Manchu rulers of the time and exposed the Chinese to the power of Western knowledge, technology, and science. The broadening of cultural horizons and the broadening of medical inquiry combined to shake the classical underpinnings of Chinese medical thought. In 1822 acupuncture was formally eliminated from the Imperial Medical College (Qiu, 1993).

By the close of the Qing dynasty in 1911 political and cultural institutions were in a state of decline. The scattered practitioners of traditional Chinese medicine found themselves increasingly under fire from the advocates of a new and modern China and a new and modern medicine.

The collapse of the Qing and the formation of the Republic laid traditional medicine open to the conquering influence of Western medicine. The Imperial College of Physicians was eliminated (Wong & Wu, 1985), and the Western-educated proponents of reform began to work toward the elimination of the traditional medicine of China and the establishment of Western medicine as the dominant medical system.

From 1914 through 1936 a series of encounters and clashes over the regulation, establishment, or elimination of practitioners of Chinese medicine occurred (Wong & Wu, 1985). The traditional medicine of China, or "medicine" (yi) as it had been known, came to be termed "Chinese medicine" (Zhong Yi). Both nationalist and marxist reformers disliked Chinese medicine with a passion.

SO-CALLED CHINESE MEDICINE

Initially the external threat reduced the internal spectrum of competing Chinese interpretations of the classics. The great diversity of individual efforts to reconcile insights from personal experience with the ancient theories of yin yang and the five phases, as well as with other older views about the structure of the body, disappeared behind the illusion of a so-called Chinese medicine (chung-I [zhong yi]), supposedly well defined and with theory easily converted into practice. This situation, in turn, has given rise to the historically misleading impression that these diverse elements, like the concepts and practices of Western medicine, constituted a unified, coherent system (Unschuld, 1985).

A critical feature of this new Chinese medicine was its rejection of practices that were manifestly "unscientific," represented in the creation of Zhong Yi. This disciplined form of medicine has emerged today as traditional Chinese medicine.

The aspects of the traditional medicine of China that were secured in Zhong Yi were later appropriated by the Chinese Marxists in an effort to build a strong medical infrastructure for substantial populations in the face of economic and technical limitations. Chairman Mao's declaration in 1958 that "Chinese medicine is a great treasure house! We must uncover it and raise its standards!" (Unschuld, 1985) inspired efforts to rehabilitate the traditional medicine of China and to "discover" a primitive dialectic within the theoretical underpinnings of the system. The Revised Outline of Chinese Medicine stated that "Yin-yang and the five

phases (wu-hsing [wu xing]) are ancient Chinese philosophical ideas. They are spontaneous, naive materialist theories that also contain elementary dialectic ideas" (Sivin, 1987).

The development of Chinese medicine as a system parallel to Western medicine was under way by the time of Mao's declaration. In 1956 four colleges of Chinese medicine were created, with many more to follow. Today Zhong Yi exists as a parallel medical system, integrating necessary biomedical elements while retaining fidelity to the traditional concepts of Chinese medicine. Educational programs emphasize acupuncture and herbal medicine and range from an undergraduate technical certificate to doctoral programs. Most independent practitioners enter the field with a 5-year medical baccalaureate degree (MB/BS) that is earned after high school (Ergil, 1994). In this system both inpatient and outpatient medical care is delivered from large, well-equipped hospitals, as well as private clinics and pharmacies.

FUNDAMENTAL CONCEPTS

Yin and Yang

The philosophy of Chinese medicine begins with yin and yang. These two terms can be used to express the broadest philosophical concepts, as well as the most focused perceptions of the natural world. Yin and yang express the idea of opposing but complementary phenomena that exist in a state of dynamic equilibrium. The most ancient expression of this idea seems to have been that of the shady and sunny sides of a hill (Unschuld, 1985, p. 55; Wilhelm, 1967, p. 297). The sunlit southern side was the yang and the shaded northern side was the yin. The contrast between the bright and dark sides of a single hill portrayed the yang and the yin, respectively. If you imagine, for a moment, the different environments that exist on either side of this one hill you can begin to get an idea of yin and yang. On the bright, sunny side, plants and animals that enjoy light are more prevalent, the air is drier, and the rocks are warm; on the dim, shaded side, the air seems moist and cool.

Yin and yang are always present simultaneously. The paired opposites observed in the world gave tangible expression to the otherwise uncontemplatable Dao of ancient Chinese thought (Box 18-1).

BOX 18-1

Origins of Yin and Yang

Out of Tao, One is born;
Out of One, Two;
Out of Two, Three;
Out of Three, the created universe.
The created universe carries the yin at its back and
   the yang in front;
Through the union of the pervading principles it
   reaches harmony (Laozi in Lin, 1942).

BOX 18-2

Yang and Yin Correspondences

Yang	Yin
Light	Dark
Heaven	Earth
Sun	Moon
Day	Night
Spring	Autumn
Summer	Winter
Hot	Cold
Male	Female
Fast	Slow
Up	Down
Outside	Inside
Fire	Water
Wood	Metal

The *Book of Changes (Yi Jing)*, which sought to explore the myriad manifestations of yin and yang, expressed the idea thusly, "That which lets now the dark, now the light appear is tao" (Wilhelm, 1967).

The *Yellow Emperor's Inner Classic*, the oldest text to discuss the medical application of yin and yang in a comprehensive way (Unschuld, 1985, p. 56), tells us that "yin and yang are the way of heaven and earth" (Wiseman et al., 1985). This text showed how yin and yang were to be used to correlate the body and other phenomena to the human experience of health and disease.

THE *INNER CLASSIC ON YIN AND YANG*

As to the yin and yang of the human body, the outer part is yang and the inner part is yin. As to the trunk, the back is yang and the abdomen is yin. As to the organs, the viscera are yin whereas the bowels are yang. The liver, heart, spleen, lung, and kidney are yin; the gallbladder, stomach, intestines, bladder, and triple burner are yang (Wiseman et al., 1993).

It is important to note that the preceding quote is taken from the translation of an important contemporary textbook of Chinese medicine. Many ideas expressed in the *Yellow Emperor's Inner Classic* are taught and applied routinely in the contemporary clinical practice of Chinese medicine.

Yin and yang were used to express ideas about both normal physiology and pathological processes. They were applied to the organization of phenomena in many ways, for example, to organize phenomena in terms of the emergence of its dominant yin or yang character. Summer was yang within yang, fall was yin within yang, winter was yin within yin, and spring was yang within yin. Thus the coldest, darkest, and most yin period was yin within yin, whereas spring,

when the yang began to emerge from the yin, was yang within yin.

There is a distinctly ecological orientation to the world view that is supported by yin and yang; each phenomenon is seen in relation to its surroundings, and it is expected that each phenomenon will exert an influence on its surroundings that is balanced by an equal but opposing influence (Box 18-2). Just as the language of ecology is the language of interrelation and interdependence, the language of Chinese medicine is a language of interrelation and interdependence. The external landscape, or human environment, is understood to be in profound and dynamic relationship with the internal landscape, or human organism. We will see this idea even more clearly when we explore the idea of disease causation.

The ancient Chinese understood human beings to have a nature and structure inseparable from yin and yang, and as such, inseparable from the world around us—a structure that is to be understood by the same rules that guide us in understanding the world in which we live. Life on the shaded side of a mountain has characteristics that differ from those on the sunny side. Finally, the comprehension and adjustment of life in relation to yin and yang would support life itself. Thus it was said "To follow (the laws of) yin and yang means life; to act contrary to (the laws of yin and yang) means death" (Unschuld, 1985).

Within the traditional medical community of contemporary China, there is debate over the actual nature of yin and yang. Some exponents of a more scientific, less traditional, perspective on Chinese medicine would like yin and yang to be used as concepts to organize phenomena. Others who express a less modern perspective will emphatically state that yin and yang are actually tangible phenomena (Farquhar, 1987). Although it is probably easiest for us to think about *yin* and *yang* as descriptive terms that help the Chinese physician organize information, it should be remembered—and this is especially true in traditional pharmaceutics—that the yin and yang constituents of the body are actual things that can be reinforced by specific substances or actions.

An analogy that is useful for thinking about yin and yang in this way is that of a candle. If one considers the yin aspect of the candle to be the wax and the yang aspect to be the flame, it can be seen how the yin nourishes and supports the yang, how the yang consumes the yin and, in doing so, burns brightly. When the wax is gone, so is the flame. Yin and yang exist in dependence on each other.

The Five Phases

Another idea that has played a significant part in the development of some aspects of Chinese medicine is that of the five phases *(wu xing)*. The five phases are earth, metal, water, wood, and fire. In Chinese *wu*

means "five" and *xing* expresses the idea of movement, to go. For a period of time the *wu xing* were translated as the five elements. This translation conveys little of the dynamism of the Chinese concept, instead focusing on the apparent similarities between the *wu xing* and the elements of medieval alchemy. This is an example of the translation problem in which we use the familiar to understand the new. However useful this method may be at first, it can lead to some confusion in the long run. *Wu xing* may include the implication of material elements, but in general, the five phases speak to a set of dynamic relations occurring among phenomena that are organized in terms of the five phases. This philosophy can cover almost every aspect of phenomena from seasons to the weather (Table 18-1).

Qi and the Essential Substances of the Body

Apart from the ideas of yin and yang and the five phases, there is no concept more crucial to Chinese medicine than qi—the idea that the body is pervaded by subtle material and mobile influences that cause most physiological functions and maintain the health and vitality of the individual. This idea is not common to biomedical thinking about the body. It is not unusual to see the idea of qi translated with the term *energy*, but this translation conceals its distinctly

TABLE 18-1

Five Phase Correspondences

Category	Wood	Fire	Earth	Metal	Water
Viscus	Liver	Heart	Spleen	Lungs	Kidney
Bowel	Gallbladder	Small intestine	Stomach	Large intestine	Urinary bladder
Season	Spring	Summer	Late summer	Autumn	Winter
Time of day	Before sunrise	Forenoon	Afternoon	Late afternoon	Midnight
Climate	Wind	Heat	Damp	Dryness	Cold
Direction	East	South	Center	West	North
Development	Birth	Growth	Maturity	Withdrawal	Dormancy
Color	Cyan	Red	Yellow	White	Black
Taste	Sour	Bitter	Sweet	Pungent	Salty
Sense organ	Eyes	Tongue	Mouth	Nose	Ears
Odor	Goatish	Scorched	Fragrant	Raw fish	Putrid
Vocalization	Shouting	Laughing	Singing	Weeping	Sighing
Tissue	Sinews	Vessels	Flesh	Body hair	Bones
Mind	Anger	Joy	Thought	Sorrow	Fear

material attributes. Furthermore, although energy is defined as the capacity of a system to do work, the character of qi extends considerably further.

The Chinese character for qi is traditionally composed of two radicals; the radical that symbolizes breath or rising vapor is placed above the radical for rice (Figure 18-2). Qi is linked with the concept of "vapors arising from food" (Unschuld, 1985). Over time this concept broadened but never lost its distinctively material aspect. Unschuld favors the use of the phrase "finest matter influences" or "influences" to translate this concept. Wiseman points out that some phenomena labeled as qi do not fit conventional definitions of substance or matter, further confusing the issue (Wiseman et al., 1995). It is for this reason that many authors prefer to leave the term *qi* untranslated.

The idea of qi is extremely broad, encompassing almost every variety of natural phenomena. Many different types of qi are in the body. In general, the features that distinguish each type derive from its source, location, and function. There is considerable room for debate in this area, and exploration of a wide range of materials can suggest a variety of different ideas about categories of qi. In general, qi has the functions of activation, warming, defense, transformation, and containment (Box 18-3).

The qi concept is important to many aspects of Chinese medicine. Organ and channel qi are influenced by acupuncture. In fact, one characteristic feature of acupuncture treatment is the sensation of obtaining the qi or *de qi*. *Qigong* is a general term for the many systems of meditation, exercise, and therapeutics that are rooted in the concept of mobilizing and regulating the movement of qi in the body. Qi is sometimes compared with wind captured in a sail; we cannot observe the wind directly, but we can infer its presence as it fills the sail. In a similar fashion, the movements of the body and the movement of substances within the body are all signs of the action of qi.

In relation to qi, blood and fluids constitute the yin aspects of the body. Blood is produced by the construction qi, which in turn is derived from food and water. Blood nourishes the body. Blood is understood to have a slightly broader and less definite range of actions in Chinese medicine than it does in biomedicine. Within the body qi and blood are closely linked because blood is considered to flow with qi and to be conveyed by it. This relationship often is expressed by the Chinese saying "qi is the commander of blood and blood is the mother of qi," and it has been suggested that qi and blood are linked in the manner of a person and their shadow.

Fluids are a general category of thin and viscous substances that serve to moisten and lubricate the body. Fluids can be conceptually separated into humor and liquid. Humor is thick and related to the body's organs; among its functions is the lubrication of the joints. Liquid is thin and is responsible for moistening the surface areas of the body, including the skin, eyes, and mouth.

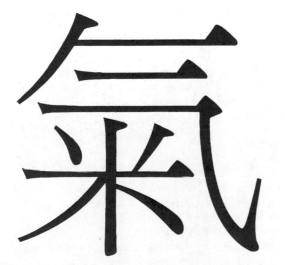

Figure 18-2 The character *qi*.

BOX 18-3

Types of Qi

Ying qi	Construction qi	Supports and nourishes the body
Wei qi	Defense qi	Protects and warms the body
Jing qi	Channel qi	Flows in the channels (felt during acupuncture)
Zang qi	Organ qi	Flows in the organs (physiological function of organs)
Zong qi	Ancestral qi	Responsible for respiration and circulation

Essence and Spirit

Together with qi, essence and spirit make up what are known in Chinese medicine as the *three treasures*. In brief, essence is the gift of one's parents and spirit is the gift of heaven. Essence is the most fundamental source of human physiological processes, the bodily reserves that support human life and that must be replenished by food and rest, and the actual reproductive substances of the body. Spirit is the alert and radiant aspect of human life. We encounter it in the luster of the eyes and face in a healthy person, as well as in their ability to think and respond appropriately to the world around them. The idea expressed by *spirit,* or *shen* in Chinese, encompasses consciousness and healthy mental and physical function.

The relation of the mind to the body in Chinese medicine does not include the notion of a distinct separation. It is understood that the psyche and soma interact with each other and that aspects of mental and emotional experience can have an impact on the body, and vice versa. In this sense, spirit is linked both to the health of the body and to the health of the mind. Similarly, aspects of human experience that are understood as predominantly mental in a biomedical frame of reference are linked to specific organs in Chinese medicine. Anger is related to the liver, obsessive thought is related to the spleen, and joy to the heart.

Viscera and Bowels (*Zang* and *Fu*)

The anatomy of human beings was understood by the ancient Chinese in ways that are not too distant from their European contemporaries, up to the seventeenth century. There are instances of systematic dissection in Chinese history, but none of these reached the extensive explorations into the structure of the body that characterized European medicine by the fifteenth century. Instead the Chinese medical perspective of the body, although rooted in familiar anatomical structures, represented a system in which organs serve as markers of associated physiological functions rather than actual physical structures.

The physician of Chinese medicine encounters a body in which 12 organs function. These organs are divided into the viscera, which includes six *zang* or solid organs and the bowels, including six *fu* or hollow organs. These organs often are related to the physical structures that we associate with conventional biomedical anatomy. The heart, lungs, liver, spleen, kidneys, and pericardium are the six viscera. The six bowels are the small intestine, large intestine, gallbladder, stomach, urinary bladder, and the "triple burner" *(san jiao)*. These organs have physiological functions that often are similar to those associated with them in biomedicine but that also might be very different. The liver is said to store blood and to distribute it to the extremities as needed. The spleen is understood as an organ of digestion. The Chinese understood the physical structure and location of most of the organs, but because systematic dissection was not extensively pursued, the close observation of physiological function was more often the basis of medical thought.

For example, circulation and elimination of fluids was observed and attributed to an organ that was said to have a name, but no form was established. This organ, the "triple burner," is considered alternatively to be the combined expression of the activity of other organs in the body, or a group of spaces in the body. This example clearly expresses the idea that physiological function, rather than substance, establishes an organ in Chinese medicine. At the same time the triple burner has always been surrounded by debate because it does not have a clear anatomical structure.

The organs of viscera and bowel are paired in what is known as the *yin* and *yang,* or *interior-exterior relationship*. The heart is linked with the small intestine, the spleen with the stomach, and so on. Each viscera and each bowel have an associated channel that runs through the organ, the paired organ, within the body, and across the body's surface, and then connects with the channel of the related organ.

Historical evidence suggests that the idea of channels is more ancient than the idea of specific acupuncture points. There has been disagreement about the locations of specific points, and efforts have been made to systematize knowledge of them. Recent research in the People's Republic of China has led to the publication of a number of texts dedicated to resolving historical, philological, and anatomical questions about acupuncture points. At this time there are understood to be 12 primary channels and 8 extraordinary vessels. The 12 channels are classically organized in terms of a sixfold yin and yang organizational scheme, although they can also be organized in terms of five-phase theory. Qi is understood to flow in these channels, making a rhythmic circuit.

Along the pathways of 14 of these channels (the 12 regular channels and 2 of the extra channels) lie 361 specific points. In addition, there are a large number of "extra" points that have been derived from clinical experience but are not traditionally considered part of the major channel systems. Beyond this, various individual elaborations of acupuncture theory suggest new points. There are also local microsystems of acupuncture points that have postulated numerous points on the ear, scalp, hand, foot, and other areas of the body.

Acupuncture points appear at many locations on the body. Most often they are located where a gentle and sensitive hand can detect a declivity with slight pressure on the skin surface. Points are located at the margins or bellies of muscles, between bones, and over distinctive bony features that can be detected through the skin. Methods used to locate points vary. In general, points are found by seeking anatomical landmarks, by proportionally measuring the body, and by using finger measurements. The first method is considered the most reliable. With time and clinical experience some practitioners can be less formal in their approach to locating acupuncture points, but this topic interests even advanced practitioners. In Japan clinicians gather regularly to hone their point location skills, and in China point location in relation to classical sources, anatomical study, and empirical evidence is an area of advanced study.

As with qi, the actual term and use of the Chinese expression that we translate as "point" is important. The character *xue,* which has been translated as "point," actually means "hole" in Chinese. A hole often is part of the clinician's subjective experience of the acupuncture point. *Xue* are holes in which the qi of the channels can be influenced by inserting a needle or by other means. If one imagines the channel system as a vast subcutaneous waterway with caves and springs punctuating its course as it flows to the surface, one will have a concept of the holes that is not far from the way the Chinese thought of them for many centuries (Box 18-4).

Holes, or points along the channels, have been categorized and organized in myriad ways. One of the oldest and most well known is a system of categories based on the idea of *shu,* or transport points. This system of point categories applies exclusively to points on the forearm and lower leg, which embody the image of qi welling gently forth from a mountainous source at the fingertips and gradually gaining

BOX 18-4

Leg Three Li

- *Location:* 3 cun (body inch) below the depression below the patella, one fingerbreadth from the anterior crest of the tibia
- *Indications:* stomach pain, vomiting, abdominal distension, indigestion, diarrhea, constipation, dizziness, mastitis, mental disorders, hemiplegia, pain in knee joint and leg
- *Depth of needle insertion:* 0.5-1.3 inches

strength and depth as it reaches the seas located at the elbow and knee joints.

What has been presented in the preceding is a brief discussion of the essential anatomy and physiology of Chinese medicine. It is important to remember that this anatomy forms a general reference for physiological function rather than an anatomy of direct links between discrete categories of tissue and specific physiological processes. A strength of Chinese medicine is that its theory allows for generalizations about complex physical processes in addition to responding to signs and symptoms whose origins are obscure. Finally, the distinction between mind and body is not present in Chinese medicine. Although Chinese physicians may display a disconcerting lack of interest in contemporary psychotherapy or its patients, they are quick to posit a link between affect and physiological process, in a manner that might intrigue a contemporary psychobiologist. On this basis then we can proceed to examine how illness manifests in the body.

The Causes of Disease

Ultimately all illness is a disturbance of qi within the body. Its expression as a pathological process displaying specific signs and symptoms depends on the location of the disturbance. Contemporary formal discussions on the cause of disease make use of the ideas of Chen Yen (1161-1174), who wrote *Prescriptions Elucidated on the Premise That All Pathological Symptoms Have Only Three Primary Causes (San Yin Qi Yi Bing Cheng Fang Lun),* and an additional idea of Wu You Ke, that each disease has its own qi.

BOX 18-5

The Three Causes of Disease (San Yin)

- *External causes,* or "the six evils": wind, cold, fire, damp, summer heat, and dryness
- *Internal causes,* or internal damage by the seven affects: joy, anger, anxiety, thought, sorrow, fear, and fright
- *Nonexternal, noninternal causes:* dietary irregularities, excessive sexual activity, taxation fatigue, trauma, and parasites

The three categories of disease are organized in terms of external causes of disease, internal causes, and causes that are neither external nor internal (Wiseman et al., 1995) (Box 18-5). The first category includes six influences that are distinctly environmental: wind, cold, fire, dampness, summer heat, and dryness. When they cause disease, these six influences are known as *evils.* If the defense qi is not robust or the correct qi is not strong, or if the evil is powerful—the evil may enter the surface of the body and, under certain conditions, penetrate to the interior.

The nature of the evil and its impact on the body were understood through the observation of nature and the observation of the body in illness. The clinical meaning of the causes of disease does not lie, for the most part, in the expression of a distinct etiology but in the manifestation of a specific set of clinical signs. In this sense, the biomedical distinction between etiology and diagnosis is somewhat blurred in Chinese medical theory.

For example, the evils of wind and cold often are implicated in the sudden onset of symptoms associated with the common cold: headache, pronounced aversion to cold, aching muscles and bones, fever, and a scratchy throat. Wind is expressed in the sudden onset of the symptoms and in their manifestation in the upper part of the body, and cold is displayed in the pronounced aversion to cold and the aching muscles and bones. Whether the patient had a specific encounter with a cold wind shortly before the onset of the symptoms is not particularly relevant. Although it is not unusual for a patient to announce that he or she was abroad on a chilly and windy day before the onset of a cold, such exposure could easily result in signs of wind heat as well, that is, a less marked aver-

sion to cold, a distinctly sore throat, and a dry mouth. The six evils are not agents of specific etiology but agents of specific symptomatology. These ideas developed in a setting where the possibility of investigating a bacterial or viral cause was nonexistent. Rather, careful observation of the body's response to disease provided the information necessary for treatment.

Each of the evils affects the body in a fashion similar to its behavior in the environment. Images of these processes observed in nature and society were inscribed on the body to permit its processes to be readily understood. The human body stood between heaven and earth and was subject to all their influences in a relationship of continuity with its environment. Although these six evils are identified as environmental influences that attack the body's surface, it also is clearly understood they may occur within the body, causing internal disruption.

Internal damage by the seven affects refers to the way in which mental states can influence body processes. However, such a statement expresses a separation not implied in Chinese medicine. Each of the seven affects can disturb the body if it is strongly or frequently expressed. As was discussed earlier each of the mental states—joy, anger, anxiety, thought, sorrow, fear, fright—is related to a specific organ.

Finally, nonexternal, noninternal causes encompass the causes of disease that do not arise specifically as a result of environmental influences or mental states. These include dietary irregularities, excessive sexual activity, taxation fatigue, trauma, and parasites. The role that most of these have in producing disease is obvious to us, with the exceptions of excessive sexual activity and taxation fatigue. Excessive sexual activity suggests the possibility that too frequent emission of semen by the male can cause illness. This can occur because semen is directly related to the concept of essence, which is considered to be vital to the body's function and difficult to replace. This category also includes possible damage that can occur to the essence through excessive childbearing or bearing a child at too young or too old an age.

Taxation fatigue is an intriguing category. This category expresses the dangers of engaging in a variety of activities for a prolonged period. This category includes both the idea of overexertion and the idea of inactivity as possible causes of disease. All of the concepts included within taxation fatigue reflect the essential thought of Chinese medicine that moderation is the key to health. Lying down for prolonged periods damages the qi and prolonged standing damages the bones. From the moment that the Yellow Emperor asks Qi Bo why people now die before their time and receives his answer, the images of balance, harmony, and moderation have informed Chinese medicine.

Each of the causes of disease—from prosaic ones, such as dietary irregularities, to somewhat exotic notions, such as wind evil—disrupt the balance of yang and yin within the body and disrupt the free movement of qi. The next step is to determine the precise pattern of imbalance.

Diagnosis

Diagnostics in Chinese medicine is traditionally expressed within four categories: inspection, listening and smelling, inquiry, and palpation. The fundamental goal is to collect information that reflects the status of physiological processes and then to analyze this information to determine which impact a disorder has on that process.

The first of the four diagnostic methods, inspection *(wang)*, refers to the visual assessment of the patient, particularly their spirit, form and bearing, the head and face, and substances excreted by the body. Inspection makes use of a large body of empirically derived information and theoretical considerations. The color, shape, markings, and coating of the tongue are inspected. In the case of our patient who had been attacked by wind and cold, one would expect to see a moist tongue with a thin white coating, signaling the presence of cold. If heat were present, we might expect a dry mouth and a red tongue. The observation of the spirit, which is considered very important in assessing the patient's prognosis, relies on assessing the overall appearance of the patient, especially the eyes, the complexion, and the quality of the patient's voice. Good spirit—even in the presence of serious illness—is thought to bode well for the patient.

The second aspect of diagnosis, listening and smelling *(wen)*, refers to listening to the quality of speech, breath, and other sounds, as well as to being aware of the odors of breath, body, and excreta. As is the case with each aspect of diagnosis, the five-phase theory can be incorporated into the assessment of the patient's condition. Each phase and pair of viscera and bowel has a corresponding vocalization and smell.

The third aspect of diagnosis, inquiry *(wen)*, is the process of taking a comprehensive medical history. This process has been presented in many ways, but perhaps best known is the system of 10 questions described by Zhang Jie Bin in the Ming dynasty. The questions were presented as an outline of diagnostic inquiry and included querying the patient about sensations of hot and cold, perspiration, head and body, excreta, diet, chest, hearing, thirst, previous illnesses, and previous medications and their effects.

One might, for example, expect the patient who has wind and cold symptoms to report an aversion to any sort of exposure to cold, headache, body aches, and an absence of thirst.

This step is considered critical to a good diagnosis. Although pulse diagnosis is sometimes regarded as a central feature of Chinese medicine and is rightly regarded as an art, it should not form the sole basis of a complete diagnosis.

The *simple questions* expresses the following idea: If, in conducting the examination, the practitioner neither inquires as to how and when the condition arose nor asks about the nature of the patient's complaint, about dietary irregularities, excesses of sleeping and waking, and poisoning, but instead proceeds immediately to take the pulse, he will not succeed in identifying the disease (Wiseman et al., 1995).

Contemporaries of Li Shi Zhen, the author of *The Pulse Studies of Bin Hu (Bin Hu Mai Xue)*, placed tremendous emphasis on the pulse. He was considered an expert himself but rejected the notion that one would place an unequal emphasis on any aspect of the diagnostic process.

Palpation *(qie)*, the fourth diagnostic method, includes pulse examination, general palpation of the body, and palpation of the acupuncture points. Pulse diagnosis offers a range of approaches and can provide a remarkable amount of information about the patient's condition. The process of pulse diagnosis is carried out on the radial arteries of the left and right wrists. The patient may be seated or lying down and should be calm. The pulse is divided into three parts: the middle part is adjacent to the styloid process of the radius, in what is called the *bar position*. The inch is distal to it and the cubit is proximal. The inch position, which is nearest the wrist, can indicate the status of the body above the diaphragm; the bar indicates the status of the body between the diaphragm and the navel; and the cubit, the area below the navel. Beyond this simple conceptual structure, each pulse position can be interpreted to shed light on the status of the organs and the channels. Table 18-2 presents two models of what can be felt at each pulse position. The first chart is derived from the *Classic of Difficult Issues,* where this type of pulse diagnosis was first presented in a systematic way, and the second chart shows a less elaborate, contemporary pattern. Some authors have suggested that the pattern associated with the *Classic of Difficult Issues* is related more to the use of pulse diagnosis in the practice of acupuncture, whereas the later pattern is of more relevance to the herbalist (Maciocia, 1989). Not all herbalists or acupuncturists make use of the pulse, but certain styles of acupuncture rely quite heavily on it. There are many possible approaches to the pulse, making it a very rich area for the clinician and a somewhat vexing one for the biomedically oriented researcher (Birch, 1994).

The pulse allows the clinician to feel the quality of the qi and blood at different locations in the body. Table 18-3 provides a list of 29 pulse qualities and some possible associations (Wiseman, 1993). Pulse qualities are organized on the basis of the size, rate, depth, force, and volume of the pulse. The overall quality of the pulse and the variations in quality at certain positions can, after several years of patient attention, become quite meaningful to the clinician. The patient who has been afflicted with a wind cold evil might display a pulse that was floating and tight, signaling the presence of a cold evil on the surface of the body.

Once the practitioner of Chinese medicine has carried out the diagnostic process, he or she must make sense of the information derived. The practitioner constructs an appropriate image of the configuration of the disease so that it can be addressed by effective therapy. Central to this process is the notion of pattern identification *(bian zheng),* the process of gathering signs and symptoms through the diagnostic process and using traditional theory to understand how they have made an impact on the fundamental substances of the body, the organs, and the channels. Many intellectual aspects of the diagnostic processes of Chinese medicine, especially when applied to the practice of herbal medicine, are as analytical as a biomedical clinical encounter. The physician must elicit signs and symptoms from the patient and then use them to understand the disruption of underlying physiological processes.

The first step of pattern identification is the localization of the disorder and the assessment of its essential nature, using the eight principles that are an expansion of yin and yang correspondences: yin, yang, cold, hot, interior, exterior, vacuity, and repletion.*

Like many other aspects of contemporary Chinese medicine, the eight principles originated in the Sung dynasty. Kou Zong Shi proposed a structure that organized disease into eight essentials: cold, hot, interior, exterior, vacuity, repletion, evil qi, and right qi

---

*Although many authors continue to use the terms *excess* and *deficiency* to express the Chinese expressions *shi* and *xu,* I prefer Wiseman's "repletion" and "vacuity" as a translation. The use of *excess* simply is incorrect because of the existence of other Chinese terms that convey this idea exactly. *Deficiency* is problematic because it implies measurable quantity, which is not a consideration in the Chinese concept (Wiseman & Boss, 1990). Unschuld uses *depletion* and *repletion* instead.

TABLE 18-2

Pulse Positions

	Position	Left		Right	
		Deep	Superficial	Deep	Superficial
Nan Jing	Inch	Heart	Small intestine	Lung	Large intestine
	Bar	Liver	Gallbladder	Spleen	Stomach
	Cubit	Kidney	Urinary bladder	Pericardium	Triple warmer
Contemporary Chinese sources	Inch	Heart		Lung	
	Bar	Liver	Gallbladder	Spleen	Stomach
	Cubit	Kidney	Urinary bladder	Kidney	Urinary bladder

TABLE 18-3

Pulse Types

English	Chinese	General Association
1 Normal	zheng chang mai	Normal pulse
2 Floating	fu mai	Exterior condition
3 Deep	chen mai	Interior condition
4 Slow	chi mai	Cold and yang vacuity
5 Rapid	shuo mai	Heat
6 Surging	hong mai	Exuberant heat, hemorrhage
7 Faint	wei mai	Qi and blood vacuity desertion
8 Fine	xi mai	Blood and yin vacuity
9 Scattered	san mai	Dissipation of qui and blood, critical
10 Vacuous	xu mai	Vacuity
11 Replete	shi mai	Exuberant evil with right qi strong
12 Slippery	hua mai	Pregnancy, phlegm, abundant qi and blood
13 Rough	se mai	Blood stasis, vacuity of qi and blood
14 Long	chang mai	Often normal
15 Short	duan mai	Vacuity of qi and blood
16 Stringlike	xian mai	Liver disorders, severe pain
17 Hollow	kou mai	Blood loss
18 Tight	jin mai	Cold, pain
19 Moderate	huan mai	Slower than normal not pathological
20 Drumskin	ge mai	Blood loss
21 Confined	lao mai	Cold, pain
22 Weak	ruo mai	Vacuity of qi and blood
23 Soggy	ru mai	Vacuity of qi and blood with dampness
24 Hidden	fu mai	Deep lying internal cold
25 Stirred	dong mai	High fever, pregnancy
26 Rapid, irregular	cu mai	Debility of visceral qi or emotional distress
27 Slow, irregular	jie mai	Debility of visceral qi or emotional distress
28 Regularly intermittent	dai mai	Debility of visceral qi or emotional distress
29 Racing	ji mai	Heat, possible vacuity

Data from Wiseman N, Ellis A, Zmiewski P, Li C. 1995. In Wiseman N, Ellis A (trans) Fundamentals of Chinese Medicine. Paradigm. Brookline.

(Bensky & Barolet, 1990). These were improved on in 1732, in the text *Awakening the Mind in Medical Studies (Yi Xue Xin Wu)* (Sivin, 1987). The original source was written, in the spirit of the times, to create a formal diagnostic structure for herbs that could be conceptually integrated with the ideas already in use for acupuncture. Today this formal structure is applied to both acupuncture and herbal medicine.

The wind cold patient came to us with these symptoms: marked aversion to exposure to cold, headache, body aches, absence of thirst, a moist tongue with a thin white coating, and a floating and tight pulse. In terms of the eight principles this would be an exterior, cold, repletion pattern. The principles of yin and yang would not directly apply.

What does this mean? The eight principles serve fundamentally to localize a condition. When the Chinese physician says that a condition is external, he means that it has not yet penetrated beyond the skin and channels to the deeper parts of the body. In this case a cold condition betrays itself through the body's expression of cold signs. To say a condition is replete is to say that the evil attacking the body is strong or that the body itself is strong.

Typically the eight principles are the first step in developing a clear pattern identification, especially if there

Types of Diagnostic Patterns

- Eight principles
- Six evils
- Qi and blood and fluids
- Five phases
- Channel patterns
- Viscera and bowels
- Triple burner
- Six channels
- Four levels

Methods of Treatment

- Diaphoresis
- Clearing
- Ejection
- Precipitation
- Harmonization
- Warming
- Supplementation
- Dispersion
- Orifice opening
- Securing astriction
- Settling and absorption

is organ involvement. The eight principles are the application of a yin and yang–based theoretical structure.

A single biomedical disease entity can be associated with a large number of Chinese diagnostic patterns (Box 18-6). For example, viral hepatitis is associated with at least six distinctive diagnostic patterns, and lower urinary tract infection might be related to one of four distinct diagnostic patterns (Ergil, 1995a, b). Each of these patterns would be treated in different ways, as it is said, "one disease, different treatments." Our patient whose clinical pattern is wind cold has the common cold and a headache, but the same disease could manifest in other patterns.

Also many different diseases may be captured within one pattern, hence the saying, "different diseases, one treatment." One contemporary text lists such diverse entities as nephritis, dysfunctional uterine bleeding, pyelonephritis, and rheumatic heart disease under the diagnostic pattern of "disharmony between the heart and kidney" (Huang et al., 1993, p. 79).

This comparatively precise diagnostic linkage begins to be broadly appreciated in the historical trends of the Sung, Jin, and Yuan dynasties. The six-channel pattern identification proposed by Zhang Zhong Jing is one among many patterns currently used. The patient who has encountered a wind cold evil would, under Zhang Jong Jing's system, be categorized as having tai yang disease. There is considerable room for overlap within the available methods of pattern identification.

Therapeutic Concepts

Once a diagnosis has been determined and, when relevant, a pattern has been differentiated, therapy be-

gins. Therapeutics in Chinese medicine is fundamentally allopathic; that is, it addresses the pathological condition with opposing measures.

Cold is treated with heat, heat is treated with cold, vacuity is treated by supplementation, and repletion is treated by drainage (Inner Classic [Wiseman et al., 1985]).

Within the realm of acupuncture, moxibustion, and herbal medicine, three fundamental principles of therapy are understood: treating disease from its root, eliminating evil influences and supporting the right, and restoring the balance of yin and yang. These refer, respectively, to approaches that are appropriate to the patient's condition. It would be appropriate to eliminate the cold evil and support the right qi of the wind cold patient. In a patient in whom the symptoms reflect a complex underlying pattern, one might attempt to treat the root of the patient's condition. For instance, functional uterine bleeding caused by a disharmony of the heart and kidney would be addressed primarily by harmonizing the heart and kidney; treating the root of the condition would adjust its symptoms. Treatment methods vary widely. The simplest expression of their organization is given in Box 18-7.

THERAPEUTIC METHODS

Acupuncture and Moxibustion

Acupuncture and moxibustion certainly can be used independently of each other but are so deeply wedded to each other in Chinese medicine that the term for this therapy is *zhen jiu,* meaning "needle moxibustion." To capture the distinctively composite character of this phrase, some authors translate the expression as "acumoxa therapy." The basis of their close linkage lies in the ancient origins of these methods and the fact that moxibustion appears to have been the form of therapy that first was applied to the channels and holes to treat problems on or within the body. Both techniques are used to provide a discrete stimulus to points that lie along channel pathways or to other appropriate sites. I will begin by discussing acupuncture and then move on to moxibustion.

The therapeutic goal of acupuncture is to regulate the qi. Qi and blood flow through the body, its organs, and the channel pathways. When it flows unimpeded, the body is in a state of health. When some cause—such as an evil, mental state, or trauma—interrupts the flow of qi, illness results and pain can occur. Pain is directly linked to an injury or an interruption of the flow of qi. Acupuncture is used to remove the obstruction. The technique may be used to remove the evil, to direct qi to where it is insufficient, or to cause qi to flow where it previously had been obstructed.

The *Spiritual Axis* of the *Inner Classic* described nine needles (Figure 18-3) for use in acupuncture. With the exception of one that appears to have had a specifically surgical application, the remaining needle types are still in use, either in original or adapted form. Acupuncture is performed today with a wider variety of tools and methods. The filiform or fine needle is the typical acupuncture tool, and it can vary significantly in terms of structure, diameter, and length.

A typical acupuncture needle has a body or shaft that is 1 inch long and a handle of approximately the same length (Figure 18-4). The distinctive part of an acupuncture needle is its tip, which is rounded and moderately sharp, much like the tip of a pine needle. The acupuncture needle is solid and gently tapered; it does not have the lumen or cutting edge of the hypodermic needle used for injection. Its diameter typically is 0.25 mm.

Once the site for insertion has been determined, the needle is inserted rapidly through the skin and then adjusted to an appropriate depth. Although a substantial number of considerations affect the angle and depth of insertion, methods of manipulation, and the length of retention, this is the basic procedure. A twelfth century text, *Ode of the Subtleties of Flow,* states, "Insert the needle with noble speed then proceed (to the point) slowly, withdraw the needle with noble slowness as haste will cause injury" (Shanghai College of Traditional Chinese Medicine, 1981).

The essential aim of the acupuncturist is to obtain qi at the needling site. The physician seeks either an objective or subjective indication that the qi has arrived. Qi can become manifest to the practitioner through sensations experienced by the hands as the needle is manipulated through observation or through reports from the patient. The sensation of the arrival of qi often is felt by the practitioner as a gentle grasping of the needle at the site, as if one is fishing, and one's line has suddenly been seized by the fish. The patient senses the arrival of qi as a sensation of itching, numbness, soreness, or a swollen feeling. The patient might experience local temperature changes or a distinct "electrical" sensation. Acupuncture points in different areas of the body respond differently; these variations in response can be an important diagnostic indicator. It is not unusual for a clinician to retain a needle in an acupuncture point where the qi has not arrived until the characteristic sensation occurs.

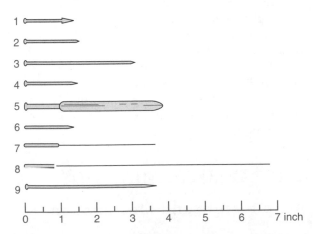

Figure 18-3 The nine needles according to the *Spiritual Pivot.* (From Qiu M-L. 1995. Chinese Acupuncture and Moxibustion. Churchill Livingstone. Edinburgh. p. 184.)

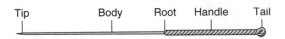

Figure 18-4 The structure of the filiform needle. (From Qiu M-L. 1995. Chinese Acupuncture and Moxibustion. Churchill Livingstone. Edinburgh. p. 186.)

Once a point has been correctly located, needled, and qi obtained, the clinician may choose to manipulate the needle to achieve a desired therapeutic effect. Styles of needle manipulation have inspired extensive discussions both in ancient and modern texts. Methods may range from simply putting the needle in place and leaving it there to engaging in complex manipulations that involve slow or rapid insertion of the needle to greater or more shallow depths. These techniques might create a distinctive sensation along the channel pathway. This needle may be withdrawn promptly after qi arrives, or a short fine needle (known as an *intradermal*) may be retained in the site for several days. In all instances the goal of the clinician is to influence the movement of qi.

One simple style of needle manipulation involves adjusting the direction of the needle to supplement or drain the qi at the particular channel point. If one thinks of the acupuncture point as a hole where the channel qi can be touched and moved, this operation can either cause the qi to become secure and increased in the channel (supplementing) or cause the qi to spill out (draining).

For our patient who is experiencing the symptoms of wind cold, an acupuncturist might choose to needle a number of acupuncture points, including Wind Pool (*Feng Chi* GB 20), located on the back of the neck below the occipital bone; Union Valley (*He Gu* LI 4), located in the fleshy area between the base of the thumb and forefinger; and Broken Sequence (*Lie Que* LU 7), on the forearm just above the styloid process of the radius. These particular points could all be treated with a draining method because, in this case, the channels are replete with the influences of the external evils of wind and cold. Wind Pool, as its name indicates, often is used to drain wind from the surface of the body and to relieve headache and neck pain. Union Valley is an important acupuncture point that often is used to influence the upper part of the body and to control pain. In this case the point is used because of its ability to course wind, resolve the exterior, and treat headache and sore throat. Broken Sequence is said to dispel cold and to diffuse the lung. It courses the channels and can be used to treat sore throat and headache.

Practitioners use various methods to select acupuncture points for treating a particular patient. One of the most traditional methods is an empirically derived understanding of what points work best for a given condition. Each acupuncture point has numerous indications associated with it based on the accumulated experience of generations of acupuncture practitioners.

Ancient and contemporary texts abound with descriptions of specific sets of acupuncture points that may be used to treat a condition successfully. Broken Sequence and Leg Three Li (*Zu San Li* St 36) are described by the Song of Point Applications for Miscellaneous Disease as useful for rapid breathing and dyspnea (Ellis et al., 1991, p. 84).

Besides choosing points on the basis of their indications and the experience and descriptions accumulated in texts, acupuncturists also can apply specific theoretical considerations to traditional acupuncture point categories. For example, they can choose acupuncture points on the basis of their theoretical associations with the five phases. An inference concerning the relative status of the five phases and the organs is made on the basis of the pulses and presenting symptoms. If the patient displayed signs of vacuity of the water phase, a choice of points could be made from the transport points along the kidney channel associated with water to supplement the water phase.

Points also may be chosen on the basis of the actual trajectory of the channel on which they lie. Union Valley is considered an important point for the head and face because the pathway of the large intestine channel on which it lies traverses that area of the body. Similarly, points on the lower extremity that lie on the urinary bladder channel, which traverses the entire back, often are used for back pain (Figure 18-5).

Finally, points often are selected entirely on the basis of their sensitivity to palpation or on the basis of a variation in texture that can be perceived by the practitioner. Often a number of suitable acupuncture points in a specific area may be assessed to determine which would be most suitable for needling. In some cases points that do not lie on specific channels or form part of the collection of recognized extra points can be identified by their tenderness. These points are known as *ah shi*, or "ouch, that's it," points, and are an important part of clinical acupuncture's traditional history and contemporary practice.

With many acupuncture points to choose from and a multiplicity of methods on which to base that choice, it is not surprising that many clinicians focus on a few specific methods or a particular collection of points. Some clinicians restrict their approach so that they can focus on adjusting the application of treatment.

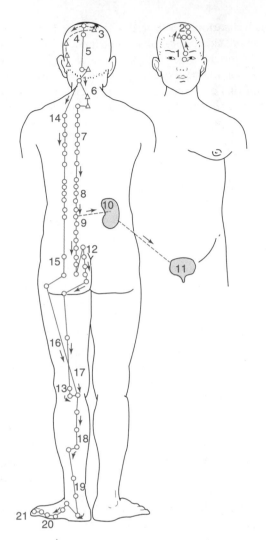

Figure 18-5 The course of the urinary bladder channel of the foot taiyang. (From Qiu M-L. 1995. Chinese Acupuncture and Moxibustion. Churchill Livingstone. Edinburgh. p. 103.)

Moxibustion *(Jiu Fa)*

Moxibustion (jiu) refers to the burning of the dried and powdered leaves of artemesia vulgaris *(ai ye)*, either on or in proximity to the skin, to affect the movement of qi in the channel, locally or at a distance. Artemesia is said to be acrid and bitter and, when used as moxa, to have the ability to warm and enter the channels. References to moxa appear in very early materials, such as the texts recovered from the excavated tombs at Ma Wang Dui (Unschuld, 1985). These texts discuss a number of therapeutic methods, including moxibustion, but do not mention acupuncture. One of them, the *Treatise on Moxibustion of the Eleven Vessels of Yin and Yang (Yin Yang Shi Yi Mai Jiu Jing)*, describes the application of moxa to treat illness by doing moxibustion on the channels (Auteroche et al., 1992).

Moxibustion can be applied to the body in many ways—directly, indirectly, pole moxa, and the warm needle method. Direct moxa involves burning a small amount of moxa, perhaps the size of a grain of rice, directly on the skin. Depending on the desired effect, larger or smaller pieces of moxa can be used, and the moxa fluff can be allowed to burn directly to the skin causing a blister or a scar, or it can be removed before it has burnt down to the skin. Techniques such as these are used to stimulate acupuncture points where the action of moxibustion is traditionally indicated or where warming the point seems to be the most appropriate response. Older texts described the use of direct moxibustion on Leg Three Li and other acupuncture points as a method of health maintenance and prevention.

Indirect moxibustion involves the insertion of a mediating substance between the moxa fluff and the patient's skin (Figure 18-6). This gives the practitioner greater control over the amount of heat applied to the patient's body and offers the patient increased protection from burning, allowing for the treatment of delicate areas such as the face and back. Popular substances include ginger slices, garlic slices, and salt. The mediating substance often will be chosen on the basis of its own medicinal properties and how they combine with the properties of moxa. Ginger might be selected in cases in which vacuity cold is present, whereas garlic is considered useful for treating hot and toxic conditions. The photo shows a patient being treated for facial paralysis with indirect moxibustion using ginger slices.

During pole moxa a cigar-shaped roll of moxa wrapped in paper is used to gently warm the acupuncture points without touching the skin. This is a very safe method of moxibustion that can be taught to patients for self-application. The warm needle method is accomplished by first inserting an acupuncture needle into the point and then placing moxa fluff on its handle. After the moxa is ignited, it burns gradually, imparting a sensation of gentle warmth to the acupuncture point and channel. This

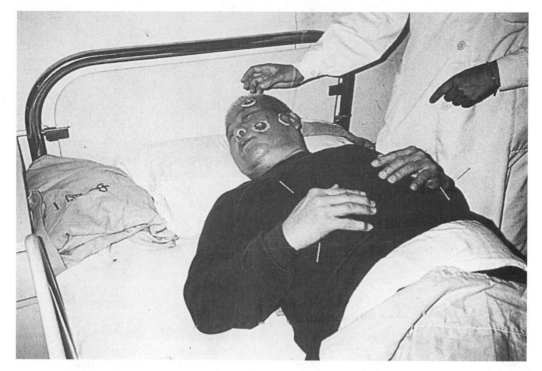

Figure 18-6 Patient receiving indirect moxa. (Courtesy Wind Horse, Marnae Ergil.)

method is especially useful for patients with arthritic joint pain.

Together, acupuncture and moxibustion are used to treat, or at least ameliorate, a wide range of conditions and symptoms. On the basis of the simple premise that all disease involves the disruption of the flow of qi and that acupuncture and moxibustion regulate the movement of qi, there is, at least theoretically, no disease that cannot benefit from these methods. A brief review of acupuncture texts will provide ample evidence of the range of conditions in which acupuncture is considered appropriate. Box 18-8 reproduces a list of "diseases that lend themselves to acupuncture treatment" developed in the late 1970s by a World Health Organization Interregional Seminar (Bannerman, 1979). The list is not based on controlled clinical research, and the specific disease names are not meant to indicate acupuncture's efficacy in treating them. The list is comparatively short if compared with a clinical manual or acupuncture

textbook, but it is informative in terms of the routine application of acupuncture in China.

Cupping and Bleeding

Two methods that are very important to the practice of Chinese medicine are cupping and bleeding. These may be used separately or together and are often used in conjunction with other methods such as moxibustion and acupuncture. Cupping involves inducing a vacuum in a small glass or bamboo cup and promptly applying it to the skin surface. This therapy brings blood and lymph to the skin surface under the cup, increasing local circulation. The method is often used to drain or remove cold and damp evils from the body or to assist blood circulation. Bleeding is done to drain a channel or to remove heat from the body at a specific location. Unlike the bloodletting practiced by Western physicians throughout the nineteenth

BOX 18-8

Diseases That Lend Themselves to Acupuncture

- Upper respiratory tract
  - Acute sinusitis
  - Acute rhinitis
  - Common cold
  - Acute tonsillitis
- Respiratory system
  - Acute bronchitis
  - Bronchial asthma
- Disorders of the eye
  - Acute conjunctivitis
  - Central retinitis
  - Myopia (in children)
  - Cataract (without complications)
- Disorders of the mouth
  - Toothache, postextraction pain
  - Gingivitis
  - Acute and chronic pharyngitis
- Gastrointestinal disorders
  - Spasms of esophagus and cardia
  - Hiccough
  - Gastroptosis
  - Acute and chronic gastritis
  - Gastric hyperacidity
  - Chronic duodenal ulcer (pain relief)

- Acute duodenal ulcer (without complications)
- Acute and chronic colitis
- Acute bacillary dysentery
- Constipation
- Diarrhea
- Paralytic ileus
- Neurologic and musculoskeletal disorders
  - Headache and migraine
  - Trigeminal neuralgia
  - Facial palsy (early stage, i.e., within 3 to 6 months)
  - Pareses after a stroke
  - Peripheral neuropathies
  - Sequelae of poliomyelitis (early stage, i.e., within 6 months)
  - Meniere's disease
  - Neurogenic bladder dysfunction
  - Nocturnal enuresis
  - Intercostal neuralgia
  - Cervicobrachial syndrome
  - Frozen shoulder, tennis elbow
  - Sciatica
  - Low back pain
  - Osteoarthritis

century, this method expresses comparatively small amounts of blood, from a drop to a few centiliters. Figure 18-7 shows a patient receiving cupping and bleeding at an acupuncture point on the urinary bladder channel associated with the lungs.

Chinese Massage (Tui Na)

Tui Na, literally "pushing and pulling," refers to a system of massage, manual acupuncture point stimulation, and manipulation that is vast enough to warrant a chapter of its own. These methods have been practiced at least as long as moxibustion, if not longer, but the first massage training class was created in Shanghai in 1956 (Wang et al., 1990, p. 16). Today, this field of study can serve as a minor component of a traditional medical education or an area of extensive clinical specialization.

A distinct aspect of Tui Na is the extensive training of the hands necessary for clinical practice. The practitioner's hands are trained to accomplish focused and forceful movements that can be applied to various areas of the body. Techniques such as pushing, rolling, kneading, rubbing, and grasping are practiced repetitively until they become second nature (Figure 18-8). Students practice on a small bag of rice until their hands develop the necessary strength and dexterity.

Tui Na often is applied to limited areas of the body, and the techniques can be quite forceful and intense. Tui Na is applied routinely to orthopedic and neurological conditions. It also is applied to conditions that might not be thought of as susceptible to treatment through manipulation, such as asthma, dysmenorrhea, chronic gastritis, and other conditions. Tui Na is used as an adjunct to acupuncture treatment to increase the range of motion of a

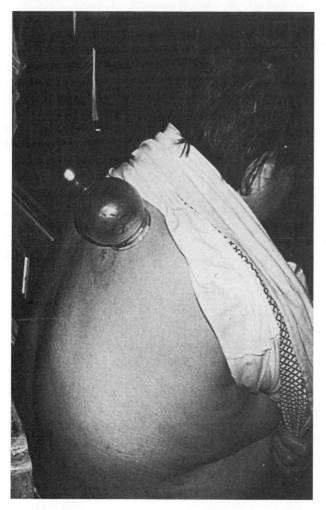

Figure 18-7 Cupping and bleeding. (Courtesy Wind Horse, Marnae Ergil.)

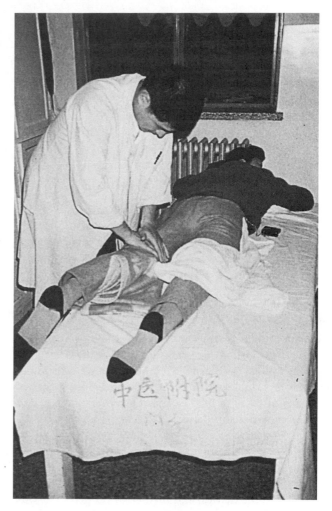

Figure 18-8 Tui Na in clinical practice. (Courtesy Wind Horse, Marnae Ergil.)

joint or instead of acupuncture when needles are uncomfortable or inappropriate, such as pediatric applications.

As with all aspects of Chinese medicine, regional styles and family lineages of practice abound. The formal curriculum available in Chinese programs is extensive but probably not a complete expression of the range of possibilities.

Qi Cultivation *(Qigong)*

Qigong is a term that literally embraces almost every aspect of the manipulation of qi by means of exercise,

breathing, and the influence of the mind. The second part of this chapter is devoted to this topic, so only a few points need to be made here. Qigong includes practices ranging from the meditative systems of Daoist and Buddhist practitioners to the martial arts traditions of China. Qigong is relevant to medicine in three specific areas: The first is to allow the practitioner to cultivate demeanor and stamina to enable him or her to engage in performing the strenuous activities of Tui Na, to sustain the constant demands of clinical practice, and to quiet the mind to facilitate diagnostic perception. The second involves cultivating the practitioner's ability to safely transmit qi to the patient. Practitioners may direct qi to the patient either through the needles or directly through their hands. This activity may be the main focus of treatment or an adjunctive aspect, in which case the qi paradigm is expanded to include direct interaction between the patient's qi and that of the clinician. Finally, patients may be taught to do specific Qigong practices that are useful for their illness.

Chinese Herbal Medicine
(Zhong Yao)

Since the legendary emperor Shen Nong tasted herbs and guided the Chinese people in their use, diet, and therapeutics, herbal medicine has been an integral part of Chinese culture and medical practice. The traditional Chinese materia medica includes far more than herbs: minerals and animal parts are listed as well. The number of substances currently identified numbers 5767, as recorded in the *Encyclopedia of Traditional Chinese Medicinal Substances (Zhong Yao Da Ci Dian)* published in 1977 by the Jiangsu College of New Medicine (Bensky & Gamble, 1986). This publication is the latest in a long line of definitive discussions of materia medica that have been produced in China over the millenia. The earliest known is the *Divine Husbandman's Classic of the Materia Medica*, which we obtained from its reconstruction by Tao Hong Jing (452-536 CE). This text classified upper, middle, and lower grade herbs and discussed the tastes, temperatures, toxicities, and medicinal properties of 364 substances.

Today substances are categorized systematically as expansions of the eight methods of therapy discussed earlier (Box 18-9). Although a comprehensive discussion of the organization of the materia medica is beyond the scope of this chapter, it should be mentioned that within the basic categories into which substances are organized, there are further subcategories. Beyond these are prescribing rules that take into account the compatibilities and incompatibilities of substances, the traditional pairings of substances, and their combination for specific symptoms.

Recommendations for the therapeutic combination of substances are given by both the Ma Wan Dui texts and the *Inner Classic*. Zhang Zhong Jing's work in systematizing herbal prescriptions as therapeutic approaches to specific diagnostic patterns on the ba-

sis of the system of yin and yang correspondences was unusual for its time. It was not until physicians of the Sung dynasty became interested in relating herbal practice to a systematic theory and organizing diagnostics accordingly that interest in the *Treatise on Cold Damage* picked up. Today this book remains a significant resource for the practitioner of Chinese herbal medicine. One of the most comprehensive English language compilations of Chinese herbal prescriptions derives approximately 20 percent of its formula from this source (Bensky & Barolet, 1990).

Not all herbal prescriptions or texts discussing their application followed the lead of Zhang Zhong Jing. Many texts offered herbs or prescriptions for specific symptoms without reference to distinct theoretical structures or diagnostic principles. Very likely, the masses applied herbs in exactly this fashion. Even today, despite the fact that the prescription of herbal formula is primarily driven by traditional diagnostic theory and pattern diagnosis, extensive compilations of empirically derived herbal formulas with symptomatic indications are published.

Contemporary compilations of formulas are organized in a fashion similar to substances. The result

---

BOX 18-9

Chinese Materia Medica
Fundamental Categories

- Exterior-resolving
- Heat-clearing
- Ejection
- Precipitant
- Wind-dispelling
- Water-disinhibiting dampness-percolating
- Interior-warming
- Qi-rectifying
- Food-dispersing
- Worm-expelling
- Blood-rectifying
- Phlegm-transforming cough-suppressing panting-calming
- Spirit-quieting
- Liver-calming wind-extinguishing
- Orifice-opening
- Supplementing
- Securing and astringing
- External use

is that both substances and formulas are organized in a fashion that makes them accessible in terms of traditional theories (Box 18-10).

Let us examine the formula and its constituent substances that might be provided to our patient who has encountered a wind cold evil or who, in the pattern identification system described in the *Treatise on Cold Damage,* would be said to have a tai yang stage pattern. In either case ephedra decoction *(Ma Huang Tang)* would be an appropriate choice, particularly if the patient had a slight cough as well. The constituents and dosage of the formula are 9 g of ephedra *(ma huang),* 6 g of cinnamon twig *(gui zhi),* 9 g of apricot kernel *(xing ren),* and 3 g of licorice *(gan cao).* These ingredients are cooked together in water to make a slightly concentrated tea, which is drunk in successive doses. The tea is taken warm to induce sweating, a sign that the qi of the surface of the body that had been impeded by the cold evil is free to move and throw off the evil. The patient stops drinking the tea once sweat arrives.

A traditional system of organizing formula is to identify ingredients as the ruler, minister, adjutant, and emissary. In this case the ruler of the formula is ephedra. The ruler sets the therapeutic direction of the formula. Acrid and warm, ephedra promotes sweating, dispels cold, and resolves the surface. (We examine ephedra again in the discussion of herbal research.) Cinnamon twig is the minister, working to assist the ruler in carrying out its objectives. In addition to the effects described for ephedra, it also is said to warm the body. Apricot kernel is the adjutant, so it addresses the possible involvement of the lung and moderates the acrid flavor of the two other substances. Because the lung is the organ most immediately affected by wind cold or wind heat, the formula addresses the organ. Finally, licorice is the emissary, serving both to render the action of the other herbs harmonious and to distribute it through the body.

The foregoing example is brief and simple but illustrates fundamental concepts. Chinese herbal therapeutics can be complex. Its practice is quite broad and the range of conditions addressed is more extensive than acupuncture. In terms of complexity and the diagnostic acumen required of the practitioner, it resembles the practice of internal medicine. Herbal therapy also encompasses the external applications of herbs and a variety of methods of preparation. Besides the traditional water decoction, or tea, substances may be powdered or rendered into pills, pastes, or tinctures.

BOX 18-10
Formulas

- Exterior-resolving
- Heat-clearing
- Ejection
- Precipitant
- Harmonizing
- Dampness-dispelling
- Interior-warming
- Qi-rectifying
- Dispersing
- Blood-rectifying
- Phlegm-transforming cough-suppressing panting-calming
- Spirit-quieting
- Tetany-settling
- Orifice-opening
- Supplementing
- Securing and astringing
- Oral formulas for sores
- External use

Dietetics

Traditional dietetics encompasses the practice of herbal therapy but also addresses traditional Chinese foods in terms of the theoretical constructs of Chinese medicine. Five-phase theory has been applied to foods since the time of the *Inner Classic.* It is not unusual to see a classroom in a college of Chinese medicine equipped as a kitchen. In larger cities special restaurants prepare meals with specific medicinal purposes. The practices of this field are deeply rooted in the cultural practices of China and that culture's beliefs concerning diet. Many of the foods that are organized for use in therapy also are routinely prepared by families when seasons change, when illness strikes, to strengthen a woman after birth, to cause milk to fill the breasts of a new mother, or to nourish the elderly in their declining years.

CHINESE MEDICINE IN OTHER COUNTRIES

Today China's traditional medicine is practiced, in various forms, all over the world. Sometimes its practice follows the contemporary patterns of traditional Chinese medicine (TCM, or *zhong yi*). Sometimes its practice is deeply informed by local custom, preference, or regional elaborations.

Chinese Medicine in Korea

The relationship between China and Korea is a close one. Chinese medicine arrived in Korea during the Qin dynasty (221-207 BCE). However, the textual basis of Korean medicine in the literary tradition of Chinese medicine seems to have been established during the Han and Tang dynasties (Hsu & Peacher, 1977), during a period of political domination by the Chinese. A close relationship between China and Korea during the Kingdom of Silla (400-700 CE) facilitated this exchange of ideas. Formal medical instruction by government-appointed physicians began in 693 CE. Texts such as the *Systematic Classic of Acupuncture* were important to the development of the tradition. With the formation of the Liao dynasty (907-1168), Korea established its independence from Chinese rule, but cultural and medical exchange continued. During the Li dynasty (1392-1910) many texts, including the *Illustrated Classic of Acupuncture Points as Found on the Bronze Model,* reached Korea (Chuang, 1982). Widely used techniques of acupuncture point selection based on five-phase theory have emerged from Korea, including those of the Buddhist priest Sa-am (1544-1610).

At least two comparatively recent innovations based on Chinese medicine have been developed in Korea and have become well known in other parts of the world. Korean constitutional diagnosis was developed initially by Jhema Lee (1836-1900) and based a system of herbal therapeutics on a system of diagnostic patterning that used the four divisions of yin and yang. It was elaborated subsequently by Dowon Kuan who, in 1965, expanded the system to an eightfold classification and applied it to acupuncture (Hirsch, 1985).

Another influential contemporary system is that of *Koryo Sooji Chim,* the system of Korean hand and finger acupuncture developed by Yoo Tae Woo and published in 1971. The system maps the chan-

nel pathways and acupuncture points of the entire body onto the hands, where they are stimulated using very short, fine needles and magnets. This system has gained a significant level of international exposure.

Chinese Medicine in Japan

The history of cultural exchange between China and Japan dates back to at least 57 CE. Kon Mu was the first physician to use Chinese methods to come to Japan. He was sent in 414 CE by the king of Silla, in southeast Korea, to treat the emperor Inkyo Tenno. This interaction continued. In 552 a Korean delegation brought a selection of Chinese medical texts to Japan (Bowers, 1970). In 562 Zhi Cong came from southern China with more than 100 books on the practice of Chinese medicine (Huard & Wong, 1968), including the *Systematic Classic of Acupuncture* (Chuang, 1982). By the early eighth century the influence of Chinese medicine was well established. With the adoption of the Taiho code in 702, provision was made for a ministry of health composed of specialists, physicians, students, and researchers (Lock, 1980). In 754 a Buddhist priest, Chien Chen, brought many medical texts from China to Japan. His influence was memorialized in a shrine in Nishinokyo (Chuang, 1982).

Chinese influences on Japanese medicine were derived primarily from the *Classic of Difficult Issues* and *Systematic Classic of Acupuncture*. A revisionist movement in the late seventeenth century established *The Treatise on Cold Damage (Shokanron)* as the core text of herbal medicine, or *kanpo* (Chinese method), in Japan (Lock, 1980).

Several factors have influenced the development of Chinese medicine in Japan, giving it a somewhat unique appearance. The scarcity of ingredients for the preparation of Chinese herbal formulas has led to an emphasis on lower doses in herbal prescriptions than are typical in China. An emphasis on palpatory diagnosis involving channel pathways and the abdomen also became well established. The use of somewhat finer gauge needles and shallow insertion became typical of Japanese acupuncture.

In the mid-seventeenth century, Waichi Sugiyama, a blind man, began to train the blind in acupuncture using very fine needles and guide tubes. Because it had become customary in the earlier part of the Edo period for the blind to do massage, both massage and acupuncture now became associated with blind practitioners. This contributed to a lower social position for acupuncture practitioners and to the specialization in medical practice. Kanpo physicians became primarily practitioners of herbal medicine (Lock, 1980).

This trend toward specialization has continued to the present day, with the division of acupuncture, moxibustion, and massage into separately licensed practices (although many individuals hold all three licenses) and the actual practice of herbal medicine being retained in the hands of medical doctors. Interestingly a large number of Chinese herbal prescriptions are recognized as appropriate therapy for certain medical conditions according to regulations governing health care in Japan.

Japan has seen both focused specialization in and the innovative exploration and expansion of traditional acupuncture. The *Classic of Difficult Issues* often has been the focus for movements to revive the practices of traditional acupuncture. Its influence has contributed heavily to the comparatively recent development of groups of acupuncturists advocating meridian therapy *(keiraku chiryo)* based on the application of concepts in the *Classic of Difficult Issues* and their subsequent interpretation by later Chinese authors. A distinctive feature of meridian therapy is the application of five-phase theory to the transport points, a practice that has influenced the perception and adoption of five-phase theory by European practitioners (Kaptchuk, 1983).

The pioneering work of Yoshio Manaka also has contributed dramatically to the practice of acupuncture. Manaka, a physician who experimented with acupuncture principles during a period when medical supplies were absent during World War II, became convinced of the efficacy and physiological relevance of traditional theories and continued to experiment and develop them throughout his life.

The range of practices and interests of Japanese acupuncture practitioners is quite broad. Although some are particular partisans of specific schools of thought, including some based on contemporary Chinese medicine perspectives, many practitioners have adopted a comparatively eclectic approach.

Chinese Medicine in Europe

The history of Chinese medicine, particularly acupuncture, in Europe is both longstanding and broadly developed. The medical use of acupuncture in Europe dates from the middle of the sixteenth century (Peacher, 1975). The work of Willem Ten Rhyne (1647-1690) in this area culminated in the publication in 1683 of *Dissertatio de Arthritide: Mantissa Schematica: de Acupunctura: et Orationes Tres,* based on information gathered during his service in Japan as a physician for the Dutch East India Company. The German physician Kampfer who also traveled with the Dutch East India Company and spent time in Japan, contributed his observations.

In France the Jesuit Du Halde published a text that included a detailed discussion of Chinese medicine in 1735 (Hsu, 1989). Soulie de Morant's publication of *L'acupuncture Chinoise* was an extensive discussion of the practice of acupuncture based on direct translation, observation, and actual practice by the author. Published in 1939, the text was rooted in de Morant's exposure to the medicine of China in that country from 1901 to 1917.

England saw the publication of JM Churchill's *A Description of Surgical Operations Peculiar to Japanese and Chinese* in 1825. Among early notable English acupuncturists are Drs. Felix Mann and Sidney Rose-Neil, both of whom began their explorations of acupuncture in the late 1950s and who have influenced its development substantially in English-speaking countries. J.R. Worsley, a physical therapist, who began his studies of acupuncture in 1962, came to have a substantial impact on the perceptions of many practitioners in England and the United States. He visited Hong Kong and Taiwan for a brief period and then became a part of the study group established by Rose-Neil (Hsu & Peacher, 1977). Worsley went on to create the British College of Traditional Chinese Acupuncture and two schools in the United States.

Chinese Medicine in the United States

In 1826 Bache became one of the first American physicians to use acupuncture in his practice (Haller, 1973). Ten Rhyne's text was a part of Sir William Osler's library (Peacher, 1975), and in his *Principles and Practice of Medicine* Osler prescribes acupuncture for lumbago (Osler, 1913).

Apart from occasional explorations by the conventional medical community in the United States, the traditional medicine of China has been practiced in the United States since the middle of the nineteenth century. Herbal merchants, entrepreneurs, and physicians accompanied Chinese who sold their labor in the United States. The practice of the China Doctor of John Day, Oregon, Doc Ing Hay probably is one of the most famous (Barlow & Richardson, 1979). Ah Fong Chuck, who came to the United States in 1866, became the first licensed practitioner of that medicine in the United States in 1901, when he successfully won a medical license through legal action in Idaho (Muench, 1984). With the strengthening of medical practice acts throughout the United States, the interruption of the herb supply from China, and the advent of World War II, these practices disappeared or retreated into Chinatowns nationwide.

Substantial attention was focused on acupuncture, the traditional medicine of China, and its regional variants, as a result of James Reston's highly publicized appendectomy and postoperative care in 1971 and the subsequent opening of China by Nixon. This caused varieties of medical practice that had been largely confined to Asia and the Chinatowns of America to gain visibility throughout the United States. Increased visibility led to substantial public interest in acupuncture and gradually to the licensure and development of training programs in many states. Today 30 states (including the District of Columbia) license, certify, or register the practice of acupuncture and a range of other activities, including herbal medicine by nonphysicians. There are at least 35 programs in the United States offering training in what is often understood as acupuncture and Oriental medicine.

In America there has been a clear interest in the available range of expressions of the medical tradition of China. In the United States, European interpretations of the application of five-phase theory, Korean constitutional acupuncture, traditional Chinese medicine (acupuncture, herbs, Qigong, and Tui Na), Japanese meridian therapy, and special family lineages within the Chinese tradition all are taught and practiced. This willingness to accept and explore the traditional and contemporary interpretations of traditional Chinese medicine has led to the emergence of the concept of "Oriental medicine" as an umbrella term for the global domain of practice in this area.

Practice Settings

In general, traditional Chinese medicine is practiced in a range of clinical settings. Large hospitals entirely devoted to its practice are common in China. In this setting acupuncture, herbal medicine, and Tui Na are provided both on an inpatient and outpatient basis. It is not unusual to see a large outpatient facility treating 20 patients simultaneously in the same space. Smaller practices and even roadside stands also are not unusual. Herbal prescriptions can be obtained from a Chinese herb store in almost any country that has a significant Chinese population. In Japan small hospitals, large clinics, and private offices are typical settings.

Wherever the medicine is practiced, the settings in which it is delivered do not appear significantly different from the environment in which biomedical services are provided—unless the practitioner has a desire to emphasize the distinctive character of his or her practice, or if the practice is marginalized through lack of regulation. In the United States record-keeping processes, insurance billing, the use of biomedical screening processes, and concerns surrounding office hygiene often produce a setting that—except for the presence of such peculiarities as acupuncture needles, moxa fluff, or herbs—looks very much like a typical physician's office.

RESEARCH AND EVALUATION

Many aspects of Chinese medicine have been the focus of concerted research efforts in China and Japan since the early part of the twentieth century. Recently substantial research initiatives in this area have been undertaken in Europe and the United States as well, and these have developed rapidly in terms of quality and quantity in the last decade. The actual and perceived quality of such research, in both east and west, can vary widely. As is the case for medical systems, research standards—even scientific research—are subject to cultural influences. Where the randomized, placebo-controlled, and double-blind clinical trial is the definitive standard for an unambiguous biomedical recognition of efficacy, not all societies require or encourage their medical communities to secure knowledge in this fashion. In addition, the simple accessibility of research data is influenced by the language and location of publication. These problems can inhibit the availability and use of information concerning research. Therefore research that is meaningful to the scientific communities of China, Japan, Europe, or the United States does not have the same influence among other communities within that same group, and particularly on the biomedical communities of the United States or Europe.

Another problem that emerges in relation to clinical research in Chinese medicine is study design. Problems surrounding research methods have come into focus as the Chinese medicine community within the United States and Europe has participated more in research and as the biomedical community has become better educated about various modalities of Chinese medicine.

Efforts by the Office of Alternative Medicine (OAM), which was created in 1991, under the National Institutes of Health (NIH) in the United States, have substantially contributed to this process within the United States. The OAM has hosted several conferences dealing with methodological considerations in the field of alternative medicine, and each of these events has come to grips with aspects of the traditional medicine of China.

Other projects supported by the OAM have included funding of numerous small research grants, many of which have been in the area of Chinese or Oriental medicine (Box 18-11).

The OAM also sponsored a workshop on acupuncture in cooperation with the U.S. Food and Drug Administration (FDA). On April 21 and 22, 1994, members of the acupuncture medical and scientific community gave presentations detailing the safety and the apparent clinical efficacy of acupuncture needles. These presentations became the core of a petition that led, in March of 1996, to the reclassification of acupuncture needles by the FDA from a class III or experimental device to a class II or medical device for use by qualified practitioners with special controls (sterility and single use).

In November of 1997 the NIH convened a Consensus Development Conference on acupuncture that involved 2 days of presentations of the evidence for the safety and efficacy of acupuncture for the treatment of specific conditions. This evidence was presented by experts in the field to a scientific panel that reviewed reports of research on the use of acupuncture in the treatment of a wide variety of conditions. They reached the formal conclusion that:

Acupuncture as a therapeutic intervention is widely practiced in the United States. While there have been many studies of its potential usefulness, many of these studies provide equivocal results because of design, sample size, and other factors. The issue is further complicated by inherent difficulties in the use of appropriate controls, such as placebos and sham acupuncture groups. However, promising results have emerged, for example, showing

BOX 18-11

OAM-funded Studies

Studies in areas related to Chinese medicine funded in 1993-1994 through the Office of Alternative Medicine

Medical Condition	Modality
Unipolar depression	Acupuncture
Osteoarthritis	Acupuncture
Premenstrual syndrome	Traditional Chinese medicine
Common warts	Chinese herbal therapy
Balance disorders	*Tai Ji*
Menopausal hot flashes	Chinese herbs
Postoperative oral surgery pain	Acupuncture
Breech version	Acupuncture and moxibustion
Chronic sinusitis in HIV infection	Traditional Chinese medicine
Hyperactivity	Acupuncture
Intractable reflex sympathetic dystrophy	Qi Gong

efficacy of acupuncture in adult postoperative and chemotherapy nausea and vomiting and in postoperative dental pain. There are other situations such as addiction, stroke rehabilitation, headache, menstrual cramps, tennis elbow, fibromyalgia, myofascial pain, osteoarthritis, low back pain, carpal tunnel syndrome, and asthma, in which acupuncture may be useful as an adjunct treatment or an acceptable alternative or be included in a comprehensive management program. Further research is likely to uncover additional areas where acupuncture interventions will be useful (NIH Consensus Statement, 1997).

Considering that less than 2 years previously acupuncture needles had still been considered an experimental device in the United States, this finding marked a significant degree of progress.

In late 1998 the OAM was established as the National Center for Complementary and Alternative Medicine and provided with a significant increase in funding. Since its inception the OAM had continued to refine and develop its approach to fostering research into complementary and alternative therapies. One strategy that it has used is the funding of complementary and alternative medicine research centers or specialty centers that bring developed institutional resources to bear on research in specific areas. At present the specialty centers number 13. Many of the centers have developed or proposed research that touches on many aspects of China's traditional medicine (Box 18-12) or some such Complementary and Alternative Medicine Specialty Centers doing Research in aspects of Chinese Medicine. Some centers such as Center for Addiction and Alternative Medicine Research at the University of Minnesota Medical School and Hennepin County Medical Center or Center for Alternative Medicine Pain Research and Evaluation at the University of Maryland School of Medicine have built their centers around long-term and sustained research efforts in specific areas, which has allowed them to make substantial strides as increased funding became available through current interest in complementary and alternative therapies.

Other organizations, in addition to those mentioned in Box 18-12, such as the Society for Acupuncture Research (SAR), have emerged out of the broad-based community of acupuncturists, physicians, and researchers interested in the range of research issues posed by this field. The SAR holds annual meetings and publishes its proceedings. Among its objectives are scholarly exchange between researchers in the area

of acupuncture, and other modalities related to Oriental medicine, the encouragement of research activities by acupuncturists, and the clarification of methodological issues related to research in these areas. In 1996 two officers of the SAR Stephen Birch and Richard Hammerschlag compiled a summary of the most successful and well-designed controlled clinical trials.

Research in Relation to Specific Areas of Chinese Medicine

Research on fundamental concepts, or what might be called *fundamental theory*, includes the exploration of whether concepts such as qi, the channels, acupuncture points, the diagnostic aspects of the pulse, and aspects of pattern diagnosis actually can refer to a reproducibly identifiable and quantifiable phenomenon. All of these areas have been or are being actively pursued in a number of countries. This research in these areas resembles basic research in physiology and relies on the development of sophisticated models and the design of instrumentation to test those models.

Research questions formed by seeking the physiological basis of Chinese medical concepts have been pursued for some time in China. One such study pursued the nature of kidney yang and reached the conclusion that patients displaying a diagnostic pattern associated with kidney yang vacuity showed low levels of 17-hydroxy corticosteroids in their urine, ultimately suggesting a relationship between the concept of kidney yang and the adrenocortical system (Hao, 1983).

Research on the correlation between the force and waveforms of the radial artery and the diagnostic perceptions of clinicians and the physical status of the patient has gone on for sometime now in China, the United States, Japan, and Korea (Broffman & McCulloch, 1986; Takashima, 1995; Zhu, 1991). Typically this research depends on the use of pressure sensors that are pressed against the skin overlying the radial artery in a manner and location that replicates that of the finger position of the traditional clinician. Pulse patterns are recorded and correlated to observations made by the clinician in an effort to determine the physical basis that must be present for a diagnostic perception. Preliminary results are intriguing, but methodological questions concerning population size and standardization of measurement remain.

BOX 18-12

CAM Research Specialty Centers

Center for Addiction and Alternative Medicine
  Research
University of Minnesota Medical School & Hennepin
  County Medical Center
Minneapolis, MN
  Addictions
  Treatment of hepatitis C with Chinese herbal med-
    icine, acupuncture, and relief of the symptoms
    of alcohol withdrawal

Complementary and Alternative Medicine Program
  at Stanford
Stanford University
Palo Alto, CA
  Aging
  Review of traditional Chinese medicine approach
    to the problems of aging

Center for Alternative Medicine Research
Harvard Medical School
Boston, MA
  General medical conditions, acupuncture and
    back pain, acupuncture and postsurgical emesis

Center for Alternative Medicine Pain Research and
  Evaluation
University of Maryland School of Medicine
Baltimore, MD
  Pain, acupuncture and antiemesis, basic sci-
    ence research on acupuncture (animal
    model), acupuncture as an adjunctive ther-
    apy for osteoarthritis of the knee, acupunc-
    ture for dental pain

Center for Research in Complementary and
  Alternative Medicine for Stroke and Neurological
  Disorders
Kessler Institute for Rehabilitation
West Orange, NJ
  Stroke and neurological conditions, Gingko
    biloba in the treatment of stroke, Qi gong in
    the treatment of stroke, acupuncture in the
    treatment of dysphagia after stroke

Center for Complementary and Alternative Medicine
  Research in Women's Health
Columbia University
New York, NY
  Traditional Chinese medicine in relation to
    women's health

Research concerning channels and acupuncture points has relied on a variety of techniques, including the measurement of electrical resistance, thermography, tracing the pathways of injected radioisotopes, and dissection. This last has not produced particularly interesting results. The so-called Bonghan corpuscles, identified on dissection by Kim Bong Han in Korea, once were proposed as the anatomical basis of acupuncture points. This research has not been replicated, and although reference is occasionally made to it in contemporary materials (Burton Goldberg Group, 1993), it generally is not perceived as credible.

More interesting are the discussions that propose or demonstrate an archaic or cellularly mediated signaling system that uses the bioelectrical properties of the body to propagate information. Early contributors in this area include Robert O. Becker, an orthopedist whose interest in the body's bioelectric properties and bone healing led him to explore the electrical

properties of acupuncture points and channel pathways (Becker, 1985; Reichmanis et al., 1975). A component of this hypothesis is the measurable, lowered electrical resistance of the skin at acupuncture points. This unusual electrical property is characteristic of many acupuncture points (Pomeranz, 1988).

Yoshio Manaka, a Japanese surgeon and acupuncturist, hypothesized the presence of an archaic signaling system he called the X-signal system, based on information theory concepts of biological systems, his reading of texts such as the *Inner Classic* and the *Classic of Difficult Issues,* and experimental observations in his acupuncture clinic (Manaka & Itaya, 1994). His perspective grew out of exploration of both Chinese and Japanese needling methods and the use of the gentler needling techniques associated with the school of meridian therapy that arose in Japan.

In his extensive discussion of the biophysical basis of acupuncture phenomena, James Oschman observes that the solid-state phenomena and the piezoelectric properties of the body's connective tissues provide a potential structure and mechanism that would allow for the existence of a signaling system similar to the role of the channels and points described in traditional literature (Oschman, 1993). Oschman goes on to explore a rich range of topics, including the measurable emission of electromagnetic fields from the hands of qigong practitioners (Seto et al., 1992).

All of these discussions are preliminary. Even in cases in which research has been carried out and replicated, as in the case of lowered electrical resistance over acupuncture points, there is a need for continued exploration. It is unlikely that we will see a precise validation of the concepts of Chinese medicine in these areas but rather a validation of the physiological basis for the existence of such concepts. It may be that the genius of Chinese medicine in these areas lies in its ability to generalize about the manifestations of incredibly complex biological phenomena in an articulate and useful fashion. Given the preliminary findings concerning the possible nature of acupuncture points and channels or the variety of mechanisms that seem to be involved in acupuncture as a therapeutic phenomena, it seems increasingly likely that a concept such as "qi," or the therapeutic effects of an acupuncture point, must represent the action of many discrete and identifiable physiological processes. The likelihood is that aspects of these processes, observed as a whole, are the basis of the traditional concept.

Materia Medica and Traditional Pharmacology

Investigations of materia medica and traditional pharmacology have been ongoing since the early part of the twentieth century, in both China and Japan. This is an area where the quality of research work is generally high, and the availability of translated literature is comparatively extensive. This is because research in this area can be divided into two areas: the examination of the pharmacological properties of traditional materia medica and the clinical efficacy of traditional pharmacology. The first area does not differ from the typical concerns of pharmacological research. In vitro studies and exploration of traditional use can suggest the potential usefulness of certain substances. If one becomes aware of a substance that

is alleged to have pharmacological properties, it is comparatively easy to conduct studies to assess the presence of these properties and to isolate apparently active compounds.

A famous case in point is the first herb listed in the Chinese materia medica: *Herba Ephedra,* known botanically as *Ephedra Sinica* Stapf *(ma huang).* Herba Ephedra is recorded in the *Divine Husbandman's Classic of Materia Medica.* Its chief active component was isolated in 1887 in Japan but remained largely unexplored for 35 years, until C.F. Schmidt and K.K. Chen began to explore its pharmacological effects at the Peking Union Medical College, where the department of pharmacology was beginning a systematic exploration of the Chinese materia medica (Chen, 1977).

These explorations revealed that ephedrine was a sympathomimetic with properties of epinephrine, causing an increase in blood pressure, vasoconstriction, and bronchodilation. Clinically it had several distinct advantages over epinephrine: it could be used orally, it had a long duration of action, and it was less toxic. It also was found to be useful in the management of bronchial asthma and hay fever and to support the patient's vital signs during the administration of spinal anesthesia. In subsequent years it became possible to synthesize ephedrine. Today we encounter this product of the Chinese materia medica in a number of pharmaceuticals, including over-the-counter products such as Sudafed and Actifed.

Historically and clinically *Herba Ephedra* has been applied in a similar fashion in Chinese medicine, except for spinal anesthesia. As we saw earlier, it is a principal ingredient in the herbal formula Ephedra Decoction. This herb also figures prominently in formulas that are applied to presentations that relate to asthma and allergy. *Herba Ephedra* represents an early and impressive example of pharmacological research in the Chinese materia medica. Other examples in which the traditional clinical applications of single herbs is supported in recent clinical experimentation include *Herba Artemisiae (yin chen hao)* for hepatitis and *Caulis Mu Tong (mu tong)* for urinary tract infections. Extensive compilations discussing identified active constituents, clinical studies, and toxicity of large numbers of substances have been prepared (Chang, 1986).

Explorations of traditional pharmacology are somewhat more complex, although they too are amenable to the methods of double blinding and placebo control that are critical to recognition in the biomedical world. However, given the breadth of possible substances that may be applied clinically (more than 5000) and the number of possible permutations for their combination in formula, the scope of the inquiry becomes quite large. In addition, there is the question of whether to include the traditional considerations that surround diagnosis and pattern identification in the process of prescription and selection of herbal formulas for investigation. Some contemporary studies are designed to take this into account, with the traditional clinician being able to assign individuals to specific treatment groups on the basis of symptoms while still being blinded in relation to the actual constituents of the substances administered to the patient. A recent example of this approach can be seen in a randomized clinical trial of Chinese herbal medicine for the treatment of irritable bowel syndrome conducted by Alan Bensoussan under the auspices of the Research Unit for Complementary Medicine, University of Western Sydney Macarthur. This study, in which patients were randomized to three treatment groups: placebo, standard formula, and individualized formula, showed that Chinese herbal medicine provided significant reduction in the symptoms of irritable bowel syndrome (Bensoussan et al., 1998). Research in this area has been extensive both in China and Japan and is emerging in the United States, as can be seen from the list of OAM-funded studies and specialty centers.

Acupuncture

Disappointingly little has been achieved by literally hundreds of attempts to evaluate acupuncture. Major methodological flaws are apparent in the vast majority of studies (Vincent, 1993).

Although the pessimism of Vincent's statement is captured in the Consensus Panel's conclusions concerning the methodological problems that continue to plague acupuncture studies, the Panel's remarks concerning the range of promising results in specific areas speaks to the development of research standards in the last several years.

Vincent was speaking to a concern that continues to be shared by many individuals working in the area of acupuncture research. Despite the relatively early interest in acupuncture as a form of alternative and complementary medicine, comparatively few studies have been designed in a fashion that renders their results useful to other researchers, clinicians, or policy makers.

Over time an increasing number of well-designed studies has emerged. Many of the studies presented at the Workshop on Acupuncture sponsored by the OAM were also presented to the Consensus Panel of Acupuncture convened by the NIH. For the most part the best clinical research can be clustered into five specific areas that seem to represent the best and most positive research related to acupuncture. These areas were antiemesis treatment, the management of acute and chronic pain, substance abuse treatment, the treatment of paralysis caused by stroke, and the treatment of respiratory disease. In addition, there are areas such as female infertility, breach version, menopause, depression, and urinary dysfunction in which acupuncture can show good clinical results (Birch & Hammerschlag, 1996).

The use of acupuncture for the treatment of pain is an area of longstanding medical interest. Pain control is the one application of acupuncture that has been used repeatedly by the traditional medical community in Europe and the United States for many years. This area became visible in the 1970s as a result of Chinese reports on acupuncture anesthesia. As a result this is one of the most widely researched applications of acupuncture. However, it also is one of the most problematic.

Some of the problems that are typical of researching acupuncture treatments for pain, as well as acupuncture therapy in general, are exemplified by the results of two meta-analyses* studies examining acupuncture in the management of chronic pain. The first was conducted by pooling data from 14 studies that used randomized and controlled trials of acupuncture to treat chronic pain and that measured their outcomes in terms of the number of patients whose condition was improved (Patel et al., 1989). This study reached a number of conclusions concerning the relationship of study design to research outcomes and concluded that acupuncture compared favorably with placebo and conventional treatment.

---

*A meta-analysis is a research method that pools the results of many studies in an effort to try to reach a more powerful conclusion than an individual study might provide.

A second meta-analysis reviewed 51 studies and compared the quality of published controlled clinical trials on the basis of research designs and specific factors, including randomization, single and double blinding, and numbers of subjects. This meta-analysis concluded that of the studies reviewed those favorable to acupuncture were more poorly designed than those that associated negative results with acupuncture. The evidence suggested that the efficacy of acupuncture as a treatment for chronic pain is doubtful (ter Riet et al., 1990).

A careful review of the ter Reit meta-analysis by Delis and Morris suggested that its authors had "included studies which did not meet their criteria," such as a study that was not controlled or in which laser light was used instead of acupuncture needles (Delis & Morris, 1993). This finding prompted them to conduct their own analysis and to reanalyze the studies examined by ter Riet in relation to a number of factors, including investigator training and the appropriateness of treatment. Their meta-analysis showed a trend toward improvement in study design over time, suggesting that many poorly designed acupuncture studies might be viewed best as preliminary efforts by investigators who were sufficiently familiar with the modality to design effective studies.

All three of these meta-analyses pointed out significant issues in relation to acupuncture study design. Besides questions concerning randomization, blinding, placebo control, and sample size, a variety of questions emerged pertinent to the practice of acupuncture as a distinct modality. Is the investigator trained in acupuncture? Is the acupuncture treatment appropriate for the condition? Does the study allow for adjusting the treatment to the individual patient's needs according to traditional diagnostics? Are outcome measures clear? Is placebo or sham acupuncture used, and how will it be administered?

Of all the debated areas in acupuncture research, this last may receive the most attention. The problem of how to provide a sham treatment in acupuncture is a vexing one. In herbal studies a capsule of inert material that appears similar to the capsule of the medication being investigated can be provided to the patient. Because the patient cannot tell the difference between the two capsules, he or she is effectively blind to the use of a placebo. In acupuncture the problem is more complex because patients receiving treatment definitely know whether they have been stuck with needles or not. Solutions that have been proposed vary from comparing real acupuncture to other modalities to carefully selecting a treatment with few effects (Vincent, 1993) or selecting acupuncture points that are entirely irrelevant (BRITS method) to the conditions being treated (Birch, 1995).

The potential importance of traditional diagnostic and therapeutic considerations in trial design have been raised by a number of authors (Coan et al., 1980; Ergil, 1995a, b; Jobst, 1995). At the same time some researchers and physicians reject the potential importance of these ideas. Vincent tells us that traditional ideas need to be understood in outline but that questions about efficacy can be asked without considering them in detail. The treatment may be effective whether the theory is valid or not (Vincent, 1993). Hans Agren attempted to make this distinction more than 20 years ago to identify suitable research agendas, arguing that only the simple empirical observations of Chinese medicine should be an object of medical inquiry (Agren, 1975). The question emerging from some clinical researchers is whether some aspects of traditional theory are relevant to the delivery of effective treatment and, consequently, the inquiry.

The control of pain is considered to be a major area for the clinical application of acupuncture, and although some of the research in this area has been problematic, a number of studies strongly indicate the importance of acupuncture in pain management. As we have seen, one of the conclusions of the Consensus Panel was that acupuncture could be demonstrated as efficacious for postoperative dental pain. One study showed that acupuncture patients required less postoperative analgesia after oral surgery than a group receiving a sham acupuncture treatment (Lao et al., 1995).

Among some of the more notable studies in the area of pain management are a clinical trial involving 43 women with menstrual pain, in which women receiving acupuncture treatment had considerably less pain than the placebo and control groups (Helms, 1987). A controlled trial of acupuncture in the management of migraines involved 30 patients who had chronic migraines. Acupuncture was significantly effective in controlling the pain of migraine headaches (Vincent, 1989). Several studies of the management of various types of back pain with acupuncture also have shown it to be helpful. A number of studies suggest that pain of osteoarthritis seems to respond well to acupuncture (Dickens & Lewith, 1989; Junnila,

1982; Thomas et al., 1991), and one study suggests that there may be a significant cost benefit when the use of acupuncture removes the need for surgical intervention (Christensen et al., 1992).

The Consensus Panel concluded that acupuncture had been demonstrated to be efficacious for the treatment of adult postoperative and chemotherapy nausea and vomiting. Research in the area of antiemesis revolves around the use of the acupuncture point Inner Gate (*neiguan,* P6) to control nausea and vomiting. The use of this point in acupressure to control nausea and vomiting is well known, and its use to control the nausea of pregnancy with pressure bands has been determined to be effective (Aloysio & Penacchioni, 1992). There even are consumer products available that exploit this effect. The point also has been investigated in relation to its use in controlling perioperative emesis that resulted from premedication and anesthetic agents (Ghaly et al., 1987) and in relation to cancer chemotherapy (Dundee et al., 1989).

On the basis of clinical experiences in China, acupuncture is used extensively in the United States for the management of symptoms associated with withdrawal from a variety of substances, including alcohol and cocaine. The summary conclusion reached by presenters at the Workshop on Acupuncture panel on substance abuse suggested that early trial and empirical findings suggest positive treatment effects (Kiresuk & Culliton, 1994).

Acupuncture has been studied clinically in the West in relation to the management of a variety of specific medical conditions, among them pulmonary disease and paralysis subsequent to stroke. An extensive review of acupuncture in pulmonary disease led the author to conclude that acupuncture produced favorable effects in the management of patients with bronchial asthma, chronic bronchitis, and chronic disabling breathlessness (Jobst, 1995). A recent study involving 16 patients with right-sided paralysis who had experienced an ischemic infarction of the left hemisphere showed acupuncture produced a good response in patients whose lesion affected no more than half the motor pathway areas (Naeser et al., 1992).

It should be pointed out that although the volume of published research on acupuncture in the West is relatively low—by one count there were only 200 randomized controlled trials, 42 review articles, and 4 meta-analyses (Foreman, 1995) available in

1995 and although there has been substantial growth in the last several years—the amount of research conducted in China and Japan in the areas discussed previously and in many other areas is vast. Although study and publication quality can be a problem and design issues are still present, acupuncture research in China must be regarded as a significant resource. One English compilation contains 117 Chinese studies on acupuncture and moxibustion (Research on Acupuncture, Moxibustion, and Acupuncture Anesthesia, 1986). Recent shifts in study design and analysis displayed at conferences in China and in newer publications suggest that the trend toward improved research design observed by Delis in the West might be at work in the East as well.

Qi Cultivation

Considerable numbers of intriguing studies of qi cultivation have been conducted in China and are beginning to be explored in the United States. Qi cultivation has been examined in relationship to an increase in immunocompetence as measured through lymphocyte profiles (Ryu et al., 1995) and by changes in electroencephalography patterns. Qi cultivation has been explored as a tool for managing gastritis, and numerous Chinese studies have suggested that it might be a promising method for treating hypertension.

Unfortunately many of the problems that have confronted acupuncture research also surround research into qi cultivation. In addition, although there is great interest in qi cultivation in the West, there has not been the equivalent enthusiasm for resolving methodological problems and beginning to establish strong research initiatives.

Research in qi cultivation that investigates the role of the practice of qi cultivation exercises in the beneficial alteration of physiological processes is similar, in many respects, to the investigation of the effects of meditation, yoga, guided imagery, and what Benson termed the *relaxation response.* The challenge here is developing an effective control and ruling out other variables that may influence the results.

Where attempts have been made to examine the effects of externally transmitted qi special problems are encountered. In some cases (as discussed earlier) it is believed that this phenomenon involves measurable portions of the electromagnetic spectrum. In cases in which investigators hypothesize qi as an existent, but presently unmeasurable, phenomenon they seek to establish the presence and effect of externally transmitted qi by examining its apparent effects on other systems that can be directly observed.

Given the extensive range of phenomena under investigation and the range of claims for the healing potential of qi cultivation, there is a certain amount of skepticism concerning the field as a whole. Even in China there is some question as to whether qi cultivation should be established as a standard method of treatment within the corpus of Chinese medicine and there is the belief that some of the practices associated with qi cultivation have the potential for abuse and charlatanism (Tang, 1994).

Qi cultivation remains a challenging part of the broad fabric of China's traditional medicine. Researchers within the field hope that as time goes on it will be possible to increase the availability of well-designed and accessible studies in the filed (Sancier, 1996).

Qigong

Given the fundamental importance of qi to health and well-being it is not surprising that one important aspect of the practice of Chinese medicine is the systematic cultivation of qi. The methods and practices that are undertaken to achieve this are myriad. It can be said that *Qigong* is a term that literally embraces almost every aspect of the manipulation and development of qi by means of exercise, breathing, and creative visualization. Qigong can also be considered to encompass practices such as *dao yin* or conduction and Tui Na or exhalation and inhalation, both of which are applied to patterning and guiding the qi in the body.

Thus the expressions *qi cultivation* or *Qigong* can refer to an extraordinarily broad range of practices and activities, ranging from the meditative systems of Daoist and Buddhist practitioners through the health-giving exercises developed by ancient physicians to the martial arts traditions of China. The unifying aspect is the intention of the practice to increase the quantity, smooth movement, and volitional control of the practitioners qi and in so doing strengthen the body.

Although the practice of Daoist and Buddhist qi cultivation is aimed ultimately at spiritual realization, the practice of medical qi cultivation addresses three specific areas. The first is self-cultivation in terms of the practitioner's own health and stamina. Training in performing the strenuous activities of Tui Na, sustaining the constant demands of clinical practice, and quieting the mind to better engage in diagnosis would all pertain to this. The second involves the cultivation of the practitioner's ability to safely transmit qi to the patient. It is understood by some practitioners that their qi may be directed to the patient either through the needles or directly through their hands. This activity may be the main focus of treatment or an adjunctive aspect. In this case the qi paradigm is expanded to include direct interaction between the patient's qi and that of the clinician. Finally, patients may be taught to do specific Qigong practices that may help treat their illness or strengthen their qi.

Qi cultivation makes extensive use of the principles of China's traditional medicine, and its history is intertwined with that of famous physicians. The history of qi cultivation practices is considered to extend back into antiquity and to point to the early recognition of the importance of exercise to the health of the body. In Lu's Spring and Autumn annals a famous aphorism relates the importance of movement to the maintenance of health and function (Engelhardt, 1989).

Flowing water will never turn stale, the hinge of the door will never be eaten by worms. They never rest in their activity: that's why.

Within this text Lu described the role of dance and movement in correcting the movement of qi and yin within the body and benefiting the muscles (Zhang, 1990).

Descriptions of qi cultivation practices and exercises are attributed to the early Daoist masters. Zhuang Zi writing in the fourth century BCE reveals the role of breathing and physical exercise in promoting longevity and describes a sage intent on extending his life (Despeux, 1989).

To pant, to puff, to hail, to sip, to spit out the old breath and draw in the new, practicing bear hangings and bird-stretches, longevity his only concern (Watson, 1968).

Among the texts recovered at Ma Huang Dui are a series of illustrated guides to the practice of conduction (*dao yin*) that provide guidance to the physical postures and therapeutic properties of this form of qi cultivation (Despeux, 1989, p. 226).

The famous physician of second century China Hua Tou is credited with the creation of a series of exercises. These were based on the movements of the tiger, the deer, the bear, the monkey, and a bird and were to be practiced to ward off disease.

Zhang Zhong Jing in his Golden Cabinet Prescriptions recommended the practices of *dao yin* or conduction and Tui Na or exhalation and inhalation to treat disease.

A wide variety of forms of qi cultivation were developed over the centuries, and many have achieved great popularity. From the 1950s on, Qigong training programs were implemented and sanatoria were built, specializing in the therapeutic application of Qigong to the treatment of disease.

Fundamental Concepts

Qi cultivation rests on several fundamental principles intended to support activity to enhance the movement of qi and to increase health. Most discussions of qi cultivation address the relaxation of the body, the regulation or control of breathing, and the calming of the mind. Qi cultivation generally is performed in a relaxed standing, sitting, or lying posture. Once the correct position is achieved, the practitioner begins to regulate breathing in concert with specific mental and physical exercises.

For example, one form of Qigong involves the action of visualizing the internal and external pathways of the channels and imagining the movement of the qi along these channels in concert with the breath. As the practice develops, the practitioner begins to experience the sensation of qi traveling along the channel pathways. Traditionally it is considered that the mind guides the qi to a specific area of the body and that the qi then guides the blood there as well, improving circulation in the area. From this point of view this particular exercise trains the qi and blood to move freely along the channel pathways, leading to good health.

Another exercise involves the use of breath, visualization, and simple physical exercises to benefit the qi of the lungs. This therapeutic exercise is recommended for bronchitis, emphysema, and bronchial asthma. It is begun by assuming a relaxed posture, whether sitting, lying, or standing. The exercise is be-

gun by breathing naturally and allowing the mind to become calm. The upper and lower teeth are then clicked together by closing the mouth gently 36 times. As saliva is produced, it is retained in the mouth, swirled with the tongue, and then swallowed in three parts while one imagines that it is flowing into the middle of the chest and then to an area about three fingerbreadths below the navel (the *dan tian,* or cinnabar field). At this point one imagines that one is sitting in front of a reservoir of white qi that enters the mouth on inhalation and is transmitted through the body as one exhales, first to the lungs, then to the *dan tian,* and finally out to the skin and body hair. This process of visualization is repeated 18 times.

This process makes use of the relationship between the mind and qi to strengthen the function of the lungs and to pattern areas of the body associated with the area where the qi that governs the lungs and respiration is stored. This area is associated with the acupuncture point *dan zhong,* or chest center (ren 17), which is located in the middle of the chest. Next the qi is directed to the cinnabar field, which is associated with another location on the ren channel *qi hai,* or sea of qi (ren 6), just below the umbilicus. This area is considered to be important in the production and storage of the body's qi and to the lungs on exhalation.

This exercise typifies the three aspects of a Qigong exercise described previously; it induces relaxation through mental concentration because the exercise of focusing on breathing and the visualized process help remove distracting thoughts from the mind and the patterning of the breath with visualization controls and regulates the breathing.

It should be stressed that although many forms of Qigong exist, they share general principles of application and a relationship to Chinese medicine concepts.

Acknowledgments

As is apparent from the text, this presentation owes a heavy debt to the work of Paul Unschuld and Nigel Wiseman. The scholarship and enterprise of these two individuals is reflected in their work and the help that they have provided to students of Chinese medicine such as myself. My wife and colleague Marnae Ergil contributed enormously by reviewing text, answering questions, and being willing to check technical points in Chinese language materials at any hour of the day or night. This project would not have been possible without the institutional commitment to scholarship and the support provided of the Pacific College of Oriental Medicine.

References

Agren H. 1975. A new approach to Chinese traditional medicine. Am J Chin Med 3(3):207-212

Aloysio DD, Penacchioni P. 1992. Morning sickness control in early pregnancy by Neiguan point acupressure. Obstet Gyenecol 80(5):852-854

Auteroche B, Gervais G, Auteroche M, et al. 1992. Acupuncture and Moxibustion: A Guide to Clinical Practice. Churchill Livingstone. Edinburgh

Bannerman RH. 1979. The World Health Organization viewpoint on acupuncture. World Health, December, pp. 24-29

Barlow J, Richardson C. 1979. China Doctor of John Day. Binford and Mort. Portland

Becker RO. 1985. The Body Electric: Electromagnetism and the Foundation of Life. Quill William Morrow. New York

Bensky D, Barolet R. 1990. Chinese Herbal Medicine: Formulas and Strategies. Eastland Press. Seattle

Bensky D, Gamble A. 1986. Chinese Herbal Medicine: Materia Medica (Revised Edition). Eastland Press. Seattle

Bensoussan A, Talley NJ, Hing M, Menzies R, Guo A, Ngu M. 1998. Treatment of irritable bowel syndrome with Chinese herbal medicine: A randomized clinical trial. JAMA 280(18):1585-1589

Birch S. 1994. A historical study of radial pulse six position Diagnosis: naming the unnameable. J Acupun Soc NY 1(3&4):19-32

Birch S. 1995. A biophysical basis for acupuncture. In Birsh S (ed). Proceedings of the Second Symposium of the Society for Acupuncture Research. Society for Acupuncture Research. Boston, pp. 274-294

Birch S, Hammerschlag R. 1996. Acupuncture Efficacy: A Summary of Controlled Clinical Trials; The National Academy of Acupuncture and Oriental Medicine; Tarrytown, New York

Bowers JZ. 1970. Western Medical Pioneers in Feudal Japan. Johns Hopkins Press. Baltimore

Broffman M, McCulloch M. 1986. Instrument-assisted pulse evaluation in the acupuncture practice. Am J Acupuncture 14(3):255-259

Burton Goldberg Group. 1993. Acupuncture. In Alternative Medicine: The Definitive Guide. Strohecker J (ed). Future Medicine Publishing, Inc. Puyallup. pp. 37-46

Chang HM. 1986. Pharmacology and Applications of Chinese Materia Medica. Hson-Mou Chang HM, Pui-Hay But P (eds). Yao S-C, Wang L-L, Chang-Shing Yeung S (trans). World Scientific Publishing Co. Singapore. pp. 1-773

Chen KK. 1977. Half a century of ephedrine. In Kao FF, and Kao JJ. (eds). Chinese Medicine—New Medicine. Neale Watson Academic publications. New York. pp. 21-27

Christensen BV, Iuhl IU, Vilbe KH, et al. 1992. Acupuncture treatment of severe knee osteoarthritis. Acta Anaesthesiol Scand (36):519-525

Chuang Y. 1982. The Historical Development of Acupuncture. Oriental Healing Arts Institute. Los Angeles

Coan R, Wong GT, Ku S-L, et al. 1980. The acupuncture treatment of low back pain: a randomized controlled study. Am J Chin Med 8(2):181-189

Delis K, Morris M. 1993. Clinical Trials in Acupuncture. In Birch S (ed). Proceedings of the First Symposium of the Society of Acupuncture Research. Society for Acupuncture Research. Boston. pp. 68-71

Despeux C. 1989. Gymnastics: The Ancient Tradition. In Kohn L (ed). Taoist Meditation and Longevity Techniques. Ann Arbor: Center for Chinese Studies The University of Michigan. pp. 225-262

Dickens W, Lewith G. 1989. A single-blind, controlled and randomised clinical trial to evaluate the effect of acupuncture in the treatment of trapeziometacarpal osteoarthritis. Comp Med Res 3:5-8

Dundee JW, Ghaly RG, Fitzpatrick KTJ, et al. 1989. Acupuncture prophylaxis of cancer chemotherapy induced sickness. J R Soc Med 82:268-271

Ellis A, Wiseman N, Boss K. 1991. Fundamentals of Chinese Acupuncture. Paradigm. Brookline

Engelhardt U. 1989. Qi for life: Longevity in the Tang. In Kohn L (ed). Taoist Meditation and Longevity Techniques. Ann Arbor: Center for Chinese Studies The University of Michigan. pp. 263-296

Ergil KV. 1995a. Chinese specific condition review: urinary tract infections. Protocol J Botan Med 1(1):130-133

Ergil KV. 1995b. Where tradition matters: identifying epistemological and terminological issues in research design. Proc 2nd Sym Soc Acupunc Res pp. 59-69

Ergil MC. 1994. Medical education in China. CCAOM News 1(1):3-5

Farquhar J. 1987. Problems of knowledge in contemporary Chinese medical discourse. Soc Sci Med 24(12):1013-1021

Foreman J. 1995. What the research shows. The Boston Globe, 22/5, 25, 27

Ghaly RG, Fitzpatrick KTJ, Dundee JW. 1987. Anesthesia 42:1108-1110

Haller JS. 1973. Acupuncture in nineteenth century western medicine. NYS J Med

Hao LZ. 1983. An attempt to understand the substance of kidney and its disorders. Cheung CS (trans). J Am Coll Tradit Chin Med 1983(3):82-97

Helms JM. 1987. Acupuncture for the management of primary dysmenorrhea. Obstet Gynecol 69(1):51-56

Hirsch RC. 1985. Korean constitutional nutrition. J Am Coll Tradit Chin Med 1985(1):24-37

Hsu E. 1989. Outline of the history of acupuncture in Europe. J Chin Med (29, January):28-32

Hsu H, Peacher W. 1977. Chen's History of Chinese Medical Science. Modern Drug Publishers. Taipei

Huang B, Di F, Li X, et al. 1993. Syndromes of Traditional Chinese Medicine. Huang B (ed). Ma D, Guo'en W, Sun S, Cao H (trans). Heilongjiang Education Press. Heilongjiang

Huard P, Wong M. 1968. Chinese Medicine. McGraw Hill, World University Library. New York

Jobst K. 1995. A critical analysis of acupuncture in pulmonary disease: efficacy and safety of the acupuncture needle. J Altern Comple Med (1, January):57-86

Junnila SYT. 1982. Acupuncture superior to Prioxicam in the treatment of osteoarthritis. Am J Acupunct 10: 341-346

Kaptchuk TJ. 1983. The Web That Has No Weaver: Understanding Chinese Medicine. Congdon and Weed. New York

Kiresuk TJ, Culliton PD. 1994. Overview of Substance Abuse Acupuncture Treatment Research. Workshop on Acupuncture. pp. 1-17, 21/4

Kleinman A. 1986. Social Origins of Distress and Disease: Depression, Neurasthenia, and Pain in Modern China. Yale University Press. New Haven

Lao L, Bergman S, Langenberg P, Wong RH, Berman B. 1995. Efficacy of Chinese acupuncture on postoperative oral surgery pain. Oral Surg Oral Med Oral Pathol Oral Radiol Endod 79:423-428

Lee JK, Bae SKB. 1981. Korean Acupuncture Ko Mun Sa

Lin Y. 1942. Laotse, the Book of Tao. In Lin Y (ed). The Wisdom of China and India. The Modern Library. New York. pp. 578-624

Lock M. 1980. East Asian Medicine in Urban Japan. Comparative Studies of Health Systems, vol. 4. University of California Press. Berkeley

Maciocia G. 1989. The Foundations of Chinese Medicine. Churchill Livingstone. Edinburgh

Manaka Y, Itaya K. 1994. Acupuncture as intervention in the biological information system. J Acupunct S NY 1(3&4):19-32

Muench C. 1984. One Hundred Years of Medicine: The Ah-Fong Physicians of Idaho. In Schwarz HG (ed). Chinese Medicine on the Golden Mountain: An Interpretive Guide. Washington Commission for the Humanities. Seattle. pp. 51-80

Naeser MA, Michael PA, Stiassny-Eder D, et al. 1992. Real versus sham acupuncture in the treatment of paralysis in acute stroke patients: a CT scan lesion study. J Neurol Rehab (6):163-173

NIH. 1997. Acupuncture. NIH Consensus Statement. Nov 3-5; 15(5):1-34

Oschman J. 1993. A Biophysical Basis for Acupuncture. In Birch S (ed). Proceedings of the First Symposium of the Society for Acupuncture Research. Society for Acupuncture Research. Boston. pp. 141-220

Osler W. 1913. The Principles and Practice of Medicine. D. Appleton and Co. New York

Patel M, Gutzwiller F, Paccand F, Marazzi A. 1989. A meta-analysis of acupuncture for chronic pain. Int J Epidemiol 18(4):900-906

Payer L. 1988. Medicine and Culture: Varieties of Treatment in the United States, England, West Germany, and France. Henry Holt and Company. New York

Peacher W. 1975. Adverse reactions, contraindications and complications of acupuncture and moxibustion. Am J Chin Med 3(1):35-46

Pomeranz B. 1988. Scientific Basis of Acupuncture. In Stox G (ed). The Basics of Acupuncture. Springer-Verlag. New York. pp. 4-37

Qiu XI. 1993. Chinese Acupuncture and Moxibustion. Churchill Livingstone. New York

Reichmanis M, Marino AA, Becker RO. 1975. Electrical correlates of acupuncture points. IEEE Trans Bio Engineer November, 533-535 Intern J Acupunct Electrother 17:75-94

Ryu H, Jun CD, Lee BS, Choi BM, Kim HM, Chung HT. 1995. Effect of qigong training on proportions of T lymphocyte subsets in human peripheral blood. Am J Chin Med, 23:27-36

Sancier K. 1996. Medical Applications of qigong alternative therapies. 2(1):40-46

Seto A, Kusaka S, Nakazatio W, et al. 1992. Detection of extraordinary large bio-magnetic field strength from human hand.

Shanghai College of Traditional Chinese Medicine. 1981. Acupuncture: A Comprehensive Text. O'Connor J, Bensky D (trans). Eastland. Seattle

Sivin N. 1987. Traditional Medicine in Contemporary China. Science, Medicine and Technology in East Asia, vol. 2. Center for Chinese Studies The University of Michigan. Ann Arbor

Takashima M. 1995. Pulse Research. Personal Communication

Tang KC. 1994. Qigong therapy—its effectiveness and regulation. Am J Chin Med 22:235-242

ter Riet G, Kleijnen J, Knipschild P. 1990. Acupuncture and chronic pain: a criteria-based meta-analysis. J Clin Epidemiol 43:1191-1199

Thomas M, Eriksson SV, Lundeberg T. 1991. A comparative study of diazepam and acupuncture in patients with osteoarthritis pain: a placebo controlled study. Am J Chin Med 19:95-100

Unschuld P. 1979. Medical Ethics in Imperial China: A Study in Historical Anthropology. University of California, Berkeley

Unschuld P. 1985. Medicine in China: A History of Ideas. University of California. Berkeley

Veith I. 1972. The Yellow Emperors's Classic of Internal Medicine. Veith I (trans). University of California Press. Berkeley

Vincent CA. 1989. A controlled trial of the treatment of migraine by acupuncture. Clin J Pain 5:305-312

Vincent CA. 1993. Acupuncture as a treatment for chronic pain. In Lewith GT, Aldridge D (eds). Clinical Research Methodology for Complementary Therapies. Hodder and Stoughton. London. pp. 289-308

Wang G, Fan Y, Guan Z. 1990. Chinese Massage. In Zhang E (ed). WenPing Y (trans). A Practical English-Chinese Library of Traditional Chinese Medicine. Publishing House of Shanghai. College of Traditional Chinese Medicine. Shanghai

Wang X. 1986. Research on the Origin and Development of Chinese Acupuncture and Moxibustion. In Xiangtong Z (ed). Research on Acupuncture, Moxibustion and Acupuncture Anesthesia. Springer-Verlag. New York. pp. 783-799

Watson B. 1968. The Complete Works of Chuang-tzu. New York. Columbia University Press

Wilhelm R. 1967. The I Ching. Third. Baynes CF (trans). Princeton University Press. Princeton

Wiseman N. 1993. A List of Chinese Formulas. Unpublished paper, Taiwan

Wiseman N, Boss K. 1990. Glossary of Chinese Medical Terms and Acupuncture Points. Paradigm Publications. Brookline

Wiseman N, Ellis A, Zmiewski P, Li C. 1985. Fundamentals of Chinese medicine. In Zmiewski P (ed). Wiseman N, Ellis A (trans). Fundamentals of Chinese Medicine. Paradigm. Brookline

Wiseman N, Ellis A, Zmiewski P, Li C. 1993. Fundamentals of Chinese Medicine. SMC Publishing. Taipei

Wiseman N, Ellis A, Zmiewski P, Li C. 1995. In Wiseman N, Ellis A (trans). Fundamentals of Chinese Medicine. Paradigm. Brookline

Wong CK, Wu TL. 1985. History of Chinese Medicine: Being a Chronicle of Medical Happenings in China from Ancient Times to the Present Period. Southern Materials Center, Taipei

Xianytong Z. 1986. Research on Acupuncture, Moxibustion, and Acupuncture Anesthesia. Springer-Verlag. New York

Zhang E. 1990. Clinic of Traditional Chinese Medicine (I). Enqin Zhang, ed. Jilong Zou, trans. A Practical English-Chinese Library of Traditional Chinese Medicine, no. first English. Shanghai: Publishing Hourse of Shanghai College of Traditional Chinese Medicine

Zhu B. 1991. Pulse Research in China. Personal communication

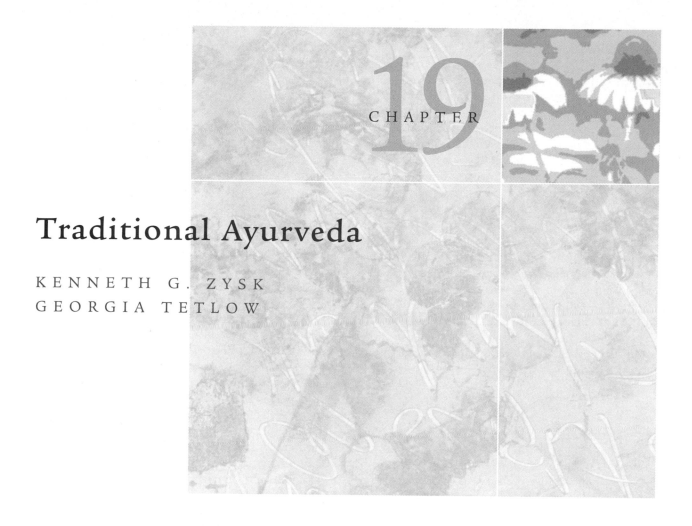

CHAPTER 19

Traditional Ayurveda

KENNETH G. ZYSK
GEORGIA TETLOW

As the health care professions look seriously at complementary and alternative modalities of medicine, a growing interest in traditional Indian medicine is emerging simultaneously. As with any popular development, aspects of the Indian medical system and its cures have sometimes been appropriated by individuals not wholly familiar with the basics of Ayurveda or the science of longevity. Over the past decade, however, a group of dedicated scholars has undertaken serious study of this ancient healing tradition. In this book it is appropriate to present the fundamental principles and practices of traditional Ayurveda as they may be understood from classical Sanskrit sources and traditional Indian practitioners.

HISTORY

On the basis of available literary sources, the history of Indian medicine occurred in four main phases. The first, or Vedic, phase dates from about 1200 to 800 BCE. Information about medicine during this period is obtained from numerous curative incantations and references to healing that are found in the *Atharvaveda* and the *Rigveda*, two religious scriptures that reveal a "magico-religious" approach to healing. The second, or classical, phase is marked by the advent of the first Sanskrit medical treatises, the *Caraka* and *Sushruta Samhitas*, which probably date from a few centuries before to several centuries after the start of the common era. This period includes all subsequent medical treatises dating from before the Muslim invasions of India at the beginning of the eleventh century, because these works tend to follow the earlier classical compilations closely and provide the basis of traditional Ayurveda. The third, or syncretic, phase is marked by clear influences on the classical paradigm from Islamic or Unani, South Indian Siddha, and other nonclassical medical systems. Bhavamishra's sixteenth century *Bhavaprakasha* is one text that reveals the results of these influences, which included diagnosis by examination of pulse or urine. This phase extends from the Muslim incursions to the present era. I would term the final phase as "New Age Ayurveda," wherein the classical paradigm is being adapted to the world of modern science and technology, including quantum physics, mind-body science, and advanced biomedical science. This recent manifestation of Ayurveda is most visible in the Western world, although there are indications that it is filtering back to India. These four phases of Indian medical history provide a chronological grid necessary to understanding the development of this ancient system of medicine.

THEORETICAL FOUNDATIONS

From its beginnings during the Vedic era Indian medicine always has adhered closely to the principle of a fundamental connection between the microcosm and macrocosm. Human beings are minute representations of the universe and contain within them everything that makes up the surrounding world. Comprehending the world is crucial to comprehending the human, and conversely, understanding the world is necessary to understanding the human.

The Human Body

According to Ayurveda the cosmos consists of five basic elements: earth, air, fire, water, and space. Certain forces cause these to interact, giving rise to all that exists. In human beings these five elements occur as the three *doshas,* forces that, along with the seven *dhatus* (tissues) and three *malas* (waste products), make up the human body.

The Three Doshas
When in equilibrium the three doshas maintain health, but when an imbalance occurs among them,

they defile the normal functioning of the body, leading to the manifestation of disease. An imbalance indicates an increase or decrease in one, two, or all three of the doshas. The three doshas are *vata, pitta,* and *kapha.*

Vata or *Vayu* meaning "wind," is composed of the elements air and space. It is the principle of kinetic energy and is responsible for all bodily movement and nervous functions. It is located below the navel and in the bladder, large intestines, nervous system, pelvic region, thighs, bone marrow, and legs; its principal seat is the colon. When disrupted, its primary manifestation is gas and muscular or nervous energy, leading to pain.

Pitta, or bile, is made up of the elements fire and water. It governs enzymes and hormones and is responsible for digestion, pigmentation, body temperature, hunger, thirst, sight, courage, and mental activity. It is located between the navel and the chest and in the stomach, small intestines, liver, spleen, skin, and blood; its principal seat is the stomach. When disrupted, its primary manifestation is acid and bile, leading to inflammation.

Kapha or *Shleshman,* meaning "phlegm," is made up of the elements of earth and water. It connotes the principle of cohesion and stability. It regulates Vata and Pitta and is responsible for keeping the body lubricated and maintaining its solid nature, tissues, sexual power, and strength. It also controls patience. Its normal locations are the upper part of the body, the thorax, head, neck, upper portion of the stomach, pleural cavity, fat tissues, and areas between joints; its principal seat is the lungs. When it is disrupted, its primary manifestation is liquid and mucus, leading to swelling, with or without discharge.

The attributes of each dosha help determine the individual's basic bodily and mental makeup and to isolate which dosha is responsible for a disease. The qualities of *Vata* are dryness, cold, light, irregularity, mobility, roughness, and abundance. Dryness occurs when Vata is disturbed and is a side effect of motion. Too much dryness produces irregularity in the body and mind. *Pitta* is hot, light, intense, fluid, liquid, putrid, pungent, and sour. Heat appears when Pitta is disturbed, resulting from change caused by Pitta. The intensity of excessive heat produces irritability in the body and mind. *Kapha* is heavy, unctuous, cold, stable, dense, soft, and smooth. Heaviness occurs when Kapha is disturbed and results from firmness caused by Kapha. The viscosity of excessive heaviness and stability produces slowness in body and mind.

The Seven Dhatus

The seven dhatus or tissues are responsible for sustaining the body. Each dhatu is responsible for the one that comes next in the following order.

1. Rasa, meaning sap or juice, includes the tissue fluids, chyle, lymph, and plasma, and functions as nourishment. It comes from digested food.
2. Blood includes the red blood cells and functions to invigorate the body.
3. Flesh includes muscle tissue and functions as stabilization.
4. Fat includes adipose tissue and functions as lubrication.
5. Bone includes bone and cartilage and functions as support.
6. Marrow includes red and yellow bone marrow and functions as filling for the bones.
7. Shukra includes male and female sexual fluids and functions in reproduction and immunity.

The Three Malas

The malas are the waste products of digested and processed food and drink. Ayurveda delineates three principal malas, urine, feces, and sweat. A fourth category of other waste products includes fatty excretions from the skin and intestines, ear wax, mucus of the nose, saliva, tears, hair, and nails. According to Ayurveda an individual should evacuate the bowels once a day and eliminate urine six times a day.

Ayurveda considers digestion to be the most important function that takes place in the human body. It provides all that is required to sustain the organism and is the principal cause for all maladies from which an individual suffers. The process of digestion and assimilation of nutrients is discussed under the topics of the Agnis (enzymes), Ama (improperly digested food and drink), and the Srotas (channels of circulation).

The Three Agnis

The Agnis, or enzymes, assist in the digestion and assimilation of food and are divided into three types.

Jatharagni is active in the mouth, stomach, and gastrointestinal tract and helps break down food. The waste product of feces results from this activity.

Bhutagnis are five enzymes located in the liver. They adapt the broken down food into a homologous chyle according to the five elements and assist the chyle to assimilate with the corresponding five elements in the body. The homologous chyle circulates in the blood channels as rasa, nourishing the body and supplying the seven dhatus.

Dhatvagnis are seven enzymes that synthesize the seven dhatus from the assimilated chyle homologized with the five elements. The remaining waste products result from this activity.

Ama

Ama, the chief cause of disease, is formed when there is a decrease in enzyme activity. A product of improperly digested food and drink, it takes the form of a liquid sludge that travels through the same channels as the chyle. Because of its density, however, it lodges in different parts of the body, blocking the channels. It often mixes with the doshas that circulate through the same pathways and it gravitates to a weak or stressed organ or to a site of a disease manifestation. Because all diseases invariably come from Ama, the word *Amaya*, meaning "coming from Ama," is a synonym for disease. Internal diseases begin with Ama, and external diseases produce Ama. In general, Ama can be detected by a coating on the tongue; turbid urine with foul odor; and feces that is passed with undigested food, an offensive odor, and abundant gas. The principal course of treatment in Ayurveda involves the elimination of Ama and the restoration of the balance of the doshas.

The Thirteen Kinds of Srotas

The srotas are the vessels or channels of the body through which all substances circulate. They are either large, such as the large and small intestines, uterus, arteries, and veins, or small, such as the capillaries. A healthy body has open and free-flowing channels. Blockage of the channels, usually by Ama, results in disease.

1. Pranavahasrotas convey vitality and vital breath *(prana)* and originate in the heart and alimentary tract.
2. Udakavahasrotas convey water and fluids and originate in the palate and pancreas.
3. Annavahasrotas convey food from the outside and originate in the stomach.
4. Rasavahasrotas convey chyle, lymph, and plasma and originate in the heart and in the 10 vessels connected with the heart. Ama primarily accumulates within them.
5. Raktavahasrotas convey red blood cells and originate in the liver and spleen.
6. Mamsavahasrotas convey ingredients for muscle tissue and originate in the tendons, ligaments, and skin.

7. Medovahasrotas convey ingredients for fat tissue and originate in the kidneys and fat tissues of the abdomen.
8. Asthavahasrotas convey ingredients for bone tissue and originate in hip bone.
9. Majjavahasrotas convey ingredients for marrow and originate in the bones and joints.
10. Shukravahasrotas convey ingredients for the male and female reproductive tissues and originate in the testicles and ovary.
11. Mutravahasrotas convey urine and originate in the kidney and bladder.
12. Purishavahasrotas convey feces and originate in the colon and rectum.
13. Svedavahasrotas convey sweat and originate in the fat tissues and hair follicles.

This broad outline exhibits that Ayurveda understands that the human body's anatomical parts are composed of the five basic elements, which have undergone a process of metabolism and assimilation in the body. Human beings differ, depending on their normal bodily constitution *(prakriti),* which is determined at the moment of conception and remains until death. The four factors that influence constitutional type include the father, the mother (particularly her food intake), the womb, and the season of the year. A large imbalance of the doshas in the mother will affect the growth of the embryo and fetus, and a moderate excess of one or two of the doshas will affect the constitution of the child.

Prakriti

There are seven normal body constitutions based on the three doshas: *vata, pitta, kapha, vata-pitta, pitta-kapha, vata-kapha,* and *sama.* The latter is balanced, which is best, but extremely rare. Most people are a combination of doshas, in which one dosha predominates. In general, Vata-type people tend to be anxious and fearful, exhibit light and "airy" characteristics, and are prone to vata-diseases. Pitta-type people are aggressive and impatient, exhibit fiery and hot-headed characteristics, and are prone to pitta-diseases. Kapha-type people are stable and entrenched; exhibit heavy, wet, and earthy characteristics; and are prone to kapha-diseases.

These are the principal factors that help the Ayurvedic physician determine the correct course of treatment to be administered to a patient for a particular ailment.

Three Mental States

In addition to physical constitution, Ayurveda understands that an individual is influenced by three mental states, based on the three qualities *(gunas)* of balance *(sattva),* energy *(rajas),* and inertia *(tamas).* In the state of balance the mind is in equilibrium and can discriminate correctly. In the state of energy the mind is excessively active, causing weakness in discrimination. In the state of inertia the mind is excessively inactive, also creating weak discrimination.

Ayurveda always has recognized that the body and the mind interact to create a healthy, normal *(prakriti)* or unhealthy, abnormal *(vikriti)* condition. A good Ayurvedic physician will determine both the mental and physical condition of the patient before proceeding with any form of diagnosis and treatment.

DISEASE

Aspects of the Ayurvedic understanding of disease have been mentioned in the previous section. Here we shall focus specifically on the Ayurvedic classification of disease, the naming of disease, and the manifestations of disease.

Classification of Disease

Ayurveda identifies three broad categories of disease on the basis of causative factors.

Adhyatmika diseases originate within the body and may be subdivided into hereditary diseases, congenital disease, and diseases caused by one or a combination of the doshas.

Adhibhautika diseases originate outside the body and include injuries from accidents or mishaps, and in the terminology of the modern era, from germs, viruses, and bacteria.

Adhidaivika diseases originate from supernatural sources, including diseases that are otherwise inexplicable, such as maladies stemming from providential causes, planetary influences, curses, and seasonal changes.

Disease Names

In Ayurveda diseases receive their names in one of six ways. A disease is named for the misery it produces (fever, or *Jvara*), its chief symptom (diarrhea, or *Atisara*), its chief physical sign (jaundice, or *Pandu*), its principal nature (piles, or *Arshas*), the chief dosha(s) involved (wind-disease, or *Vata-roga*), or the chief organ involved (disease of the duodenum, or *Grahani*). Regardless of its given name, most diseases will involve one or more of the doshas.

Manifestation of Disease

During the course of a disease an Ayurvedic physician seeks to identify its site of origin, its path of transportation, and its site of manifestation. The site of manifestation of a disease usually differs from its site of origin. Recognizing this distinction enables the physician to determine the correct course of treatment.

Ayurveda describes the manifestation of all diseases in the same fundamental way. Causative factors (e.g., food, drink, regimen, season, mental state) suppress enzyme activity in the body, leading to the formation of Ama. The circulating Ama blocks the channels. The site of the disease's origin is where the blockage occurs. The circulating Ama, often combining with one or more of the doshas, then takes a divergent course, referred to as the *path of transportation*. Finally, the dosha(s) and Ama mixture comes to rest in and afflicts a certain body part, which is known as the *site of disease manifestation*. Treatment entails correction of all the steps in the process resulting in disease manifestation, thus restoring the entire person to his or her particular balanced state.

THERAPEUTICS

In Ayurveda restoring a person to health is not viewed simply as the eradication of disease. It entails a complete process of diagnosis and therapeutics that takes into account both mental and physical components integrated with the social and physical worlds in which the patient lives. I shall therefore briefly explain Ayurvedic diagnosis, examination of the disease, and types of therapeutics.

Ayurvedic Diagnosis

Ayurveda established a detailed system of diagnosis, involving examination of pulse, urine, and physical features.

After a preliminary examination by means of visual observation, touch, and interrogation, the Ayurvedic physician undertakes an eightfold method of detailed examination to determine the patient's type of physical constitution and mental status and to get an indication of any abnormality.

Pulse Examination

Pulse examination is first mentioned in a medical treatise from the late thirteenth or early fourteenth century of the common era. It is a highly specialized art. Not every Ayurvedic physician uses pulse examination. The diagnostic process involves evenly placing the index, middle, and ring fingers of the right hand on the radial artery of the right hand of men and the left hand of women, just at the base of the thumb. A pulse resembling the movement of a snake at the index finger indicates a predominance of Vata; a pulse resembling the movement of a frog at the middle finger indicates a predominance of Pitta; a pulse resembling the movement of a swan or peacock at the ring finger indicates a predominance of Kapha; and a pulse resembling the movement of a woodpecker indicates a predominance of all three doshas. To get an accurate reading, the physician must keep in mind the times when each of the doshas are normally excited and should take the pulse at least three times early in the morning when the stomach is empty, or 3 hours after eating in the afternoon, making sure to wash his or her hands after each reading.

Urine Examination

Like pulse examination, urine examination probably was formalized in the syncretic phase. After collecting the morning's midstream evacuation in a clear glass container, the physician submits the urine to two kinds of examination after sunrise. First, the physician studies it in the container to determine its color and degree of transparency. Pale-yellow and unctuous urine indicates Vata; intense yellow, reddish, or blue urine indicates Pitta; white, foamy, and muddy urine indicates Kapha; urine with a blackish tinge indicates a combination of doshas; and urine resembling lime juice or vinegar indicates Ama. The physician also puts a few drops of sesame oil in the urine and examines it in sunlight. The shape, movement, and diffusion of the oil in the urine indicate the prognosis of the disease. The shape of the drops also reveals which dosha(s) is involved. A snakelike shape indicates Vata; umbrella shape, Pitta; and pearl shape, Kapha.

Examination of Bodily Parts

The physician concludes his diagnostic examination with careful scrutiny of the tongue, skin, nails, and physical features to determine which dosha(s) is affected. Using the basic characteristics of each of the doshas, the physician will examine the different parts of the body. Coldness, dryness, roughness, and cracking indicate Vata; hotness and redness indicate Pitta; and wetness, whiteness, and coldness indicate Kapha.

Having completed this phase of the diagnosis, the Ayurvedic physician proceeds to examine any malady present.

Examination of the Disease

A detailed examination of the disease involves a five-step process, leading to a complete understanding of the abnormality.

Etiology

A disease results from one or several of the following factors: mental imbalances resulting from the effects of past actions *(karma);* unbalanced contact between the senses and the objects of the senses affecting the body and the mind; effects of the seasons on the mental and doshic balance; and the immediate causes of diet, regimen, and microorganism; doshas and Ama; and the combination of interaction of individual components such as doshas and tissues or doshas and microorganisms.

Early Signs and Symptoms

Early signs and symptoms that appear before the onset of disease provide clues to the diagnosis. Proper diet and administration of medicine can avert disease if it is recognized early enough.

Manifest Signs and Symptoms

The most crucial step in the diagnostic process is manifest signs and symptoms. It involves determining the site of origin and of manifestation and of the path of transportation of the Ama and dosha(s). Most signs and symptoms are associated with the site of disease manifestation, from which the physician must work his or her way back to the site of the origin of disease to effect a complete cure. Although symptomatic treatment was largely absent in traditional Ayurveda, modern medicine in India has intro-

duced Ayurvedic physicians to techniques of symptomatic treatment in cases of acute disease.

Exploratory Therapy

Exploratory therapy involves 18 different experiments that use drugs, diet, and regimens to determine the precise nature of the malady and suitable therapy by allopathic and homeopathic means.

Pathogenesis

Pathogenesis is a six-step process that determines the manner by which a dosha becomes aggravated and moves through the different channels to produce disease. An accumulation of a dosha leads to its aggravation, which causes it to spread through the channels until it lodges in a particular organ of the body, bringing about a manifestation of disease. Once a general form of the disease appears, it progressively splits into specific varieties. As in systems of medicine the world over, many patients consult the Ayurvedic physician only after the disease appears.

Ayurveda delineates seven basic varieties of disease on the basis of the doshas: diseases involving a single dosha, diseases involving two doshas, and diseases involving all three doshas together.

Prognosis is the final step in the Ayurvedic diagnostic process. Because Ayurvedic physicians traditionally did not treat persons with incurable diseases, it was important for the physician to know precisely the patient's chances of full recovery. Therefore disease is one of three types. It is easily curable, palliative, or incurable or difficult to cure. In general, if the disease type (Vata, Pitta, Kapha) is different from the person's normal physical constitution, the disease is easy to cure. If the disease and constitution are the same, the disease is difficult to cure. If the disease, constitution, and season correspond to doshic type, the disease is nearly impossible to cure.

Having determined the patient's normal constitution, diagnosed his or her illness, and established a prognosis for recovery, the Ayurvedic physician can begin a proper course of treatment.

Ayurvedic Treatment

Ayurveda recognizes two courses of treatment on the basis of the condition of the patient. The first is prophylaxis, for the healthy person who wants to maintain a normal condition based on his or her physical constitution and to prevent disease. The second is therapy, for an ill person who requires health to be restored. Once healthy, Ayurveda recommends continuous prophylaxis based on diet, regimen, medicines, and regular therapeutic purification procedures.

When a person is diagnosed with a doshic imbalance, either purification therapy, alleviation therapy, or a combination of these is prescribed.

Purification Therapy

Purification therapy involves the fundamental *Pañchakarma*, or Five Action treatment. The fivefold process varies slightly in different traditions and regions of India, but a standard regimen generally is followed. All five procedures can be performed, or a selection of procedures can be chosen on the basis of different factors such as the physical constitution of the patient, his or her condition, the season, and the nature of the disease. Before any action is taken, the patient is given oil internally and externally (with massage) and is sweated to loosen and soften the dosha(s) and Ama. An appropriate diet of food and drink is prescribed. After this twofold preparatory treatment, called *Purvakarma*, the five therapies are administered in sequence over the period of about a week. Because of the profound effects on the mind and body, the patient is advised to set aside time for treatment. First, the patient might be given an emetic and vomits until bilious matter is produced, thus removing Kapha. Second, a purgative is given until mucus material appears, thus removing Pitta. Third, an enema, either of oil or decocted medicines, is administered to remove excess Vata. Fourth, head purgation is given in the form of smoke inhalation or nasal drops to eradicate the dosha(s) that have accumulated in the head and sinuses. Fifth, leeches may be applied and bloodletting performed to purify the blood. Some physicians do not consider bloodletting in the five therapies of *Pañchakarma*, instead counting oily and dry (decoated medicine) enemas as two separate forms.

Alleviation Therapy

Alleviation therapy uses the basic condiments honey, butter or ghee, and sesame oil or castor oil to eliminate Kapha, Pitta, and Vata, respectively. This therapy and *Pañchakarma* often are used in conjunction with one another.

PHARMACEUTICS

Ayurveda prescribes a rich store of natural medicines that have been collected, tested, and recorded in medical treatises from ancient times. The tradition of collecting and preserving information about medicines in recipe books called *Nighantus* continues to the present day. The most traditional source of Ayurvedic medicine is the kitchen. It is likely that, at an early stage of its development, Indian medical and culinary traditions worked hand in hand with each other.

Because of the close association between food and medicine, Ayurveda classifies foods and drugs (usually vegetal) by the tongue, potency, and taste after digestion.

Rasa, taste by the tongue, is categorized into six separate tastes, with their individual elemental composition and doshic effect as follows:

1. Sweet, composed of earth and water, increases Kapha and decreases Pitta and Vata.
2. Sour, composed of earth and fire, increases Kapha and Pitta and decreases Vata.
3. Saline, composed of water and fire, increases Kapha and Pitta and decreases Vata.
4. Pungent, composed of wind and fire, increases Pitta and Vata and decreases Kapha.
5. Bitter, composed of wind and space, increases Vata and decreases Pitta and Kapha.
6. Astringent, composed of wind and earth, increases Vata and decreases Pitta and Kapha.

Virya, potency, comprises eight types that are divided into four pairs: hot-cold, unctuous-dry, heavy-light, and dull-sharp.

Vipaka, postdigestive taste, identifies three kinds of aftertaste: sweet, sour, and pungent.

Contrary foods and drugs are to be avoided always. For instance, clarified butter and honey should not be taken in equal quantities, alkalies and salt must not be taken for a long period, milk and fish should not be consumed together, and honey should not be put in hot drinks.

Four important criteria are considered when compounding plant substances and other ingredients into medical recipes. The substances that make up the recipe should have many attributes that enable it to cure several diseases; they should be usable in many pharmaceutical preparations, they should be suitable for the recipe and not cause unwanted side effects, and they should be culturally appropriate to the patients and their customs. Every medicine should be able to treat the disease's site of origin, site of manifestation, and its spread simultaneously.

A brief survey of the different kinds of medical preparations indicates the depth and content of Ayurvedic pharmaceuticals. The botanically based medicines derive largely from the Ayurvedic medical tradition, whereas the mineral and inorganic-based drugs derive from the Indian Alchemical traditions, called *Rasashastra.*

1. Juices are cold-presses and extractions made from plants.
2. Powders are prepared from parts of plants that have been dried in the shade and other dried ingredients.
3. Infusions are parts of plants and herbs that have been steeped in water and strained.
4. Cold infusions are parts of plants and herbs that were soaked in water overnight and filtered the next morning.
5. Decoctions are vegetal products boiled in a quantity of water proportionate to the hardness of the plant part and then reduced by a fourth. It is then filtered and often used with butter, honey, or oils.
6. Medicated pastes and oils. Often the plant and herbal extracts are combined with other ingredients and formed into pastes, plasters, and oils. Used externally, pastes and plasters are applied for joint, muscular, and skin conditions, and oil is used for hair and head problems. Medicated oils also are used for massages and enemas.
7. Large and small pills and suppositories. Plant and herbal extracts are also formed into pills and suppositories to be used internally.
8. Alcoholic preparations are made by fermentation or distillation. Two preparations are delineated: One requires the drug to be boiled before it is fermented or distilled, and in the other, the drug is simply added to the preparation. Fifteen percent is the maximum allowable amount of alcohol content in a drug.

Several Ayurvedic medicines are prepared from minerals and metals and are derived ultimately from ancient traditions.

9. Sublimates are prepared by an elaborate method leading to the sublimation of sulfur in a glass container. They are found in recipes *(Rasayanas)* used in rejuvenation therapies.
10. *Bhasmas* are ash residues produced from the calcination of metals, gems, plants, and animal products. Most are metals and minerals that are first detoxified and then purified. An important bhasma is prepared from mercury, which undergoes an 18-stage detoxification and purification process. Ayurveda maintains that bhasmas are quickly absorbed in the blood and increase the red blood cells.
11. *Pishtis* are fine powders made by trituration of gems with juices and extracts.
12. Collyrium is made from antimony powder, lead oxide, or the soot from lamps burned with castor oil. Collyrium is used especially to improve vision.

Space does not allow a discussion of the individual plants used in Ayurvedic recipes. It is safe to say, however, that of the hundreds of plants mentioned in various Ayurvedic treatises, only a small portion are commonly used by most Ayurvedic physicians.

AYURVEDIC CLINICAL APPROACH

The first step undertaken in clinical Ayurveda is proper diagnosis of the patient and his or her condition. The general diagnostic procedure determines the individual's overall health and strength and the specific morbidity from which the person is suffering. The first, *Rogipariksha,* focuses on establishing the patient's Prakriti and assessing his or her mental and physical strength. The second, *Rogapariksha,* aims at identifying the illness from which the patient suffers in terms of the dosha(s) involved and the dhatus involved and srotas in which it is located. A specific name of a disease is not necessary if the twofold process of diagnosis is executed properly. The Ayurvedic doctor, Vaidya, now knows the patient's strength and weakness and the anatomical and physiological areas affected. Correct therapeutic treatment follows from this diagnosis.

Ayurvedic therapies are designed to rebalance and reintegrate the individual. They are classified as tonifying and reducing and are intended either to nourish deficiencies and tissue weakness or to detoxify and reduce aggravated doshas. Reduction usually comes first, followed by rejuvenation therapies to rebuild the body's strength.

Reduction is often prescribed for Kapha disorders and tonification for Vata disorders, whereas Pitta disorders normally require a mixture of both therapies. Reduction therapy itself is divided into two parts: palliation and purification. Palliation consists of strengthening the digestive fire, reducing Ama, and calming the excess doshas so that they can be removed during purification. Purification therapy involves five cleansing therapies, *Panchakarma*: medicated enemas, nasal medications, therapeutic purgation, therapeutic vomiting, and therapeutic release of toxic blood.

An example of a specific disease will illustrate the traditional Ayurvedic clinical approach. In Sanskrit terminology, the malady *Amavata* refers approximately to arthritic and rheumatic conditions.

Amavata (Arthritis)

As the word itself indicates, *Amavata* involves Ama and the dosha Vata (wind). Traditional Ayurveda does not distinguish types of arthritis. This disease is caused by all factors that lead to the formation of Ama: unwholesome foods and regimens, bad digestive power, insufficient exercise, and excessive intake of unctuous foods and meat. The site of origin is principally the colon, but the entire alimentary canal is involved. Contrary foods and mental disturbance aggravate Vata and lead to the formation of Ama in the colon. Ama, propelled by Vata, leaves the site of origin and affects the enzymes, causing Ama to form at every level. Ama then becomes lodged in the joints and the heart, the sites of manifestation. The path of transport is the *Rasavahasrotas*, the vessels transporting chyle, lymph, and plasma.

Vata is the principal dosha affected. With the aggravation of Vata, symptoms include severe pain in the joints, rough skin, distension of the stomach, and indigestion. If Pitta is involved, a burning sensation spreads all over the body, especially in the joints. If Kapha is involved, the patient gradually becomes crippled. Little pain is experienced in the early morning because Ama is just beginning to move. The Ayurvedic treatment of Amavata involves actions, medicines, and procedures to reduce Ama and alleviate Vata. The first course of action is to put the patient on a mild fast and to administer medicines that have a bitter taste, hot potency, and pungent postdigestive taste, all of which help to reestablish the digestive powers. Sweating might be recommended to aid the digestive process.

The second step of the treatment involves the purification therapy of *Panchakarma*. The two preparatory actions, oleation and sweating, are administered first to dislodge and soften the Ama. The remaining five procedures are performed over the course of a week, during which time the patient maintains a strict diet. These actions will eradicate the dislodged Ama from the system and restore the balance of the doshas, especially Vata. One of two types of enema will be used, depending on the amount of Ama present. If Ama persists, an enema with decoctions is administered until Ama is removed when an oily enema is given.

After the *Panchakarma* therapy, the patient should assume a regimen that includes avoiding sleep during the day and after meals, as well as heavy foods that hinder digestion. Effective treatment of arthritic conditions, especially in children, has included wet massage therapy in conjunction with the enemas of *Panchakarma*. The affected areas are patted with a cloth bag filled with rice that has been cooked with milk and herbs. Massages with oils also are routinely prescribed.

Cancer (No Sanskrit equivalent in classic Ayurveda)

Under the influence of cancer, the three doshas destroy rather than preserve and nourish the body. Vata causes normal cells to proliferate and become cancerous. Pitta steals nutrients from other dhatus to feed cancerous cells, and Kapha allows these cells to increase unchecked. Although cancer regulates the activities of all three doshas, it usually begins by domination in one. A doshic imbalance, accompanied by an overaccumulation of Ama and insufficient digestive fire, sets the stage for cancer. In addition, Ayurveda recognizes an intimate link between suppressed emotion and suppressed immunity. Other proposed factors include devitalized foods, a sedentary lifestyle, long-term exposure to radiation or chemical carcinogens, and a lack of spiritual purpose or effort in life.

Because Ama is one of the primacy causes and enablers of cancer, detoxification is the primary therapy. *Panchakarma* rids the body of both Ama and any excessive accumulation of doshas. Cancer is classified into Vata, Pitta, and Kapha varieties, according to the nature of the tumors themselves, the color of the patient's skin, the patient's demeanor, and other symptoms. Patients are put on powerful blood-cleansing herbs, strong circulatory stimulants, immune strengthening tonics, and special Kapha-dispelling herbs. Specific anticancer herbs are administered differently for Vata, Pitta, or Kapha to obtain maximum assimilation. Vata cases are advised to imbibe fresh ginger tea with their herbs; Pitta patients should use aloe gel; and Kapha cases take honey and black pepper.

Jvara Roga (Fever)

Ayurveda views fever as both a disease and a symptom. It is considered a positive sign because it helps loosen and release Ama. It is often left to run its course unless one of the following is involved: fever is both high and prolonged, a child has had a febrile seizure in the past, or the individual is rapidly becoming depleted. Causes other than infection include the wrong combination of foods (e.g., hot with cold, fruit with starch, bananas with milk), emotions such as excessive anger or fear, or overwork.

Vata fever is more likely to occur during the vatic time of day (i.e., dawn or dusk) or during the fall. Pitta fever appears more often at midday and midnight and during the summer months. Kapha fever is noticed frequently in morning and evening and during late winter and spring.

In terms of pathogenesis Vata fever begins in the colon, as is often the case in Vata disorders. An excess of Vata in the colon cools the digestive fire of the stomach (Jatharagni) and pushes it into the channels for transporting lymph, chyle, and plasma (Rasavahasrotas). Eventually this fire makes its way through the chyle into the blood and heats the blood.

Vata fever may be accompanied by shivering, tremors, extreme body ache, or headache. Constipation, insomnia, intense fatigue, and lower backache may also be present.

Pitta fever begins like a Vata fever, when the digestive fire in the stomach and small intestine are pushed out of their respective seats into the Rasavahasrotas. Symptoms include red eyes, diarrhea, nausea, vomiting, rash, nosebleeds, perspiration, and aversion to light. Pitta fever can cause severe dehydration and a significant reduction in blood pressure. It may be caused by alcohol abuse or consumption of very sour or fermented food. Aspirin is contraindicated in Pitta fever because it may damage the stomach lining.

Kapha fever occurs when the body produces excessive Kapha secretions in the stomach and dampens the digestive fire. With the fire diminished, undigested food accumulates in the stomach, Ama increases, and both Kapha and Ama are forced into the Rasavahasrotas. Presymptoms include runny nose, cold, and congestion. Causes may be overexposure to cold or improper combination of foods, especially when milk is involved. The fever itself is often low grade in nature; cough, breathlessness, or chest pain may be present. Laryngitis, hoarseness, sinus congestion, and sinus headache can be accompanying symptoms. Complete loss of appetite usually occurs during and for several days after the fever. The patient may feel heavy and dull and may have cold and clammy skin.

In addition to Vata, Pitta, and Kapha types of fevers, Ayurveda also recognizes and specifically treats fevers caused by intestinal parasites, continuous versus fluctuating fevers, and fevers that affect each of the seven Dhatus.

Dhamani Pratichaya (Hypertension)

Because the heart regulates both the venous and arterial systems, Ayurveda believes that high venous blood pressure (Sirabbinodhana) and arterial hypertension (Dhamani Pratichaya) are equally important in understanding blood pressure disorders. Arterial hypertension, the most common type, is examined here. Ayurveda considers it a tridoshic disorder (i.e., one that can be caused by imbalances in any of the three doshas). With all types of hypertension, Ayurveda recommends that the patient follow a lifestyle and diet that reduce the primary aggravating dosha. In addition, caffeine, salt, sugar, and fatty or fried foods should be eliminated. Deep breathing exercises, daily walking of 3 miles, and meditation are recommended.

The disease pathway differs in each type of hypertension. In Vata-type hypertension, an excess of Vata dosha may lead to an accumulation of toxins in the colon. They are then absorbed into the blood, causing constriction of the blood vessels, especially the arteries. Blood pressure may rise and fall suddenly, the pulse may be erratic, and the diastolic pressure is often higher than the systolic pressure. The tongue may be dry and the patient may experience insomnia. Puffiness under the eyes and constipation are also common. Colonic cleansing, often with a medicated enema, is the initial treatment, followed by a Vata-balancing diet that includes plenty of fish and the oily vitamins A, E, and D. Garlic is also recommended, especially in conjunction with milk.

In Pitta-type hypertension, toxins from undigested foodstuffs in the small intestine can cause increased viscosity of the blood. Symptoms may include a violent headache, flushed face, red eyes, nosebleeds, sensitivity to light, anger, irritability, or burning sensation. Both the systolic and diastolic pressures tend to increase. Bitter herbs are prescribed, including aloe vera gel, bayberry, and *Katuka*, and purgation is recommended. The herb gotu kola is given to calm the mind, and other special herbal formulas act to pacify the Pitta dosha.

Kapha-type hypertension originates in the stomach. Kaphic mucosal secretions responsible for the production of triglycerides can overproduce the fatty molecules and cause increased blood viscosity and eventually arterial sclerosis. Symptoms often include obesity, tiredness, edema, hypothyroidism, and elevated cholesterol. Both systolic and diastolic pressures increase somewhat, but diastolic pressure may not rise as much as in Pitta hypertension. Dairy and high fatty foods should be aggressively eliminated, and appropriate herbs include cayenne, myrrh, garlic, motherwort, and hawthorn berries. Ayurveda recommends the use of diuretics only in Kapha hypertension.

Astmya (Allergies)

Ayurveda understands allergies as "changed reactivities," whose root cause is the body's weakened metabolism in one or more of the seven tissues of the body. Categories of allergic reactions are classified according to Vata, Pitta, and Kapha. All immediate, anaphylactic reactions are classified as Pitta-type, all intermittent allergies as Vata-Pitta–type or Vata-Kapha–type, and all delayed allergies, for example, seasonal sensitivities, as Kapha-type.

Vata-type allergic symptoms include headache, coughing, sneezing, gas, aches, and pains; sensitivity to dirt, dust, and pollens; heart palpitation; muscle spasms; nightmares; and wheezing. Patients having these allergies may be sensitive to nightshades (potato, tomato, eggplant), black beans, chick peas, and other beans. Emotionally they are likely to experience anxiety, fear, insecurity, or hyperactivity. A Vata-pacifying diet is advised, along with appropriate Vata-reducing herbs.

Pitta-type symptoms include contact dermatitis, eczema, rash, acne, infections, heat and light sensitivity, insect bites, and sensitivity to foam mattresses, formaldehyde, and preservatives. Reactions to strawberries, bananas, grapefruit, eggs, carrots, onions, garlic, spicy food, pork, and some cheese products are considered Pitta allergies. A Pitta-pacifying diet and Pitta-pacifying herbs are recommended.

Kapha-type allergies include hay fever, bronchial asthma, laryngeal edema, colds, generalized edema, latent spring fever, allergic rhinitis, runny nose, teary eyes, and reactions to some pollens. Individuals may be sensitive to avocado, bananas, lemons, watermelons, cucumbers, beef, lamb, pork, peanuts, and dairy products. A Kapha-reducing diet and teas are prescribed. The thymus gland (*Jatrugranthi*) and spleen (*Pliha*) play an important role in immunity and increased allergen reactivity. The heating (*Agni*) factor of the thymus helps to maintain immunity, and its weakness may be one of the causes of Kapha-type allergies. The spleen is considered the root of the hematopoietic system and, according to Ayurvedic theory, not only acts as a blood reservoir but also contains components that destroy foreign particles and microorganisms. Any weakness in the spleen, detectable through Ayurvedic pulse diagnosis, is likely to be found in individuals prone to allergies.

Shira Shula (Headache)

According to Ayurveda theory headaches have many causes, including constipation, indigestion, colds and flu, poor posture, lack of sleep, overwork, stress, and muscle tension. Migraines specifically are thought to relate to congenital factors and are most commonly caused by Vata and/or Pitta imbalance.

Treatment for general headaches and migraines is very similar. Diagnosis is based on identification of Vata, Pitta, or Kapha symptoms. Vata headaches are characterized by extreme pain, anxiety, depression, constipation, and dry skin. The condition may worsen with lack of sleep, excessive activity, irregular lifestyle, and worry or stress. Pitta headaches involve burning sensation, red eyes and face, irritability, anger, light sensitivity, and sometimes nosebleeds. Often liver problems accompany the condition, or toxicity in the blood is detected. Kapha headaches, although usually not migraine in nature, bring feelings of tiredness, heaviness, and a dull ache. There may be nausea, phlegm, vomiting, or excess salivation. Often Kapha headaches are caused by an accumulation of Kapha in the head and may be accompanied by pulmonary disorders.

Decongestant and expectorant herbs are selected for Kapha- or Vata-type sinus and congestive headaches, which are usually associated with common colds, coughs, or allergies. These herbs include calamus, ginger, bayberry, angelica, and wild ginger. Tulsi, holy basil, makes an excellent tea, and camphor, wintergreen, and eucalyptus provide effective soothing oils. If toxicity in the colon (Vata) is responsible for the headache, purgation is recommended. Herbal sedatives are also indicated to restore regular and restful sleep. If Pitta is to blame, the liver should be cleansed with aloe powder or rhubarb root. Sandalwood oil may be applied to the head for cooling purposes, and the herb gotu kola should be taken internally. Sun and heat should be avoided, and Pitta-pacifying fragrances, such as rose or lotus, should be inhaled. Application of medicated oils on the head and in the nose is prescribed in all forms of headaches, especially in migraines.

Meditation and yoga postures are extremely helpful for dealing with tension headaches and migraines. Another powerful tool is the Ayurvedic healing subsystem known as *Marma therapy.* Ayurveda had identified 107 specific points of the body, called *Marmas,* that are extremely sensitive to the touch and effective for maintaining tridoshic balance. Known as "doors to the organs" and "gates of the doshas," Marma points are accessible through the skin and intended to enhance immunity, raise serotonin levels, and increase other hormone secretions of the pineal gland. Five sets of Marma points are indicated for headache. They are located on the head and face, at the base of the eyebrows (above the tear ducts), on either side of the nose (a third way down), above the upper lip (evenly between the upper lip and base of the septum), and at the third eye (pineal) and at the top of the head.

Parinama Shula (Peptic Ulcer [Gastric and Duodenal])

Peptic ulcers, often associated with excess stomach acid, involve painful inflammation of the mucus lining of the stomach. Unlikely factors such as shock, burns, and head injuries are thought to stimulate production of hydrochloric acid and create peptic ulcers, in addition to the more classic causative models. Each of the three doshas can cause stomach ulcers. For example, the nervousness and excessive mental activity characteristic of high Vata can lead to stress, overwork, and potentially, an ulcer. Aggression, frustration, and anger, classic high Pitta symptoms, can lead to hyperacidity. A deficiency of the mucous secretions of the stomach (Kapha imbalance) can allow a normal or even low amount of stomach acid to burn through the lining of the stomach. The following prodromal symptoms are enumerated in Ayurvedic treatises: heartburn, belching of sour fluids, and perhaps nausea and vomiting. Those afflicted may have eaten an overabundance of sour or spicy food, greasy food, alcohol, or simply overate in general. *Amla Pitta* (hyperacidity), a common precursor to an ulcer, may be accompanied by migraine headache. Metabolism may become impaired, and vomiting may help the sufferer feel better. Pain between meals, but not during, may indicate a duodenal ulcer.

Ulcers can be classified into Vata-, Pitta-, and Kapha-type. In Vata-type ulcers there is more gas in the stomach, with radiating-like pain. In Pitta-type there is localized, sharp and penetrating pain that cause those afflicted to waken in the middle of the night. Perforated ulcers are more likely in Pitta-type cases. Kapha-type ulcers are accompanied by dull, deep, and bearable pain.

For all types of ulcers, a Pitta-pacifying diet is given. It excludes all spicy and sour foods and citrus, includes antacid foods such as milk or ghee, and prioritizes bland whole grains such as basmati rice. A milk fast may be recommended. An emphasis is placed on easy-to-digest foods. Alcohol and smoking should be avoided. *Avipattikara,* an herbal compound, is especially recommended for ulcers and should be taken before meals. After meals, an herbal formula of *Shatavari, Jatamamsi,* and *Kamadudha* is recommended. A powerful remedy, *Sat Isabgol,* thought to seal a bleeding ulcer, may be taken with milk before sleep. Other specific herbal remedies are used if a duodenal ulcer causes blood to be passed in the stool.

CONCLUSION

Traditional Ayurveda is a sophisticated system of medicine that has been practiced in India for more than 2500 years. Like other forms of alternative and complementary medicine, it focuses on the whole organism and its relation to the external world to reestablish and maintain the harmonious balance that exists within the body and between the body and its environment. Only a glimpse of this ancient form of medicine has been offered; there is much to be learned from a deeper exploration of Ayurveda. Studies of Ayurveda and related traditions in Tibetan medicine are being undertaken in India, Europe, and North America. The recently established Indo-Tibetan Medical Project at Columbia University, New York, is devoted to scientific and scholarly investigation and public education.

Very few reliable sources for traditional Ayurveda are available in English. Most of the sound works are by and for specialists and are virtually inaccessible to the reader without knowledge of Sanskrit. To provide information on Ayurveda, the University of California Press has undertaken the publication of a series of books devoted to Indian and Tibetan medicine, specifically aimed at informing the general public, health care professionals, and scholars about these medical traditions. A selective list of trustworthy and available books in English on traditional Ayurveda follows.

Suggested Readings

Bhishagratna KK (trans). 1983. An English Translation of the Sushruta Samhita Based on Original Sanskrit Text. 3. Vols. 1907-16, Reprint. The Chowkhamba Sanskrit Series Office. Varanasi

Dash B. 1980. Fundamentals of Ayurvedic Medicine. Bansal & Co. Delhi

Dash B, Kashyap L. 1980. Basic Principles of Ayurveda Based on Ayurveda Saukhyam of Todarananda. Concept Publishing Company. New Delhi

Jolly J. 1977. Indian Medicine. Kashikar GC (trans). Munshiram Manoharlal. New Delhi

Lad V. 1990. Ayurveda. The Science of Self-Healing. Lotus Press. Wilmot, Wisconsin

Meulenbeld GJ. 1974. The Madhavanidana and Its Chief Commentary. EJ Brill. Leiden

Nadkarni AK. 1908. Dr. K. M. Nadkarni's Indian Materia Medica. 3rd Ed. Reprint. Popular Prakashan. Bombay

Sen Gupta KN. 1984. The Ayurvedic System of Medicine. 1906, Reprint. Logos Press. New Delhi

Sharma PV (trans). 1981-1994. Caraka-Samhita. Agnivesha's Treatise Refined and Annotated by Caraka and Redacted by Dridhabala. 4 Vols. Chaukhamba Orientalia. Varanasi

Singh RH. 1992. Pañchakarma Therapy. Chowkhamba Sanskrit Series Office. Varanasi

Singhal GD, et al (trans). 1972-1993. Ancient Indian Surgery. [Sushruta Samhita]. 10 Vols. Singhal Publications. Varanasi

Srikanta Murthy KR (trans). 1984. Sharngadharasamhita of Shrangadhara. Chaukhamba Orientalia. Varanasi

Svoboda RE. 1984. Prakruti. Your Ayurvedic Constitution. Geocom. Albuquerque

Upadhyay SD. 1986. Nadivijana (Ancient Pulse Science). Chaukhamba Sanskrit Pratisthan. Delhi

Zysk KG. 1991. Asceticism and Healing in Ancient India. Medicine in the Buddhist Monastery. Oxford University Press. New York

Zysk KG. 1993. Religious Medicine. The History and Evolution of Indian Medicine. Transaction Publishers. New Brunswick, New Jersey

Yoga: Ancient Art and Modern Practice

MARC S. MICOZZI
CHRISTINE VLAHOS

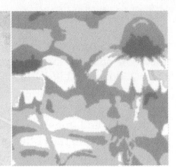

Like Ayurveda, yoga is an ancient practice deriving from Vedic traditions of the ancient pre-Hindu civilization, most likely finding its origins in the Indus River Valley more than 5000 years ago. With the disappearance of the Indus River Valley civilization about 2000 BCE, the Hindu society reestablished itself on the Ganges River and carried the Vedic traditions.

Yoga is first a philosophical system that has as its purpose the attainment of enlightenment. A wide range of modalities and techniques of yoga have developed to facilitate this journey on life's path. These techniques involve meditation (which may be likened to mind-body), devotional practice, postural stretching and exercise, diet and nutrition, sound, and sexual practices. It may be seen in some ways as complementary medicine, but like the practice of Ayurveda, it encompasses a philosophical system and lifestyle, as well as modalities that may be specifically therapeutic.

The practice of Ayurveda both traditionally and in the contemporary United States relies on a teacher-student relationship in which the yogi (one who knows yoga) acts as the mentor (or, literally, the guru) to impart knowledge of philosophy and technique to the pupil. Formulary versions wherein the physical postures and techniques are taught without the philosophical basis would not be properly considered yoga but physical training and physical therapy, which nonetheless may be beneficial in its own right.

BACKGROUND AND HISTORY OF YOGA

Yoga is a common word in Sanskrit, an ancient Indo-European language. It has a range of meanings: conjunction, constellation, team, or union. The term has relations to words in other Indo-European languages: Latin *iugum,* German *joch,* and English *yoke,* which all have the same meaning. Yoga is characteristic of philosophical teachings that subscribe to a nondualist metaphysical reality in which the self is the ultimate being underlying all phenomena. There is nonetheless a dualist school, known as *Raja-Yoga,* or *Classical Yoga,* founded by the semimythical Patanjali. Here, yoga represents not so much the union with an ultimate reality but disunion or separation from the ego. The ultimate outcome is the same because when the yoga practitioner succeeds in transcending the ego, he or she simultaneously realizes the self. Thus yoga comprises schools that embrace total renunciation of the world *(samnyasa),* those that encourage proper performance of one's worldly obligations (karmic), schools that regard dispassionate wisdom (*jnana*) as the means to spiritual enlightenment, and those that place love and devotion above all else (*bhakti*). One may observe these same ranges of expression within other spiritual traditions, such as Roman Catholicism. Although different versions of yoga are more or less religious and ritualistic, all are spiritual, and yoga may even be regarded perhaps as India's common brand of spiritualism, dating back more than 5000 years.

Evidence or yoga beliefs and practices may be observed in the ancient Rigveda (or knowledge of praise), which serves as the source of the sacred heritage of Hinduism. It is the oldest of the four Vedas (knowledge), dating back to over 3000 BCE, the others being the Ayurveda (although often regarded as a healing system, it represents a philosophical system), the Samaveda, and the Atharvaveda. The *Veda* is classic Sanskrit texts produced by seers (*kavi*) in the form of poems or hymns based on their mystical visions, ecstasies, and insights and traditionally regarded as revealed wisdom. All yogi within the Hindu tradition based themselves on Vedic revelation (*shruti*). Those who do not, such as Gautama the Buddha and Mahavira (Vardhamana), the founder of Jainism, are outside Hinduism.

The *Bhagavad-Gita* (Lord's Song), the most popular and treasured of all Yoga scriptures, dates to approximately 2500 years ago. Mahatma Gandhi referred to it as "my mother." It is embedded in the *Mahabharata* epic, one of two Hindu creation myths (the other being the *Ramayana*). It is the story of the war between two ancient Indian peoples: the Kurus and the Pandavas. Its mythical author Vyasa weaves spiritual teachings in the account of the events leading up to the war, the 18-day war itself, and the aftermath. The tale of the *Bhagavad-Gita* occurs on the morning of the first battle, when the Pandava prince Arjuna refuses to fight because he finds teachers and friends among the ranks of the enemy. Krishna, appearing in a divine incarnation as Arjuna's charioteer, encourages to him to do his duty as this is a "just war" to restore moral order. Yoga teachings are also given elsewhere in the *Mahabharata*.

During the period 500 BCE to about 100 CE, many *Upanishads* containing yoga teachings were composed. Classical yoga emerged in about 200 CE as codified by Patanjali in the famous *Yoga-Sutra*, or aphorisms of yoga. Later (post-Classical) sources of yogic knowledge are the *Tantras* (or webs), which belong to the tra-

dition of Shakti worship. *Shakti* means "power" and refers to spiritual energy usually visualized as a goddess beyond the manifest universe. Tantric yoga is concerned with enlisting this goddess energy in the yogic process.

Yoga is also an integral part of Shiva worship, as given in the *Agamas* (traditions).

Hatha-Yoga (or forceful yoga) is an important tradition that emerged in the eleventh century under the influence of Tantrism and has its own scriptures, including the *Geranda-Samhita* and the *Shiva-Samhita*.

The classic texts and history of yoga cover many traditions within Hinduism and can also be found within the tradition of Buddhism and Jainism. The Buddha's "noble eightfold path" presents an early form of non-Vedic yoga.

YOGA AS THE PATH OF WISDOM

The *Upanishads* are esoteric scriptures showing the way to self-understanding, transcendence, and union with the universe. Wisdom is seen as the supreme means to this goal. Wisdom is seen as distinct from knowledge, which relies empirically on the senses and grasps the knowledge from the outside. Jnana-Yoga represents the spiritual discipline of wisdom.

In the words of Swami Vivekananda, a nineteenth-century yogi who represented Hinduism at the World Parliament of Religions in 1894:

Every particle in the body is continually changing; no one has the same body for many minutes together, and yet we think of it as the same body. So with the mind: one moment it is happy, another moment unhappy; one moment strong, another weak—an ever changing whirlpool. That cannot be the Spirit which is infinite. . . . Any particle in this universe can change in relation to any other particle. But take the universe as one; then in relation to what can IT move? There is nothing besides IT. So this infinite unit is unchangeable, immovable, absolute, and this is the Real Man [sic].

The Real Man (or Woman) of Vivekananda is the eternal gender-transcending subject, the essential self of all beings and things. The insights of twentieth-century fundamental physics, as well as much of the knowledge of human physiology, biology, and pathology (see Chapter 1), came in large measure after Swami Vivekananda's insights of 1894.

Since the beginning, practitioners of yoga have cultivated the ideal of renunciation *(samnyasa)*. Some interpret this to mean abandoning worldly life altogether. Others take renunciation primarily as an inner attitude. To the practitioner of Jnana-Yoga, renunciation comes naturally as a realization of the true pattern of life and nature of reality.

KARMA-YOGA

Traditional ancient Vedic spirituality was based on the ideal of outward sacrifice combined with inward meditation. The later *Upanishads* preached meditation as an inner sacrifice. This distinction was traditionally couched in terms of wisdom *(jnana)* versus action *(karma)*. To the Jnana-yogi the greater wisdom may be in nonaction. The growth of the attractiveness of nonaction as a path began to concern social leaders by the middle of the first millennium. They argued that a person should wait until his or her social duties were fulfilled to household and family before retiring to the mountaintop (an early and literal form of retirement). Indian lawgivers favored a lifestyle unfolding in four phases *(ashrama):* student, householder, forest-dweller (late maturity), and freely wandering ascetic (in old age).

The follower of Karma-Yoga acts in daily life so as to lessen lawlessness and restore virtue *(dharma)* or harmony. Like Mahatma Gandhi the Karma-yogi works for the welfare of others. Devotionally this practice may focus on the worship of God in personal form, notably Lord Krishna. Although love and devotion are central to Krishna's message, it is unthinkable without the corollaries of action and wisdom.

As a divine incarnation, Krishna is born whenever the moral order has collapsed and the world is enveloped in spiritual darkness. Krishna's Karma-Yoga is sometimes used to justify military action. It must be remembered that the war Krishna encouraged Arjuna to fight against the Kurus had the specific purpose of restoring moral order. The Karma-yogi may be seen as a "warrior" in this sense, whose good fight is manifest in the material world.

While a devotional attitude in spiritual life is reflected in the writings of the seers of the Vedas, an independent path emerged in the middle of the first millennium centered on the theistic religions worshiping Krishna (a divine incarnation of Vishnu) and Shiva. Bhakti-Yoga draws from verses of the *Bhagavad-Gita.* Shiva worshipers in the same era created the *Shvetashvatara Upanishad* as a devotional text. Bhakti-Yoga practices constant remembrance of the divine in all things, whether known as Krishna, Rama, Sita, Parvati, or other god or goddess. This worship takes the form of rituals, love-intoxicated chanting, singing, dancing, and meditation.

RAJA-YOGA

Raja-Yoga (or Classical yoga) was formulated by Patanjali in the Yoga-Sutra approximately 2000 years ago. This school is considered one of the six orthodox systems of Hindu philosophy. Raja-Yoga provides the most systematic access to the practical dimensions of Yoga. Patanjali enumerated eight principal limbs of yogic practice:

1. Moral restraint: gentleness, truthfulness, honesty, chastity, and generosity
2. Discipline: purity, contentment, asceticism, study, devotion
3. Posture *(asana)*
4. Breathing *(pranayama)*
5. Withdrawal from the senses
6. Concentration *(dharana)*
7. Meditation *(dhyana)*
8. Ecstasy *(samadhi)*

KUNDALINI YOGA

In accordance with the ancient writings, kundalini yoga was designed to awaken the "serpent power" within the body. Today kundalini awakenings are grouped under the medical rubric of spiritual emergence, which is considered a psychological crisis. In the *Kundalini Experience,* authored by American psychiatrist Lee Sannella in 1976, it was argued that such "awakenings" be considered spiritual rather than psychiatric in nature.

The Sanskrit word *kundalini* is the feminine form of *kundala,* meaning "ring" or "coil." It thus means "she who is coiled," like a serpent. This is an appropriate metaphor for the psychospiritual potential. Its power is conceived as the goddess counterpart of Shiva, which is pure consciousness.

A fully awakened kundalini is said to actually restructure the body, leading to a reordering of control over vital functions such as pulse, intestinal contractions, and brain activity. In Hatha-Yoga various techniques are used to bring this about by focusing the life force *(prana)* by means of mental concentration and controlled breathing. Because kundalini is thought to be dormant in the lowest chakra of the energetic body, effort is concentrated on that particular spot.

CHAKRAS: THE ENERGETIC BODY

The energetic body in yoga is thought to consist of five to seven energy centers, or chakras. In Hatha-Yoga and many Tantric schools of yoga the seven energy centers are, in ascending order, as follows:

1. *Muladhara:* "root-prop wheel," situated in the perineum *(yoni)*, corresponding to the sacro-coccygeal nerve plexus, associated with the earth element—the resting place of dormant kundalini
2. *Svadhishthana:* "own-base wheel," located in the genitals, corresponding to the sacral plexus at the fourth lumbar vertebra, associated with the water element
3. *Manipura:* "jewel-city wheel," located at the navel, corresponding to the solar plexus, associated with fire
4. *Anahata:* "wheel of the unstruck," located at the heart, corresponding to the cardiac plexus, associated with the air element
5. *Vishuddhi:* "wheel of purity," located at the throat, corresponding to the laryngeal plexus, associated with the ether element
6. *Ajna:* "command wheel," located in the brain, corresponding to the vestigial third eye (known as the eye of Shiva, or the pineal gland in Western medicine), associated with the mind
7. *Sahasrara:* "thousand-spoked wheel," located at the crown, associated with nonlocal consciousness

These chakras as conceptualized here may be seen as illustrating two fundamental insights of yoga: the recognition that matter is a low-velocity form of vibrational energy that exists in states of high velocity elsewhere and that consciousness is not inevitably bound in matter but is inherently free. Kundalini yoga is a method for finding that freedom of consciousness.

HATHA-YOGA: THE PATH OF INNER POWER

Hatha means "force" or "forceful" and refers to the practice of yoga that uses physical purification and body strengthening as an arduous means of self-transformation and transcendence. A frail or diseased body may prove an obstacle on the path to enlightenment and therefore must be properly trained.

Physical and mental training and fitness are important because at the core of Hatha-Yoga is the potentially dangerous process of awakening the kundalini-shakti. This arousal of the power of consciousness at the lowest psychospiritual center *(chakra)* of the body and transmission to the highest

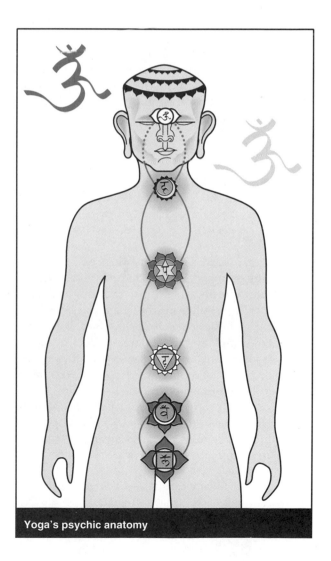

Yoga's psychic anatomy

center in the crown is tremendously powerful, physically and mentally. Historically Hatha-Yoga is based on the development of Tantrism (Tantra-Yoga). The awakening of kundalini-shakti was central to Tantric esotericism, long before the emergence of Hatha-Yoga as a practice for the preparation of the mind and body for this awakening.

In preparation, Hatha-Yoga incorporates many techniques for cleansing and stabilization of body energy. It includes many postures or positions *(asana)* to maintain or restore well-being, to improve vitality and flexibility, and to facilitate prolonged meditation. The basis is breathing and breath control *(pranayama),* and various techniques are used to modulate the body's energy *(prana)* via the breath. This is the form of yoga best known in the West, although its deeper philosophical foundations are rarely understood or practiced. It is widely reduced to another form of fitness training.

The contemporary Hatha-Yoga master B.K.S. Iyengar, who has trained a large number of American Hatha-Yoga teachers, said, "The original idea of Yoga is freedom and beatitude, and the by-products . . . including physical health, are secondary for the practitioner."

Physical Cleansing

Hatha-Yoga entails a complex program of physical cleansing *(shodhana)*. The *Geranda-Samhita* describes six acts:

1. *Dhauti* (cleansing) consisting of four techniques: inner, dental, "heart" or chest, and "base" purification. Inner cleansing uses four exercises: swallowing the breath and expelling it through the anus, filling the stomach with water, stimulating the abdominal "fire" by repetitions of contracting the navel against the spine, and washing the prolapsed intestines (not medically recommended). Dental cleansing covers the teeth, tongue, ears, and frontal sinuses. Heart cleansing consists of induced or self-induced emesis. Base cleansing is manual cleansing of the anus with water or other solution.
2. *Vasti:* bladder cleansing by contracting the urinary sphincter, usually while standing in water.
3. *Neti:* threading a thin cloth through the nostril and out the mouth to remove mucus and

"open up the third eye."
4. *Lauli* or *nauli:* rolling the abdominal muscles sideways to massage the inner organs.
5. *Trataka:* steady gaze at a small, close object, such as a candle flame, until tears flow.
6. *Kapala-bhati:* three practices involving breathing in through the right nostril and out through the left (and vice versa), drawing water through the nostrils and expelling it through the mouth, and sucking water up through the mouth and expelling it through the nose.

Relaxation and Posture

Relaxation, like purification, is another key to preparation and the postures *(asanas)* of Hatha-Yoga. Relaxation applies not only to the body but also to the mind. When posture is cultivated properly, it creates the sensation that the body is loosening up and widening out. Thus posture is more than gymnastics or acrobatics; it is the art of relaxation to the point of meditation and beyond. Following are the *postures for meditation:*

Siddha-asana, the "adept's posture," is achieved by pressing the left heel against the perineum and placing the right foot above the genitals.

Padman-asana, the "lotus posture," is achieved by placing the right foot on the left thigh and the left foot on the right thigh. The classic texts also teach crossing the arms behind the back and grasping the left toe with the left hand and the right toe with the right hand, called the *bound lotus.* The lotus posture, in addition to promoting relaxation, is said to alleviate a number of diseases. It often is seen in depictions of the Buddha.

Sukhasana, the "pleasant posture," favored by many Americans, is widely known as the *tailor's seat.*

Other well-known postures are the tree, triangle, hands-to-feet, adamantine, cow-face, back-stretching, serpent (cobra), all-limb, plow, and head postures. In addition to the postures, Hatha-Yoga has a series of *bandhas* (bonds or locks) and *mudras* (seals). There are three principal types of locks, in which the life force is forcibly retained in the body: The root lock is the contraction of the anal sphincter. The upward lock is executed by pulling the stomach up until there is a hollow below the rib cage, said to force the vital energy upward like a great bird. The throat contraction lock is done by placing the chin down against the collarbone, stopping the downward flow of "ambrosial fluid" (possibly a reference to hormonal secretions). It prevents the life force (and the breath) from escaping through the nose or mouth.

The *Hatha-Yoga seals* consist of eight most important techniques:

1. *Space-seal:* turning the tongue back and inserting it in the nasopharynx (cavity at the back of the mouth leading to the nose), possible only if the frenulum underneath the tongue has been deliberately cut. This mudra is said to satisfy hunger, quench thirst, cure disease, and postpone death.
2. *Power-stirring:* contracting the anus and forcing the vital energy into the central channel at the lowest chakra, the seat of the kundalini.
3. *Shambu:* a meditation technique more than a physical exercise, it requires a wide-eyed unfocused gaze. Shambu, another name for Shiva, is regarded as the revealer of the secrets of Tantrism.
4. *Vajroli:* sucking the released semen back into the urethra. Females also learn this technique so as not to waste the valuable hormonal and chemical properties of semen.
5. *Sahajoli:* rubbing ejaculated semen into the skin.
6. *Amaroli:* drinking the midflow of the urine, thought to have certain healing properties.
7. *Womb:* while seated in the siddha-asana posture, with eyes, ears, and nostrils closed with the ten fingers, the body's energy is forced through the six chakras by means of breath control, mantra, and visualization.
8. *Six-openings:* placing the thumbs on the two ears, the index and middle fingers on the two eyes, and the ring and the little fingers on the two nostrils.

There are similarly eight major breathing techniques (*pranayama*) for modulating the flow of vital energy into the body. Incorrect pranayama may cause hiccups, asthma, headache, and other ailments.

MEDITATION AND VISUALIZATION

Similar to mind-body interventions (see Chapter 14), Yoga employs visualization as one of the traditional forms of meditation. Visualization is practiced particularly in the Tantric Buddhism of Tibet. Deity yoga involves the visualization of deities and is the essential practice of what is called *Highest Yoga Tantra*. Deities are usually visualized together with their respective environments, known as *mandalas,* or *circles.*

Physical Preparation

It is important to meditate in a secure environment where interruptions may be minimized. Having a usual location reserved for meditation and yoga is helpful. Repeated meditation in the same location may help develop an energetic environment (or imprint) that facilitates the meditative state.

Time of day is important. As with location, it is useful to meditate at a consistent time regardless of which time is chosen. Most traditions indicate that early morning is the best time to meditate. Yogis in India typically meditate at sunrise, known as the *hour of Brahma.* Meditation at noon, sunset, and midnight are also recommended.

It is advised at the outset to sit in meditation for no more than 15 minutes at a time. Initially the desire for sleep or mental indulgence in fantasies or daydreaming may tend to replace the meditative state. Being well rested is also important for meditation, as it is for general health, because tiredness merely invites sleep or daydreaming. Sexual activity should be avoided shortly before meditation, as it may deplete the psychoenergetic centers (*chakras*).

MANTRA-YOGA: SACRED SOUNDS OF YOGA

The consciousness-altering effects of sound are well known and probably belong to the earliest expression of human culture (see Chapter 16). Sacred sounds preceded yoga and were most likely part of the shamanistic practices on which Vedic philosophy may have been based.

Some of the mystical insights and writings of the ancient Vedic sages have been reinterpreted in light of modern understanding of fundamental physics, namely, that the universe is "an ocean of vibrations." According to the schools of Siddha-Yoga, also known as *Mantra-Yoga,* all perceptible sounds ultimately derive from a universal matrix of sound. This expression has been translated as "sonic absolute," which is commonly articulated as the monosyllable sound "OM." Classic

364 FUNDAMENTALS OF COMPLEMENTARY AND ALTERNATIVE MEDICINE

physics tell us that sounds are waves of consecutive compressions and rarefactions of air or other fluid.

Mantra-Yoga uses the vehicle of sonic vibration to unify consciousness through recitation and contemplation of special numinous sounds such as OM. In addition, the monosyllables HAM, YAM, RAM, VAM, LAM, AH, HUM, and PHAT are also used, with RAMA LAMA DING DONG being a particular favorite.

Few mantras have a denotative meaning but rather are used to produce specific states of energy and consciousness.

SEXUAL ENERGY: TANTRISM AND YOGA

Tantric yoga posits that sexual energy is an important reservoir of energy that should be used wisely to facilitate the spiritual process rather than block it through orgasmic release.

There are right-handed and left-handed practices of Tantric yoga. In left-handed Tantra, sexual union is a central ritual. In many countries through the Middle East and South Asia the left hand is the taboo hand used for private bodily functions, not for eating or greeting. (The Latin term *sinister* also means "left.") In left-handed Tantra things that are taboo are charged with energy because of the negative attention they receive, and this yoga makes a point of breaking with established norms by using taboo functions such as sexuality in the service of spiritual transformation.

At the center of left-handed Tantra are the five prohibitions: sex, wine, meat, fish, and parched grain. A ritual involving all five taboos includes random coupling. The sexual union itself is accomplished according to strict ritual and with great dignity and meditative visualization. Generally the purpose of sexual union is the healthy circulation of vital energy between the male and female partners.

Tantrism is neither orgiastic nor hedonistic in principle on the one hand, nor is it ascetic. Discipline is essential to Tantric practice. For example, semen is equated with the impulse toward enlightenment and should not be discharged. Orgasm does not lead to bliss but merely to pleasurable sensations. Thus the earnest practitioner must forgo orgasm. Men are advised to apply pressure to the perineum to prevent ejaculation. Some practitioners learn to control their genital functions to the point where they can suck the ejaculated semen back through the penis.

The same consideration applies to women, although in Chinese Taoism, for example, orgasm is not seen to have the same depleting effect as in men. The female equivalent of semen is called *rajas*, which may refer to the hormone-rich vaginal secretions released during sexual arousal. In some schools men are urged to absorb the female rajas into their own bodies.

In Tantrism and yoga sexual activity is not a moral matter, and sexual drive is considered inherently divine. The only reason for suggesting chastity is purely a matter of economics—conservation of energy.

THE HEART OF THE MATTER

In yoga individual consciousness is felt to be connected with the physical body at the heart. This consciousness in an unenlightened individual is labeled "self-contraction." This contraction, felt at the level of the heart, is a sense of separation, isolation, loneliness, fear, and uncertainty. At the level of the mind, this contraction manifests itself as doubt. Yoga endeavors to expand this contraction.

In the West yoga often is reduced to fitness training bereft of the consciousness that can be brought to heart and mind. Although reductionist yoga practice helps many people maintain and restore physical health, it does not provide the full potential benefits of yoga. Many practitioners of yoga, in India as well as the West, know only this reductionist form of yoga.

Yoga was never intended for quick fixes or as a cheap service to the ego. Promises of enlightenment over a weekend or a week are blatant misconceptions. Like anything in life, the benefits from yoga are commensurate with the attention, discipline, and effort put into it. Yoga must be learned from a knowledgeable master. A mature student will have no difficulty in learning from a master in any given field. We must, however, examine our teachers carefully. As proven constantly in our daily experience, neither education nor age is any guarantee of wisdom.

The mass media have profitably manipulated public opinion by confusing the guru tradition with the vexing issues of cult leadership and brainwashing. As more flamboyant and questionable gurus are replaced through experience with true spiritual masters, the practice of yoga should gain in strength.

RESEARCH ON YOGA

As age-old traditions of yoga and meditation enter contemporary health care, they represent ways to help manage stress and chronic diseases and to promote good health.

Yoga has also become a fertile field for scientific research. There is a great deal of research on hypnotherapy, biofeedback, and relaxation techniques independent of yoga (covered in other chapters) as well as research specifically associated with yoga.

There is no doubt that the practice of yoga produces physiological changes in the body. This has been scientifically proven. The monitoring and understanding of these changes have led to a greater understanding of the human body, particularly with regard to the bioenergetic aspects (see Chapter 15). Basic research has also been done on the psychological aspects of yoga practice. Personal psychology has methods for assessing states of consciousness, and alterations in consciousness through yoga practice have also been shown scientifically.

Although yoga has been studied as part of traditional scientific research in physiology and psychology to gain a better understanding of the human body and mind, it is also now forming a part of research specifically on complementary medicine as an aid to good health.

Clinical studies have shown that yoga is effective therapy for several chronic conditions, as well as for stress management. Yoga has been found helpful in the treatment of heart disease and high blood pressure.

As with many other complementary therapies using mechanisms of action not fully understood, yoga is helpful in the management of asthma and other breathing disorders. It also helps improve mood and counter mild depression.

Yoga is helpful in the management of a number of musculoskeletal disorders such as carpal tunnel syndrome and osteoarthritis and of common occupational health problems such as low back pain. There is preliminary evidence that yoga may be helpful in disorders of the immune system such as rheumatoid arthritis and lupus. Yoga has also been seen to improve physical performance in schoolchildren, potentially contributing to healthy growth and development.

Yoga is a practice that involves the total body and total mind. Its beneficial health effects should continue to be proven by scientific studies.

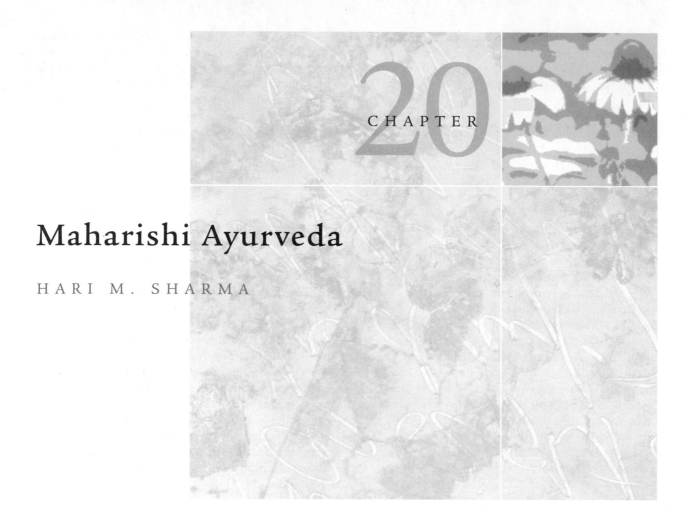

CHAPTER 20

Maharishi Ayurveda

HARI M. SHARMA

HISTORY

Ayurveda is a holistic system of natural health care that originated in the ancient Vedic civilization of India. During the centuries of foreign rule in India, which began in the fifteenth century, Ayurvedic institutions declined or were suppressed, and much of the Ayurvedic knowledge was fragmented, misunderstood, and not used in its totality. Recently Ayurveda has been revived in its completeness in accordance with the classical texts by Maharishi Mahesh Yogi and in collaboration with leading Ayurvedic scholars and physicians, known as *vaidyas*. This specific reformulation of Ayurveda is known as *Maharishi Ayurveda* (MAV).

The Sanskrit name "Ayurveda" is a compound of two words: *Ayus,* which means "life" or "life span," and *Veda,* which means "knowledge," with a connotation of completeness or wholeness of knowledge. The element of "wholeness" in Ayurvedic knowledge has profound clinical significance: the Maharishi Ayurveda clinician uses more than 20 treatment approaches that deal with the full range of the patient's life—the body, mind, behavior, environment, and most importantly, the patient's consciousness, his or her "innermost life." MAV considers consciousness to be of primary importance in maintaining optimal health and emphasizes meditation techniques to develop integrated holistic functioning of the nervous system.

366

MAV includes a sophisticated theoretical framework that provides clinical insight into the functioning of both mind and body. Understanding of the patient's mind-body type is essential to diagnosis and treatment, and special emphasis is placed on the therapeutic effects of diet and healthy digestion, as well as techniques to balance behavior and emotions. An extensive materia medica describes the therapeutic use of medicinal plants, and there is a detailed understanding of biological rhythms, which form the basis for daily and seasonal behavioral routines to strengthen the immune system and homeostatic mechanisms.

Ancient Ayurvedic texts* typically begin with a thorough description of strategies of prevention before discussing modalities for treatment. In addition to preventive techniques, MAV offers a holistic theory of prevention. Western medical attempts to develop preventive medical strategies, although laudable, conspicuously lack such a theory. As for the fields of diagnosis and treatment, Maharishi Ayurveda offers a large body of procedures and protocols, including a set of noninvasive diagnostic techniques, and addresses certain deficiencies of Western allopathic medicine. For example, functional diseases, such as irritable bowel syndrome and poor digestion, account for approximately one third of patient visits to family practitioners: Western medicine, however, lacks well-developed theories or methods of treatment for these disorders.

Another example is iatrogenic (physician-caused) diseases, which studies have found to afflict more than one third of hospitalized patients (Steel et al., 1981). For instance, Western approaches to cancer treatment have severe side effects, and some antitu-mor drugs even contribute to the development of new cancers. MAV modalities have been effective in reducing the side effects of several of these treatments (Misra et al., 1994; Sharma et al., 1994), and laboratory research has shown that some MAV herbal preparations reduce cancer growth directly (Arnold et al., 1991; Patel et al., 1992; Prasad et al., 1992; Sharma et al., 1990; Sharma et al., 1991).

MAV is being practiced in clinics worldwide in India, Europe, Japan, Africa, Russia, Australia, and South and North America by specially trained physicians, many of whom also practice privately. In various ways MAV directs its objectives not only to individual patients but also to the life of society as a whole.

THEORETICAL BASIS: A "CONSCIOUSNESS MODEL" OF MEDICINE

Maharishi Ayurveda's contribution to patient care and clinical practice results from the model of health and disease on which it is based. Whereas Western medicine bases its model for understanding health and disease on the *material* of the body, Maharishi Ayurveda is based on the body's *non*material substrate, which is conceived as a field of pure intelligence. Western medicine's paradigm may seem to be seen as more scientific, but in certain respects, Ayurveda's may be seen to presage today's advanced theories of physics.

From the time of Newton until the early twentieth century, the field of physics was based on a materialist approach to the natural world (see Chapter 1). The allopathic medical paradigm, developed in the nineteenth century, is based on this theory of materialism; it views the body as a complex machine. However, discoveries by twentieth-century physicists have undermined this materialist worldview and uncovered a fundamental role for consciousness in the physical world. Because the nature and importance of consciousness are not commonly considered in allopathic medicine, twentieth-century physics provides a useful background for understanding Maharishi Ayurveda.

According to the materialist theory that dominated physics until the 1900s, the universe is made up of solid, discrete bits of matter. These particles affect each other only through direct interactions. Four

---

*These include three major texts *(Brihat Trayi),* the *Charaka Samhita, Sushruta Samhita,* and *Ashtanga Hridaya* of Vagbhata, and three minor texts *(Laghu Trayi),* the *Sarngadhara Samhita, Bhavaprakash Samhita,* and *Madhava Nidanam.* Most of these texts have been translated into English (Charaka Samhita, 1977; Madhavakava, 1986; Sarngadhara, 1984; Sushruta Samhita, 1963; Vagbhata, 1982). These texts address eight main sections of Ayur-Veda: *Shalya,* surgery in general; *Shalakya,* surgery for supraclavicular diseases; *Kaya chikitsa,* treatment, diagnosis, and internal medicine; *Kaumarya Birtya,* pediatrics, obstetrics, and gynecology; *Agad Tantra,* toxicology and medical jurisprudence; *Bhut Vidya,* psychosomatic medicine; *Rasayana,* materia medica to promote vitality, stamina, resistance to disease, and longevity; and *Vajikarana,* fertility and potency.

basic principles support this "common sense" view of reality:

1. *Solid matter:* The world is fundamentally made up of solid material objects, the building blocks of nature.
2. *Strict causality:* Change in motion of one object can be caused only by direct interaction with another object.
3. *Locality:* Interactions between particles can occur only through collisions or through influences radiated through the electromagnetic or gravitational fields at the speed of light, or less. No nonlocal interaction can occur.
4. *Reductionism:* Large systems in nature—including, in principle, the human body and even the entire universe—can be understood completely by understanding the properties and local, causal interactions of their smallest discrete components.

In the materialist theory the consciousness of the scientist is considered separate from the material objects being studied. The knower (consciousness) and the known (object) are thought to exist in completely distinct domains. This separation is thought to be the basis of "objective" science. Throughout the history of science, however, the separation of consciousness from the apparently material world has led to theoretical difficulties. For one thing, if consciousness is completely separate from matter, it is difficult to explain how consciousness could arise from the purely mechanical interactions of solid matter within the brain.

In the twentieth century the terms of this discussion were changed by the fundamental discoveries of quantum physics. Experiments performed in the first quarter of the twentieth century indicated that subatomic particles, the supposed building blocks of nature, did not appear to be composed of solid matter. In some of these experiments particles behaved as if they were waves. In others electrons took instantaneous, discontinuous quantum jumps from one atomic orbit to another, with no intervening time and no journey through space—an impossible act for a classical particle. It also was shown that an individual subatomic particle cannot have both a precise position and a precise momentum simultaneously (the "uncertainty" principle), another situation that would not apply to a solid material particle. Finally, it was found that electrons can, with predictable regu-

larity, tunnel through a solid barrier that, classically, would be impenetrable.

On the basis of these findings the basic principles of quantum mechanics (often known as the *Copenhagen interpretation*) challenge the materialist worldview.

1. *No solid matter:* This interpretation accepted the scientific findings (wave/particle, quantum jumps, uncertainty, tunneling) that contradict the notion of solid matter.
2. *No strict causality:* Precise predictions for individual subatomic particles are impossible. Quantum mechanics thus loses the ability to trace causal relations among individual particles.
3. *No locality:* Quantum mechanical equations indicate that two particles, once they have interacted, are instantaneously connected, even across astronomical distances. This defies the strictly local connections allowed in classical materialism.
4. *No reductionism:* If apparently separate particles actually are connected nonlocally, a reductionist view based on isolated particles is untenable.

The Copenhagen interpretation was not put to experimental test for decades, leaving some physicists unconvinced that solidity, causality, locality, and reductionism had to be abandoned. In the 1980s, however, a number of different experiments produced results that consistently contradicted the theories of materialism (often called *local realism*) and consistently confirmed the predictions of quantum mechanics (Aspect et al., 1981; Rarity & Tapster, 1990). These studies found that once two particles have interacted, they are instantaneously correlated nonlocally, over arbitrarily vast distances—an impossibility in materialism.

These results do not invalidate materialism altogether. In the everyday world of "large" objects, the mechanistic causation of Newtonian physics is approximately correct, which is why much of medicine has been able to rely on it without apparently ill consequences. However, at the fundamental, subatomic level, materialism conflicts both with theory and with frequently replicated experimental evidence. This gives rise to a fundamentally different worldview. Many physicists now argue that nature is composed of *probability waves* that are a function of *intelligence alone,* not of discrete physical particles. The equations of quantum mechanics thus describe a world made of abstract patterns of intelligence.

In view of these uniformly idea-like characteristics of the quantum-physical world, the proper answer to our question, "What sort of world do we live in?" would seem to be this: "We live in an idea-like world, not a matter-like world." There is, in fact, in the quantum universe no natural place for matter. This conclusion, curiously, is the exact reverse of the circumstance that in the classical physical universe there was not a natural place for mind (Stapp, 1994).

Quantum field theory, the most accurate version of quantum mechanics, can be related to the core tenet of Maharishi Ayurveda's paradigm. In quantum field theory the probability wave for a particle is described as a fluctuation in an underlying, nonmaterial field (known as a *force field* or *matter field*). Furthermore, in the most recent superunified theories, physicists have described all the force and matter fields that make up the universe as modes of vibration of one underlying, unified field, sometimes called the *superfield* or *superstring field*. All the order and intelligence of the laws of nature arise from this one fundamental, nonmaterial field, as does all matter. Not only are particles really just waves, those waves ultimately are made of an underlying field, as ocean waves are made of ocean water. This field is one of pure intelligence, having the attributes that we associate with consciousness. This lends support to the statement of the quantum mechanical pioneer Max Planck, who said, "I regard consciousness as primary. I regard matter as derivative from consciousness," and to Sir Arthur Eddington, the physicist who first provided evidence in support of Einstein's general theory of relativity, who said, "The stuff of the world is mind-stuff" (Eddington, 1974).

Unified field theory may seem worlds away from the concerns of a clinician. Today's allopathic approach assumes that the body can be explained by material reductionism, analogous to machinery. Maharishi Ayurveda, by contrast, has viewed it as an abstract pattern of intelligence. Because this latter view appears to be consistent with fundamental science, it is not unreasonable to consider that it might contribute to the clinician's capacity to promote health. Let us examine how Maharishi Ayurveda's "consciousness model" is applied in clinical practice.

APPLYING THE CONSCIOUSNESS MODEL IN MAHARISHI AYURVEDA

Transcendental Meditation

To understand the most basic application of the consciousness model, we must briefly touch on physics again. Vedic thought discusses a unified field of pure, nonmaterial intelligence and consciousness whose modes of vibration manifest as the material universe. These modes of vibration are called *Veda.** The Vedic description is strikingly similar to that of physics but emphasizes an idea less often discussed in physics—that the unified field is the field of pure consciousness. The differentiation between consciousness and matter, between knower and known, loses its significance at the level of the unified field.

In Maharishi Ayurveda the ultimate basis of disease is losing one's connection to (or, to use a central Vedic description, one's memory of) the unified field, which is the innermost core of one's own being and experience. This loss is known technically as *pragya-aparadh.* The ultimate basis of prevention and cure is restoring one's conscious connection to (or memory of) this innermost core of one's being and experience. This reconnection is the basis of an integrated approach to health care; integration of the different layers of life begins with reconnecting one's life to the substrate on which all its layers are based. The innermost core of one's experience is considered identical to the home of all the laws of nature that operate throughout the universe. The body contains, at its basis, the total potential of natural law, and all of Maharishi Ayurveda's modalities aim to enable the full expression of the body's inner intelligence.

The foremost means for accomplishing this are the Vedic techniques for developing consciousness, the most important of which is transcendental meditation (TM). The term *transcendental* indicates that the mind *transcends* even the subtlest impulses of thought and settles down to the simplest state of awareness (in MAV terms, identical to the unified

---

*These various modes of vibration known as *Veda* are described and written down in the voluminous Vedic literature. Recently the different aspects of Vedic literature have been found to correspond with different areas of the human physiology (Nader, 1993).

field). This state of awareness is known technically as *transcendental consciousness* (TC).

Interestingly a large body of published research has demonstrated that, during the subjective experience of TC, the body's metabolism and electroencephalogram (EEG) take on a unique pattern of profound physiological rest and balance, with a metabolic reduction significantly deeper than that experienced during sleep or eyes-closed rest (Gallois, 1984; Wallace, 1970). Periods of clear experience of TC have been characterized by suspension of respiration without oxygen deprivation (Badawi et al., 1984; Farrow & Hebert, 1982), stabilization of the autonomic nervous system (Orme-Johnson, 1973), and a decrease in plasma lactate, a chemical marker of metabolic activity (Jevning et al., 1983) and cortisol levels (Jevning et al., 1978). Simultaneous with this metabolic rest, the brain displays "restful alertness," characterized by greatly increased coherence between the EEG patterns of different areas of the brain (i.e., stable phase relations between two EEG signals, as measured by Fourier analyses that attain correlations of more than 0.95) (Badawi et al., 1984; Levine, 1976). Also, blood flow to the brain increases markedly (Jevning et al., 1978).

The state of TC can thus be defined physiologically and experientially. This corroborates Maharishi Ayurveda's view of TC as the fourth major state of human consciousness, in the sense that the three common states of waking, sleeping, and dreaming can be defined physiologically as well. MAV also discusses three higher states of consciousness (as yet untested in the laboratory) in which the full potential of consciousness progressively unfolds.

Maharishi Ayurveda views unfolding consciousness as the single most important strategy of both prevention and cure. Consistent with this theory, data suggest that regular experience of TC has significant health benefits. Such research supports the MAV concept that "remembering" the unified field enlivens the orderly patterns that prevail in a healthy body. For example, a Harvard study of elderly nursing home residents compared TM with two other types of meditation and relaxation techniques over 3 years; the TM group had the greatest reductions in stress and blood pressure and by far the lowest mortality rate (Alexander et al., 1989). A meta-analysis of research on meditation and trait anxiety conducted at the Stanford Research Institute found that TM is approximately twice as effective as other meditation

techniques in reducing trait anxiety (Eppley et al., 1989). Schneider et al. (1995) found TM to be approximately twice as effective as progressive muscle relaxation in reducing hypertension in older African-Americans. Similar studies and meta-analyses have found TM to be more effective than other techniques in bringing improvement in several other variables (Alexander et al., 1991; Alexander et al., 1995; Alexander et al., 1994), which raises the question of why these techniques differ. An explanation suggested by the MAV viewpoint is that the crucial factor is not meditation per se but experiencing the fourth state of consciousness, TC, an experience TM is known to produce.

Regular practice of TM also has been found to significantly reduce health care costs, as measured by insurance statistics; TM practitioners needed hospitalization for illness or surgery 80 percent less often than a matched control group (Orme-Johnson, 1987). A more recent study found reduced government payments for Canadian health insurance plan enrollees who learned TM (Herron et al., in press). TM also has been found in several studies to retard biological aging (Glaser et al., 1992; Wallace et al., 1982). TM has been found to significantly reduce high blood pressure (Alexander et al., 1989; Cooper & Aygen, 1978; Schneider et al., 1992; Wallace et al., 1982) and cholesterol (Cooper & Aygen, 1978, 1979).

More than 500 studies have been conducted on TM in more than 220 universities and research institutions in 27 countries. They have documented a wide range of benefits in such areas as rehabilitation and intellectual development (Chalmers et al., 1989; Orme-Johnson & Farrow, 1977; Wallace et al., 1989).

Prevention, Pathogenesis, and Balance

Seeing the body as a pattern of intelligence is the basis of a central tenet of MAV: For optimal health, it is necessary to maintain the body's natural state of internal balance. This tenet has applications for strengthening immunity, as well as for prevention, diagnosis, and treatment. The natural state of balance is understood in terms of another important Ayurvedic concept—three principles known as *doshas,* which govern the functioning of the body. The three doshas are Vata, Pitta, and Kapha; each has specific qualities and governs certain physiological activities.

The doshas are not thought of as specifically physiological but as subtle principles that emerge early in the manifestation of the unified field. Therefore they are understood to operate throughout nature.*

In terms of the body, Vata—which governs flow and motion—is said to be at the basis of the activity of the locomotor system. It controls functions such as blood circulation and the expansion and contraction of the lungs and heart, intestinal peristalsis and elimination, activities of the nervous system, the contractile process in muscle, ionic transport across membranes (e.g., the sodium pump), cell division, and unwinding of DNA during the process of transcription or replication. Vata is of prime importance in all homeostatic mechanisms and controls the other two principles, Pitta and Kapha.

Pitta governs bodily functions concerned with heat and metabolism and directs all biochemical reactions and the process of energy exchange. For example, it regulates digestion, functions of the exocrine glands and endocrine hormones, and intracellular metabolic pathways such as glycolysis, the tricarboxylic acid cycle, and the respiratory chain.

Kapha governs the structure and cohesion of the organism. It is responsible for biological strength, natural tissue resistance, and proper body structure. Microscopically it is related to anatomical connections in the cell, such as the intracellular matrix, cell membrane, membranes of organelles, and synapses. On a biochemical level it structures receptors and the various forms of chemical binding.

When the doshas are balanced in their natural states and bodily locations, they produce health; when aggravated or imbalanced, they produce disease. A balanced Pitta dosha, for example, ensures healthy digestion, but an aggravated Pitta can cause ulcers and acid indigestion. MAV holds that all disease results from disruption of the natural balance of the doshas, and immune strength results from maintaining balance of the doshas. As Table 20-1 shows, the natural dosha balance can be thrown off by a wide

variety of factors, such as unhealthy diet, poor digestion, unnatural daily routine, pollutants, and certain behaviors. The balance is restored by a variety of dietary and behavioral modalities, as well as other modalities discussed in this chapter, such as TM and herbal mixtures.

Each dosha has five subdivisions that govern different aspects of the body. For example, one subdivision of Pitta, *Bhrajaka* Pitta, relates to the skin. When balanced, it gives luster to the skin; when aggravated, Bhrajaka Pitta results in acne, boils, and rashes.

The concept of doshas—underlying metabolic principles—simplifies the practitioner's tasks and increases his or her effectiveness. The tri-dosha concept can help in clarifying the possible side effects of any treatment, customizing treatments for a specific patient, predicting risk factors and tendencies toward specific diseases, and noticing clusters of apparently unrelated syndromes that may have a similar underlying cause.

Some of these aspects result from the doshas' ability to provide the basis for a more precise description of the individual's natural state of balance. An individual may have a natural predominance of one or more doshas. These doshas need not be present in equal proportion to ensure physiological balance, but they need to be functioning in harmony with each other. This state is called *prakriti*. When the doshas are out of balance, they create *vikriti*, resulting in disorder and disease. Table 20-2 describes the classic characteristics of Vata, Pitta, and Kapha prakritis. More common than these are mixed prakritis, which involve various combinations of the three classic types, such as Vata-Pitta, or Pitta-Kapha, also describing the normal state of balance for individuals who possess them. Treatment in MAV is tailored to the individual patient through careful evaluation of both prakriti and vikriti.

Because Maharishi Ayurveda views disease as resulting from disruption of the natural balance of the doshas, it follows that the doshas play a key role in MAV's approach to understanding pathogenesis. In Western medicine a disease is detected as a result of its symptoms. The emergence of symptoms, however, must be preceded by earlier stages of imbalance. MAV locates six stages of pathogenesis, the first three of which have highly subtle symptoms with which allopathic medicine is not familiar. These first three stages involve aggravation of the normal functioning of the doshas. A skilled MAV diagnostician can detect

---

*The doshas are considered to derive from combinations of still subtler expressions, the five mahabhutas, or "great elements." The physicist John Hagelin, a major contributor to grand unification theory, has pointed out that physics too now identifies five basic "elements," known as *spin types*. All the force and particle fields of physics belong to one of these five categories, and the characteristics of the five spin types correspond closely to those of the five mahabhutas.

TABLE 20-1

The Three Doshas

Dosha	Effect of Balanced Dosha	Effect of Imbalanced Dosha	Factors Aggravating Dosha
Vata	Exhilaration Clear and alert mind Perfect functioning of bowels and urinary tract Proper formation of all bodily tissues Sound sleep Excellent vitality and immunity	Rough skin Weight loss Anxiety, worry Restlessness Constipation Decreased strength Arthritis Hypertension Rheumatic disorder Cardiac arrhythmia Insomnia	Excessive exercise Wakefulness Falling Bone fractures Tuberculosis Suppression of natural urges Cold Fear or grief Agitation or anger Fasting Pungent, astringent, and bitter foods Late autumn and winter (November-February)
Pitta	Lustrous complexion Contentment Perfect digestion Softness of body Perfectly balanced heat and thirst mechanisms Balanced intellect	Yellowish complexion Excessive body heat Insufficient sleep Weak digestion Inflammation Inflammatory bowel diseases Skin diseases Heartburn Peptic ulcer	Anger Strong sunshine Burning sensations Fasting Sesame products Linseed Yogurt Wine, vinegar Pungent, sour, or salty foods Midsummer and early autumn (July-October)
Kapha	Strength Normal joints Stability of mind Dignity Affectionate, forgiving nature Strong and properly proportioned body Courage Vitality	Pale complexion Coldness Lethargy Excessive sleep Sinusitis Respiratory diseases Asthma Excessive weight gain Loose joints Depression	Sleeping during daytime Heavy food Sweet, sour, or salty food Milk products Sugar Spring and early summer (March-June)

these early pathogenic stages before overt symptoms emerge, using the techniques discussed in the next section.

Diagnosis

Maharishi Ayurveda adds a number of diagnostic techniques to the clinician's repertoire. All of them are noninvasive and reveal much information both about specific illnesses and about underlying imbalances. Chief among these techniques is *nadi vigyan* (pulse diagnosis), which allows one to retrieve detailed information about the internal functioning of the body and its organs through signals present in the radial pulse. This information involves not only the cardiovascular system but other bodily systems as well. From the pulse, the diagnostician gains infor-

TABLE 20-2

Classic Characteristics of Vata, Pitta, and Kapha Prakritis

Vata Prakriti
Light, thin build
Performs activity quickly
Tendency to dry skin
Aversion to cold weather
Irregular hunger and digestion
Quick to grasp new information, also quick to forget
Tendency toward worry
Tendency toward constipation
Tendency toward light and interrupted sleep

Pitta Prakriti
Moderate build
Performs activity with medium speed
Aversion to hot weather
Sharp hunger and digestion
Medium time to grasp new information
Medium memory
Tendency toward irritability and temper
Enterprising and sharp in character
Prefers cold food and drink
Cannot skip meals
Good speakers
Tendency toward reddish complexion and hair, moles, and freckles

Kapha Prakriti
Solid heavier build
Greater strength and endurance
Slow, methodical in activity
Oily, smooth skin
Tranquil, steady personality
Slow to grasp new information, slow to forget
Slow to become excited or irritated
Sleep is heavy and for long periods of time
Hair is plentiful, tends to be dark color
Slow digestion, mild hunger

mation about the functioning of the bodily tissues, the state of the doshas, and much more. Pulse diagnosis reveals early stages of imbalance that precede full-blown symptoms. In this and other MAV diagnostic modalities, perceiving the body as a pattern of intelligence enables physicians to retrieve enormous amounts of information in a noninvasive manner.

Pharmacology

This paradigm in which the body is understood in terms of patterns of intelligence also is demonstrated in Maharishi Ayurveda's approach to pharmacology, which makes sophisticated use of thousands of herbs and other plants.

Western pharmacology—applying the mechanistic model of the body—isolates and then synthesizes single active ingredients from herbs and plants. For example, the Ayurvedic remedy willow bark was the source of acetylsalicylic acid, and the Ayurvedic remedy rauwolfia was the source of reserpine. The active-ingredient model reflects a weakness of the scientific method—its inability to deal with complex systems, and its requirement that the researcher radically simplify a process to evaluate it (Sharma, 1995). By contrast, Ayurvedic pharmacology, called *dravyaguna,* uses the synergistic cooperation of substances as they *co*exist in natural sources. It uses either single plants or, more often, mixtures of plants whose effects are complementary. Such synergistic effects are gaining consideration in Western medical research, which is finding, for example, that *combinations* of antioxidants may stop oxidation damage and cancer cell growth more effectively than these substances acting alone. In terms of MAV's consciousness model, the effectiveness of herbal mixtures relative to active ingredients can be explained by the idea that plants, especially herbs, are concentrated repositories of nature's intelligence, which, when used properly, can increase the expression of that intelligence in the body. Research and experience with Maharishi Ayurveda herbal mixtures, known as *rasayanas,* shows that synergism enhances the free radical-scavenging properties of herbs and mitigates the harmful side effects that often accompany Western drugs.

According to Maharishi Ayurveda rasayanas promote longevity, stamina, immunity, and overall well-being (Sharma, 1993). Research has shown several of them to have significant antioxidant properties (Dwivedi et al., 1991; Engineer et al., 1992; Fields et al., 1990; Hanna et al., 1994; Niwa, 1991; Sharma et al., 1992; Sharma et al., 1995; Tomlinson & Wallace, 1991). The rasayana known as *Maharishi Amrit Kalash* (MAK) is approximately 1000 times more effective at scavenging free radicals than such active ingredients as vitamins C and E and is a commonly used pharmaceutical antioxidant (Sharma et al., 1992). Research also has found these herbal mixtures to be effective in clinical use. For example, in angina patients using MAK, the angina frequency and systolic blood pressure were reduced significantly, and exercise tolerance was improved (Dogra et al., 1994). MAK also increased resistance of low-density lipoprotein to oxidation in hyperlipidemic patients, which is important for the prevention of atherosclerosis (Sundaram et al., 1995). As mentioned earlier, MAK also is effective in protecting against the side effects of chemotherapy (Misra et al., 1994). MAK has been found to improve age-related visual discrimination, which also might involve attentional capacity and alertness (Gelderloos et al., 1990). Another MAV herbal mixture known as Student Rasayana improved the performance of children on a test of nonverbal intelligence (Nidich et al., 1993).

MAK was found in laboratory research to have anticancer and anticarcinogenic properties (Arnold et al., 1991; Dileepan et al., 1993; Patel et al., 1992; Prasad et al., 1992; Sharma et al., 1990; Sharma et al., 1991); to prevent atherosclerosis and human platelet aggregation (Lee, 1995: Sharma et al., 1989); to improve immunity (Dileepan et al., 1990, 1993); and to protect against the toxic effects of toluene, an industrial chemical that can cause brain damage (Bondy et al., 1994; Sharma et al., 1995).

Diet and Digestion

Western medical research is accumulating more and more evidence that diet plays a critical role in the development of heart disease and cancer. For example, researchers now suspect that diet plays a role in at least 35 percent of cancer deaths. Ayurveda has long considered problems of diet and digestion to be among the central causes of all disease and has considered improvement of diet and digestion to be crucial to almost any therapeutic regimen. Ayurveda views faulty diet as not only contributing to specific degenerative diseases but also to throwing off the body's natural balance, thus weakening immunity.

MAV's approach to diet rests on the "consciousness model"; food is viewed as not only providing matter and energy to the body but also intelligence, order, and balance. This brings to mind the observations of the Nobel Laureate physicist Erwin Schrödinger that food helps the body resist the Second Law of Thermodynamics, which normally leads any complex system into chaos (Schrödinger, 1967).

By this view, when we eat, we are eating not only nutrients but also orderliness. MAV dietetics considers not only the nutritional value and caloric content of food but also the food's impact on the body's underlying state of balance; food affects the doshas, and diet must be suited to the individual vikriti and prakriti. It also must reflect the climate and season, as well as specific health conditions.

The influence of food on the doshas is specific to the food but usually can be determined by knowing in which generic categories of tastes and qualities the food belongs. According to MAV the six categories of taste are sweet, sour, salty, pungent, astringent, and bitter. The six major categories of quality are heavy, light, cold, warm, oily, and dry. Table 20-3 summarizes how taste and food qualities affect the doshas, and Table 20-4 gives examples of foods that possess these various qualities and tastes.

TABLE 20-3

Taste and Food Quality Effects on the Doshas

Tastes	
Decrease Vata	Increase Vata
Sweet	Pungent
Sour	Bitter
Salty	Astringent
Decrease Pitta	Increase Pitta
Sweet	Pungent
Bitter	Sour
Astringent	Salty
Decrease Kapha	Increase Kapha
Pungent	Sweet
Bitter	Sour
Astringent	Salty

Major Food Qualities	
Decrease Vata	Increase Vata
Heavy	Light
Oily	Dry
Hot	Cold
Decrease Pitta	Increase Pitta
Cold	Hot
Heavy	Light
Oily	Dry
Decrease Kapha	Increase Kapha
Light	Heavy
Dry	Oily
Hot	Cold

To give an example of how this information would be applied clinically, a patient with Kapha syndromes (e.g., sinusitis, certain types of obesity) would be told to minimize eating cold, oily, and heavy foods, as well as foods with sweet, sour, and salty tastes. The patient would be advised instead to give predominance to foods exhibiting the remaining qualities and tastes.

Maharishi Ayurveda recommends a lactovegetarian diet for optimal health. Meat is more difficult to digest and has been linked to numerous diseases, including heart disease and cancer. MAV also recommends the use of fresh produce. These emphases map well with emerging Western findings on diet, which have shown significant health benefits from a meatless diet and from increasing consumption of plant-based foods.

Maharishi Ayurveda focuses not only on what one eats but also on how one digests it. The emphasis on digestion contrasts with Western allopathic medicine, which deals with digestion only when it is significantly disrupted. In MAV excellent digestion is critical to robust health. MAV contains a number of techniques for improving digestion and treating digestive disorders. They center around the concept of *agni*, which literally means "fire," and refers to metabolic and digestive activities that convert foodstuff into bodily substances. Ayurveda describes 13 types of agni

in the body. Their importance in Ayurvedic health care is suggested by the fact that one of the eight branches of Ayurveda, *Kaya Chikitsa* (internal medicine), focuses on the strength or weakness of the agnis.

This becomes clearer when we consider the end product of poor digestion, which Ayurveda calls *Ama*. Ama plays a key role in pathogenesis, interacting with aggravated doshas and causing them to "stick" to areas where they do not belong. Healthy digestion reduces the amount of Ama produced.

To rid the body of accumulated Ama, pollutants, and other pathogenic impurities that disrupt or block the natural expression of the body's inner intelligence, Maharishi Ayurveda emphasizes the importance of purification therapies that rid the body of these substances. Foremost among these purification therapies is *pañchakarma*, which literally means "five activities," because it includes five main treatment modalities:

1. Whole-body massage with herbalized oil *(abhyanga)*
2. Continuous flow of warm herbalized oil on the forehead *(shirodhara)*
3. Fomentation of the body with herbalized heat *(swedana)*
4. Special herbalized oil head massage and nasal administration of herbs *(nasya)*
5. Sesame oil retention or herbalized eliminative enemas *(basti)*

Daily treatments, administered for 2 to 14 days or longer, are recommended with each change of the seasons. Certain aspects of Pañchakarma can fit easily into a patient's daily preventive regimen. Preliminary research has shown that regular Pañchakarma reduces several cardiovascular risk factors, including cholesterol (Sharma et al., 1993; Waldschutz, 1994). Sesame oil, which is used topically and for colonic irrigation in pañchakarma, has been shown to inhibit in vitro malignant melanoma growth (Smith & Salerno, 1992) and human colon adenocarcinoma cell line growth (Salerno & Smith, 1991).

The central role of food and digestion is demonstrated particularly well by consideration of another central MAV concept—the importance of a substance called *ojas*. Ojas is said to be the finest manifestation of the unified field, which serves as a sort of glue to link consciousness and matter. Ojas maintains the integrity of the seven bodily tissues *(dhatus)*: plasma *(rasa)*, blood *(rakta)*, muscle *(mamsa)*, fat *(meda)*, bone *(asthi)*, bone marrow and nervous system *(majja)*, and

---

TABLE 20-4

Common Examples of the Six Tastes and the Major Food Qualities

The Six Tastes and Some Common Examples
  Sweet: sugar, milk, butter, rice, breads, honey
  Sour: yogurt, lemon, cheese
  Salty: salt
  Pungent: spicy foods, peppers, ginger, cumin
  Bitter: spinach, other green leafy vegetables
  Astringent: beans

The Six Major Food Qualities and Some Common Examples
  Heavy: cheese, yogurt, wheat products
  Light: barley, corn, spinach, apples
  Oily: dairy products, fatty foods, oils
  Dry: barley, corn, potato, beans
  Hot: hot (temperature) food and drink
  Cold: cold food and drink

sperm/ovum *(sukra)*. Most MAV therapies and behavioral advice are designed to maximize the presence of ojas, and almost all MAV proscriptions are designed to minimize the depletion of ojas. The end product of truly healthy diet and digestion is said to contain significant amounts of ojas. According to an MAV expression, "like a bee which gets honey from the flowers, we get ojas from our food." MAV also asserts that positive, loving emotions increase the abundance of ojas; food should be eaten in a warm, congenial, and uplifting atmosphere. Arguing, or any other negativity at meals, interferes with digestion, producing a harmful end product instead of ojas.

Behavior, Emotions, and the Senses

The recommendation for a positive emotional tone during meals reflects a general concept of MAV regarding behavior, speech, and emotions, and their effect on health. This concept springs naturally from the model that places consciousness at the basis of the body. Emotions can be understood as fine fluctuations of consciousness (or the unified field); as such, their impact on the more expressed physical levels of the body are immense. Recently Western medicine has begun to investigate the effect of emotions on health, with interesting findings; Ayurveda has discussed this field for millennia. Ayurvedic texts include detailed discussions of lifestyle and behavior, and their impact on health. Interestingly traditional virtues—such as respect for elders, teachers, loved ones, and family members, pardoning those who wrong you, practicing nonviolence, and not speaking ill of others—are understood to promote health for the individual's mind and body, as well as for the community and society.

In addition to emotion, sensory input is understood to have an impact on health. This idea is applied clinically, not only in terms of behavioral advice but also in the form of sensory therapies, such as aromatherapy and sound therapy involving both music (called *Gandharva-Veda*) and primordial sounds that are used for their healing qualities. A study on Maharishi Ayurveda primordial sound therapy (specifically, Vedic sounds known as *Sama Veda*) found it to reduce in vitro human tumor cell growth significantly, whereas hard rock music tended to increase growth significantly (see Chapter 19).

Biological Rhythms

In Maharishi Ayurveda attuning the patient's lifestyle to natural biorhythms is considered a crucial element of prevention and treatment. MAV gives a detailed analysis of circadian (daily) and circannual (seasonal) rhythms, with recommendations for daily and seasonal routines. These include such advice as rising and retiring early and eating one's main meal at lunchtime, when the digestive "fires" are strongest. This advice must be suited to the individual. Emerging Western data on biorhythms correlate well with Ayurvedic knowledge. Again, the idea of a connection between patterns of order in nature and in the human body was obvious to Ayurveda millennia ago.

The three-dosha concept plays a key role in understanding these connections. Different times of the day are associated with different doshas, as are different seasons and the different stages of the human life cycle (Box 20-1). For example, the summer is dominated by Pitta (the dosha that governs heat and metabolism), whereas the spring is dominated by Kapha (which has qualities of coolness and moisture). Childhood is dominated by Kapha (which governs structure, substance, and growth), old age by Vata. In fact, physicians see a preponderance of Kapha-based disorders in children, such as colds and respiratory illnesses, and an ever-increasing number of Vata disor-

---

BOX 20-1

The Seasons and Times of Day Classified According to the Doshas

- Kapha season: Spring-early summer (approximately March to June)
- Kapha time: Approximately 6 AM (sunrise) to 10 AM and 6 PM to 10 PM
- Kapha period in life cycle: Childhood
- Pitta season: Midsummer-early autumn (approximately July to October)
- Pitta time: Approximately 10 AM to 2 PM and 10 PM to 2 AM
- Pitta period in life cycle: Adulthood
- Vata season: Late autumn-winter (approximately November to February)
- Vata time: Approximately 2 AM to 6 AM (sunrise) and 2 PM to 6 PM
- Vata period in life cycle: Old age

ders in elderly patients, such as constipation and lighter, shorter, and more frequently interrupted sleep. They also see more Kapha-type disorders in spring and Pitta disorders in summer. Understanding the concept of doshas is helpful in treating these ailments.

COLLECTIVE HEALTH AND THE ENVIRONMENT

Maharishi Ayurveda holds great promise in several areas of collective health. In terms of infectious disease and epidemics, the Western approach of using antibiotics has an inherent limitation and risk caused by the process of natural selection that produces new resistant strains of microbes. As a result overreliance on antibiotics can foster the growth of serious new infectious diseases. MAV's focus on strengthening immunity and its techniques for dealing directly with epidemics offer a more effective and safer means of ensuring collective health.

In terms of chronic disease Western medicine has long recognized that preventing and treating these disorders requires changes in lifestyle, diet, and behavior. However, allopathic medicine has been at a loss as to how to effect these changes in patients for a prolonged time. Research has shown that those who practice TM are better able to give up harmful habits, such as cigarette smoking, alcohol consumption, and illegal drug use, and to incorporate healthy dietary and lifestyle changes (Alexander et al., 1994; Gelderloos et al., 1991; Monahan, 1977). MAV also offers other time-tested modalities that benefit individual patients, such as daily routine and purification procedures, which could be useful in large-scale applications. Finally, MAV offers an overall theory of prevention, involving such elements as the three-dosha concept, that could have value for future research on preventive medicine.

The most significant public health approach of Maharishi Ayurveda deals with larger social disorders and the dangers they pose. War, crime, and violence rarely are considered subjects of public health policy, but their implications for health are obvious. As with individual disease, Maharishi Ayurveda understands these as originating not in material factors but ultimately in consciousness—in this case, both individual and collective consciousness. Just as an abstract field of consciousness underlies the individual's mind and body, so such a field underlies societal trends. Society reflects the influence of its members not only in a linear, additive way—in the sense that a green forest is made of green trees—but also through a field effect—in the sense that a gravitational field's influences are not localized. If the individual consciousness of a sufficient number of members of a society is coherent, harmonious, and life-supporting, those influences spread through the "field" of the collective consciousness of the society, influencing the whole society.

This idea has been tested by a number of studies. One study found that when a sufficiently large group of practitioners of the TM and advanced TM-Sidhi techniques meditated together as a group in Israel, war deaths in Lebanon were significantly reduced compared with casualty rates on days when the number of practitioners meditating together decreased below a certain threshold (Orme-Johnson et al., 1987). Similar findings have emerged in studies of other localities, usually involving reductions in the rate of violent crime (Dillbeck et al., 1981; Dillbeck et al., 1988; Orme-Johnson & Gelderloos, 1988). For example, a 1993 study in Washington, DC, showed that when a large group of practitioners of the TM and TM-Sidhi programs assembled to meditate during the summer, it produced an 18 percent reduction in violent crime compared with levels that had been predicted on the basis of the previous years' crime and weather trends (Hagelin et al., 1994). There has been much discussion and debate regarding these observations and the validity of what has been called the *Maharishi effect.*

FUTURE DIRECTIONS

Many central elements of Ayurveda—such as the ideas that diet and emotions play a crucial role in disease and in prevention—were not taken seriously by Western medicine a generation ago but are now major themes of research. Other concerns of MAV might prove to be of value both in clinical work and in research. Already, Maharishi Ayurveda's Transcendental Meditation technique and herbal preparations have produced bodies of significant research findings whose implications have yet to be fully explored. Other areas, such as prakriti and vikriti, will likely prove equally interesting to researchers.

The clinical use of Maharishi Ayurveda has appeared to be most dramatic when applied to diseases that Western medicine finds difficult to treat, such as poor digestion, cancer, and chronic disease (Janssen, 1989; Orme-Johnson, 1987). Its clinical value extends to other areas not discussed previously, such as pediatrics, where it has been found to significantly reduce the incidence of childhood ailments such as frequent colds, or gynecology, where it has been able to reduce the severity of menstrual and premenstrual problems.

Hundreds of physicians worldwide have been trained in Maharishi Ayurveda and have incorporated its principles into their practice. Maharishi Ayurveda schools, institutions, and universities are being opened in each state of the United States to train physicians, technicians, and nurses and to teach the general public various areas of health care management. Several medical institutions have incorporated this teaching into their curriculums. Maharishi Ayurveda continues to make significant contributions to the health care profession in the United States and around the world.

References

Alexander CN, Langer EJ, Davies JL, et al. 1989. Transcendental Meditation, mindfulness and longevity: an experimental study with the elderly. J Pers Soc Psychol 57:950-964

Alexander CN, Rainforth MV, Gelderloos P. 1991. Transcendental Meditation, self-actualization, and psychological health: A conceptual overview and statistical meta-analysis. J Soc Behav Pers 6:189-247

Alexander CN, Robinson P, Orme-Johnson DW, et al. 1995. The effects of Transcendental Meditation compared to other methods of relaxation and meditation in reducing risk factors, morbidity and mortality. Homeostasis

Alexander CN, Robinson P, Rainforth M. 1994. Treating alcohol, nicotine, and drug abuse through Transcendental Meditation: A review and statistical meta-analysis. Alcohol Treat Q 11:13-87

Arnold JT, Wilkinson BP, Korytynski EA, Steel VE. 1991. Chemopreventive activity of Maharishi Amrit Kalash and related agents in rat tracheal epithelial and human tumor cells. Proc Am Assoc Cancer Res 32:128 (abstract)

Aspect A, Grangier P, Roger G. 1981. Experimental tests of realistic local theories via Bell's theorem. Physical Rev Lett 47:460

Badawi K, Wallace RK, Orme-Johnson DW, Rouzere AM. 1984. Electrophysiologic characteristics of respiratory suspension periods occurring during the practice of the Transcendental Meditation Program. Psychosom Med 46:267-276

Bondy SC, Hernandez TM, Mattia C. 1994. Antioxidant properties of two Ayurvedic herbal preparations. Biochem Arch 10:25-31

Chalmers RA, Clements G, Schenkluhn H, Weinless M (eds). 1989. Scientific Research on Maharishi's Transcendental Meditation and TM-Sidhi Program: Collected Papers, Vols. 2, 3, 4. MVU Press. Vlodrop, The Netherlands

Charaka S. 1977. Sharma RK, Dash B, (trans.) Chowkhamba Sanskrit Series Office, Varanasi, India

Cooper MJ, Aygen MM. 1978. Effect of Transcendental Meditation on serum cholesterol and blood pressure. Harefuah 95(1):1-2

Cooper MJ, Aygen MM. 1979. A relaxation technique in the management of hypercholesterolemia. J Hum Stress 5:24-27

Dileepan KN, Patel V, Sharma HM, Stechschulte DJ. 1990. Priming of splenic lymphocytes after ingestion of an Ayurvedic herbal food supplement: evidence for an immunomodulatory effect. Biochem Arch 6:267-274

Dileepan KN, Varghese ST, Page JC, Stechschulte DJ. 1993. Enhanced lymphoproliferative response, macrophage mediated tumor cell killing and nitric oxide production after ingestion of an Ayurvedic drug. Biochem Arch 9:365-374

Dillbeck MC, Banus CB, Polanzi C, Landrith III G. 1988. Text of a field model of consciousness and social change: the transcendental meditation and TM-Sidhi program and decreased urban crime. Mind Behav 9(4):457-486

Dillbeck MC, Landrith III G, Orme-Johnson DW. 1981. The Transcendental Meditation program and crime rate change in a sample of 48 cities. J Crime Justice 4:24-45

Dogra J, Grover N, Kumar P, Aneja N. 1994. Indigenous free radical scavenger MAK 4 and 5 in angina pectoris: Is it only a placebo? J Assoc Physicians India 42(6):466-467

Dwivedi G, Sharma HM, Dobrowki S, Engineer F. 1991. Inhibitory effects of Maharishi Amrit Kalash (M-4) and Maharishi Amrit Kalash (M-5) on microsomal lipid peroxidation. Pharmacol Biochem Behav 39:649-652

Eddington A. 1974. The Nature of the Physical World, University of Michigan Press, Ann Arbor, p. 276

Engineer FN, Sharma HM, Dwivedi C. 1992. Protective effects of M-4 and M-5 on Adriamycin-induced microsomal lipid peroxidation and mortality. Biochem Arch 8:267-272

Eppley KR, Abrams A, Shear J. 1989. Differential effects of relaxation techniques on trait anxiety: a meta-analysis. J Clin Psychol 45:957-974

Farrow JT, Hebert JR. 1982. Breath suspension during the transcendental meditation technique. Psychosom Med 44(2):133-153

Fields J, Rawal P, Hagen J, et al. 1990. Oxygen free radical (OFR) scavenging effects of an anti-carcinogenic natural product, Maharishi Amrit Kalash (MAK). Pharmacologist 32:A155 (abstract)

Gallois P. 1984. Modifications neurophysiologiques et respiratoires lors de la practique des techniques de relaxation. L'encephale 10:139-144

Gelderloos P, Ahlstrom HHB, Orme-Johnson DW, et al. 1990. Influence of a Maharishi Ayur-vedic herbal preparation on age-related visual discrimination. Int J Psychosom 37:25-29

Gelderloos P, Walton KG, Orme-Johnson DW, Alexander CN. 1991. Effectiveness of the Transcendental Meditation program in preventing and treating substance misuse: A review. Int J Addic 26:293-325

Glaser J, Brind J, Vogelman J, et al. 1992. Elevated serum dehydroepiandrosterone sulfate levels in practitioners of the Transcendental Meditation (TM) and TM Sidhi programs. J Behav Med 15(4):327-341

Hagelin JS, Orme-Johnson DW, Rainforth M, et al. 1994. Results of the national demonstration project to reduce violent crime and improve governmental effectiveness in Washington, D.C. Institute of Science, Technology, and Public Policy Technical Report ITR-94:1

Hanna AN, Sharma HM, Kauffman EM, Newman HAI. 1994. In vitro and in vivo inhibition of microsomal lipid peroxidation by MA-631. Pharmacol Biochem Behav 48:505-510

Herron R, Hills S, Mandarino J, et al. 1995. Reducing medical costs: the impact of transcendental meditation on government payments to physicians in Quebec. Am J Health Promotion

Janssen GWHM. 1989. The application of Maharishi Ayur-Ved in the treatment of ten chronic diseases: a pilot study. Ned Tijdschr Geneeskd 5:586-94

Jevning JR, Wilson AF, Davison JM. 1978. Adrenocortical activity during meditation. Horm Behav 10:54-60

Jevning JR, Wilson AF, O'Halloran JP, Walsh RN. 1983. Forearm blood flow and metabolism during stylized and unstylized states of decreased activation. Am J Physiol 245:R110-R116

Lee JY. 1995. The antioxidant and antiatherogenic effects of MAK-4 in WHHL rabbits. Ph.D. dissertation, The Ohio State University, Columbus, Ohio

Levine JP. 1976. The Coherence Spectral Array (COSPAR) and its application to the study of spatial ordering in the EEG. Proc San Diego Biomed Symp 15:237-247

Madhavakava. 1986. Madhava Nidanam. Srikanta Murthy KR (trans). Chaukambha Orientalia. Delhi, India

Misra NC, Sharma HM, Chaturvedi A, et al. 1994. Antioxidant adjuvant therapy using a natural herbal mixture MAK during intensive chemotherapy: reduction in toxicity—A prospective study of 62 patients. In: Rao RS, Deo MG, Sanghvi LD (eds). Proceedings of the Sixteenth International Cancer Congress, Monduzzi Editore, Bologna, Italy, pp. 3099-3102

Monahan RJ. 1977. Secondary prevention of drug dependence through the transcendental meditation program in metropolitan Philadelphia. Int J Addict 12:729-754

Nader T. 1993. Human Physiology: Expression of Veda and the Vedic Literature. MVU Press. Vlodrop, The Netherlands

Nidich SI, Morehead P, Nidich RJ, et al. 1993. The effect of the Maharishi Student Rasayana food supplement on non-verbal intelligence. Person Individ Diff 15:599-602

Niwa Y. 1991. Effect of Maharishi-4 and Maharishi-5 on inflammatory mediators—with special reference to their free radical scavenging effect. Indian J Clin Prac 1:23-27

Orme-Johnson DW. 1973. Autonomic stability and transcendental meditation. Psychosom Med 35:341-349

Orme-Johnson DW. 1987. Medical care utilization and the transcendental meditation program. Psychosom Med 49:493-507

Orme-Johnson DW, Alexander CN, Davies JL, et al. 1987. International peace project in the Middle East: The effects of the Maharishi Technology of the Unified Field. J Conflict Resolution 32(4):776-812

Orme-Johnson DW, Farrow JT (eds). 1977. Scientific Research on the Transcendental Meditation Program: Collected Papers, Vol. 1. MERU Press. Rheinweiler, Germany

Orme-Johnson DW, Gelderloos P. 1988. The long term effects of the Maharishi Technology of the Unified Field on the quality of life in the United States (1960-1983). Soc Sci Per J 2(4):127-146

Patel VK, Wang J, Shen RN, et al. 1992. Reduction of metastases of Lewis Lung Carcinoma by an Ayurvedic food supplement in mice. Nutr Res 12:667-676

Prasad KN, Edwards-Prasad J, Kentroti S, et al. 1992. Ayurvedic (science of life) agents induce differentiation in murine neuroblastoma cells in culture. Neuropharmacology 31:599-607

Rarity JG, Tapster PR. 1990. Experimental violation of Bell's inequality based on phase and momentum. Physical Rev Lett 64:2495

Salerno JW, Smith DE. 1991. The use of sesame oil and other vegetable oils in the inhibition of human colon cancer growth in vitro. Anticancer Res 11:209-216

Sarngadhara. 1984. Sarngadhara Samhita. Srikanta Murthy KR (trans). Chaukhambha Orientalia. Delhi, India

Schneider RH, Alexander CN, Wallace RK. 1992. In search of an optimal behavioral treatment for hypertension: a review and focus on transcendental meditation. In Johnson EH, Gentry WD, Julius S (eds). Personality, Elevated Blood Pressure, and Essential Hypertension. Hemisphere. Washington, DC, pp. 123-131

Schneider RH, Staggers F, Alexander CN, et al. 1995. A randomised controlled trial of stress reduction for hypertension in older African Americans. Hypertension 26(5):820-827

Schrödinger E. 1967. What is Life? Cambridge University Press. Cambridge

Sharma H. 1993. Freedom from Disease: How to Control Free Radicals, a Major Cause of Aging and Disease. Veda Publishing. Toronto

Sharma HM. 1995. The fallacy of the active ingredient. In: Chesworth J (ed). Alternative Perspectives on Health: An Ecological Approach. Sage Publications. Thousand Oaks, California

Sharma HM, Dwivedi C, Satter BC, Abou-Issa H. 1991. Antineoplastic properties of Maharishi Amrit Kalash, an Ayurvedic food supplement, against 7, 12-dimethylbenz(a)anthracene-induced mammary tumors in rats. J Res Educ Indian Med 10(3):1-8

Sharma HM, Dwivedi C, Satter BC, et al. 1990. Antineoplastic properties of Maharishi-4 against DMBA-induced mammary tumors in rats. Pharmacol Biochem Behav 35:767-773

Sharma HM, Feng Y, Panganamala RV. 1989. Maharishi Amrit Kalash (MAK) prevents human platelet aggregation. Clin Ter Cardiovasc 8:227-230

Sharma H, Guenther J, Abu-Ghazaleh A, Dwivedi C. 1994. Effects of Ayurvedic food supplement M-4 on cisplatin-induced changes in glutathione and glutathione-S-transferase activity. In: Rao RS, Deo MG, Sanghvi LD, (eds). Proceedings of the Sixteenth International Cancer Congress, Vol. 1. Monduzzi Editore, Bologna, Italy pp. 589-592

Sharma HM, Hanna AN, Kauffman EM, Newman HAI. 1992. Inhibition of human LDL oxidation in vitro by Maharishi Ayur-Veda herbal mixtures. Pharmacol Biochem Behav 41:1175-1182

Sharma HM, Hanna AN, Kauffman EM, Newman HAI. 1995. Effect of herbal mixture Student Rasayana on lipoxygenase activity and lipid peroxidation. Free Radic Biol Med 18:687-697

Sharma HM, Nidich SI, Sands D, Smith DE. 1993. Improvement in cardiovascular risk factors through Panchakarma purification procedures. J Res Educ Indian Med 12(4):2-13

Smith DE, Salerno JW. 1992. Selective growth inhibition of a human malignant melanoma cell line by sesame oil in vitro. Prostaglandins Leuko Essen Fatty Acids 46:145-150

Stapp HP. 1994. Mind, Matter and Quantum Mechanics. Springer-Verlag. New York, pp. 220-221

Steel K, Gertman PM, Crescenzi C, Anderson J. 1981. Iatrogenic illness on a general medical service at a university hospital. N Engl J Med 304:638-642

Sundaram V, Hanna AN, Lubow G, et al. 1995. Increased resistance of human LDL to oxidation in hyperlipidemic patients supplemented with oral herbal mixture MAK-4. FASEB J 9(3):A141 (abstract)

Sushruta S. 1963. Ghisagrantne KL (trans). Chowkhamba Sanskrit Series Office. Varanasi, India

Tomlinson PF, Wallace RK. 1991. Superoxide scavenging of two natural products, Maharishi-4 (M-4) and Maharishi-5 (M-5). FASEB J 5(5):A1284 (abstract)

Vagbhata. 1982. Ashtanga Hridayam. In: Upaohyaya VY (ed). Chaukambha Sanskrit Sansthan. Varanasi, India

Waldschütz R. 1994. Influence of Maharishi Ayur-Veda purification treatment on physiological and psychological health. Translation; original German version appeared in 1988, Erfahrungsheilkunde-Acta medica empirica 11:720-729

Wallace RK. 1970. Physiological effects of transcendental meditation. Science 167:1751-1754

Wallace RK, Dillbeck MC, Jacobe E, Harrington B. 1982. The effects of the transcendental meditation and TM-Sidhi program on the aging process. Int J Neurosci 16:53-58

Wallace RK, Orme-Johnson DW, Dillbeck MC (eds). 1989. Scientific Research on Maharishi's Transcendental Meditation and TrMSidhi Program: Collected Papers, Vol. 5. MIU Press, Fairfield, Iowa

Suggested Readings

Carr T. 1991. Medicine at the mind-body interface: The approach of Maharishi Ayur-Ved. Int Clin Nutr Rev 11(4):190-220

Lonsdorf N, Butler V, Brown M. 1993. A Woman's Best Medicine: Health, Happiness and Long Life Through Ayur-Veda. Jeremy P. Tarcher/Putnam. New York

Sharma HM, Kauffman EM, Dudek A, Stephens RE. 1995. In press. Effect of different sounds on growth of human cancer cell lines in vitro. J Res Educ Indian Med

Wallace RK. 1993. The Physiology of Consciousness. MIU Press, Fairfield, Iowa

21

The Islamic Sufi Tradition and Healing

HOWARD HALL

HISTORICAL BACKGROUND

The history of Sufism can be traced back 15 centuries to the time of the Prophet Muhammad. The foundation of Sufism is based on belief in the mystical aspects of the spirituality of the Prophet (Hussein et al., 1997). During his lifetime, pious individuals from different nations learned under his guidance the Spiritual Laws of Islam, because these laws lead toward direct experience of the Divine or **Allah,** the Arabic word for the One God (Ansha, 1991).

The spiritual leader of a Sufi school is known as a *Shaikh.* The spiritual knowledge of the Shaikh can be traced back to the Prophet Muhammad. Allah revealed the Holy Qur'an to the Prophet who later converted his cousin and son-in-law 'Ali bin abi Talib. 'Ali is considered a spiritual heir to the Prophet and the

one who inherited his spiritual knowledge and power. Thus all Sufi Masters are his students, directly or indirectly, and this is the origin of his title "Shaikh of the Shaikhs." Through a line of succession, each Shaikh would initiate a successor. Thus this maintains a direct spiritual link or attachment with the Prophet Muhammad to the present spiritual leader (Chishti, 1991). This chain from the Prophet Muhammad down to the present Master of a Sufi school is known as a *silsila* (Hussein et al., 1997). Today there are more than 150 orders or schools of Sufism.

If the Shaikh did not find among his students someone with the attributes that qualify him to be a Shaikh, the Shaikh would not name a successor, and the silsila of that particular tariqa (way) would discontinue. In this case the dervishes would have to join another tariqa after the departure of their

381

Shaikh to maintain the spiritual link necessary for the attainment.

The unifying factor and ultimate aim of the Sufi way is the attainment to Allah by means of following a chain of masters who have already attained to Allah and who reached the status of becoming themselves a means of attainment to Allah. The process of drawing near to Allah includes the acquisition of paranormal powers and paranormal knowledge, including Qur'anic knowledge. One of the great Sufi Masters, Shaikh "Abdul Qadir al-Gaylani," used to describe what the dervish would obtain as being something that no eye has ever seen, no ear has ever heard, and has never occurred to any human heart. In Sufi terms the attainment to Allah means the transformation into light by becoming absorbed or extinct in the Light (i.e., Allah). Allah describes Himself in the Holy Qur'an as being "nur" (light): "Allah is the Light of the heavens and the earth" (24:35). The nearer the dervish draws to Allah, the more he acquires of Allah attributes. When the dervish achieves the ultimate goal of total "extinction" (Arabic: "fana") in Allah, he will lose his own will and become an instrument in the hands of Allah.

Sufism is a mystical spiritual tradition within Islam. The Sufi musician Hazrat Inayat Khan (1983) provides the following description of spiritual development:

The word "spiritual" does not apply to goodness or to wonder-working, the power of producing miracles, or to great intellectual power. The whole of life in all its aspects is one single music; and the real spiritual attainment is to tune oneself to the harmony of this perfect music.

It should be pointed out that the Sufi spiritual viewpoint is not generally accepted by traditional Muslims and has even been met with hostility from other Muslim schools of thought (Hussein et al., 1997).

THE WAY

An integral part of Sufism is the notion of a "path" or "way" toward Allah through self-understanding, certain practices, and discipline (Ansha, 1991). Many great spiritual traditions use the concept of a "path" or "way" toward the experience or knowledge of the divine. For example, Buddhism is known as a path toward Nirvana or enlightenment (Clarke, 1993). In the Holy Bible, 25:4, it is written: "Show me thy ways,

O Lord; teach me thy paths." Continuing with verses 9-10, "The meek will he guide in judgment: and the meek will he teach his way, All the paths of the Lord are mercy and truth unto such as keep his covenant and his testimonies." In the New Testament, 14:6, Jesus said: "I am the way, the truth, and the life; no man cometh unto the Father, but by me." Similarly, in the beginning chapter of the Holy Qur'an, *Al Fatihah* (The Opening) 1:6-7, Allah teaches the people how to pray to Him in the above verses: "Show us the straight way, The way of those on whom Thou hast bestowed Thy Grace, Those whose portion is not wrath, and who go not astray."

The idea of a spiritual path has a corollary within the Western philosophy concept of "means" versus an "end." As John Dewey (1922) noted when discussing "means" and "end" concerning an activity:

The distinction of means and end arise in surveying the course of a proposed line of action, a connected series in time. The "end" is the last act thought of; the means are the acts to be performed prior to it in time. To reach an end we must take our mind off from it and attend to the act which is next to be performed. We must make that the end.

Dewey's concept of means and end were greatly influenced by the mind-body movement therapy work of F. Matthias Alexander (1910). Alexander observed that many postural problems people encountered were due to unconscious movements to gain some end such as sitting or standing without much thought as to the means, way, or path of accomplishing this goal. Alexander taught individuals to focus on the "means whereby" of doing a simple act such as the process of moving from sitting to standing versus focusing on the end results or "end gaining" as he termed it (Alexander, 1910). The process of attending to the "means" or "way" resulted in increased conscious guidance and control of the self. As Alexander (1910) noted:

This triumph is not to be won in sleep, in trance, in submission, in paralysis, or in anaesthesia, but in a clear, open-eyed, reasoning, deliberate consciousness and apprehension of the wonderful potentialities possessed by mankind, the transcendent inheritance of a conscious mind.

From this perspective, following a path or way or attending to a means may be associated with increased awareness or consciousness or perhaps even a higher consciousness. This is comparable to the increased consciousness or awareness found in one's body movements following instructions with the Alexander method (Alexander, 1910) (see Chapter 8).

ISLAMIC TRADITIONS AND HEALTH

As a spiritual tradition within Islam, Sufism follows the orthodox spiritually based (and healthy) Islamic practices such as prayer five times a day (early morning, noon, midafternoon, sunset, and evening), fasting, and prohibition against the consumption of pork products and intoxicating liquors. There are also prohibitions against gambling, sexual relations outside of marriage, and behavior or dress that is indecent (Abdalati, 1996). There are obvious health benefits for avoiding such high-risk behaviors such as multiple sexual relationships, the use of intoxicants, and gambling as prescribed by Islamic tradition. Avoiding alcohol intoxication also helps prevent the disinhibition effects of this substance and the accompanying social problems. One researcher indicated: "It has been said that the super-ego is the alcohol-soluble portion of the personality" (Friend, 1957, p. 84). Avoiding pork would also provide protection against swine-related foodborne diseases, such as salmonella typhimurium gastroenteritis (Gessner & Beller, 1994), *Yersinia* enterocolitis (Tauxe, 1997), viral illnesses from pork or pork products, including foot and mouth disease, classical swine fever (hog cholera), African swine fever, and swine vesicular viral diseases (Farez & Morley, 1997; McKercher et al., 1978). Even the use of modern microwave ovens may fail to protect against pork-related illness such as salmonellosis (Gessner & Beller, 1994). Of course, pork is not the only source of foodborne diseases, and such pathogens in general are emerging as a major public health challenge (Tauxe, 1997).

PRAYER

The healing benefits of prayer are now becoming recognized within the disciplines of science and medicine (Dossey, 1996). As Dossey (1996) noted:

Prayer works. More than 130 controlled laboratory studies show, in general, that prayer or a prayer like state of compassion, empathy, and love can bring about healthful changes in many types of living things, from humans to bacteria. This does not mean prayer always works, any more than drugs and surgery always work, but that, statistically speaking, prayer is effective.

FASTING

Being hungry is better than the maladies that come with satiety. Subtlety and lightness and being true to your devotion are some of the advantages of fasting.

—RUMI (1991)

During the lunar holy month of Ramadan, Muslims all over the world fast from sunrise to sunset. This fasting means abstaining completely from foods, drinks, and sexual intercourse from dawn to sunset (Abdalati, 1996). Fasting is done for spiritual purposes in Islam. As stated in the Qur'an (23:183) "O ye who believe! Fasting is prescribed to you as it was prescribed to those before you, so that ye may learn self-restraint and become Allah-fearing." One writer noted: "Fasting is thought to purge the body of passion and sin and reduce the risk of disease. Once passion has been controlled, it is possible to clear the mind (an element of the spiritual body) of conscious thought. This allows the mystic to establish contact with saints, spirits, sources of magical power and ultimately with Allah" (Woodward, 1985). Fasting also teaches patience and unselfishness, for when a person fasts, he or she can identify with the pains and deprivations of others less fortunate (Abdalati, 1996).

In naturopathic medicine (see Chapter 11), fasting is used as a method of detoxifying the body (Murray & Pizzorno, 1991). It is a very rapid way to increase the elimination of wastes within the body so as to facilitate healing (Murray & Pizzorno, 1991). Also, a number of medical conditions have been treated with fasting, ranging from obesity, allergies, and chemical poisoning to irritable bowel syndrome (Murray & Pizzorno, 1991).

MEDITATION

When you neglect your meditation, you contract with pain. This is God's way of telling you that your inner pain can become visible. Don't ignore it.

—RUMI (1991)

Worshipful meditation is an integral part of Sufism and is known as Divine Remembrance, *Dhikr,* or *Zekr* (Chishti, 1991). As noted within the Qur'an: "Then do ye remember ME, I will remember you" (2:152). Such meditation practices involve a prescribed number of repeated recitations of verses from the Qur'an such as: "la illaha illa Allah" or, "there is no other god but Allah" (Ansha, 1991) or other remembrances such as "The Beautiful Names" of Allah. For some Tariqa (e.g., Tariqa Casnazaniyyah) this recitation is done aloud with accompanying head movements symbolizing a hammer slamming the heart itself as becoming a stone because of its remoteness from the remembrance of Allah. As noted in the Qur'anic verse 2:74, "Thenceforth were your hearts hardened: they became like a rock and even worse in hardness." Other tariqas use silent remembrance or use different movements all together. Meditation has been suggested to help treat diseases (see Chapter 14). It has been suggested that the number of recitations to treat diseases end with a zero at the end of the number (e.g., 100, 300) (Chishti, 1991). Again, from the Sufi perspective, worshipful meditation is a means of connecting with Allah.

Research has documented the many health and physiological benefits of meditation, including decreasing blood pressure, rate of breathing, heart rate, and oxygen consumption (Benson, 1975). The positive effects of meditation are associated with the production of a physiological "relaxation response" that is opposite to the "fight-or-flight response" (Benson, 1975). Thus the regular worshipful meditative practice of Sufism may also contribute to increased health.

THE PSYCHOLOGY OF SUFISM

The notion of the heart and the ego or lower self (Arabic: *nafs*) has played a prominent role in Sufi psychology (Ansha, 1991; Chishti, 1991). The spiritual path of Sufism is geared toward inner spiritual development by helping the follower in the extinction (*fana`*) of the ego/lower self (*nafs*) or more basic appetitive aspects of the body. The health benefits of a system that helps manage the excessive appetitive motives would have positive implications for a number of disorders of overindulgence such as weight problems and addictions.

The heart, in Sufism, is related to one's spiritual self. As mentioned earlier, the head movement that accompanies the recitation meditation, Dhikr practice, symbolizes a hammer slamming the heart that has become a stone so that its true luster can shine through. The Prophet indicated that: "There is a polish for everything that taketh away rust; and the polish of the Heart is the invocation of Allah (Ling, 1977).

FAITH

Faith has also been suggested as an important factor in the psychology of healing from a Sufi perspective as it is in other healing traditions. As noted by a contemporary Sufi, M. R. Bawa Muhaiyaddeen (1991):

Illnesses can be treated in many ways, but no matter how many different treatments are used, they may still fail to heal the patient. In order for a treatment to work, first of all, even if the patient does not have faith in God, he must have faith in the doctor and in whatever treatment he suggests. Secondly, the doctor who is performing the treatment must have faith in God; he must have God's qualities, His love, and His patience. The doctor must give all responsibility to God, instead of thinking that he is the one who is responsible for curing the patient.

When these conditions exist, when the patient has faith in the doctor and the doctor has faith in God, then treatment becomes very easy and the illness will be cured, at least to a certain extent.

PAN ISLAMIC SUFISM AND HEALING TRADITIONS

Although the primary focus of Sufism is on attainment to Allah, some Sufis have developed a particular focus on healing (Chishti, 1991). Often there is a blend of Sufi philosophy with other healing traditions, as well as incorporating the use of herbs, food, and other practices (Chishti, 1991).

The Sufi Healing Order, currently under the guidance of Himayat Inayati, offers both training and services in spiritual healing. Some healing services are conducted within a group prayer circle, where Divine help is requested for healing. Members also visit the ill, offering spiritual support. Himayat Inayati incorporates a number of different traditions within his Sufi healing approach (website: www.sufihealingorder.org).

Sufi philosophy has played a major role in influencing traditional medical practices in the Indonesian island of Java (Woodward, 1985). This author noted:

> The Javanese medical system draws on a wide variety of symbols, roles and interactional patterns, none of which may be understood as uniquely medical. Concepts of personhood, cosmology, power and knowledge are melded into a corpus of closely related theories explaining the origins of disease and motivating highly diverse treatment strategies. Medical pluralism is, therefore, an inherent feature of Javanese traditional medicine. There are two primary modes of medical practice. One practiced by Sufi saints (wali) is based on Islamic mystical concepts of miracles and gnosis. The other, practiced by dukun (curers), involves the use of morally suspect forms of magical power.

THE METAPSYCHOLOGY OF SUFISM

Extraordinary feats of healing have been reported of some Sufi Masters (Hussein et al., 1997). One of the largest Sufi schools in the Middle East has followers who have been observed to deliberately cause bodily damage (DCBD phenomena) without subsequent harm to the body and with complete control over pain, bleeding, infection, and rapid wound healing within 4 to 10 seconds (Hussein et al., 1994). This Sufi school is known as *Tariqa Casnazaniyyah,* an Arabic-Kurdish name that means "the way of the secret that is known to no one" (Hussein et al., 1997). Such extraordinary abilities are reported to be accessible to anyone and are not restricted to only a few talented individuals who have years of special training. The ability to accomplish DCBD is believed to be an "others-healing phenomena." This ability is alleged to be transferable based on a spiritual link from the practitioner to the current Shaikh Master of the Tariqa Casnazaniyyah Sufi school (Hussein et al., 1997).

Similar healing phenomena have been observed by Brazilian trance surgeons who often cut into a patient's body for therapeutic purposes. Despite the lack of anesthesia or sterile procedures, there is apparently no postoperative infection, absence of pain, and minimal bleeding, and the patient often claims that he or she was healed.

These phenomena do not appear to be related to hypnosis, relaxation, altered states of consciousness, or trance states such as relaxation or meditative states (Hussein et al., 1996; Hussein et al., 1997). Electroencephalographic recordings reflect the absence of a meditative state during DCBD. Similarly, electroencephalographic recordings of Brazilian trance surgeons confirm that they are not in a meditative state but demonstrate brain activity reflecting hyperarousal. Although such phenomena receive scant attention from the Western scientific community, they may have profound implications for healing serious diseases. There is much to be understood within the metapsychology of the healing field.

CONCLUSION

Sufism is a mystical tradition within Islam and is based on the spirituality of the Prophet Muhammad. Masters of present Sufi schools trace their origins back to the Prophet through a chain of Masters. Sufism can be described as a path or way of attainment to Allah with its possible paranormal powers and knowledge. The psychology of Sufism is also geared toward this attainment. The Sufi way involves following orthodox Islamic practices such as daily prayer, fasting, and some dietary prohibition, as well as frequent worshipful meditation. These practices may have not only spiritual purposes but also many positive health implications. Although Sufism generally is focused on spiritual development, some Sufi schools have focused on healing. This healing is a blend of Sufi philosophy with other Islamic healing traditions. Finally, paranormal Sufi healing abilities have been observed and explained on the basis of a spiritual link with the Sufi Master back to the Prophet and Allah. Such phenomena from the Sufi way do not appear to be due to meditative or altered states of consciousness, but may perhaps be due to a higher consciousness.

Acknowledgments

This research was supported in part by a NIDA Grant #DA07957.

References

Abdalati, H. (1996). Islam in focus. Plainfield: American Trust Publications.

Alexander, F. M. (1910). Man's supreme inheritance: Conscious guidance and control in relation to human evolution in civilization. London: Chaaterson LTD.

Ansha, N. (1991). Principles of sufism. Fremont: Asian Humanities Press.

Benson, H. (1975). The relaxation response. New York: Avon.

Chishti, H. M. (1991). The book of sufi healing. Rochester: Inner Traditions International.

Clarke, P. B. Ed. (1993). The World's religions: Understanding the living faiths. Pleasantville, New York: Reader's Digest.

Dewey, J. (1922). Human nature and conduct. New York: Henry Holt and Company.

Dossey, L. (1996). Prayer is good medicine. San Francisco: Harper.

Farez, S., & Morley, R. S. (1997). Potential animal health hazards of pork and pork products. Revue Scientifique et Technique, 16(1), 65-78.

Friend, M. B. (1957). Group hypnotherapy treatment. Hospital treatment of alcoholism: A comparative, experimental study, Menninger Clinic Monograph series no. 11, 77-120.

Gessner, B. D., & Beller, M. (1994). Protective effect of conventional cooking versus use of microwave ovens in an outbreak of salmonellosis. American Journal of Epidemiology, 139(9):903-909.

Hussein, J. N., Almukhtar, N., Fatoohi, L. J., & Al-Dargazelli, S. S. (1996). The role of ambiguous terminology of consciousness in misunderstanding healing phenomena. Frontier Perspectives, 6(1):27-32.

Hussein, J. N., Fatoohi, L. J., Al-Dargazelli, S., & Almuchtar, N. (1994). The deliberately caused bodily damage phenomena: Mind, body, energy or what? Part 1). International Journal of Alternative and Complementary Medicine, 12:9-11.

Hussein, J. N., Fatoohi, L. J., Hall, H., & Al-Dargazelli, S. (1997). Deliberately caused bodily damage phenomena. Journal of the Society for Psychical Research. 62:97-113.

Khan, H. I. (1983). The music of life. New Lebanon: Omega Publications.

Lings, M. (1977). What is sufism? Berkeley: University of California Press.

McKercher, P. D., Hess, W. R., & Hamdy, F. (1978). Residual viruses in pork products. Applied & environmental microbiology, 16(1):65-78.

Muhaiyaddeen, M. R. B. (1991). Questions of life, answers of wisdom by the contemporary sufi M. R. Bawa Muhaiyaddeen: Volume 1. Philadelphia: The Fellowship Press.

Murray, M. & Pizzorno, J. (1991). Encyclopedia of natural medicine. Rocklin, California: Prima Publishing.

Rumi, J. (1991). Feeling the shoulder of the lion. Putney, Vermont: Threshold Books.

Tauxe, R. V. (1997). Emerging foodborne diseases: An evolving public health challenge. Emerging Infectious Diseases, 3(4):425-434.

Woodward, M. R. (1985). Healing and morality: A javanese example. Social Science & Medicine. 21:1007-1021.

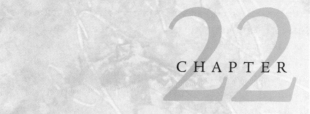

CHAPTER 22

Native American Healing: A Pan-Indian Perspective

RICHARD W. VOSS

VICTOR DOUVILLE

GAYLA TWISS

It is this loss of faith that has left a void in Indian life—a void that civilization cannot fill. The old life was attuned to nature's rhythm—bound by mystical ties to the sun, moon, stars; to the waving grasses, flowing streams and whispering winds. It is not a question (as so many white writers like to state it) of the white man "bringing the Indian up to his plane of thought and action." It is rather a case where the white man had better grasp some of the Indian's spiritual strength. I protest against calling my people savages. How can the Indian, sharing all the virtues of the white man, be justly called a savage? The white race today is but half civilized and unable to order his life into ways of peace and righteousness (Luther Standing Bear, 1931).

These preceding words of Luther Standing Bear provide a sobering orientation toward understanding a pan-Indian perspective of medicine and health. Long

before Columbus landed in what he thought was Hindustan the indigenous peoples of the Americas practiced a highly advanced medicine that was effective in combating diseases then common in the Americas (Iron Shell, 1997; Little Soldier, 1997; Looking Horse, 1997; Red Dog, 1997; Standing Bear, 1933). These medicine ways emphasized the "right order of things" and viewed human beings not as some higher intellectual being above lower animal and inanimate beings but as a kindred partner in the universe (creation), reliant on the other beings in creation for life itself.

However, the world view of the new European visitors to the Americas prompted misunderstandings and exploitation of the peoples they called *Indios*, a corruption of the Spanish, derived from Columbus' perception of the people he encountered in the New

World whom he described as *"una gente en dio,"* which literally means "a people in with God" (Means, 1995).

Tragically this early perception of the natural peacefulness, harmony, and ease of temperament of these "Indians" prompted Columbus to conclude that "they would make excellent slaves" (Means, 1995), setting the stage for the subsequent historical events that led to the degradation of the indigenous or natural people of the Americas who were called *Indians*. The "natural" style of these people was to be perceived as "brutish" and "savage"; their attentiveness to primal experience would be perceived as "primitive"; their understanding of the creation (all of the universe) as infused with life and spirit would be seen as "animistic." In all these assessments what was "Indian" was evaluated as inferior to the European cultural standards, including advanced technology and "higher" (theistic) religion(s).

The term *Indian* was imposed on the indigenous peoples of the Americas erroneously, because they were not a homogeneous group but rather distinct "nations" or "peoples" with different languages, beliefs, customs, social and political structures, and historical rivalries. The term *American Indian* is used today to talk about common values and a certain shared identity among many Native American people, and it is also used as the legal title of federally recognized tribes holding jurisdiction on reservation lands in the United States. The indigenous people of Canada and the Six Nations' People (Iroquois) preferred the term *Natives,* which is the official term used by the Canadian government to identify indigenous people. The terms *American Indian, Native American,* and *Indian People* are used interchangeably throughout this chapter, aware of the historical and political complexity associated with these terms (Means, 1995).

HISTORY

To understand American Indian health care and approaches to medicine, one needs to "get the history right" and take a critical look at the "other" American history that most Americans were never taught and was never included in their textbooks and which, today, continues to be glossed in mainstream American classrooms—the largely invisible history of Native Americans in the United States. Non-Indian people need to learn both sides of American history, to understand the "bad medicine" that has infected relations between Indians and non-Indian people. Recall the interaction between Tosawi, chief of the Comanches and General Sheridan after Tosawi brought the first band of Comanches in to surrender. Addressing Sheridan, Tosawi spoke his own name and two words in English. "Tosawi, good Indian." Sheridan responded with the, now infamous, words: "The only good Indians I ever saw were dead" (Brown, 1970; Ellis, 1990).

Beyond the larger cultural-historical context one also needs to take into consideration the distinctive Indian tribal culture. It is important to know how each tribe dealt with its own survival in the wake of U.S. expansionism, policies of extermination, and the extent to which each tribe was exposed to racial and cultural genocide. It is also important to understand how its tribal leadership related with the U.S. government and to assess the degree of broken trusts and treaties. With this background information one can then develop an awareness of, and sensitivity to, the issues that have an impact on the consciousness and sense of well-being or disease and distrust of government and other social institutions by many Native American people today. One needs to be informed about the issues of loss of land and culture, repeated broken trusts, and unenforced treaties and be sensitive about the forced assimilation policies, programs, and depersonalizing attitudes directed toward Indian people both formally and informally by the U.S. government, missionaries, and other social institutions that were embedded in the "progressive American consciousness" and committed to civilizing and incorporating the Indian into this larger consciousness.

Although some Indian people claim to have benefited from their boarding school experience, the greater number of Indian people are beginning to speak out about the cultural trauma of the boarding school systems. Through assimilation programs, what was "natural" and basic to Indian self-identity was suppressed, discouraged, and literally "beaten out" of them through systematic resocialization. Indian children were separated from their families and their traditional ceremonial practices, which were intimately linked to the extended family and reinforced by social, moral, political, and spiritual life, and introduced to what was perceived as a more civilized (materialistic) view of life, which devastated Indian society (Clark, 1997; Clifford, M., 1997; Douville, 1997;

Little Soldier, 1997; Mestheth, 1993; White Hat, Sr., 1997). For Indian people, all aspects of life were intimately connected to good health and well-being. The interconnections between family, tribe or clan, moral, political, and ceremonial life all contributed to a sense of harmony and balance that was called *wicozani* (good total health) by the Lakota and *hozhon* (harmony, beauty, happiness, and health) by the Navajo. For Indian people, life is like a circle, continuous, harmonious, cyclical, with no distinctions. Medicine was a coming together of all the elements in this circular pattern of life. The circle of healing was formed by the interconnections between the sick person, his or her extended family or relatives, the spirits, the singers who helped with the ceremonial songs, and the medicine practitioner (Figures 22-1 and 22-2).

Therefore, as ceremonial practices were suppressed and as government policies undermined the integrity of traditional Indian practices, the cultural fabric of

Indian peoples was also torn. Official U.S. government assimilation policies forced many traditional Indian medicine practitioners "underground" for risk of being cited for committing actions prohibited by government regulation or being accused of "devil worship" and held up to public ridicule. Archie Fire Lame Deer and Richard Erdoes note that "Between 1890 and 1940, the Sundance, as well as all other native ceremonies, were forbidden under the Indian Offenses Act." They continue, recalling the following:

One could be jailed for just having an Inipi [a sweatlodge ceremony] or praying in the Lakota way, as the government and the missionaries tried to stamp out our old beliefs in order to make us into slightly darker, "civilized" Christians. Many historians believe that during those fifty years no Sundances were performed, but they are wrong. The Sundance was held every year . . . but it had to be done in secret, in lonely places where no white man could spy on us (1992, p. 230).

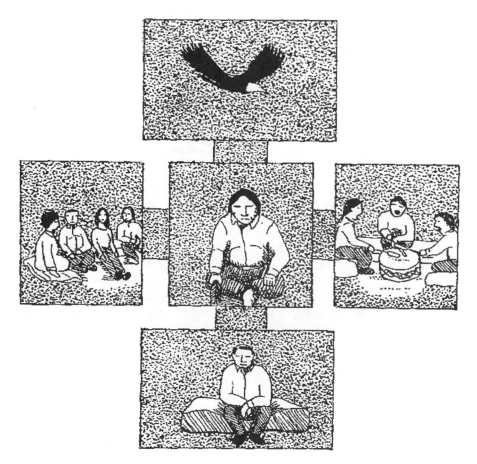

Figure 22-1 Spirits, relatives, singers, and sick person in the shape of two intersecting lines. (Courtesy Sinte Gleska University.)

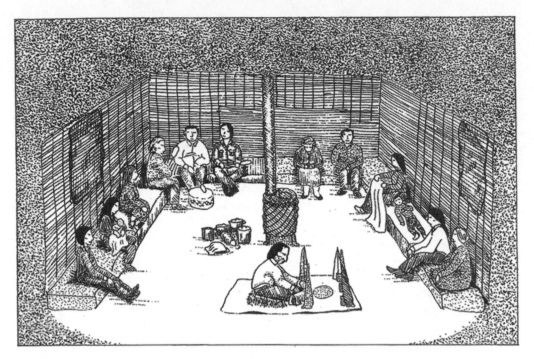

Figure 22-2 All of the elements from Figure 22-1 are depicted in this ceremony of the extended family in the healing process. The drawing shows a quiet gathering of people in a darkened room. (Courtesy Sinte Gleska University.)

Clyde Holler notes the official ban of the Sundance beginning on April 10, 1883, with the enforcement of "Rules for Indian Courts," which were in effect until 1934, with the ban on piercing up until 1952 or later, depending on interpretation (Holler, 1995; see also Commissioner of Indian Affairs, 1883).

Luther Standing Bear reflected on the profound shift that was occurring as he recalled his experience traveling to the Carlisle Indian School as a boy. He wrote:

It was only about three years after the Custer battle, and the general opinion was that the Plains people merely infested the earth as nuisances, and our being there simply evidenced misjudgment on the part of Wakan Tanka. Whenever our train stopped at the railway stations, it was met by great numbers of white people who came to gaze upon the little Indian "savages." The shy little ones sat quietly at the car windows looking at the people who swarmed on the platform. Some of the children wrapped themselves in their blankets, covering all but their eyes. At one place we were taken off the train and marched a distance down the street to a restaurant. We walked down the street between two rows of uniformed men whom we called soldiers, though I suppose they were policemen. This must have been done to protect us, for it was surely known that we boys and girls could do no harm. Back of the rows of uniformed men stood the white people craning their necks, talking, laughing, and making a great noise. They yelled and tried to mimic us by giving what they thought were war-whoops. We did not like this (Standing Bear, 1933).

To this day many older Indian people are reluctant to talk about the older traditional ways, and many middle-age Indian people who were educated in the boarding school system were literally removed from their tribes and forced to assimilate white man's ways. Resocialized in often abusive environments, many never learned the older traditions and their native languages. Often students from western tribes were sent east to the Carlisle Indian School at Carlisle, Pennsylvania, and students from eastern tribes were sent west (e.g., the Nanticokes of Delaware were sent to the Haskell Indian School in Kansas) (Clark, 1997).

Other Indians whose behavior seemed odd or troublesome were sent to the infamous Hiawatha Insane Asylum for Indians, also known as the *Canton In-*

sane Asylum, which was the only segregated asylum built exclusively for American Indians in the United States, located in Canton, South Dakota (Hoover, 1997; Iron Shield, 1992; Putney, 1984). This institution was opened in 1902 as the second federal institution for the insane (predated by St. Elizabeth's Hospital in Washington, DC) to provide psychiatric care exclusively to Indian people by an act of Congress, despite opposition from the Department of the Interior and the Superintendent of St. Elizabeth's Hospital when the bill was first passed by Congress in 1898 (Iron Shield, 1988, 1992). Under the abusive administration of Dr. Harry Hummer, the institution would become the subject of a 150-page report filed by Dr. Samuel Silk in 1929 detailing the abhorrent conditions endured by the patient-residents there.

As a result of Dr. Silk's report, Dr. Hummer was dismissed, and in December of 1933, after further study, the Hiawatha Asylum for Indians was closed, its remaining 71 Indian patients transferred to St. Elizabeth's Hospital. Over the 31 years of operation, the asylum housed 370 Indians. There are 121 Indians buried on the grounds of the former asylum; the causes of these deaths are unknown. Although the asylum was founded "as a place to alleviate the suffering of mentally ill tribesmen from the Indian reservations; it ended as an institution that itself caused genuine human misery" (Putney, 1984). The asylum has since been turned into a community hospital in the 1950s and is now the Canton-Inwood Memorial Hospital. The Indian burial ground is now located next to a public golf course, named the Hiawatha Golf Course, which sits adjacent to the grounds of the asylum in Canton, South Dakota (Iron Shield, 1991, 1994, 1997). Harold Iron Shield is currently leading a movement to identify relatives of those buried at the Canton (Hiawatha) Asylum and is seeking to repatriate their remains to their respective tribes, where possible, and preserve the Cemetery as a National Historic Site.

Medical treatment and health care for American Indians was historically grossly inadequate and often seen as antagonistic with traditional Indian medicine ways (DeMallie & Jahner, 1991). There was no supervision of agency doctors, and "not until 1891 were physicians placed in a classified service and required to pass examinations in addition to having a medical degree" (DeMallie & Jahner, 1991). Charles Alexander Eastman, a Lakota Sioux Indian who served as an agency physician at Pine Ridge from 1890 to 1892,

observed the practice of government-sponsored medical care. He wrote:

> The doctors who were in the service in those days had an easy time of it. They scarcely ever went outside of the agency enclosure, and issued their pills and compounds after the most casual inquiry. As late as 1890, when the Government sent me out as a physician to ten thousand Ogallalla Sioux and Northern Cheyennes at Pine Ridge Agency, I found my predecessor still practicing his profession through a small hole in the wall between his office and the general assembly room of the Indians. One of the first things I did was to close that hole; and I allowed no man to diagnose his own trouble or choose his pills (DeMallie & Jahner, 1991).

Physicians in the Indian Service had to use their own funds and gifts of money from friends to buy medicines and supplies. Drugs supplied to the Indians were "often obsolete in kind, and either stale or of the poorest quality" (DeMallie & Jahner, 1991). In 1893 Dr. Z.T. Daniel recommended that the procedures for Indian Service doctors be reappraised, modernized, and compiled in serviceable form. He also recommended that an agency physician be sent annually as a representative of the American Medical Association, and he urged that Indian Service doctors be supplied with medical textbooks and medical journals (DeMallie & Jahner, 1991).

In light of the inadequate health care provided to Indian people, it is important to keep in mind the decimation Indian people faced by the exposure to Old World diseases. Henry Dobyns estimated that Native people faced serious contagious diseases that caused significant mortality at approximately 4-year intervals from 1520 to 1900 (1983). The pandemics affecting Indian people are often treated by white historians and others as kinds of "natural disasters," never intended by Europeans (Jaimes, 1992). However, Indian people are cognizant of their history and remember their oral history where forms of germ warfare were conducted by military operations against them. One example often cited was the distribution of smallpox-infected blankets by the U.S. Army to Mandan (Indians) at Fort Clark on June 19, 1837, thought to be the causative factor in the smallpox pandemic of 1836-1840 (Chardon, 1932; Jaimes, 1992).

The shame nurtured by decades and centuries of efforts to "civilize the heathen Indian" has taken its toll on our American consciousness. One cannot begin to appreciate traditional Indian medicine ways without a profound awareness at a "gut level" of how much effort went into the eradication of what is now being perceived as "alternative medicine." This is the uneasy starting point of understanding traditional Indian medicine. Within this historical context, one can better perceive the basis for many Indian peoples' objections to the growing "popularity" of their traditional spirituality and healing practices among non-Indians—by the *wasicun* (a Lakota word that described the early white hunter's propensity to take the fatty, choice portion of the buffalo, and leave the rest to rot; Buechel translates it as "One who takes things"). It is a term still used today to express their perception of the narrow, materialistic, and destructive worldview of mainstream white culture. Interest among whites in seeking out "Indian medicine men and shamans" and the resultant exploitation of Indian ceremonies, through buying Indian spirituality in weekend or half-day workshops, seminars, and paying fees for sweatlodge ceremonies, and so on, has prompted some Lakota leaders to issue a "declaration of war" against such exploitation (Mestheth et al., 1993). There are strong feelings about the contemporary curiosity of whites about Indian medicine ways.

WILLIAM PENN'S ACCOUNT OF TENOUGHAN'S SWEATBATH

One of the earliest accounts of a European observing an American Indian healing ceremony is in William Penn's Own Account of the Lenni Lenape or Delaware Indians (Meyers, 1970). The account portrays a number of things relevant to understanding Indian medicine ways and the quality of interaction of Indian people with Europeans. The account cited here is Penn's observation of a Lenape man named Tenoughan involved in a healing sweatbath.

I called upon an Indian of Note, whose Name was Tenoughan, the Captain General of the Clan of Indians of those Parts. I found him ill of a Fever, his Head and Limbs much affected with Pain, and at the same time his Wife preparing a Bagnio for him: The Bagnio resembled a large Oven, into which he crept, by a Door on the one side, while she put several red hot Stones in a small Door on the other side thereof, and fastened the Doors as closely from the Air as she could. Now while he was Sweating in this Bagnio, his Wife (for they disdain no Service) was, with an Ax, cutting her Husband a passage into the River,

(being the Winter of 83 the great Frost, and the Ice very thick) in order to the Immersing himself, after he should come out of his Bath. In less than half an Hour, he was in so great a Sweat, that when he came out he was as wet, as if he had come out of a River, and the Reak or Steam of his Body so thick, that it was hard to discern any bodies Face that stood near him. In this condition, stark naked (his Breech-Clout only excepted) he ran into the River, which was about twenty Paces, and duck'd himself twice or thrice therein, and so return'd (passing only through his Bagnio to mitigate the immediate stroak of the Cold) to his own House, perhaps 20 Paces further, and wrapping himself in his woolen Mantle, lay down as his length near a long (but gentle) Fire in the midst of his Wigwam, or House, turning himself several times, till he was dry, and then he rose, and fell to getting us Dinner, seeming to be as easie, and well in Health, as at any other time (Surveyor General Thomas Holme's letter, dated 5th Month [May] 7, 1688, concerning the running of a survey line) (Meyers, 1970).

Penn made this observation when he was on a surveying expedition of the "farthest northern region of his Provence," which was actually near Monocacy, Berks County, Pennsylvania, today about a 45-minute commute from Philadelphia. The river would be the Schuylkill River, now polluted by a century of industrial contaminants and washoff from coal mines and agriculture farther north. This old account provides a powerful illustration of the cultural chasm that separated Penn from Tenoughan's world of medicine and health care. What this story conveys is the tremendous gap in appreciating what was happening during the observation. Penn was intent on buying land from the Lenape people, so it was on an economic venture that he stumbled on a healing bath taken by Tenoughan, a Lenape leader of some stature.

The story provides a model for understanding the complexity and the obstacles that confront non-Indian people, embedded in Eurocentrism, in non-comprehending Indian medicine ways. Penn was struck by the exotic and the unusual nature of the event he witnessed, as well as the apparent efficacy of the sweatbath on Tenoughan, but the observation lacks any real personal encounter between Penn and Tenoughan, although we read that *Tenough* served dinner for his guests after the sweatbath. As old and as minimally detailed as this account is, it illustrates a number of important insights into American Indian medicine and health care.

First of all, the sweatbath was located near Tenoughan's home. It was familiar, literally, in his back yard. Second, the practice included the assistance by a family member, Tenoughan's wife who actually prepared the sweatbath for him, carried the red hot stones into the Bagnio, and assisted in closing the door securely. Much of Indian medicine is family-oriented. It is not something that is done by strangers. It is a family matter; family is intimately involved and plays a significant role in the healing process. Later Tenoughan's wife assisted in the arduous task of cutting a path through the ice for the "patient" to plunge into the river. Indian medicine often brings the patient into close interaction with the natural world and the elements. After the sweatbath Tenoughan rests by the fire in his wigwam, and he then serves dinner to his guests. For many Indian people stone, fire, air, water, food, spirits, and social and familial relationships are seen as medicine.

CULTURE

Sutton and Broken Nose cite a powerful clinical vignette about how the cultural differences can create real tension between expectations of clinical practitioners from the dominant culture and Indian sensibilities and practices. Although they cite the experience of a social worker sent to run an alternative school program on a Montana Indian reservation, the setting could be any health care or service-oriented setting. The vignette is quoted in the following:

One day I came into work and no one was there. There were no teachers, students, or counselors. At first I thought it was Saturday or some holiday I had forgot about. I checked my calendar and the one the tribe printed to see if it was some special kind of Indian holiday, but it was not. Finally, I went riding around in my car. I saw one of the counselors and asked where everyone was. He said Albert Running Horse had died. I found out later that Albert was one of the oldest men in the tribe and was somehow related to almost everyone at school. When I tried to find out when everyone would be back at work, I couldn't get a definite answer because they weren't sure when some of Albert's relatives would come in from out of state. I was upset because I felt we had been making progress with some particularly difficult cases. I was concerned about the continuity of therapy and the careful schedule we had all worked out. When I expressed my frustration to one of my counselors she just shrugged her shoulders and said we all have to grieve. All I could think of is how am I going to explain this to my superiors (in McGoldrick et al., 1996).

This example illustrates the fundamental difference in worldview between Indian and non-Indian Americans and presents a common "clinical dilemma" that is likely to occur between mainstream approaches to health care and the "natural" approach to healing and human relationships typical among Indian people. Which is the better medicine, following the prescribed treatment plan or attending to the sense of community loss and grief on the death of an esteemed elder? Health care practitioners need to look for ways to affirm and support the values, beliefs, and needs of Indian people. Conversely, these values, beliefs, and needs may well be the same for non-Indian people as well, but denied in the face of economic expediency. Appreciating the impact of diverse cultures on medical and health care practice is essential and is perhaps the most important thing the health care practitioner needs to address in developing cultural competence with Indian people or with any group not often credited or valued by the larger, dominant culture.

First, the concept of "professional helper/healer" is foreign to traditional Indian peoples and has no precedent in prereservation Lakota society. The idea of "paid professionals" conflicts with the tradition that "helping other people" is a social responsibility for everyone, not just for a few. Professional/paid health care practitioners are often viewed with suspicion by some traditionalists as governmental "agents of forced assimilation." Along with government-sanctioned missionary activity, the legacy of Indian boarding schools, and psychiatric hospitalization, health care professionals were associated with oppressive social structures that were intended to "civilize the Indian." So, a Lakota-centric view of health care starts with the awareness of the power of the institutionalized systems (e.g., social, health care, educational systems) to influence and assert social control, which although aimed at "improved health care" or social well being, may also reflect and enact the larger, more pervasive oppression of racist attitudes, policies, and procedures of "civilizing the Indian."

Although there were no permanent or paid professional "health care providers" as such among the Lakota bands or tribes in prereservation days, various individuals, groups, and societies within Lakota bands provided health care functions to the people. In effect, every tribal member was expected to follow the "natural law of creation" or the *Wo-ope*, the unwritten natural law that guides Lakota life, which emphasizes unselfishness and generosity. The *Wo'ope* embodies the philosophy of *mitakuye oyas'in,* which, according to White Hat Sr. "is what keeps us together." It is the knowledge "that we come from one source, and we are all related." However, to make this work, "we must identify the good and evil in us, and practice what is good" (White Hat, Sr., 1997). Lakota philosophy does not separate good and evil, sickness and health, right and wrong as distinct realities, they coexist in each person, in every creation, even in the most sacred thing there is good and evil. The important thing is to understand that there is the negative and the positive within everyone and everything, and to be responsible in one's life to live in a good, moral, healthy way, in balance with all creation.

The natural law is the way nature acts. Understanding Lakota philosophy begins with understanding the natural law or the seven laws of the Creator (Iron Shell, 1997; Looking Horse, M., 1997; Lunderman, 1997). The "natural law" or the *Wo'ope* required each person to exercise shared values, which, if acted on in one's life, gave the person and the extended family *(tios'-paye)* and the tribe *wicozani,* which was understood as total or perfect health, balance and harmony, good social health, and well being (Iron Shell, 1997); it implies physical and spiritual health (White Hat, Sr., 1997).

Another orienting value of helpers and healers among the Lakota is *Nagi'ksapa,* or self-wisdom is the awareness of your aura/spirit (Iron Shell, 1997). White Hat, Sr., translates and explains the *nagi'ksapa* as "one's spirit, the wise spirit in a person." White Hat, Sr., notes that "The Lakota are very much aware of the spirit within [us]—we talk to our spirit—we ask our spirit to be strong and to help us in our decisions" and life (1997). *Iha'kicikta* is the ability to look out for one another. If you move camp, you should be concerned that everyone is going to move together. You want to make sure there is enough water and food for everyone (Iron Shell, 1997). *Wo'onsila* is the ability to have pity on each other (Iron Shell, 1997). Albert White Hat, Sr., explains the word as "recognizing a specific need of someone or something, and you address that (specific) need." According to White Hat, Sr., Lakota philosophy does not encourage people to "stay stuck" or dependent. *Iyus'kiniya* is the ability to go do things with a happy attitude (Iron Shell, 1997). *Wi'ikt ceya* is the measure of wealth by how little one has; it is the capacity to give to others; it is one's capacity for self-sacrifice (Iron Shell, 1997). *Teki'ci'hilapi*

is the ability to cherish, esteem, and treasure each other (Iron Shell, 1997). Practicing these social values ensured good social functioning.

The primary orientation of traditional Indian medicine was universalistic. Health and welfare resources were made available to everyone through their family and community. Prereservation Lakota society emphasized tribalism over individualism, social harmony over self-interest, and a commitment or loyalty to the people or the larger extended family relations over individual success. Health care functions were accomplished by one's extended family *(tios'paye);* it was the extended family that provided for the social support and material assistance of all its members. Wealth was distributed through the practice of the give-away ceremony *(wopila),* which is still practiced by traditional Lakotas. This practice ensured that no one person's or one family's wealth or resources dominated.

Mental and physical health are viewed as inseparable from spiritual and moral health. The good balance of the one's life in harmony with the *Wo'ope* or natural law of creation, brings about *wicozani* or good health, which was both individual and communal. Rather than viewing the individual as a mind-body split, which has influenced much of western psychiatric thinking, traditional Lakota philosophy viewed the individual person as an unexplainable creation with four constituent dimensions of self, which included the following: *nagi* or one's individual soul. Buechel translates the word as "The soul, spirit; the shadow of anything, as of a man *(wicanagi)* or of a house *(tinagi)*" (1983). The *nagi la* is the divine spirit immanent in each human being; *niya* or "the vital breath" gives life to the body and is responsible for the circulation of the blood and the breathing process. The fourth element of the person is the *sicun* or "intellect" (Goodman, 1992, p. 41). Albert White Hat, Sr., however, describes the *sicun* as "your (spirit's) presence [that] is felt on something or somebody." Beuchel translated the word as "That in a man or thing which is spirit or spiritlike and guards him from birth against evil spirits" (1983). Often a person appeals to his *nagi la* for assistance. This is a power within each person that can help him or her overcome obstacles. When one goes on the *hanbleceya* or pipe-fast, one leaves the physical world as a *nagi.*

According to Gene Thin Elk, "we are not humans on a soul journey. We are nagi, 'souls,' who are making a journey through the material world,"

(Goodman, 1992). The *nagi la* has been described as the "little spirit," which is the "divine spirit immanent in each being" (Goodman, 1992). Existence in the material world is tenuous for the newborn, according to Lakota philosophy: Ms. Edna Little Elk commented: "The most important things for infants and little children are to eat good, sleep good and play good" and by doing so, the *nagi* of the child is persuaded to become more and more attached to its own body (Goodman, 1992). Traditional Lakota philosophy sees abuse, rejection, or neglect affecting the child's *nagi*, where it may detach from the child's body and not come back. In this case ceremonies are conducted by a medicine man to find the child's *nagi* and bring it back (Goodman, 1992). Such a condition has been called *soul loss*. So, good mental or emotional health is intimately related to good spiritual, moral, and physical health; these cannot be separated out.

CONTRIBUTIONS OF INDIAN PEOPLE TO MEDICINE AND HEALTH CARE

Despite the fact that Native American people have ancient oral traditions of healing and helping tribal members in need during reservation times, prereservation times, and the traumatic transition periods in between (Douville, 1997; Lunderman, 1997; Red Dog, 1997), much of the health care literature reviewed focused on practice issues concerning Native American people where they were viewed primarily as a special client or health care risk-group in need of a specialized approach to treatment (DuBray, 1985, 1992; Garrett & Garrett, 1994; Good Tracks, 1973; Williams & Ellison, 1996). This literature generally treats "Native Americans" as a generic, homogeneous group and does not examine specific tribal traditions or practices of help and healing indigenous to specific tribal traditions.

DuBray calls for a more holistic approach to treatment intervention based on Native American (Lakota) practices. DuBray (1992) discusses the use of the vision quest, the importance of food as a symbol of love and respect, the role of cultural healing ceremonies, and the importance of the collective unconscious in Indian experience of reality. The contributions of Native American practices, philosophies, and traditions of help and healing have also been discussed in anthropological studies

(Wallace, 1958), rehabilitation medicine (Braswell & Wong, 1994; Hodge, 1989), nursing (Reynolds, 1993; Turton, 1995), and psychiatric literatures (Garro, 1990; Hammerschlag, 1988, 1992; Lewis, 1982, 1990). There is a growing use of traditional medicine ways in alcohol treatment programs for American Indians, both on and off the reservation (Hall, 1985, 1986; Red Dog, 1997; Thin Elk, 1995), as well as in health programs for Indian children and youth (e.g., Healthy Nations Program at the Cheyenne River Sioux Tribe, Red Dog, 1997).

The timing is ripe for health care and medical educators to look carefully at how native practices, traditions, and values can shape theory, practice, and policy at a foundational level, particularly important as tribal governments develop strategies and responses to welfare reform with the implementation of the Temporary Assistance to Needy Families (TANF) program, which is being met with great concern by many Native American tribal leaders and health care providers (Goldsmith, 1996).

ORIENTING CONCEPTS TO INDIAN MEDICINE

In a report to the National Institutes of Health, *Alternative Medicine: Expanding Medical Horizons* (1992), the Lakota (Sioux Tribe) were cited for the use of healing ceremonies by specialists who are essentially shamanic in their approach to treatment. Although the report cites key ceremonies and practices used by healers and helpers, the report reflects a number of important inaccuracies. To understand Indian medicine ways, one cannot rely solely on written accounts. Although written ethnographical studies may provide a wealth of descriptive data, it is best to talk to authoritative sources personally.

Although the sweatlodge, Sundance, and vision quest are all used by Lakotas for health, help, and healing, not all were always conducted by "medicine women" or "medicine men." The report tends to project an exclusivity of these ceremonies when in fact there is considerable variation and scope for these practices, most of which were family-oriented (Douville, *Personal communication*, September 5, 1997).

The sweatlodge or "purification ceremony," for example, is very common and may be conducted by anyone who has "been on the hill" or completed the *hanbleceya*, often called the "vision quest" (Figure 22-3).

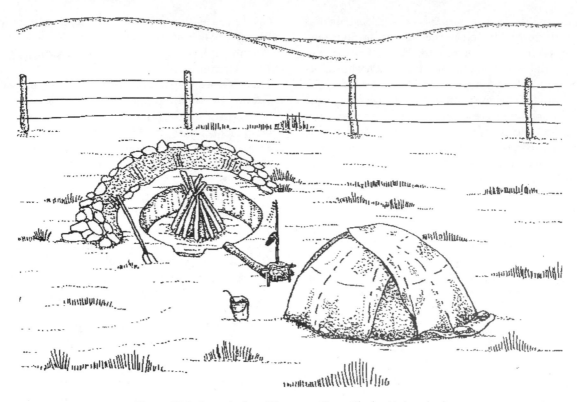

Figure 22-3 Sweatlodge. (Courtesy Sinte Gleska University.)

Although the English name emphasizes the physiological reaction of the "sweat," this ceremony of the common man (Lakota: *ikce wicasa*), it is really an encounter with one's spiritual self and one's spirit relatives. This is a purification that "gives life" (*inipi'kogapi,* that which gives life) to the participants and represents a kind of rebirth. This is a family-oriented ceremony and is an integral part of all other Lakota ceremonies. Participants enter a small lodge made of willow saplings (for support) and covered with heavy-darkening canvas. Between 7 and 16 or more red-hot stones are brought into this little lodge, which can be 10 to 15 feet in diameter. The stones represent the "first creation" and have deep spiritual meaning in this ceremony. Water is poured over the stones by someone who is permitted to conduct this ceremony, and the steam from this generates intense heat. There is deep spiritual significance to this.

Family members usually participate in this ceremony on a regular basis. Often, sweatlodges are located behind one's home. There is a prohibition that excludes menstruating women from ceremonies out of respect for the ceremony the woman's body is undergoing (i.e., menstruation, which is seen by Lakota people as a purification with its own proper spiritual power). This is often viewed by white culture as "discriminatory," but the tradition is not intended to be discriminatory. It is an affirmation of the natural feminine power, which white culture tends to minimize (e.g., menstruation is often viewed as a handicap or a problem [e.g., PMS]).

There are also different kinds of "medicine" people among the Lakota. It is hard to generalize the diverse functions by the English term "medicine man/woman." The Lakota practiced common medicines that included herbal remedies that were known to families whose primary medical care was prevention and geared to building up the immune system (Douville, *Personal communication,* September 5, 1997). The various common medicines included teas, ointments, and smudging (smoke from burning certain herbs, e.g., prairie sage or "flat cedar"). This first line of medical care was performed by knowledgeable family members or friends. When required, more spiritual consultations were sought from a shaman medicine man or an interpreter for the *Wakantanka* (the great mystery in all creation), which represents sacred medicine.

A "ceremony" may be requested by the patient and is usually held at night with family members, close friends, and singers (see Figure 22-2). Usually the patient presents a sacred pipe to the medicine man who will smoke it if he accepts the request. The ceremony (which usually describes a *Lowanpi* or a spirit ceremony) takes place in a darkened room in the home. All furniture is removed and the windows are covered. Certain ceremonial objects are used (e.g., various colored flags, tobacco offerings, and earth). During the ceremony the Spirits instruct the medicine man or interpreter on what remedies would be provided by *Unci Maka* (Grandmother Earth) to heal the patient. This process is done with the support of the *tios'paye* or the extended family for the *wicozani* (good health) of the patient.

Along with these practices, family members actively participated in a ceremonial life, which revolved around the *wo'ope* or "natural law of creation," which included the behaviors and attitudes for right living. The *wo'ope* is embodied in the philosophy of *mitakuye oyas'in,* which recognizes that all things, persons, and creations (both animate and inanimate, seen and unseen) are related (White Hat, Sr., 1997). These laws are not written down anywhere; they are learned through observing the creation. These behaviors for right living were reinforced by the ceremonial life of the extended family system or *tios'paye.*

Health care was primarily an extended family matter. Medical care was common and free to everyone who needed it, because the herbs or materials for ceremonies used natural elements that could be harvested from nature's bounty. Although medical care was "free," it was not provided without cost, because in Lakota philosophy when someone gives you something, you are expected to return it fourfold the value. When treated by healers, the people who received help gave something back. The concept of receiving "something for nothing" is not part of Indian philosophy (White Hat, Sr., 1997). The Lakota philosophy encourages self-reliance *and* mutual relations. Something changed when white man's medicine became institutionalized in the United States, emphasizing intervention over prevention; the individual over the tribe or extended family; materialism over spirituality; the physical body-self over the spirit-body-self.

TRENDS IN CONTEMPORARY INDIAN MEDICINE AND HEALTH CARE

Today many of the old Indian healing traditions are experiencing a renaissance and are beginning to be viewed with a renewed sense of respect and credibility as an alternative and complement to more invasive or secular Western medical models of treatment (Hall, 1985, 1986; NIH Report, 1992; Thin Elk, 1995a, b, c). For example, on the Cheyenne River Indian Reservation at Eagle Butte, the tribal council approved alcohol treatment programs and delinquency prevention programs based on traditional methods and approaches to helping people with alcoholism (viewed as a problem with social, emotional, physical, and spiritual dimensions) (Red Dog, 1997; Thin Elk, 1995). These traditional methods include the *Inipi* or purification ceremony (popularly called the *sweatlodge*), the *Hanbleceya* or pipe fast (often called the *vision quest*), and the *Wiwang Wacipi* or the gazing-at-the-sun dance. The infusion of these ceremonies within the treatment process, collectively, has been called the *Red Road Approach* (Thin Elk, 1995a, b, c).

A number of medical facilities on various reservations include medicine men as consultants on a formal and informal basis (Clifford, 1997; Douville, 1997; Erickson, 1997; Twiss, 1997) and the use of traditional ceremonies in health care settings is encouraged and respected (Erickson, Rosebud Indian Health Services Hospital, 1997; Richards, Rapid City Regional Hospital, 1997). Where the ceremonial burning of sage (a common medicinal herb burned for purification) had been discouraged in the past, hospital staff report increased acceptance of this practice and now arrange appropriate space for traditional ceremonial practices both within the health care facility and outside on hospital grounds (Erickson, 1997; Richards, 1997). One Lakota friend commented on his recent hospitalization at an allopathic hospital. He was visited by a medicine man who placed a bundle of sage under his pillow. This made him feel better and showed how simple cooperation between allopathic medicine and health care practices, and alternative health care practices, can be.

Rapid City Regional Hospital has initiated a Diversity Committee to discuss cultural sensitivity in both employee-administration and staff-patient relationships and credits this committee for improved retention rates of Indian staff (Montgomery, 1997).

The Diversity Committee, which meets monthly, provides an opportunity to surface areas of cultural awareness, tension, and misperception, whereby understanding across culture can take place. Conflicts in cultural views and values are inevitable, but there are growing opportunities for understanding and joint efforts.

Mike Richards, Discharge Planner and Liaison with the tribes at Rapid City Regional Hospital, noted one situation in which a Lakota client was discharged to his extended family. The plan was for the child to live in a tent in the backyard. This plan was challenged by State Social Services, failing to recognize that it is not uncommon for Lakota children to share close space in the family home or relative home. During my visits and stays with Lakota friends, it was not uncommon to see many children from an extended family share a small space in the family dwelling, or outbuildings or tents on the family compound or community *(tios'paye)* during the summer months. Although this practice might be considered "inappropriate" based on middle-class white standards, it affirms the Lakota value of close kinship bonds and enjoyment of children and is illustrative of the "bifurcating-merging family structure," a traditional Lakota kinship structure that considered parallel family relationships (e.g., one's aunts and uncles as "mothers" and "fathers"). Close kinship among all family members was reinforced by this family structure, whereby households and family resources were shared generously (Douville, 1997; also in Driver, 1969).

The mental health liaison to the tribe advocated the child's return to his extended family, and the plan was eventually approved. The case illustrates how simple cultural misunderstanding can occur when service delivery is not centered on the values, family system organization, and beliefs of the traditional Indian perspective. Further illustrating this cultural insensitivity at a structural level is the fact that reservation housing financed by HUD grants are on a lottery basis and "invent" communities that are not based on natural extended family relationships. This social invention (i.e., building housing developments and populating them on the basis of governmental criteria) often conflicts with the natural, familial basis of the *tios'paye* or extended family system of Lakota people (Lunderman Jr., 1977). Such practices undermine the natural sense of community among Indian people and unwittingly create community tensions.

There is active cooperation between medical practitioners and traditional medicine men on Lakota reservations. Referrals are made both ways; medicine men will refer patients to medical doctors when they have exhausted their repertoire of remedies, and medical doctors will refer to medicine men when they have exhausted their treatment repertoire. The relations between traditional and medical health care providers appear cooperative and fluid. Antagonism between these distinct and complementary approaches to health care is not apparent presently.

Although traditional Western psychiatric thought has emphasized the mechanics of the mind, traditional American Indian philosophy looks at the "natural" flow of the individual's spirit-body-mind-self in relation to everything that is. The Lakota term *mitakuye oyas'in* is often heard during ceremonies reminding and reaffirming the participants of their relationships to ancestral spirits, powers, and energies of creation, and their kinship relatives or *tios'paye,* the extended family and community. All of these elements are considered essential for *wicozani* or good health. The notion of *mitakuye oyas'in* is consistent with family systems' theory that looks at the impact of intergenerational family dynamics on the present functioning of family members.

Shamanic traditions and healing practices are very active among traditional American Indians today and seem to be gaining ground after generations of official and unofficial prohibitions and sanctions. There is diversity among traditional Indian tribal practices. Unlike the tribes of the Southwest in which the repetition of specific prayer formulas are required in ceremony and in which traditions have long been rigorously insulated from encroachments by the dominant white culture, the Lakotas have been much more open and receptive to sharing knowledge and technology with others, and they have a much more fluid ceremonial practice where the Lakota medicine people rely on their spirit helpers to "give them permission" to treat people and conduct ceremonies (Holler, 1995; Little Soldier, 1997; Running, 1987; Smith, 1987; Twiss, 1997). This permission is very specific (e.g., a medicine man may be instructed to use certain herbal medicines for men only or women only or people in general). The spirits work through the healer. The medicine man is only as effective as the spirits "working through him." He is responsible and accountable to the spirits for everything. This is a grave responsibility that these people accept.

Perhaps one of the most important trends in Indian health care today is the concern about the impact of welfare reform on Indian peoples, along with the national trend of individual states to reduce welfare rolls and move Medicaid services under managed care providers. An article that appeared in *JAMA (The Journal of the American Medical Association)* noted that American Indians know a lot about government program reforms. "If some people had had their way, Native American tribes would have been reformed out of existence a century ago. So it's not surprising that members of some 500 federally recognized tribes that remain are wary when talk in their locality turns to 'health care reform' " (Goldsmith, 1996, p. 1786).

At present, the Indian Health Service (IHS), a federally administered Indian health care program that is accredited by the Joint Commission on Accreditation of Healthcare Organizations (JCAHO), is facing severe budget deficits, overall receiving only 50% to 75% of what it needs to operate (Goldsmith, 1996, p. 1787). At the same time IHS Director Michael H. Trujillo, MD, MPH, reported that the service population has increased by more than 2 percent per year. It is safe to say that although there have been increasing federal appropriations for IHS over the years, the actual amount of "real money" has gone down (Goldsmith, 1996). For many Indian people the IHS is the only medical provider in their often remote areas, serving a population with disproportionately higher incidence rates of diabetes and cervical cancer, for example, than the general American population (Goldsmith, 1996). In the wake of anticipated health care reform, Dr. Gerald Hill, the Director of the Center for American Indian and Minority Health in the Institute for Health Services Research at the University of Minnesota, reminds health care planners of the statistic that in the American Indian population 31% of the people die before their forty-fifth birthday (Goldsmith, 1996). The present situation of Indian health care is at another critical crossroad.

CONCLUSION

A pan-Indian perspective of health care and medicine challenges the intervention model and offers a prevention model as the starting place for social health and assistance. A Lakota-centric view of health and wellness prioritizes a universal approach to health care opposed to an exceptional approach typical of most Western medicine today in the United States. Traditional Lakota values emphasize the participation of the family in the healing process, including the extended family, as well as the larger kinship community to bring about *wicozani* or good health. The help and healing process is not impersonal, but rather is highly personalized and individualized around specific needs. This personal dimension touches on all of reality (creation) as fundamentally relational and ecological, challenging the mechanism of Cartesian dualism. For the Lakotas and other Indian peoples there is no split or dualism in reality or creation. Health and sickness, good and evil, mind and body are intrinsic, interrelated, and unified. The roles of medicine practitioners include that of healer, counselor, politician, and priest (Figure 22-4).

Another important contribution of a pan-Indian perspective of health is that it provides a rich topology of spirit. The human creation, like all creations, is a spirit-being composed of multilayered aspects of spirit. "Spirit" here is not some "supernatural" reality outside the human being, but it is an intrinsic dimension of everything that is, including the human creation (person). To speak of human beings is to speak about spiritual reality. Medical treatment or any kind of social or human/mental health service is first and foremost a spiritual endeavor. A pan-Indian view of medicine and health care forces us to look at a broader, more encompassing view of the human person. Rather than taking a narrow biomedical approach, a pan-Indian view of health and well-being looks at the human being as part of a lively and interacting bio-psycho-social-spiritual creation, in which the human person is viewed as a peer to other beings in a highly personalized universe and is intimately related to all creation (i.e., the natural world of plants, animals, insects, fish, stone, earth, fire, air, water, wind, and spirit entities).

The human being, or to use the Lakota term, the *ikce wicasa,* is the common (wo)man—a peer to all other beings. He or she is not above creation and as a peer depends on good relations with all the other creations for survival and good health. If anything, the human creation is the most needy of all the created beings and depends on the medicine of other beings (e.g., plant nations and various animal nations) to overcome sickness. The Lakota view of life is based on a radical mutuality, interrelationships, and respect among all the members or peoples of creations. They have no word for "animal," the birds belong to a na-

WHAT IS A MEDICINE MAN?

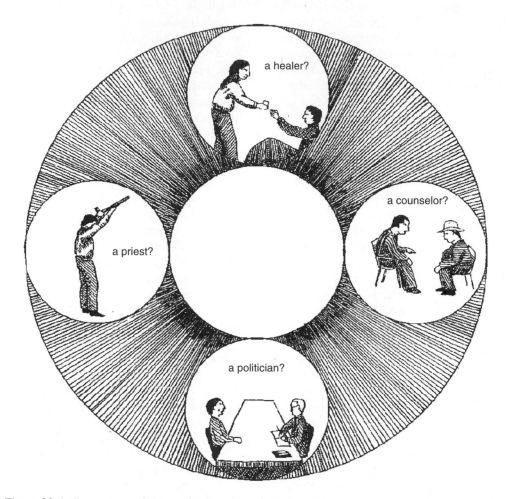

Figure 22-4 Illustration of the multiple roles of the medicine man: healer, priest, counselor, politician. (Courtesy Sinte Gleska University.)

tion and have status as everything does (Smith, 1989; White Hat, Sr., 1997).

The most obvious implication of a pan-Indian perspective of health care and medicine is that it compels health care educators and practitioners to begin "indigenizing" our own consciousness, not only about the "missing chapter" in our introductory textbooks but also the fundamental influence of Western materialism and Eurocentrism on our thinking.

As we begin to take multicultural perspectives seriously, the Eurocentrism of our epistomologies, pedagogies, and professional practice of medical and health services will come under greater scrutiny, and we may even question some long-held beliefs about how to provide medical and health services. There will be a greater awareness of the role and importance of spirituality, shamanic practices, and the role of common or herbal remedies as a complement to clinical practice. Finally, there will be a reaffirmation of the importance of grass-roots community development in health care delivery services and an expanding awareness of the prescribed limitations of our dominant Eurocentric models of help and healing in the United States, and the increasing need, as well as opportunities, to incorporate alternative and complementary models of health care in our mainstream health care services (see Chapter 1).

The increasing cooperative relations between medical and health care service personnel and traditional Indian medicine practitioners provides ground for encouragement that a multicultural approach is not only possible but is also actually taking root in Indian country. It is time for the diverse medical and health care disciplines to learn more about Native American and pan-Indian ways of healing and health. The benefits of this cross-cultural collaboration not only affect Indian people but everyone in the larger culture who will benefit from greater access to a more holistic health care model recognizing both the physiological and spiritual causes of disease and sickness, as well as the efficacy of both biological and spiritual remedies.

Endnote

Indian people are understandably wary of the written word. Some may criticize the inclusion of this chapter in this edition. This criticism is understandable, because often the written word objectifies understandings and can be manipulated outside of the relationship in which the understanding was shared. This is a concern and a risk in contributing this chapter to the second edition of *Fundamentals of Complementary and Alternative Medicine*. However, not to include a chapter about American Indian views about medicine and health care is also a concern, because it helps perpetuate the invisibility of Indian people amidst the dominant social, political, and religious factions. The untold history of Native American people is a sobering context through which one must view contemporary concerns. The purpose of this chapter is to honor the continuing journey of understanding between medical science practitioners and traditional Indian medicine practitioners to see how these two medicine paths can help restore health to the people and to bring about increased understanding—*wo'wableza*—among peoples. This chapter is not intended to encourage "mixing" Indian medicine with allopathic or "alternative" medicines, but rather to emphasize the importance of respecting the integrity of each of these paths in bringing health and help to people in need.

Hecetu'yelo! *(Lakota: "the way it is")*

References

Alternative Medicine: Expanding Medical Horizons. (1992). A Report to the National Institutes of Health on Alternative Medical Systems and Practices in the United States. Washington, DC: U.S. Government Printing Office.

Black Elk. (1953). The Sacred Pipe: Black Elk's Account of the Seven Rites of the Oglala Sioux, Recorded and Edited by Joseph Epes Brown, Norman, Oklahoma: University of Oklahoma Press.

Braswell, M. Ellen and Henry D. Wong. (1994). Perceptions of rehabilitation counselors regarding Native American healing practices. The Journal of Rehabilitation, April-June 1994, v60, 2, pp. 33-43.

Brown, Dee. (1970). Bury My Heart at Wounded Knee: An Indian History of the American West. New York: Henry Holt and Company.

Chardon, Francis A. (1932). Journal at Fort Clark. 1834-39. State Historical Society of South Dakota, Pierre.

Clark, Charles, Jr. (1997). Personal Communication, Member and Tribal Historian of the Nanticoke Tribe, Millsboro, Delaware.

Clifford, Berdette. (1997). Personal Communication, Dean, Human Services Department, Sinte Gleska University, Mission, South Dakota, June 21.

Clifford, Marvin. (1997). Personal Communication, member of Pine Ridge Sioux Tribe, Rapid City, South Dakota, June 10.

Commissioner of Indian Affairs. (1872-92). Annual Report of the Commissioner of Indian Affairs to the Secretary of the Interior. Washington, DC: Government Printing Office.

Deloria, Ella Cara. (1988). Waterlily, Afterword by Raymond J. DeMallie, Lincoln, Nebraska: University of Nebraska Press.

DeMallie, Raymond, and Elaine A. Jahner, editors. (1991). Lakota Belief and Ritual: James R. Walker. Lincoln, NB: University of Nebraska Press.

Dobyns, Henry F. (1983). Their Numbers Become Thinned: Native American Population Dynamics in Eastern North America. Knoxville, Tennessee: University of Tennessee Press, p. 24.

Douville, Victor. (1997). Personal Communication, member of Rosebud Sioux Tribe, Sinte Gleska University, Mission, South Dakota, June 12.

Driver, Harold E. (1969). Indians of North America (Second Edition, Revised), Chicago: The University of Chicago Press.

DuBray, Wynne Hanson. (1992). Human Services and American Indians, Minneapolis/St.Paul: West Publishing Company.

DuBray, Wynne Hanson. (1985). American Indian Values: Critical Factor in Casework, Social Casework, 66,1, pp. 30-37.

Ellis, Edward S. (1900). The History of Our Country. Indianapolis, p. 1483.

Erikson, Jill. (1997). Personal Communication, Intake Social Worker, Indian Health Services Hospital, Rosebud, South Dakota.

Garrett, J.T. and Michael Walkingstick Garrett. (1994). The Path of Good Medicine: Understanding and Counseling Native American Indians, Journal of Multicultural Counseling and Development, Vol. 22, pp. 134-144.

Garro, L.D. (1990). Continuity and change: the interpretation of illness in Anishnaabe (Ojibway) community. Culture, Medicine and Psychiatry, 14, pp. 417-454.

Goldsmith, Marsha F. (1996). First Americans face their latest challenge: Indian health care meets state Medicaid reform. JAMA, The Journal of the American Medical Association, June 19, 1996 v275, n23, p. 1786.

Good Tracks, J.G. (1973). Native American non-interference, Social Work, 18,6, pp. 30-34.

Goodman, Ronald. (1992). Lakota Star Knowledge: Studies in Lakota Stellar Theology, (Second Edition), Rosebud, South Dakota: Sinte Gleska University.

Hall, Roberta. (1985). Distribution of the Sweat Lodge in Alcohol Treatment Programs, Current Anthropology 26,1, pp. 134-135.

Hall, Roberta. (1986). Alcohol Treatment in American Indian Populations: An Indigenous Treatment Modality Compared with Traditional Approaches, Annals of the New York Academy of Sciences, Vol. 472, Alcohol and Culture: Comparative Perspectives from Europe and America, edited by Thomas F. Babor, New York: The New York Academy of Sciences, pp. 168-178.

Hammerschlag, Carl A. (1988). The Dancing Healers: A Doctor's Journey of Healing with Native Americans. New York: HarperSanFrancisco.

Hammerschlag, Carl A. (1992). The Theft of the Spirit: A Journey to Spiritual Healing. New York: Fireside, Simon and Schuster.

Holler, Clyde. (1995). Black Elk's Religion: The Sun Dance and Lakota Catholicism. Syracuse, New York: Syracuse University Press.

Hoover, Herbert. (1997). Personal Communication about the Canton File. University of South Dakota, Vermillion, South Dakota, September 26.

Iron Shell, James "Tony". (1997). Personal Communication, member Rosebud Sioux Tribe, Public Relations/Cultural Resource Coordinator, Mission, South Dakota, June 19.

Iron Shield, Harold. (1997). Personal Communication. Coordinator of the Native American Reburial Restoration Committee, 116 12th Street, Moorhead, Minnesota 56560. Telephone: (218) 236-5434.

Iron Shield, Harold. (1994). Journalist talks about Indian asylum. Minnesota Daily, May 20, 1994.

Iron Shield, Harold. (1992). The legacy of an infamous institution: Hiawatha Insane Asylum for American Indians, Native American Press, Vermillion, South Dakota, November 13, 1992, p. 3.

Iron Shield, Harold. (1991). Indian activist wants 119 bodies reburied, Sioux City Journal, November 11, 1991.

Iron Shield, Harold. (1988). Research indicates asylum wasn't in Indians' best interest. Different Voices, Argus Leader, Sioux Falls, South Dakota, August 8, 1988.

Jaimes, M. Annette, Editor. (1992). The State of Native America: Genocide, Colonization, and Resistance. Race and Resistance Series, Boston: South End Press.

Lame Deer, Archie Fire and Richard Erdoes. (1992). Gift of Power: The life and teachings of a Lakota medicine man, introduced by Alvin M. Josephy, Jr. Santa Fe, New Mexico: Bear & Company.

Lewis, Thomas. (1982). Group Therapy Techniques in Shamanistic Medicine, Group Psychotherapy, Psychodrama and Sociometry, 35,1, pp. 24-30.

Lewis, Thomas. (1990). The Medicine Men: Oglala Sioux Ceremony and Healing. Lincoln, Nebraska: University of Nebraska Press.

Little Soldier, Alex. (1997). Personal Communication, elder of Rosebud Sioux Tribe, Ring Thunder, South Dakota, June 12 and June 15.

Little Soldier, Alex, aka Alex Lunderman, Sr. (1992). Federal Policy and Social Disparity on Indian Reservations: Problems and Solutions for the 1990s. (A Study of the Rosebud Sioux Tribe Social Structure), unpublished paper.

Looking Horse, Martina. (1997). Personal Communication, member of Cheyenne River Sioux Tribe, Green Grass, South Dakota, June 24.

Lunderman, Alex, Jr. (1997). Personal Communication, Rosebud Sioux tribal member and Lakota student, Mission, South Dakota.

McGoldrick, Monica, Joe Giordano, and John K. Pearce (editors). (1996). Ethnicity and Family Therapy, (Second Edition), New York: The Guildford Press.

Means, Russell. (1995). Where White Men Fear to Tread: The Autobiography of Russell Means, with Marvin J. Wolf. New York: St. Martin's Press.

Mestheth, Wilmer, Darrell Standing Elk, and Phyllis Swift Hawk. (1993). Declaration of War Against Exploiters of Lakota Spirituality, http://maple.lemoyne.edu/~bucko/war.htm.

Meyers, Alber Cook. (1970). William Penn's Own Account of the Lenni Lenape or Delaware Indians, with a foreword by John E. Pomfret, Tercentenary Edition. Wilmington, Delaware: The Middle Atlantic Press.

Montgomery, Jean. (1997). Personal Communication, licensed practical nurse and member of cultural diversity committee at Rapid City Regional Hospital. Rapid City, South Dakota, June 16.

Putney, Diane. (1984). Canton Insane Asylum for Indians, South Dakota History, Vol. 14(1), pp. 1-30.

Red Dog, Gilbert. (1997). Personal Communication, member of Cheyenne River Sioux Tribe and Tribal Council, Eagle Butte, South Dakota, June 25.

Red Dog, Leon. (1997). Personal Communication, member of Cheyenne River Sioux Tribe, On the Tree, South Dakota, June 24.

Reynolds, C. (1993). The nature of health promotion with Ojibwe culture [dissertation] Detroit: Wayne State University.

Richards, Michael. (1997). Personal Communication, Social Worker and Discharge Planner, also clinical tribal liaison at Psychiatric Unit, Rapid City Regional Hospital, Rapid City, South Dakota, June 16.

Smith, Henry (Program Director). (1987). Wokiksuye: Live and Remember, includes an interview with a traditional medicine man and elders [Videotape], New York: Solaris Lakota.

Standing Bear, Luther. (1933). Land of the Spotted Eagle, with a Foreword by Richard N Ellis, Lincoln, Nebraska: University of Nebraska Press.

Thin Elk, Gene. (1995a). The Red Road Approach, Appendix, Wounded Warriors: A Time for Healing, as told to Doyle Arbogast, Minneapolis/St. Paul: Little Turtle Publications, pp. 319-320.

Thin Elk, Gene. (1995b). The Red Road to Sobriety [Videotape], written and directed by Chante Pierce, San Francisco: Kifaru Productions.

Thin Elk, Gene. (1995c). The Red Road to Sobriety Video Talking Circle [Videotape], written and directed by Chante Pierce, San Francisco: Kifaru Productions.

Turton, C.L.R. (1995). Spiritual needs of hospitalized Ojibwe people. Michigan-Nurse, May, v68, n5, pp. 11-2.

Twiss, Gayla J. (1997). Personal Communication, Administrator, Rosebud Public Health Services Indian Hospital.

Wallace, A. C. (1958). Dreams and the Wishes of the Soul: A Type of Psychoanalytic Theory among the Seventeenth Century Iroquois, American Anthropologist, 60, pp. 234-248.

White Hat, Sr., Albert. (1997). Personal Communication, member of Rosebud Sioux Tribe, Sinte Gleska University, Mission, South Dakota, June 11.

Suggested Readings

Attneave, C.L. (1982). American Indians and Alaska Native families: Emigrants in their own homeland. In M. McGoldrick, J. Pearce, and J. Giorando (Eds.), Ethnicity and Family Therapy, New York: Guilford, pp. 55-83.

Brown Wolf, Oliver. (1997). Personal Communication, elder of Cheyenne River Sioux Tribe.

Canda, Edward R., Sun-in Shin, and Hwi-Ja Canda. (1993). Traditional Philosophies of Human Service in Korea and Contemporary Social Work Implications, Social Developmental Issues, Vol. 15, 3, pp. 84-104.

Catches, Pete and Peter Catches. (1997). Oceti Wakan: Sacred Fireplace, Pine Ridge, South Dakota: Oceti Wakan Press.

D'Andrea, Michael. (1994). The Concerns of Native American Youth, Journal of Multicultural Counseling and Development, 22, pp. 173-181.

Dauphinais, P., Dauphinais, L., and Rowe, W. (1981). Effects of race and communication style on Indian perceptions of counselor effectiveness, Counselor Education and Supervision, 21, pp. 72-80.

DeMallie, Raymond. (Ed.), (1984). The Sixth Grandfather: Black Elk's Teachings Given to John G. Neihardt, with a Foreword by Hilda Neihardt Petri, Lincoln, Nebraska: University of Nebraska Press.

Erikson, Erik Homburger. (1937). Observations on Sioux Education, The Journal of Psychology, 7, pp. 101-156.

Gross, Emma R. (1995). Deconstructing Politically Correct Practice Literature: The American Indian Case, Social Work, Vol. 40,2, pp. 206-213.

Gross, Gregory. (1996). Postmodern Social Work: No Truths Outside the Gates of Eden?, The Journal of Baccalaureate Social Work, Vol. 2, 1, pp. 63-77.

Hartman, A. (1992). In Search of Subjugated Knowledge [Editorial], Social Work, 37, pp. 483-484.

Herring, Roger D. (1994). The Clown or Contrary Figure as a Counseling Intervention Strategy with Native American Indian Clients, Journal of Multicultural Counseling and Development, 22, pp. 153-164.

Keith, Shirley. (1997). Personal Communication. Elder Cheyenne River Sioux Tribe, Rapid City, South Dakota, June 16.

Kelley, Mary Louise, Sharon McKay, and Connie H. Nelson. (1985). Indian Agency Development: An Ecological Practice Approach, Social Casework, 66, 10, pp. 594-602.

Lakota Cultural Center and Manual Productions. (1997). Lakota: land of survivors [Videotape], Eagle Butte, South Dakota: HVJ Lakota Cultural Center.

Looking Horse, Stanley. (1997). Personal Communication, elder of Cheyenne River Sioux Tribe, Green Grass, South Dakota, June 24.

Mehl-Madrona, Lewis. (1997). Call me Coyote: Stanford-trained Cherokee physician talks of coyote medicine and other Native American healing techniques. Natural Health, May-June, v27, no3, p. 96.

Morales, et al. (1995). Social Work: A Profession of Many Faces, (Seventh Edition), Needham Heights, Massachusetts: A Simon & Schuster Company.

Neihardt, John G. (1932). Black Elk Speaks: Being the Life Story of a Holy Man of the Ogalala Sioux. New York: William Morrow. Reprints. Lincoln, Nebraska: University of Nebraska Press, 1961, 1979 (with new preface, introduction, illustrations, appendixes).

Niess, Ron. (1997). Personal Communication, member of Rosebud Sioux Tribe, Ring Thunder Wacipi, Mission, South Dakota, Alliance of Tribal Tourism Advocates, June 14.

Porterfield, K. Marie. (1997). Sitting Bull Pipe returns. Indian Country Today, November 10-17, B Section, p. B1 and B3.

Powers, William K. (1982). Yuwipi: Vision and Experience in Oglala Ritual, Lincoln, Nebraska: University of Nebraska Press.

Red Bird, Stanley. (1997). Personal Communication, member of Rosebud Sioux Tribe, Rosebud, South Dakota, June 19.

Red Dog, Leon. (1995). Leon Speaks, Wounded Warriors: A Time for Healing, as told to Doyle Arbogast, editor, Omaha, Nebraska: Little Turtle Publications, pp. 146-170.

Smith, Wilfred Cantwell. (1979). Faith and belief, Princeton, New Jersey: Princeton University Press.

St. Pierre, Mark. (1997). Personal Communication, author and educator, Cheyenne River Sioux Cultural Center, Eagle Butte, South Dakota, June 17.

St. Pierre, Mark, and Tilda Long Soldier (1995). Walking in the Sacred Manner: Healers, Dreamers, and Pipe Carriers—Medicine Women of the Plains Indians. New York: A Touchstone Book.

St. Pierre, Mark. (1991). Madonna Swan: A Lakota Woman's Story as told through Mark St. Pierre, Norman, Oklahoma: University of Oklahoma Press.

Schacht, A.J., Tafoya, N., and Mirabla, K. (1989). Home-based therapy with American Indian families, American Indian and Alaska Native Mental Health Research. 3.2, pp. 27-42.

Simms, Thomas E. (1987). Otokahekagapi (First Beginnings): Sioux Creation Story, Lakota translations by Ben Black Bear, Jr., Chamberlain, South Dakota: Tipi Press.

Standing Bear, Luther. (1931). "The Tragedy of the Sioux," American Mercury 24, no. 95.

Sutton, CharlesEtta T. and Mary Anne Broken Nose. (1996). American Indian Families: An Overview. Ethnicity and Family Therapy (Second Edition), Monica McGoldrick, Joe Giordano, and John K. Pearce. (editors), New York: The Guilford Press.

Thomason, Timothy C. (1991). Counseling Native Americans: An Introduction for Non-Native American Counselors, Journal of Counseling and Development, 69, pp. 321-327.

Walker, James R. (1980). Lakota Belief and Ritual, Edited by Raymond J. DeMallie and Elaine A. Jahner, Lincoln, Nebraska: University of Nebraska Press.

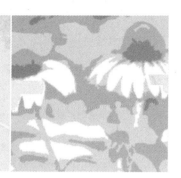

APPENDIX

Native American Medicinal Plants

DANIEL E. MOERMAN

Native American peoples developed a sophisticated plant-based medical system in the millennia before the European arrival in America. Many of the plants used by them are familiar medicinal species and have taken a role in contemporary medicine.

- *Echinacea* is well known in Europe and increasingly in North America as a treatment for colds and particularly as an "immune system stimulant." The cone flowers, native American species, were used more than 100 ways by a dozen Midwestern tribes (Blackfoot, Cheyenne, Dakota, Omaha, Pawnee, and Paiute, among others) to treat a variety of diseases and conditions, including headaches, burns, and toothaches. The Winnebago used *Echinacea* in an interesting way: fire handlers used the plant to make themselves insensitive to hot coals that they put in their mouths.

- Another very interesting plant—*Podophyllum peltatum,* the mayapple—is less well known to the public but is probably more important medically than *Echinacea*. The plant was used in many ways by American Indians, but the most common use was as a laxative or purgative, a common use of the plant in early American medicine, too. For many years, podophyllum resin has been a standard treatment for venereal warts. And etoposide (VePesid), a semisynthetic derivative of podophyllotoxin, another may apple constituent, is an effective treatment for refractory testicular tumors and for small cell lung cancer.

- Plants used by Native Americans as medicinal species can also be quite dangerous. This is fairly obvious with toxic species like *Datura meteloides* (jimsonweed) and *Heracleum maximum* (cow parsnip). Others are less obviously dangerous. A classic case is ephedrine, derived from several species of the genus *Ephedra,* notably *E. sinica*. The American species, *E. viridis,* contains less ephedrine than the Asian species, but does contain some. It was used by many native American groups for internal illnesses. It has a long use in the American Southwest as a stimulating drink known variously as "teamster's tea" or "Mormon tea," and the drug and various synthetic variations (particularly pseudoephedrine) is a useful decongestant. In the past few years, herbal drug companies have made capsules containing from 7 to more than 40 mg of ephedrine along with other *Ephedra* alkaloids and sold them under names like "Herbal Ecstacy," "Ultimate Xphoria," and "Cloud 9." These drugs presumably mimic the action of the street drug MDMA (4-methyl-2, dimethoxyamphetamine)—illegal in the United States—which produces euphoria; the street name of the drug is "Ecstacy." In a number of cases, people taking 6 or 8 of these "herbal highs" have died of heart attack, stroke, and various sorts of seizures.[1] Just because a drug is "natural" does not mean it is safe.

There are many such interesting stories about native American drug plants and their modern uses, and accounts of them of this sort are easy to find. There are, however, other approaches to the medicinal plants of native North America, which I will describe now. Although there were significant differences between the systems developed by the many native

405

groups,[2] there were also many broad similarities that will be detailed here. There are approximately 21,000 species of plants in North America. Native Americans used more than 2800 of them medicinally.[3]

Over the past 25 years, I have built a database with 44,775 entries in it listing uses of plants by Native American peoples as drugs, foods, dyes, fibers, and so on. The database contains 25,025 entries on uses of drugs representing a total of 2865 different species of plants. An additional 11,079 entries describe the uses of 3896 species that were used as food. The database was constructed by gathering together several hundred published works on the ethnobotany of Native American peoples and coding all the information in them in a systematic way. Because many of these publications were originally quite obscure and often hard to find, this database makes it much easier to make such global statements about American Indian plant use.

The used portion of the flora (the "medicinal flora") is a distinctly nonrandom assortment of the plants available. The richest sources of medicines are the sunflower family (Asteraceae), the rose family (Rosaceae), and the mint family (Lamiaceae). By contrast, the grass family (Poaceae) and the rush family (Juncaeae) produce practically no medicinal species. This remarkable volume and extraordinary selectivity demonstrate without any doubt the falseness of demeaning claims that suggest that Native American medicines were chosen at random, that they "just used everything and stumbled on something useful (like *Echinacea* or *Podophyllum*) once in a while."

HEALTH AND DISEASE

To understand the character and effectiveness of a medical system, one must understand the health status of the people who use it. Native American peoples were typically very healthy. They generally did not have the degenerative diseases of the heart and circulatory systems so common today; their diets were rich in fiber and carbohydrates and low in fats. They lived vigorous lives that provided hearty exercise on a daily basis. They experienced little cancer. Cancer is largely a modern disease of civilization; although the situation is obviously complex, an apparently necessary condition for cancer is carcinogens that are largely products manufactured by industrial societies (e.g., organic chemicals and dyes, nuclear radiation). Even

into the current day there is evidence that the traditional Navajo have lower rates of cancer than surrounding people (Csordas, 1989).

In addition, Indian people had less classic infectious diseases, which have ravaged European society over the past two millennia. In large part this seems to be because many such diseases (e.g., plague, typhoid, smallpox, cholera) are zoonoses, diseases of animals that, under conditions of domestication, underwent evolutionary change and subsequently affected the human keepers of these animals. Native Americans never domesticated animals to any significant degree (the guinea pig and llama of Peru were apparently only coming under domestication in the few hundred years before European contact). Once these diseases were introduced into North America, they devastated native populations, which had no natural immunity to them.[4] Until the sixteenth century, when Europeans underwent successive epidemics that regularly killed a quarter or half of the population, Native Americans were spared this devastation.

What medical problems *did* Native Americans face? In the Southeast and Southwest, there is evidence of a decline in health status after the invention of agriculture as the diet became simpler (less varied), which apparently led to some deficiency diseases. Hunting and gathering peoples avoided that problem, but they, like Europeans, may have experienced some zoonotic infections, particularly from beaver, and some trichinosis from bears; but these would have been "direct" zoonoses that individuals contracted directly from the infected animal, not "remote" zoonoses, which, once passed to one human being, were subsequently passed from person to person. Like rabies, a terrible disease for the individual who contracts it, these direct zoonoses are not serious threats to a whole society because they are not "contagious" in the ordinary sense of the term, from human to human.

Native Americans probably paid a price for the vigorous life they led. Accidents, sprains, broken bones, cuts, lacerations, and the like were common. There was a range of arthritic conditions, some probably the result of injury like those just mentioned, and perhaps some similar to rheumatoid arthritis. There is ample evidence that native peoples engaged in warfare; this would have been a source of serious medical problems. There was a range of occasional problems associated with menstruation, pregnancy, childbirth, and lactation that required attention. Liv-

Echinacea angustifolia

There are a total of 123 records for *Echinacea*, the coneflowers, in my database. They represent 26 distinctly different use categories, such as "analgesic," "antirheumatic," "cold remedy," and so forth. There are 18 different tribes represented in those data, and 93 combinations of tribe and use: "Pawnee analgesic," "Crow cold remedy." Nine different tribes are reported to have used Echinacea as an analgesic. Some tribes used it several different ways: The Winnebago used it in a wash for pain from burns and also put it in a smoke treatment for headaches. The Ponca used it the same two ways.

Toxicodendron radicans

Poison ivy is a common North American plant that causes serious and very unpleasant itchy rashes on many people. Children are taught "leaflets three; let it be." The toxic chemical urishol is found throughout the plant—in the soft woody stem, the leaves, and the berries. It is particularly dangerous when someone unwittingly burns it with fallen leaves in the fall—contact with the smoke can also cause serious allergic reactions. There are several other members of this genus with similarly noxious properties among them *T. diversilobum* (Pacific poison oak), *T. pubescens* (Atlantic poison oak), and *T. vernix* (poison sumac). It may be somewhat surprising then to find that Native American people found this genus to be useful as a medicine. There are 57 listings of the genus in the database. Although some of these listings indicate simply that the people recognized the plant as being poisonous, others found medicinal uses for them: The Yuki Indians of California, for example, used Pacific poison oak to treat warts, whereas the Cherokee used a decoction of the bark of Atlantic poison oak as an emetic. The Kiowa Apache rubbed poison ivy leaves over boils or other skin eruptions, and the Houma of Louisiana took a decoction of the leaves as a tonic and "rejuvenator."

Geranium maculatum

There are eight species of wild geraniums that were used medicinally by Native American peoples (note that these are not the same as the common ornamental plants often called *geraniums*, which are actually Pelargoniums). The most widely used is *Geranium maculatum*, the wild cranesbill. This plant produces a long pointed seed that has a series of small but distinct hooks on the end, which probably serve to catch the seeds in the fur of passing animals to aid in their dispersal. However, these hooks also provide for the Iroquois a rationale for using a poultice of the roots of this plant on chancre sores; the "hooklike and ensnaring qualities" of the plant (implied by its hooked seeds) are precisely the thing to use on a "loose, running, everted" sore. The plant is therefore a "meaningful" medicine for the Iroquois. The roots also contain substantial quantities of tannin, which would probably be an effective treatment for sores. Medicines almost always have this double quality of meaning and chemistry in all medical systems.

Daucus carota

The wild European carrot, or Queen Anne's Lace, is a common medicine for American Indian people. This is true of a number of introduced species; other common European plants that became widely used are mullein (*Verbascum thapsus*), curly dock (*Rumex crispus*), catnip (*Nepeta cataria*), and the common tansy (*Tanacetum vulgare*). The Delaware and Mohegan Indians used wild carrot to treat diabetes; the Iroquois used it as a diuretic; and the Cherokee used an infusion of the plant as a wash for swellings.

ing in smoky houses, it is not surprising that they had a broad range of treatments for irritated eyes and skin; they also treated colds, headaches, cold sores, and bruises, the normal insults of daily life everywhere.

HERBAL DRUGS

To address this range of problems, Native Americans inevitably resorted to drugs based on various plants.[5] Although a good deal of research has been done on this ethnobotany, much of it is hard to find and to work with. Most of the research has been done on a "tribe-by-tribe" basis. This means that if you are interested in what plants the Iroquois used for medicines and how they used them, you could look in James Herrick's doctoral dissertation, *Iroquois Medical Botany,* and find out. However, if you were interested in how different cultural groups used the same plant, it was a much more challenging proposition. My database, described earlier, makes this work much more practical.

Every Native American group for which we have any information had a botanical pharmacopoeia.

Although some were quite small (the Inuit had few plant resources on which to rely), most were quite elaborate with hundreds of plant drugs used for a broad range of conditions. This straightforward proposition raises a number of much more challenging questions. Native American healers, even into the early twentieth century, regularly knew the identity of 200 or 300 medicinal plants, which they could readily distinguish from the 3000 to 5000 species that grow in any particular area. Among 100 sophisticated and well-educated modern Americans or Europeans, it seems unlikely that very many could identify 200 species of plants of any kind unless they were professional botanists. How did nonliterate people, without reference to botanical keys or floras compiled by professionals, maintain this extraordinary amount of knowledge?[6]

If a Native American discovered by whatever means a marvelous medicinal plant that cured a child of a terrible rash and if the plant were very rare and unusual, an annual of uncertain provenience, she might be hard pressed to find it a second time, and harder pressed yet to teach her daughter or niece or neighbor where to find it. Such a plant would be unlikely to become part of the common knowledge of the community. If the situation were compounded by the fact that the plant were drab, with no particularly visible flowers or leaves—an undistinguished, rare, annual forb, for example, it is even less likely that it would become part of common knowledge. Such a proposal can lead to some testable propositions. For example, I would predict that, compared with other species, medicinal plants will *tend* to be the following:

- Abundant
- Perennial
- Large (e.g., trees rather than forbs)
- Widespread
- Distinctive, that is showy and visible

This does not mean that a tiny, drab, undistinguished, rare annual occurring in one forest in Tennessee could not be part of the Native American medicinal flora. It means it is *more likely* that a large, common, perennial tree found in 20 states will be used medicinally than the rare one.

Abundance

I cannot directly test the proposition that "medicinal plants tend to be relatively abundant" because I have no data set listing the relative abundance of North American plants. However, I can test a variation on that proposition, which states that "medicinal plants tend not to be rare and endangered."

The United States has a law called the Endangered Species Act, which seeks to protect endangered and threatened species of plants and animals. To administer the act, the Department of Agriculture maintains a list of such species (many of which are actually varieties or subspecies). Currently there are 389 species (or subspecies or varieties) on the list in four categories—proposed threatened, threatened, proposed endangered, and endangered. These are all taxa that, by definition, are found in limited areas, which are infrequent in their ranges. Two of 2572 medicinal species (0.08 percent) are on the list, whereas 387 of the remaining 28,543 taxa (species, subspecies, varieties, quads) in North America (1.3 percent) are on the list. This difference is highly statistically significant. By this admittedly flawed test, medicinal plants tend not to be rare and unusual. If it were possible to directly measure the abundance of a goodly sample of American species, a much better test of this proposition could be carried out.

Distribution[7]

In addition, evidence accumulated by the U.S. Department of Agriculture is available for the distribution of North American plant species. There is information on the presence or absence of species in 60 U.S. states and territories and 12 Canadian provinces. Species used as drugs are found in an average of 15.6 states or provinces, whereas species not used as drugs are found in an average of only 5.2. Drug plants are much more widespread than non-drug plants.

Growth Habit

Evidence indicates, first, that among native North Americans, a disproportionate share of medicinal plants have a perennial rather than annual growth habit. There are many more perennials (12,284) than annuals (3060); 16 percent of the perennials are used medicinally, whereas only 8.7 percent of the annuals are used medicinally.

Growth Form

The most commonly used growth form is trees and shrubs followed by forbs, vines, and grasses. The following table shows the numbers and percentages of each type. Although these differences may not look large, they are highly statistically significant; a given tree or shrub is 30 percent more likely to be used as a medicine than a given forb.

	Drug plants	Total plants	Percentage
Trees	340	2,213	13.32
Shrubs	598	4,002	13.00
Forbs	1,386	11,753	10.55
Vines	103	1,037	9.04
Grasses	75	2,039	3.55

Flavor

There is circumstantial evidence from a number of cases to indicate that medicinal plants often have a distinctive and, in particular, a bitter taste. This cannot be easily tested because there is no evidence anywhere on the flavors of plants *not* used as medicines (because botanists do not consider a plant's flavor to be an important characteristic of it).

Showiness

Finally, there is evidence that plants used for medicine used by Native American peoples are more showy or visible than other plants. The test for this is an indirect one. As I have become more interested in flower gardening in the past few years, I had a sense that most of the garden plants I was learning about were also in my database of medicinal plants. Why do we put this plant in a flower garden, and not that one? Generally it is because the garden species has beautiful, or unusual, or colorful flowers, or leaves, or scent, or growth habits or the like; garden plants are typically recognizable and distinctive. Of course many of our garden varieties are a far cry from their wild ancestors, but the hybridizers rarely began with nothing. I reasoned that medicinal plants would be more likely to show up in gardens than plants not used as medicinals. How to test this notion? I looked among my garden books and found *Ortho's Complete Guide to Successful Gardening*.

The book has a 122-page encyclopedic chart of plants of value in a garden, alphabetically arranged from *Abelia* to *Zoysia*. I checked genera in the gardening book, which also appeared in a standard list of the flora of North America (Kartesz, 1994). There are 3138 genera in this list, of which 852 appear in my database of medicinal plants. In addition, there were 423 genera of plants listed in the garden book that appear on the Kartesz checklist (a few items in the book were not in the checklist because they do not appear outside of gardens). If all were distributed randomly, and medicinal plants were not favored for use in the garden, we would predict that 115 of the garden plants would have appeared on the list of 852 medicinal species. But there are actually nearly twice that many, 213, again a highly statistically significant difference. Medicinal plants tend to be visible, recognizable, and showy.

CONCLUSION

The medicinal knowledge of native North American peoples is extraordinary. Just how this knowledge was developed remains a mystery. Native American peoples have been considered to have come from Asia; the flora of Asia is in many ways similar to that of North America. It is quite likely that the first migrants to the New World brought with them detailed knowledge of medical botany, much of which was applicable to this new flora.

Most remarkable, however, may be this: I am unaware of any significant medicinal use of any indigenous American plant species that was not used medicinally by one or another Native American group. An interesting example involves recent research on taxol, a substance of great potential medical value found in the common yew, *Taxus brevifolia*, and the Canadian yew, *Taxus canadensis*. Taxol has shown substantial effect in the destruction of tumors in a number of forms of cancer, particularly ovarian cancer, a highly refractory form of the disease. Native Americans did not use yew to treat cancer (see previous discussion), but they did use it for a variety of other conditions, among them skin problems, wounds, rheumatism, and colds. In general, if one is interested in finding potentially useful botanical chemicals from the North American flora, it would clearly be wise to focus first on that portion of the flora that has been used by Native Americans. Their experience and knowledge can yet guide our scientific efforts to enhance human health.

Acknowledgments

The work reported here has been generously supported by the National Science Foundation (SBR-9200674). I also wish to thank Claudine Farrand for helpful discussions about gardening, and Michael Heinrich for his wise counsel on this chapter.

Notes

1. For a recent review of this situation, see the detailed article by Blumenthal and King (1996) in *HerbalGram*.
2. Many fine works on the medical systems of particular groups are available, although sometimes hard to find. Perhaps the finest of them is by James Herrick on the Iroquois (1977). For a superb overview of the range of forms of treatment and understanding of illness, see Vogel's classic work *American Indian Medicine* (1970).
3. The most comprehensive available listing of Native American medicinal plants is Moerman's *Medicinal Plants of Native America* (1986). A more recent and much larger database is in press and should be available during 1997 under the title *Native American Ethnobotany* (Timber Press, Portland, OR, 1998). A version of the forthcoming database is available on the World Wide Web at www.umd.umich.edu/cgi-bin/herb.
4. For a fascinating and controversial review of the impact of European diseases on native Americans, see Calvin Martin's *Keepers of the Game* (1978). The classic work on the zoonotic origins of modern diseases is R.N. Fiennes' book *Zoonoses and the Origins and Ecology of Human Diseases* (1978, Academic Press, New York.)
5. There were some nonplant substances used medicinally. Castoreum from beaver was used for various conditions, and some minerals and clays were used as well. The preponderance of medicinal substances came from plants.
6. The definitive treatment of non-Western botanical knowledge is Brent Berlin's *Ethnobiological Classification* (1992); the best modern treatment of the problems of the origins of knowledge of food and drug plants is Timothy Johns' *With Bitter Herbs They Shall Eat It* (1990).
7. The next three sections on distribution, habit, and form are based on data from the United States Department of Agriculture National Plants Database. These data are available on the Internet at http://trident.ftc.nrcs.usda.gov/plants/plntmenu.html.
8. A detailed comparison of the ethnobotany of North America and China awaits scholarly attention. A preliminary account by James Duke (in Duke and Ayensu, *Medicinal Plants of China*, 1985) is provocative.

References

Berlin, Brent. 1992. Ethnobiological Classification. Principles of Categorization of Plants and Animals in Traditional Societies. Princeton, New Jersey: Princeton University Press.

Blumenthal, Mark and Penny King. 1996, "The Agony of the Ecstasy: Herbal High Products Get Media Attention." HerbalGram: The Journal of the American Botanical Council and the Herb Research Foundation. Number 37.

Brower, Lincoln P., Carolyn J. Nelson, James N. Seiber, Linda S. Fink, and Calhoun Bond. 1988. "Exaptation as an Alternative to Coevolution in the Cardinolide-Based Chemical Defense of Monarch Butterflies (Danaus plexippus L.) against Avian Predators." In Chemical Mediation of Coevolution. Ed. Kevin C. Spencer. San Diego: Academic Press, pp. 447-476.

Csordas, Thomas. 1989. "The Sore That Does Not Heal: Cause and Concept in the Navajo Experience of Cancer." Journal of Anthropological Research 45(4): 457-485.

Duke, James A. and Edward S. Ayensu. 1985. Medicinal Plants of China. Algonac, Michigan: Reference Publications Inc.

Fiennes, R. N. 1978. Zoonoses and the Origins and Ecology of Human Diseases. New York: Academic Press.

Herrick, James William. 1977. Iroquois Medical Botany. Ann Arbor: University Microfilms International.

Johns, Timothy. 1990. With Bitter Herbs They Shall Eat It. Chemical Ecology and the Origins of Human Diet and Medicine. Tucson, Arizona: The University of Arizona Press.

Kartesz, John. 1994. Synonymized Checklist of the Flora of North America. Portland, Oregon: Timber Press.

Martin, Calvin. 1978. Keepers of the Game. Indian-Animal Relationships and the Fur Trade. Berkeley: University of California Press.

Moerman, Daniel E. 1997. Native American Ethnobotany. Portland, Oregon: Timber Press.

Vogel, Virgil J. 1970. American Indian Medicine. Norman, Oklahoma: University of Oklahoma Press.

Suggested Readings

Moerman, Daniel E. 1991. "The Medicinal Flora of Native North America: An Analysis." Journal of Ethnopharmacology 31:1-42.

Wrangham, R. W. and Jane Goodall, 1987. "Chimpanzee Use of Medicinal Leaves." In Understanding Chimpanzees. Ed. Paul G. Heltne and Linda Marquardt. Chicago: University of Chicago Press.

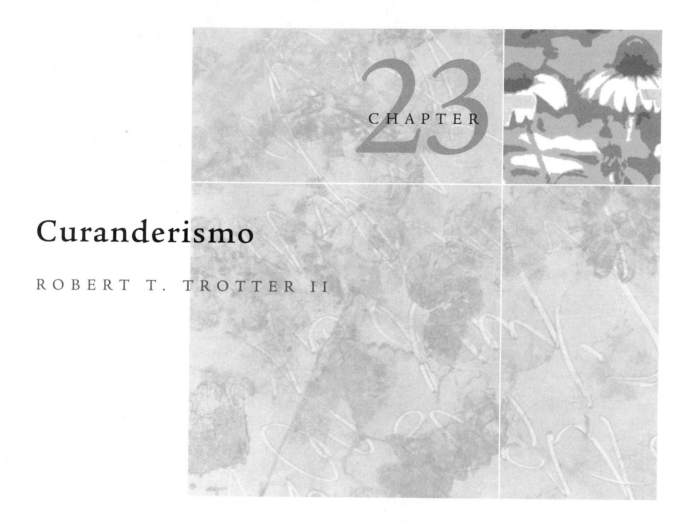

Curanderismo

ROBERT T. TROTTER II

HISTORY

Curanderismo, from the Spanish verb *curar* (to heal), is a healing tradition found in Mexican-American communities throughout the United States. Its historic roots are common with traditional healing practices in Puerto Rican and Cuban-American communities, as well as traditional practices found throughout Latin America. At the same time it has a history and a set of traditional medical practices that are unique to Mexican cultural history and to the Mexican-American experience in the United States.

Seven historic roots are embedded in modern curanderismo. Its theoretical beliefs partly trace their origins to Greek humoral medicine, especially the emphasis on balance, and the influence of hot and cold properties of food and medicines on the body.

Many of the rituals that provide both a framework and a meaningful cultural healing experience in curanderismo date to healing practices contemporary to the beginning of the Christian tradition and even into earlier Judeo-Christian writings. Other healing practices derive from the European Middle Ages, including the use of traditional medicinal plants and magical healing practices.

The Moorish conquest of Southern Europe is visible in the cultural expression of curanderismo. Some common Mexican-American folk illnesses originated in the Near East and then were transmitted throughout the Mediterranean, such as belief in *mal de ojo,* or the evil eye (the magical influence of staring at someone). Homeopathic remedies for common health conditions such as earaches, constipation, anemia, cuts and bruises, or burns were brought from Europe

411

to the New World to be passed down to the present time within curanderismo. There also is significant sharing of beliefs with Aztec and other Native American cultural traditions in Mexico. Some of the folk illnesses treated in pre-Columbian times, such as a fallen fontanelle *(caida de la mollera)* and perhaps the blockage of the intestines *(empacho)* are parts of this tradition. The pharmacopeia of the New World also is important in curanderismo (and added significantly to the plants available for treatment of diseases in Europe from the 1600s to the present). Some healers *(curanderos)* keep track of developments in parapsychology and New Age spirituality, as well as acupuncture and Eastern healing traditions and have incorporated these global perspectives into their own practices.

Finally, curanderismo is a traditional healing system, but it exists within the modern world. Biomedical beliefs, treatments, and practices are very much a part of curanderismo and are supported by curanderos. On the border between the United States and Mexico, it is not unusual for healers to recommend the use of prescription medications (which can often be purchased in Mexico over the counter) for infections and other illnesses. These healers also use information obtained from television and other sources to provide the best advice on preventive efforts such as nutrition and exercise and on explanations for biomedical illnesses. Individual healers vary greatly in their knowledge of the practices that stem from each of these seven historical sources. The overall system of curanderismo is complex and not only maintains its cultural link to the past but evolves toward accommodation with the future as well.

Cultural Context

This chapter is based partly on research that was conducted in the Lower Rio Grande Valley of Texas for more than 15 years. That information is enhanced by data from other regions near the U.S.-Mexican border, and from Mexican-American communities in Colorado, Nebraska, Chicago, and Florida. A multiplicity of research environments, both rural and urban, has affected the practice of curanderismo. Alger (1974) has described one possible outcome of urbanized curanderismo, in which the folk healing system mimics the modern medical system. Yet this mimicry does not exist to any significant extent in southern Texas, where both curanderos and their patients have

extensive knowledge of the medical system in urban and rural areas. However, unlike attitudes reported in earlier studies of the area (Madsen, 1961; Rubel, 1966), curanderos and their patients accept the use of modern medicine. These multiple environments of curanderismo practice create a complex healing system with core elements that are common to each place and modifications that respond to local cultural, political, and legal circumstances.

The earliest systematic research was done on curanderismo in the late 1950s, when modern medicine was inaccessible, or only recently available to significant segments of the Mexican-American population. Since that time, the efficacy of modern medicine has been demonstrated empirically numerous times, so it is an integrated part of the cultural system, although many access barriers still exist to prevent its full use by everyone. These barriers reflect the same reasons that the holistic health movement and the charismatic healing movements are becoming increasingly popular. Although traditional healers in Mexican-American communities believe that modern medicine is as capable in certain types of healing, their experience shows that their own practices are not recognized in hospitals and clinics and that they can accomplish those same tasks better than modern medicine. Thus curanderismo and modern medicine often assume complementary roles in the minds of the curanderos and their patients, although not necessarily in the minds of the medical professionals of the area.

Intellectual Tradition

Traditional Mexican-American healers perceive health and illness to contain a duality of "natural" and "supernatural" illnesses. This duality forms the theoretical base on which curanderismo is constructed. The natural source of illness is essentially a biomedical model of illness that includes lay interpretations of some diseases inspired by Mexican-American culture. Biomedical aspects such as the germ theory of disease, genetic disorders, psychological conditions, and dietary causes for medical conditions are accepted. These natural illnesses are treated by physicians with herbal remedies. A parallel supernatural source of illness also is recognized by this healing tradition. These illnesses are not considered amenable to treatment by the medical establishment. They can be repaired only by the supernatural manipulations of curanderos. The curanderos fault the scientific medical system for its failure to recognize the existence of magic or of supernatural causation. One curandero commented that as many as 10 percent of patients in mental institutions were really *embrujados* (hexed or bewitched), and because doctors could not recognize this condition, it went untreated.

Supernaturally induced illnesses are most commonly said to be initiated by either evil spirits *(espiritos malos)* or by *brujos* (individuals practicing antisocial magic). They form a significant part of the curanderos' work; these healers explain that any particular illness experienced by a patient could be caused theoretically by either natural or supernatural processes. For example, they believe there is a natural form of diabetes and a form that is caused by a supernatural agent, such as a *brujo*. The same is true for alcoholism, cancer, and other diseases. Identifying the nature of the causal agent for a particular illness is a key problem for the curandero. Some identify more supernatural causes for illnesses, and others take a more biomedically balanced approach. In either case there is far less dichotomizing of physical and social problems within curanderismo than within the medical care system (Holland, 1963; Kiev, 1968).

Curanderos routinely deal with problems of a social, psychological, and spiritual nature, as well as physical ailments. Many cases overlap into two or more categories. Bad luck in business is a common problem presented to curanderos. Other problems encountered were marital disruptions, alcoholism or alcohol abuse, infidelity, supernatural manifestations, cancer, diabetes, and infertility. One healer distinguishes between the problems presented by women and men. The central focus of the problems brought by women is the husband—the husband drinks too much, does not work, does not give them money, or is seeing other women. Men bring problems of a more physical nature, such as stomach pain, headaches, weakness, and bladder dysfunction. Men also bring problems that deal directly with work; they need to find a job, cannot get along with people at work, or are having trouble setting up a business. The wife rarely is the focal point of their problems. The total list of problems presented to curanderos includes nearly every situation that can be thought of as an uncomfortable human condition. Curanderismo seems to play an important, culturally appropriate

psychotherapeutic role in Mexican-American communities (Galvin & Ludwig, 1961; Klineman, 1969; Torrey, 1972).

Another element of curanderismo that forms an important intellectual foundation for its practices is the concept that healers work by virtue of "a gift of healing" *(el don)* (Hudson, 1951; Madsen, 1965; Romano, 1964; Rubel, 1966). This inherent ability allows the healer to practice his or her work, especially in the supernatural area. In the past this was believed to be a gift from God. However, a secular interpretation of the *don* is competing with the more traditional explanation. Many healers still refer to the *don* as a gift from God and support this premise with Biblical passages (Corinthians 12:7 and James 5:14), but other healers explain the *don* as an inborn trait that is present in all human beings, just like the ability to sing, run, or talk. Almost any human being can do these things, but some do them better than others, and a few people can do them extremely well. Curanderos, according to this theory, are the individuals with a better ability to heal than is normative for the population as a whole. Healers refer to this concept as "developed abilities."

Another element common to Hispanic-based folk medicine is the hot-cold syndrome (Currier, 1966; Foster, 1953; Ingham, 1940). This belief system is not common in southern Texas (Madsen, 1961), where the only indications of a hot-cold syndrome found among the patients were scattered folk beliefs such as not eating citrus during menses, not ironing barefoot on a cement floor, or taking a cold shower after prolonged exposure to the sun. None of these beliefs were organized in a systematic fashion, nor were they extensively shared within the Mexican-American population. In other areas there is extensive knowledge and use of this system of classifying foods, treatments, and elements of illnesses to provide the basis for deciding which remedies apply to specific illnesses.

THEORETICAL BASIS

The community-based theoretical structure for curanderismo has three primary areas of concentration, called *levels (niveles)* by the healers: the material level *(nivel material),* the spiritual level *(nivel espiritual),* and the mental level *(nivel mental).* More curanderos have the *don* for working at the material level, which is or ganized around the use of physical objects to heal or to change the patient's environment. This theoretical area can be subdivided into physical and supernatural manipulations. Physical treatments are those that do not require supernatural intervention to ensure a successful outcome. *Parteras* (midwives), *hueseros* (bone setters), *yerberos* (herbalists), and *sobadores* (people who treat sprains and tense muscles) are healers who work on the *nivel material* and effect cures without any need for supernatural knowledge or practices. All of the *remedios caseros* (home remedies) used in Mexican-American communities are part of this healing tradition.

The supernatural aspect of this level is involved in cures for common folk illnesses found in Mexican-American communities, such as *susto, empacho, caida de mollera, espanto,* and *mal de ojo.* These illnesses are unique to Hispanic cultural models of health and illness. This area of healing also includes the spells and incantations that are derived out of medieval European witchcraft and earlier forms of magic, such as the cabala, that have been maintained as supernatural healing elements of curanderismo. Supernatural manipulations involve prayers and incantations in conjunction with such objects as candies, ribbons, water, fire, crucifixes, tree branches, herbs, oils, eggs, and live animals. These treatments use a combination of common objects and rituals to cure health problems.

The spiritual level *(nivel espiritual)* is an area of healing that is parallel to the channeling found in New Age groups and in shamanistic healing rituals around the world (Macklin, 1967, 1974a, 1974b, 1974c; Macklin & Crumrine, 1973). Individuals enter an altered state of consciousness and, according to the curanderos, make contact with the spirit world by one or all of the following methods: opening their minds to spirit voices, sending their spirits out of the body to gain knowledge at a distance, or allowing spirits the use of the body to communicate with this world, or all three.

The mental level *(nivel mental)* is the least commonly encountered of the three levels. One healer described working with the mental level as the ability to transmit, channel, and focus mental vibrations *(vibraciones mentales)* in a way that would affect the patient's mental or physical condition directly. Both patients and healers are confident that the curanderos can effect a cure from a distance using this technique.

The three levels are discrete areas of knowledge and behavior, each necessitating the presence of a separate gift for healing. They involve different types of training and different methods of dealing with both the natural and the supernatural world. The material level involves the manipulations of traditional magical forces found in literature on Western witchcraft. Spiritualism involves the manipulation of a complex spirit world that exists parallel to our own and the manipulation of *corrientes espirituales,* spiritual currents that can both heal and provide information or diagnosis from a distance. The mental level necessitates the control and use of the previously mentioned *vibraciones mentales.* Thus the levels are separate methods of diagnosing and treating human problems that are embedded into a single cultural tradition.

Not all problems can be dealt with successfully using each level. An example of this is serious alcohol abuse (Trotter, 1979; Trotter & Chavira, 1978). Alcohol abuse and alcoholism are treated by curanderos, using techniques of both the material and the mental level. The techniques of the spiritual level, however, were considered ineffective in dealing with alcohol-related problems. So if one has the *don* for working with the spiritual level alone, he or she is excluded from the process of curing alcohol problems.

One theme that is common to the practices of all three levels is the use of energy to change the patient's health status. On the material level this energy often is discussed in relation to the major ritual of that level, known as the *barrida* or *limpia* (a sweeping or cleansing). In that ritual a person is "swept" from head to foot with an object that is thought to be able to either remove bad vibrations *(vibraciones malos)* or to give positive energy *(vibraciones positives)* to the patient. The type of object used (e.g., egg, lemon, garlic, crucifix, broom) depends on the nature of the patient's problem and whether it is necessary to remove or to replace energy. On the spiritual level the energy that is used for both diagnosis and healing is the previously mentioned *corrieiites espirituales.* The mental level is nearly totally oriented around generating and channeling *vibraciones mentales.* The following sections provide more detail on the actual practices of the curandero's work on each level.

The Material Level *(Nivel Material)*

The material level is the easiest of the three levels to describe; it is the most extensively practiced and the most widely reported. At this level the curandero manipulates physical objects and performs rituals (or trabajas, spells). The combination of objects and rituals is widely recognized by Mexican Americans as having curative powers. Practitioners of the material level use common herbs, fruits, nuts, flowers, animals and animal products (chickens, doves, and eggs), and spices. Religious symbols, such as the crucifix, pictures of saints, incense, candles, holy water, oils, and sweet fragrances are widely used, as are secular items, such as cards, alum, and ribbons. The curandero allows the patients to rely extensively on their own resources by prescribing items that either are familiar or have strong cultural significance; thus a significant characteristic of the objects used at the material level is that they are common items used for daily activities such as cooking and worship.

Natural Illnesses and Herbal Cures

Curanderos recognize that illnesses can be brought about by natural causes, such as dysfunction of the body, carelessness or the inability of a person to take proper care of himself or herself, and infection. Curanderos at the material level used large amounts of medicinal herbs *(plantas medicinales)* to treat these natural ailments. Some traditional curanderos classify herbs as having the dichotomous properties considered essential for humoral medicine, based on a hot-cold classification system common throughout Latin America (Foster, 1953). They use these dual properties to prescribe an herb or combination of herbs, depending on the characteristics of the illness. If a person's illness supposedly is caused by excessive "heat," an herb with "cold" properties is given. Conversely, if a person's illness is believed to be caused by excessive "coldness and dryness," a combination of herbs having "hot" and "wet" properties is administered.

Other curanderos recognize herbs for their chemical properties, such as poisons *(yerba del coyote, Karwinskia humboldtuna Roem. et Sch.)*, hallucinogens *(peyote, Lophaphora williams Lem.)*, sedatives *(flor de tila, Talia mexicana Schl.)*, stimulants *(yerba del trueno)*, and purgatives *(cascara sagrada)*. These individuals refer to the beneficial chemical properties of the herbs that allow them to treat natural illnesses.

Curanderos prescribe herbs most frequently as teas, baths, or poultices. The teas act as a sort of formative chemotherapy. *Borraja (borage: Borajo officialis L.)*, for example, is taken to cut a fever; *flor de tila*, a mild sedative, is taken for insomnia; *yerba de la golondrina (Euphorbia prostrate Ait.)* is used as a douche for

vaginal discharges; and *peilos de elote* are used for kidney problems. Herbal baths usually are prescribed to deal with skin diseases; *fresno* (ash tree, *Fraxinus* species) is used to treat scalp problems such as eczema, dandruff, and psoriasis; and *linaza* is prescribed for body sores. For specific sores such as boils, *malva* (probably a *Malvastrum*) leaves are boiled until soft and then applied to the sores as a poultice. Other herbs are used as decongestants. A handful of *oregano (oregano: Oregenum vulgare L.)* is placed in a humidifier to treat someone with a bad cold.

Some herbal lore is passed on as an oral tradition, and other information is available in Spanish language books for Mexico that are widely circulated among both curanderos and the public (Arias; Wagner). These works describe and classify numerous herbs. Herbal remedies are so important to Mexican-American folk medicine that their use often is confused with the art of curanderismo itself by the mass culture. Indeed, some curanderos known as *yerberos* or *yerberas*, specialize in herbs, but their knowledge and skills go beyond the mere connection of one disease to one herbal formula. For curanderos to be genuine, even at the material level, an element of mysticism must be involved in their practice. Herbs are used commonly for their spiritual or supernatural properties. Spiritual cleansings *(barridas)* often are given with *ruda (Ruta graveolens L.), romero* (rosemary, *Rosmarinus officiates L.)*, and *albacar* (sweet basil, *Ocimum basiticum L.)*, among others. Herbs are used as amulets; *verbena* (verbena, *Verbena officinalis L.)*, worn as an amulet, is used to help open a person's mind to learn and retain knowledge.

Some curanderos have successful practices on the material level without resorting to the use of herbs. Some nonherbal treatments are described in the following section.

Supernaturally Caused Illnesses and Ritual Cures

Supernatural illnesses, which occur when supernatural negative forces damage a person's health, sometimes can be confused with natural illnesses. One healer stated that these supernatural illnesses may manifest as ulcers, tuberculosis, rheumatism, or migraine headaches, but in reality, they are believed to be hexes that have been placed on the person by an enemy. Supernatural influences also disrupt a person's mental health and his or her living environment. Physicians cannot cure a supernatural illness.

The curandero commonly deals with social disruption, personality complexes, and sometimes with serious psychological disturbances. One healer gave the following description of a case that contained several of these elements:

This patient worked for the street maintenance department of (a small city in south Texas). Every day after work a voice would lead him out into the brush and sometimes keep him there until 2:00 AM. This activity was wearing out the man and his family and he was going crazy. A bad spirit was following this man and would not leave him alone. The man was cured, but it took three people to cure him: myself, a friend, and a master *(maestro)* from Mexico. This man was given three *barridas* each day for seven days, one by each of us. The tools used were eggs, lemons, herbs, garlic, and black chickens. The man was also prescribed herbal baths and some teas to drink. He was also given a charm made from the *haba mijrina* designed to ward off any more negative influences which might be directed at him. This patient regained his sanity.

There also are a number of illnesses that are both supernaturally caused and of a supernatural nature, which can be treated on the material level. The following account is an example of such an illness and cure.

My brother-in-law was working at a motel . . . in Weslaco. When he started working they laid off this other guy who had been working there for several years. This guy didn't like it, and he's been known to be messing around with black magic. I don't know what he did to my brother-in-law, but every other day he'd have to be taken home because he was sick. He started throwing up, had shaky knees, and weak joints. So my mother and I went over to see this lady in Reynosa, and she told my mother just what to do. My sister rubbed her husband with a lemon every night for three days. She also gave him some kind of tea. . . . On the third day, a big black spot appeared on the lemon, so we threw it away, and he's been fine ever since.

Rituals and the Material Level

Curanderos use several types of rituals for supernatural cures. The *barrida* is one of the most common rituals. These cleansings are designed to remove the negative forces that are harming the patient, while simultaneously giving the patient the spiritual strength necessary to enhance recovery. Patients are always "swept" from head to toe, with the curandero making sweeping or brushing motions with an egg, lemon, herb, or whatever object is deemed spiritually appropriate. Special emphasis is given to areas in pain. While sweeping the patient, the curandero recites specific prayers or invocations that appeal to God, saints, or other supernatural beings to restore health to the patient. The curandero may recite these prayers and invocations out loud or silently. Standard prayers include the Lord's Prayer, the Apostles' Creed, and *Las Doce Verdades de Mundo* (The Twelve Truths of the World).

The following description of a *barrida* illustrates how the material objects, the mystical power of these objects, the invocations, the curandero, and the patient come together to form a healing ritual designed for a specific patient and a specific illness: In this case, five eggs, four lemons, some branches of *albacar* (sweet basil), and oil were used. To begin the healing process, the lemons and eggs were washed with alcohol and water to cleanse them spiritually. Before beginning the ritual, the participants were instructed to take off their rings, watches, and other jewelry; high-frequency spiritual and mental vibrations can produce electrical discharges on the metal, which might disturb the healing process. The sweeping itself is done by interchanging an egg and a lemon successively. Sweeping with the egg is intended to transfer the problem from the patient to the egg by means of conjures *(conjures)* and invocations *(rechasos)*. The lemon is used to eliminate the *trabajo* (magical harm) that has been placed on the patient. The patient is swept once with *albacar* (sweet basil) that has been rinsed in *agua preparada* (prepared water). This sweeping purifies the patient, giving strength and comfort to his spiritual being. The ritual ends by making crosses with *aceite preparado* (specifically prepared oil) on the principal joints of the patients, such as the neck, under the knees, and above the elbow. This oil serves to cut the negative currents and vibrations that surround the patient, which have been placed there by whoever is provoking the harm. The crosses protect against the continued effect of these negative vibrations. *Agua preparada* is then rubbed on the patient's forehead and occiput *(cerebro)* to tranquilize and to give mental strength. All the objects used in the *barrida* are then burned to destroy the negative influences or harm transferred from the patient.

Another common ritual is called a *sahumerio*, or *incensing*. The *sahumerio* is a purification rite used primarily for treating businesses, households, farms, and other places of work or habitation. This ritual is executed by treating hot coals with an appropriate incense. The curandero may prepare his own incense, or he may prescribe some commercially prepared incense such as *el sahumerio maravilloso* (miraculous incense). A pan with the smoking incense is carried throughout the building, making sure that all corners, closets, and hidden spaces, such as under the beds, are properly filled with smoke. While "incensing," the healer or someone else recites an appropriate prayer. If the *sahumerio maravilioso* is used, the prayer often is one to Santa Marta, requesting that peace and harmony be restored to the household. After the *sahumerio*, the healer may sprinkle holy water on the floor of every room in the house and light a white candle that stays lit for 7 days. The *sahumerio* is an example of the curandero treating the general social environment, seeking to change the conditions of the persons who live or work there. Incensing of a house removes negative influences such as bad luck *(salaciones)*, marital disruptions, illness, or disharmony. For business and farms, incensing helps ensure success and growth and protects against jealous competitors. These rituals are designed to affect everyone in the environment that has been treated.

Another type of ritual, called a *sortilegio* (conjure), uses material objects such as ribbons to tie up the negative influences that harm the curandero's patients. These negative influences are often personal shortcomings such as excessive drinking, infidelity, rebellious children, unemployment, or any other problem believed to be imposed by antisocial magic *(un trabajo)*. One *sortilegio* that I observed required four ribbons in red, green, white, and black, each approximately 1 yard in length. The color of each ribbon represents a type of magic, which the curanderos can activate to deal with specific problems. Red magic involves domination, green deals with healing, white with general positive forces, and black with negative or debilitating forces.

When working with a specific area of magic, one uses material objects that are the appropriate color naturally or that have been made that color artificially. The color-based division of magic also is carried over into another type of ritual system used on the material level, *velacione,* or burning candles to produce supernatural results. The *velaciones* and the colored material objects used in the *sortilegios* tie into the energy theme that runs throughout curanderismo, because the colors and objects are believed to have specific vibratory power or energy that can affect the patient when activated by the incantations used in conjunction with the objects. For example, blue can-

dles are burned for serenity or tranquility; red candles are burned for health, power, or domination; pink candles are burned for good will; green candles are burned to remove a harmful or negative influence; and purple candles are burned to repel and attack bad spirits *(espiritus obscuros)* or strong magic. Once the proper color of candle has been chosen to produce the proper mental atmosphere, the candles are arranged in the correct physical formation and activated by the *conjuros y rechasos*. If a patient asks for protection, the candles might be burned in a triangle, which is considered to be the strongest formation, one whose influence cannot be broken easily. If they want to dominate someone—a spouse, a lover, or an adversary—the candles might be burned in circles. Other formations include crosses, rectangles, and squares, depending on the results desired (Buckland, 1970).

Another relatively common use of candles is to diagnose problems by studying the flame or the ridges that appear on the melted wax. A patient may be swept with a candle while the healer recites an invocation asking the spirit of the patient to allow its material being to be investigated for any physical or spiritual problems that may be affecting the person. This ritual also can be performed by burning objects used in a *barrida*. Lighting the candle or burning the object after the *barrida* helps the curandero reveal the cause and extent of the patient's problems. Similarly, if a petitioner asks for candling, the wax of the candles burned for the velacion may be examined for figures or other messages that point to the source of a patient's problems.

One of the organizing principles of the material level of curanderismo is synchronicity with Christianity in general and the Catholic Church in particular. Special invocations often are directed at saints or spirits to bring about desired results. For example, San Martin de Porres is asked to relieve poverty, San Martin Caballero is asked to ensure success in business, San Judas Tadeo is asked to help in impossible situations, and Santa Marta is asked to bring harmony to a household. Ritual materials used by the church, such as water, incense, oils, and candles, are extensively used by folk healers. The ways in which these religious objects are used and the theories for their efficacy closely mirror the concepts found within the healing ministry of the Church, which are not incompatible with European witchcraft, from which curanderismo partly derives.

The Spiritual Level
(Nivel Espiritual)

Curanderos who have the *don* for working on the spiritual level *(nivel espiritual)* of curanderismo are less numerous than those who work on the material level. These practitioners also must go through a developmental period *(desarrollo)* that can be somewhat traumatic. Spiritual practices in communities revolve around a belief in spiritual beings who inhabit another plane of existence but who are interested in making contact with the physical world periodically. Healers become a direct link between this plane of existence and that other world. In some cases the curanderos claim to control these spirit beings, and in other cases, they merely act as a channel through which messages pass. Some of these practices are carried out by individual healers, whereas other activities occur in conjunction with spiritual centers *(centros espiritistas)* that are staffed by trance mediums and other individuals with occult abilities. These centers often work through two prominent folk saints: El Nino Fidencio from Northern Mexico and Don Pedrito Jaramillo from southern Texas (Macklin, 1974a, 1974b, 1974c). This trend in visiting spiritualist centers appears to be relatively recent, having not been reported during the 1950s and 1960s by those doing research on Mexican-American folk medicine (Clark, 1959; Madsen, 1964; Rubel, 1960, 1966).

The practice of spiritualism rests on "soul concept," a belief in the existence of spirit entities derived from once-living humans. The soul is thought to be the immortal component, the life and personality force of human beings—an entity that continues to exist after physical death on a plane of reality separate from the physical world. This concept is important not only to curanderismo but also to the religions and mystical beliefs found in all Western cultures.

The soul is alternatively described by curanderos as a force field, ectoplasm, concentrated vibrations, or group of electrical charges that exist separate from the physical body. It is thought to retain the personality, knowledge, and motivations of the individual even after the death of the body. Under proper conditions the soul is ascribed the ability to contact and affect persons living in the physical world. Although souls occasionally can be seen as ghosts or apparitions by ordinary human beings, they exist more often in the spiritual realm previously mentioned. Some people view this realm as having various divisions that have positive or negative connotations associated with them, for example, heaven, limbo, purgatory, or hell. Other people see the spiritual realm as parallel to the physical world. They state that the spiritual is a more pleasant plane on which to live, but few attempt any suicidal test of this belief. One healer commented that "spirits" *[espiritos]*, "souls" *[almas]*, are the same thing. These spirits' activities closely parallel their former activities in this world. Because the personality, knowledge, and motivation of the spirits are much the same as they were for the living being, there are both good and evil spirits, spirits who heal and spirits who harm, wise spirits and fools.

These spirits might communicate with or act on the physical plane. Some have left tasks undone in their physical lives they wish to complete; others want to help or cause harm; many wish to communicate messages to friends and relatives, telling them of their happiness or discontent with their new existence. Therefore curanderos with the ability to work on the spiritual realm become the link between these two worlds. Some curanderos believe that there are multitudes of spirits who want to communicate with the physical world, and they tend to hover around those who have the *don* to become a medium, waiting for an opportunity to enter their bodies and possess them. This explains the cases of spirit possession in Western cultures. Individuals who become possessed are people with a strong potential to be trance mediums, who have not had the opportunity to learn how to control this condition.

The ability to become a medium is thought to be centered in the *cerebro,* that portion of the brain found at the posterior base of the skull. Those with the gift are said to have a more fully developed *cerebro,* whereas those who do not are said to have a weak cerebros *(un cerebro debil)*. This weakness has no relationship either to the intelligence or to the moral nature of the individual, only to his or her ability to communicate with the spiritual realm. Weak cerebros represent a danger for anyone who wishes to become a medium. Only rare individuals demonstrate mediumistic potential spontaneously and can practice as mediums without further training. So, curanderos often test their patients and friends for this gift of healing, and those with the gift are encouraged to develop their ability. The development of this ability is called *desarrollo* and is a fairly lengthy process that might last from 2 months to more than 6 months initially, with periodic refresher encounters often available from the *maestro* (teacher). *Desarrollo* is a gradual process of increasing an apprentice's contact with the spirit world, giving him or her more and more experiences in controlled trances and possessions, as well as the knowledge necessary to develop and protect himself or herself as a spiritualist. The teacher also is responsible for giving the apprentice knowledge at a safe pace. The curandero does not always explain what each sensation means; each person, as he or she develops, becomes more sensitive to his or her environment. The apprentice must expect to encounter odd sensations such as bright light, noises, changes in pressure, and other sensations associated with developing powers. At the end of these *desarrollo* sessions, the conversation reverts to social chatting for some time before the apprentice takes his leave. This developmental process continues, with variations, until the apprentice is a fully developed medium.

Fully developed mediums control how, where, and when they work, and several options are available to them. Some mediums work alone and treat only family problems (Box 23-1); others might use their

---

BOX 23-1

Curanderos

Many curanderos able to work on the spiritual level prefer to work at home, alone. Their practices tend to be less uniform than the practices of mediums working at spiritual centers, because they do not have to conform to the calendric and ritual structure found in more formalized temples. However, there is enough commonality to their actions to provide an accurate description of a lone medium. This healer is described by a student in his early 20s who was one of her patients; she had been handling problems for him and his family for several years.

R: Can you describe how this *curandera* works, in as great detail as you can?
S: We drive up into the driveway of a fairly decent-looking place. She walks out and greets us, shakes our hands, asks how we are doing and how we have been. Then we go inside. She's got a small room perhaps 8 by 10 feet. She has an altar with saints and candles and flowers on it. She has a small vase shaped like a crystal ball sitting on a table. Sometimes it has water on it and sometimes turned upside down.

You walk in there and sit down and she's talking with you. She's not in her trance; it's just social talk. Then she sits and puts her hand on that crystal-deal. She taps it, closes her eyes, and she starts asking you what kind of problem you have or whatever you want to ask her.

R: Her voice changes?
S: Yes, it does. It's a lot lower. All of a sudden her voice becomes soft, sort of like whispering. Really mild.
R: Does she keep her hands on the glass all of this time?
S: No. Sometimes she grabs a folder with papers in it and starts writing down things on it, using her finger.

R: Can she read what she has written?
S: I'm pretty sure she can.
R: How does she cure people?
S: She does it in a number of ways. Some time ago my mother had pains on both of her heels. She went to the doctor and the doctor didn't find anything wrong. So she went over to this lady again who said it was something (a *trabajo* or hex) that [a woman across the alley from his house] had put in the yard. When my mother's out hanging up clothes she's barefooted and she stepped on it. And that's what was hurting her. So the *curandera* gave her a "shot" on her arm like a regular shot. And that cured her.
R: How did she give her the shot?
S: (Simulated the action of giving an injection without a syringe or hypodermic.)
R: Could your mother feel it?
S: She told me she didn't. But it cured her.

The informant went on to tell of several other cures this curandera had performed for his family. She had prescribed herbs, suggested the use of perfumes to ward off the *envidia* (envy) of their neighbors, and suggested that the mother perform a series of *barridas* on her son-in-law to remove a hex against him that was making him ill and keeping him from work. Each of these cures could just as easily have been suggested or performed by a curandero working on the material level of curanderismo, but this curandera did it from a trance state. Therefore what sets this curandera apart from those working strictly on the material level is not the tools she uses or the rituals she suggests to her clients, but the source of her diagnosis and cure—her contact with a spirit world.

abilities only for their own knowledge and gratification. Some mediums work in groups with other mediums or with other persons whom they believe have complimentary spiritual or psychic powers. Some mediums work in elaborate spiritual centers (centros espiritistas) that are formal churches, often dedicated to a particular spirit (e.g., Fidencio, Francisco Rojas, Don Pedrito Jaramillo). The spiritual centers and the activities surrounding them take on the major aspects of a formalized religion.

Sometimes a trance session is open to more than one person at the same time. This group session can be carried out by a lone curandero but more often is found at spiritual centers. The process of the development of these centers is described elsewhere (Trotter & Chavira, 1975a). Once a temple has been established, it may house from 1 to 20 mediums. The more mediums, the better; otherwise, a medium may have to let his or her body be used by too many different spirits, exhausting them and laying them open to supernatural harm. Larger temples might have four or five videnntes (clairvoyants), as well as the mediums, and might be putting several apprentices through desarrollo at the same time. Many of the accounts provided to these authors about spiritual healing were from individuals who had had experiences with spiritual temples in Mexico. Some temples were located in Espinaso, the home of El Niño Fidencio and a center of pilgrimage for mediums practicing in his name, and others were in urban centers such as Tampico and Mexico City. Large numbers of people make pilgrimages to these healing centers in Mexico to deal with health care problems that they have not resolved in the United States.

One healing center is called Roca Blanca, after the spirit that speaks most often in that place. The owner, Lupita, founded it 25 years ago, after discovering her ability to cure. She was granted permission to practice by a spiritual association. This report is from a visitor to Lupita's healing center:

I went to this place simply because I was curious. I was swept with albacar and the medium was at my side. While I was being swept, the medium went into trance. The sister who was sweeping me asked the spirit who he wanted to talk to. He said, "with the one you are sweeping." Then, the sister finished sweeping me and directed me to talk with the person who was addressing me. When she (the medium in trance) talked to me, she sounded like a man. He asked me, "Do you know who I am?" I have a cousin who got killed in a place in Tampico. "You must be my cousin," I said. "Yes, exactly, I am your cousin." "Look," he said, "You have come here with your husband." On other occasions I really had been there with my husband, mother and different relatives. "You have come here with your husband because you think he is hexed and that is why he is sick. But that's not true. He has a physical illness that the doctor can cure. Don't believe it's anything bad."

He said, "I'm going to prove who I am by coming to your house. Tell my cousin I'm going to see her." You see, I have a sister who's not nervous at all and who isn't afraid of anything. On Tuesday, as my sister was leaning by the window watching a television show, she felt someone embrace her. She turned and saw no one.

These spiritual centers vary according to their size, their owners, and the spirits who are associated with them, yet there is considerable regularity in the services they perform. Sometimes mediums prescribe simple herbal remedies for physical problems. These recipes are virtually identical to the ones presented in the previous section on the material level, although, occasionally, it is said that a spirit will recommend a new use for an herb. The mediums might suggest that the patient perform the already familiar rituals of curanderismo, such as the barrida. The spirits are thought to be able to influence people's lives directly, in addition to imparting knowledge about remedies. The curanderos state that spirits control spiritual currents (Corrientes espirituales) and mental vibrations (vibraciones mentales); they can manipulate the patient's health by directing positive or negative forces at them from the spiritual realm.

During spiritual sessions observed at a developing spiritual center in southern Texas, a spirit repeatedly presented himself over the course of several weeks to treat several patients. One of these patients was a man with lower back pain. One week the spirit told him to buy a bandage and bring it to the next session. The man did so, but then the spirit chided him for not following instructions correctly. The bandage was too narrow and not long enough. The man was instructed to buy a new bandage and place it on the window ledge to catch the morning dew, which is thought to have healing properties. He then was to place a glass of water under the head of his bed and a jar of alcohol at the side of the bed. He was to wrap himself in the bandage according to given instructions and lie quietly on his bed for no less than 2 hours, during which time the spirit promised to visit him and complete the cure. The man followed these instructions and stated that he did gain relief from his back pain. The same spirit treated a young college girl who periodically had asthma attacks. The girl's mother, a regular member of the group, brought her to the session. The spirit, in the person of the medium, stood and clasped the girl's head with one hand on her *cerebro* and the other on her forehead, sending *Corrientes espirituales* through her brain. The spirit then told her to take a sip of *agua preparada* and sit back down in the circle. The treatment was successful in overcoming this particular attack, and the mother mentioned after the session that these cures relieved her own asthma for several months.

Another patient requested a social and emotional treatment. Her husband recently had begun to practice witchcraft *(btujeria),* and she was worried that he or his friends might attack her or members of her family. A considerable amount of tension existed between the couple's families. She felt under continual stress and had gone to a doctor for help. The doctor prescribed a mild sedative, which she had taken for 3 weeks without relief. The medium's spirit probed her mind and told her to take three sips of *agua preparada* to break any spells that had been cast on her. The spirit promised to provide her with protection and help from the spiritual realm to counteract anything that her husband might do. She appeared to be content with the spirit's activities on her behalf and was greatly relieved.

Several aspects of the spiritual level have not been covered in this brief description but are described in more detail elsewhere (Trotter, 1975). These include the actual techniques of testing for *el don,* the physical and supernatural dangers of trance mediumship, the acquisition of spiritual protectors to overcome those dangers, detailed descriptions of the trance state from the subjective perspective of the developing medium and the objective perspective of an observer, and finally, the existence and purpose of mediums' associations.

The Mental Level *(Nivel Mental)*

Conducting observational, descriptive, and experimental research on the practices of the mental level has proven to be the most difficult task in exploring all of the aspects of curanderismo. The mental level has the fewest rituals and the least outward complex behavior associated with it. To date, it has the fewest

practitioners, which severely limits the number of people who could be approached for an opportunity to investigate the phenomenon. All of the cases the author observed followed a similar pattern. For example:

After the curandero chatted with the patient and asked them about the basic problem, he asked the patient to state her complete name *(el nombre completo).* The curandero wrote the name on a piece of paper. Sitting behind the desk he used for consultations, he leaned his arms on the desk, bent forward slightly, closed his eyes, and concentrated on the piece of paper. After a few minutes, he opened his eyes, told the patient more about his or her problem, and stated that it was being resolved.

The curandero stated that he had learned to use his mind as a transmitter through *desarrollo.* He could channel, focus, and direct *vibraciones mentales* at the patient. These mental vibrations worked in two ways—one physical, one behavioral. If he was working with a physical illness, such as cancer, he channeled the vibrations to the afflicted area, which he already had pinpointed, and used the vibrations to retard the growth of damaged cells and accelerate the growth of normal cells. In a case of desired behavioral changes, he sent the vibrations into the person's mind and manipulated them in a way that modified the person's behavior. The curandero gave an example of one such case in which a husband had begun drinking excessively, was seeing other women, was being a poor father to his children, and was in danger of losing his job. The curandero stated that he dominated the man's thought processes and shifted them so that the husband stopped drinking to excess, and became a model husband and father (Trotter, 1981, p. 473).

There also are a number of syncretic beliefs drawn from other alternative healing traditions—such as New Age practices, the "psychic sciences," and Eastern philosophy—that have been incorporated into this area of curanderismo. For example, some healers state that they are able to perceive "auras" around people and that they can use these auras to diagnose problems that patients are encountering. They conduct the diagnosis on the basis of the color or shape of the patient's aura. Some state that they learned these practices from other healers, whereas others indicate that they learned them from books on parapsychology.

The mental level is practiced most often by individual healers working with individual patients, rather than in groups. It appears to be a new addition to this healing system and does not have, as yet, a codified body of ritual associated with it. It therefore constitutes an area in which additional descriptive work will be necessary to unify healers' behavior.

Theoretical Unification

The three levels of curanderismo unify the theories of disease and illness found in the Mexican-American folk medical model. They create a framework for determining the therapeutic approaches of curanderos in southern Texas. The system emphasizes a holistic approach to treatment and relies heavily on the intimate nature of the referral system and the extensive personal knowledge of the patient's social environment that is normally held by the curandero. Christian symbols and theology provide both tools (candles, incense, water) and organization models (rituals, prayers, animistic concepts) for the material and the spiritual levels, but not to a similar degree for the mental level. An energy concept is the central idea that integrates the three levels and forms a systematic interrelationship between them. This energy concept derives from belief in forces, vibration, and currents that center in the mind of those who have the gift for healing and that can be transmitted to cause healing from a distance, by affecting the patient's social, physical, spiritual, or psychological environment.

All three levels of healing are still evolving. The variations in the practices of curanderismo can be explained partly by differences in the curanderos' personality, differences in their treatment preferences or abilities, and differences in their emphasis on theoretical or experiential approaches. There also are variations produced by individual interpretations of an underlying body of theory. A study of these variations would be useful, now that the underlying theoretical system provides a common starting point and common objectives.

SETTINGS FOR CURANDERISMO HEALING SYSTEM

Curanderismo is a community-based healing system. It is complex and widespread. At one level it may be practiced anywhere that there exist Mexican Americans who know about it. Part of this healing tradition is the information that is spread throughout the Mexican-American culture on home treatments for common physical ailments (colds, flu, arthritis, asthma, or diabetes) and for common spiritual or "folk illnesses" (*susto, mal de ojo,* and *empacho*). This is analogous to the biomedical information that is spread throughout all European cultures, including the Mexican-American culture, where the home is the first line of defense and diagnosis of illnesses that eventually might necessitate a doctor or a hospital. On the other hand, some aspects of curanderismo require the use of special locations, preparations, and tools. This is especially true of spiritual practices on the spiritual level and for the effective treatment of supernatural harm on the material level.

The first setting where this knowledge is used is at home. When people become ill, they use their existing cultural model of health and illness to come up with solutions. One type of solution is home diagnosis and home treatment. Therefore both biomedical concepts and folk medical concepts are applied immediately, and home treatments are attempted. In the case of curanderismo this often results in the use of home remedies *(remedio caseros)* that have been part of the culture for generations, especially herbal cures. When the diagnosis identifies a magical or supernaturally caused illness, the illness results in a home-based ritual. These interventions are done by mothers, grandmothers, cousins, friends, or knowledgeable acquaintances.

Illnesses that appear to be too serious to handle at home, both natural and supernatural, are taken to professional healers who have a locally widespread reputation for being able to treat both biomedical and traditional health care problems. Most of these healers work in a silent, but positive, partnership with physicians, although the physicians often are unaware of the link. The curanderos interviewed in various studies of Mexican-American folk medicine are consistent in their positive regard for modern medicine. They consistently refer patients to modern health care services, where they see the efficacy of that approach to be equal to or greater than their own. At the same time they note significant differences in the models of health and illness between their own practices and modern medicine, especially in the areas of supernatural illnesses, in addressing social (marital, business, interpersonal) problems, and in dealing with psychological problems. In these cases the treatments take place either in the patient's home or work environment or in special workrooms established by the curanderos as part of their practices. The cure might call for working directly in the environment that is affected. In other cases the venue of choice is the curandero's area because the cure depends on careful preparation and protection from outside influences. These work areas contain altars, medicinal plants, tools for supernatural rituals, and other items, and the atmosphere is considered most beneficial for the healing process, particularly in the case of supernatural problems and treatments (Trotter & Chavira, 1981).

RESEARCH AND EVALUATIONS APPROACHES

The research that is available on curanderismo is broad in interest and historic depth. Unlike specific healing techniques, such as acupuncture, which can be studied in relation to specific illnesses with relative ease, curanderismo is a complex brew of both theoretical approaches to healing and an interrelated set of healing techniques. The techniques range from herbal cures, which must be approached from an ethnopharmacological perspective; to rituals, which can be studied symbolically as projective psychiatric techniques; to methods such as massages, natural birth, nutritional prescriptions, and dietary practices. Some studies have investigated the scientific efficacy of the practices of curanderismo, whereas others have approached it from a sociopolitical or symbolic viewpoint. Some practices have not been studied at all. Therefore, although the efficacy of some parts of the system are clearly defined, others remain to be explored.

Early research on curanderismo can be found in the classic anthropological works on Mexican-American folk medicine, published primarily in the 1960s (Clark, 1959a; Currier, 1966; Kiev, 1968; Madsen, 1961, 1964; Romano, 1965; Rubel, 1960, 1964, 1966). These authors produced descriptive baseline data on the prominent folk medical practices of Hispanic communities in the United States. They provide an initial view of curanderismo that is rich in descriptions of Mexican-American folk illnesses such as *susto, empacho, mal de ojo, caida de mollera, bilis,* and *espanto* (Nail & Speilberg, 1967). These works generally treat traditional healing in Mexican-American communities as a body of knowledge that is widely distributed throughout the culture, rather than as a theoretical healing system. Therefore the works consider the consensual data on what is available to a significant segment of the existing Mexican-American population but spend less time describing the professional actions of curanderos, because these mass cultural phenomena are generally thought of as having themes or unifying elements rather than a theoretical structure. This viewpoint is well represented in articles about curanderismo and its form and function within Mexican-American communities (Clark, 1959b; Edgerton, et al., 1970; Foster, 1953; Martinez & Martin, 1966; Torrey, 1969).

Later research maintains the strengths of this approach but adds folk theoretical concepts. Early epidemiological approaches to folk illnesses give an idea of the geographical spread and variation in beliefs, illnesses, and healing rituals, whereas later studies identify or discuss the common denominators that unify curanderos—their underlying perception of illness. Traditional anthropological research techniques were used to gather the data for these studies, primarily participant observation and interviewing over prolonged periods. Most of the authors used personal networks to identify individuals who were known locally as healers. Emphasis often was placed on finding individuals who were full-time healers rather than talking to those who treated only family members and neighbors. Therefore a curandero can be defined as an individual who is recognized in his community as having the ability to heal, who sees an average of five or more patients a day, and who has knowledge of and uses the theoretical structure described in this chapter. These people can be viewed as both specialists and professionals. Several areas of curanderismo have received a considerable amount of research attention.

Home Remedies

Herbal and chemical treatments for both natural and supernatural illnesses are very common in Mexican-American communities. More than 800 *remedios caseros* have been identified on the U.S.-Mexican border alone (Trotter, 1981a, 1981b). Many of the remedies have been tested for biochemical and therapeutic activities (Etkin, 1986; Trotter, 1981, 1983; Trotter & Logan, 1986). Overall, the remedies are not only biochemically active; more than 90 percent have demonstrated therapeutic actions that matched the folk medical model for their uses. At the same time only a small proportion of the herbs have been tested. This lack of information is being overcome by an ongoing project to study the efficacy of the complete range of herbal cures available in Mexican-American communities (Graham, 1994), by use of combined ethnographic and biomedical methods (Browner et al., 1988; Croom, 1983; Ortiz de Montellano & Browner, 1985; Trotter, 1985).

The exceptions to the general rule of efficacy are the use of remedies for illnesses such as the common cold, where they relieve symptoms but do not directly treat the illness. The actions of these remedies, some of which are described earlier, include diuretics, treatments for constipation, abortifacient, analgesics, sedatives, stimulants, cough suppressants, antibacterial agents, coagulants and anticoagulants, vitamin and mineral supplements, and plants with antiparasitic actions. Most have proven safe and effective when used in the manner described and recommended by the curanderos. This area, and the therapeutic, culturally competent counseling practices of the healers are the most clearly acceptable and useful for articulation with modern medicine.

Additional Information on the Epidemiology of Folk Illnesses

Of all the complex areas of Mexican-American traditional healing, the one that has received the most research attention has been the study of common folk illnesses that are experienced and treated in Mexican-American communities. The most commonly reported are *susto,* an illness caused by a frightening event; *mal de ojo,* an illness that can be traced to the Near East, which involves a magically powerful glance taking away some of the vital essence of a susceptible person; *empacho,* a blockage of the intestines caused by eating the wrong type of food at the wrong time or by being forced to eat unwanted food; and *caida de la mollera,* a condition of fallen fontanel in infants. A number of others also are well defined, if not as commonly studied, but these four take up most of the research attention.

The epidemiology and the cognitive models of these illnesses have been well documented (Rubel, 1964; Trotter, 1982, 1985; Weller et al., 1993). They have been studied both singly and in combination (Baer et al., 1989; Logan & Morrill, 1979; Rubel et al., 1984; Weller et al., 1991, 1993), in terms of their cognitive structure within and between Hispanic cultural groups, their frequency of treatment, belief and mention in various communities, and their relationships to medical conditions and to the treatment of medical conditions (Collado-Ardon et al., 1983; Trotter, 1991; Trotter et al., 1989). In the case of *susto* there is clear evidence that it is linked directly to serious morbidity patterns in Latin-American communities and acts as an excellent indicator that biomedical personnel should investigate multiple conditions and problems among patients complaining of its symptoms. *Caida de la mollera,* on investigation, is a folk medicine label that corresponds to severe dehydration in infants caused by gastrointestinal problems. It is life-threatening and, when identified by parents, is an excellent indicator that the child should be brought in immediately for medical care. *Empacho* is a severe form of constipation based on its description and is treated with numerous remedies that cause diarrhea. Because it is thought to be a blockage of the intestines, the purgative effect of these remedies signals that treatment has been effective. To date, no studies have linked *mal de ojo* to any biomedical condition; however, because the symptoms include irritability, lethargy, and crying, it is possible that some connection will be made in the future.

Healing and Psychiatry

Another area of significant endeavor in curanderismo is the identification of parallels and areas of compatibility between the processes and rituals of curanderismo and the use of psychiatry in cross-cultural settings. The time period between 1969 and the mid-1970s saw the analysis and publication of several seminal works in this area (Kiev, 1968; Klineman, 1969; Torrey, 1969: Trotter, 1979: Velimirovic, 1978). The parallels are clear, especially when healers concentrate on psychological conditions that they recognize from their knowledge of psychology and psychiatry. This is an area in which a number of successful collaborations have been conducted between traditional healers and individuals from modern medical establishments in several states.

Unexpected Consequences

It is clear that Mexican-American folk medicine contains a very high ratio of useful, insightful, and culturally competent healing strategies that work well in Hispanic communities. As seen previously, these range from proven herbal cures to therapeutic models to culturally important labeling systems that can help physicians identify the cultural labels for certain types of biomedical problems. The complexity of curanderismo ensures that these findings will increase.

At the same time no health care system exists that does not have side effects and unexpected results. With allopathic medicine, these range from the birth defects of thalidomide to dreadful side effects of chemotherapy and the limited ability of psychology to deal with chronic mental health conditions such as alcohol and drug abuse. In curanderismo conditions are not the bulk of the effects of its use, a few unexpected consequences have been discovered in treating *empacho* (Baer & Ackerman, 1988; Baer et al., 1989; Trotter, 1983b). These occurrences are rare but must be taken into account and understood within the overall cultural context of curanderismo and within the context of the far more pervasive positive benefits that the communities derive from having these alternative health care practices available. With the complexity and the diversity of practices within this traditional healing system, there remains a great deal of useful and insightful research that can be conducted beneficially in relation to curanderismo.

Acknowledgments

The initial phase of the research findings reported by the author was supported by a grant from the Regional Medical Program of Texas (RMPT Grant No. 75-108G). Further efforts at data collection were supported by the Texas Commission on Alcoholism, Pan American University, and the author himself.

References

Alger N (ed). 1974. The Curandero-Supremo. In Many Answers. West Publishing. New York

Baer R, Ackerman A. 1988. Toxic mexican folk remedies for the treatment of empacho: the case of azarcon, greta and albayalde. Ethnopharmacol 24:31-39

Baer R, Garcia de Alba DJ, Cueto LM, et al. 1989. Lead based remedies for empacho: patterns and consequences. Soc Sci Med 29(12):1373-1379

Browner CH, Ortiz de Montellano BR, Rubel AJ. 1988. A new methodology for ethnomedicine. Curr Anthropol 29(5):681-701

Buckland R. 1970. Practical Candle Burning. Llewellyn Publications. St. Paul, Minnesota

Clark M. 1959a. Health in the Mexican American Culture. University of California Press, Berkeley

Clark M. 1959b. Social functions of Mexican-American medical beliefs. California's Health 16:153-55

Collado-Ardon R, Rubel AJ, O'Nell CW. 1983. A folk illness (susto) as indicator of real illness. Lancet 2:1362

Croom EM. 1983. Documenting and evaluating herbal remedies. Economic Botany 37(1):13-27

Currier RL. 1966. The hot-cold syndrome and symbolic balance in Mexican and Spanish American folk medicine. Ethnology 4:251-263

Edgerton RB, Karno M, Fernandez I. 1970. Curanderismo in the metropolis: the diminished role of folk psychiatry among Los Angeles Mexican-Americans. Am J Psychiatry 24:124-134

Etkin N (ed). 1986. Plants Used in Indigenous Medicine: Biocultural Approaches. Redgrave Publications. New York

Foster GM. 1953. Relationships between Spanish and Spanish-American folk medicine. J Am Folklore 66:201-247

Galvin JAV, Ludwig AM. 1961. A case of witchcraft. J Nerv Men Dis 161-168

Gillin J. 1977. Witch doctor? a hexing case of dermatitis. Cutis 19(1):103-105

Gobeil O. 1973. El susto: a descriptive analysis. Int J Soc Psychiatry 19:38-43

Graham JS. 1994. Mexican American herbal remedies: an evaluation. Herbalgram 31:34-35

Holland WR. 1963. Mexican-American medical beliefs: science or magic? Arizona Med 20:89-102

Hudson WM. 1951. The healer of Los Olmos and other Mexican lore. Texas Folklore Soc XXIV

Ingham IM. 1940. On Mexican folk medicine. Am Anthropol 42:76-87

Jaco EG. 1957. Social factors in mental disorders in Texas. Soc Probl 4(4):322-328

Kiev A. 1968. Curanderismo: Mexican American Folk Psychiatry. The Free Press, New York

Klineman A. 1969. Some factors in the psychiatric treatment of Spanish-Americans. Am J Psychiatry 124:1674-1681

Macklin J. 1967. El Niño Fidencio: Un Estudio del Curanderismo en Nuevo Leon. Anuario Huminitas. Centro de Estudios Humanisticos, Universidad de Nuevo Leon

Macklin J. 1974a. Santos folk, curanderismo y cullos espiritistas en Mexico: eleccion divina y seleccion social. Anuario Indigenista 34:195-214

Macklin J. 1974b. Folk saints, healers and spirit cults in northern Mexico. Rev Interamericana 3(141):351-367

Macklin J. 1974c. Belief, ritual and healing: New England spiritualism and Mexican American spiritism compared. In Zaretsky IT, Leone MP (eds). Religious Movements in Contemporary America. Princeton University Press. Princeton, New Jersey

Macklin J, Crumrine NR. 1973. Three north Mexican folk saint movements. Comp Studies Soc History 15(1): 89-105

Madsen C. 1965. A study of change in Mexican folk medicine. Mid Am Res Inst 25:93-134

Madsen W. 1955. Shamanism in Mexico. Southwest J Anthropol 11:48-57

Madsen W. 1961. Society and Health in the Lower Rio Grande Valley. Hogg. Austin, Texas, Foundation for Mental Health

Madsen W. 1964a. The Mexican Americans of South Texas. Holt, Rinehart and Winston. New York

Madsen W. 1964b. Value conflicts and folk psychotherapy in South Texas. In Kiev A (ed). Magic, Faith and Healing. Free Press. New York, pp. 420-440

Martinez C, Martin HW. 1966. Folk diseases among urban Mexican-Americans JAMA 196:161-164

Nall FC, Speilberg J. 1967. Social and cultural factors in the responses of Mexican-Americans to medical treatment. J Health Soc Behav 7(1):299-308

Ortiz de Montellano BR, Browner CH. 1985. Chemical basis for medicinal plant use in Oaxaca, Mexico. J Ethnopharmacol 13:57-88

Romano O. 1964. Don Pedrito Jaramillo: The emergence of a Mexican-American folk saint. PhD Dissertation, University of California. Berkeley

Romano O. 1965. Charismatic medicine, folk-healing, and folk sainthood. Am Anthropol 67:1151-1173

Rubel AJ. 1960. Concepts of disease in a Mexican-American community in Texas. Am Anthropol 62:795-814

Rubel AJ. 1964. The epidemiology of a folk illness: Susto in Hispanic America. Ethnology 3:268-283

Rubel A. 1966. Across the Tracks: Mexican-Americans in a Texas City. University of Texas Press. Austin, Texas

Torrey FE. 1969. The case for the indigenous therapist. Arch Gen Psychiatry 20(3):365-373

Torrey FE. 1972. The Mind Game: Witch Doctors and Psychiatrists. Bantam Books, Emerson Hall Pub. New York

Trotter RT II. 1979a. Evidence of an ethnomedical form of aversion therapy on the United States-Mexico border. J Ethnopharmac 1(3):279-284

Trotter RT II. 1979b. Las Yerbas de Mi Abuela (Grandmother's Tea), slide series/filmstrip. Institute of Texas Cultures. San Antonio, Texas

Trotter RT II. 1981a. Don Pedrito Jaramillo. Slide series/filmstrip. Institute of Texas Cultures. San Antonio, Texas

Trotter RT II. 1981b. Folk remedies as indicators of common illnesses. J Ethnopharmac 4(2):207-221

Trotter RT II. 1981c. Remedios caseros: Mexican American home remedies and community health problems. Soc Sci Med 15B:107-114

Trotter RT II. 1982a. Contrasting models of the healer's role: South Texas case examples. Hispanic J Behav Sci 4(3):315-327

Trotter RT II. 1982b. Susto: within the context of community morbidity patterns. Ethnology 21:215-226

Trotter RT II. 1983a. Azarcon and Greta: ethnomedical solution to an epidemiological mystery. Med Anthropol Q 14(3):3-18

Trotter RT II. 1983b. Community morbidity patterns and Mexican American folk illness: a comparative approach. Med Anthropol 7(1):33-44

Trotter RT II. 1983c. Ethnography and bioassay: combined methods for a preliminary screen of home remedies for potential pharmacologic activity. J Ethnopharmac 8(1):113-119

Trotter RT II. 1983d. Greta and Azarcon. Unusual sources of lead poisoning from Mexican American folk medicine. Tex Rural Health J May-June: 1-5

Trotter RT II. 1983e. Letter to the editor: Greta and Azarcon: two sources of lead poisoning on the United States-Mexico border. J Ethnopharmac 8(1):105-106

Trotter RT II. 1985. Greta and Azarcon: a survey of episodic lead poisoning from a folk remedy. Health Care Hum Organization. 44(1):64-71

Trotter RT II. 1991. A survey of four illnesses and their relationship to intracultural variation in a Mexican American community. Am Anthropol 93:115-125

Trotter RT II, Chavira JA. 1975a. The Gift of Healing. A monograph on Mexican American Folk Healing. Pan American University. Edinburg, Texas

Trotter RT II, Chavira JA. 1975b. Los Que Curan. A 43-minute color 16 mm film of South Texas Curanderismo

Trotter RT II, Chavira JA. 1981. Curanderismo: Mexican American Folk Healing System. University of Georgia Press. Athens, Georgia

Trotter RT II, Logan M. 1986. Informant consensus: a new approach for identifying potentially effective medicinal plants. In Etkin N (ed). Plants Used in Indigenous Medicine: Biocultural Approaches. Redgrave Publications pp. 91-112

Trotter RT II, Ortiz de Montellano B, Logan M. 1989. Fallen fontanelle in the American Southwest: its origin, epidemiology, and possible organic causes. Med Anthropol 10(4):201-217

Velimirovic B (ed). 1978. Modern Medicine and Medical Anthropology in the United States Mexico Border Population. Pan American Health Organization. Washington, DC. Scientific Publication No. 359

Weller SC, Pachter LM, Trotter RT II, Baer RM. 1993. Empacho in four latino groups: a study of intra- and intercultural variation in beliefs. Med Anthropol 15(2): 109-136

Suggested Readings

Arias HyF, Costas: No date. Plantas Medicinales. Biblioteca Practica. Mexico

Baca J. 1969. Some health beliefs of the Spanish speaking. Am J Nurs 69:2171-2176

Bard CL. 1930. Medicine and surgery among the first Californians. Touring Topics

Bourke IH. 1894. Popular medicine customs and superstitions of the Rio Grande. J Am Folklore 7:119-146

Capo N. Mis observaciones clinicas sobre el limon, el ajo, y la cebolla. Ediciones Natura

Cartou LSM. 1947. Healing herbs of the Upper Rio Grande. Laboratory of Anthropology. Santa Fe

Chavez LR. 1984. Doctors, curanderos and brujos: health care delivery and Mexican immigration in San Diego. Med Anthropol Q 15(2):31-6

Comas J. 1954. Influencia indigena en la Medicina Hipocratica, en la Nueva Espana del Sigio XVI. America Indigena XIV(4):327-361

Creson DL, McKinley C, Evans R. 1969. Folk medicine in Mexican American subculture. Dis Nervous Sys 30: 264-266

Davis J. 1979. Witchcraft and superstitions of Torrance County. NM Histor Rev 54:53-58

Dodson R. 1932. Folk curing among the Mexicans. In Toll the Bell Easy. Texas Folklore Society. Southern Methodist University Press

Esteyneffer J de SJ. 1711. Florilegio medicina vide todos las enfermedades, acadodevarios, y clasicos autores, para bien de los pobres y de los que tienen falia de medicos, en particular para las provincial remotas en donde administran los RRPP. Misioneros de la Compania de Jesus. Mexico

Esteyneffer J de SJ. 1887. Florilegio Medicinal o Oreve Epidomede las Medicinas y Cirujia. La primera obra sobre esta ciencia impresa en Mexico en 1713. Mexico

Fabrega H Jr. 1970. On the specificity of folk illness. Southwest J Anthropol 26:305-315

Farfan A. 1944. Tractado breve de medicina. Obra impresa en Mexico por Pedro Orcharte en 1592 y ahora editada en facimil. Coleccion le Incinables Americanos, Vol. X. Ediciones Cultura Hispanica. Madrid

Gudeman S. 1976. Saints, symbols and ceremonies. Am Ethnologist 3(4):709-730

Guerra F. 1961. Monardes. Diologo de Hierro. Compania Fundido de Fierro y Acero de Monterrey, SA., Mexico. D.LosCronistas-Hispanoamericano.sdelaMate-riaMedicinaColonial.al Professor Dr. Teofilo Hernando por sus amigos y in Homenaje O discipulos. Libreria y Casa Editorial Hernando. SA., Madrid

Hamburger S. 1978. Profile of Curanderos: a study of Mexican folk practitioners. Int J Soc Psychiatry 24:19-25

Jaco EG. 1959. Mental health of the Spanish-American in Texas. In Upler MK (ed). Culture and Mental Health. Macmillan. New York

Johnson CA. 1964. Nursing and Mexican-American folk medicine. Nurs Forum 4:100-112

Karno M. 1965. The Enigma of Ethnicity in a Psychiatric Clinic. A paper presented at the Southwestern Anthropological Association Annual Meeting, UCLA. April 16, 1965

Karno M. 1969. Mental health roles of physicians in a Mexican-American community. Community Ment Health J 5(1)

Karno M, Edgerton RB. 1969. Perception of mental illness in a Mexican-American community. Arch Gen Psychiatry 20:233-238

Kay M. 1972. Health and illness in the Barrio: Women's Point of View. Dissertation for Ph.D. University of Arizona. Tucson, Arizona

Kay M. 1974a. The fusion of Utoaztecan and European ethnogynecology in the florilegio medicinal. Paper presented at Medical Anthropology Symposium, XLI International Congress of Americanists. Mexico City, Mexico. Proceedings XLI International Congress of Americanists (in press)

Kay M. 1974b. Florilegio Medicinal: Source of Southwestern Ethnomedicine. Paper presented to the Society for Applied Anthropology. Boston. 1978 Parallel, Alternative, or Collaborative: Curanderismo in Tucson, Arizona. In Modern Medicine and Medical Anthropology in the United States-Mexico Border Population. Boris Velimirovic (ed). Pan American Health Organization. Scientific Publication No. 359. Washington, DC

Klein J. 1978. Susto: the anthropological study of diseases of adaptation. Soc Sci Med 12:23-28

Kleinman A. 1978. Culture, illness, and care: clinical lessons from anthropological cross-cultural research. Ann Intern Med 88:251-258

Kreisman JJ. 1975. Curandero's Apprentice: a therapeutic integration of folk and medical healing. Am J Psychol 132:81-83

Langner TS. 1965. Psychophysiological Symptoms and the Status of Women in Two Mexican Communities. Approaches to Cross-Cultural Psychiatry. Cornell University Press. pp. 360-392

Macklin J. 1965. Current Research Projects. Curanderismo Among Mexicans and Mexican-Americans. Connecticut College. New London, Connecticut

Madsen N. 1966. Anxiety and witchcraft in Mexican-American acculturation. Anthropol Q 110-127

Maduro R. 1983. Curanderismo and Latino views of disease and curing. West J Med 139:868-874

Marcos LR, Alpert M. 1976. Strategies and Risks in Psychotherapy with Bilingual Patients. Am J Psychiatry 113(11):1275-1278

Marin BV, Marin G, Padilla AM. 1983. Utilization of traditional and nontraditional sources of health care among Hispanics. Hispanic J Behav Sci 5(1):65-80

Martinez C Jr, Alegria D, Guerra E. El Hospital Invisible: A Study of Curanderos. Mimeograph. Department of Psychiatry, University of Texas Health Science Center at San Antonio. San Antonio

Montiel M. 1970. The social science myth of the Mexican-American family. El Grito 3:4 Morales A. 1970. Mental health and public health issues: the case of the Mexican Americans in Los Angeles. El Grito 111(2)

Moustafa A, Weiss G. 1968. Health Status and Practices of Mexican-Americans. University of California Graduate School of Business, Berkeley

Moya B. 1940. Superstitions and Beliefs among the Spanish Speaking People of New Mexico. Masters Thesis. University of New Mexico, Albuquerque

Padilla AM. 1973. Latino Mental Health: Bibliography and Abstracts. U.S. Government Printing Office. Washington, DC

Paredes A. 1968. Folk Medicine and the Intercultural Jest in Spanish-Speaking People in the U.S. University of Washington Press. pp. 104-119

Pattison M. 1973. Faith healing: A study of personality and function, J Nerv Ment Dis 157:397-409

Press I. 1971. The urban Curandero. Am Anthropol 73: 741-756

Press I. 1978. Urban folk medicine. Am Anthropol 78(1): 71-84

Romano O. 1960. Donship in a Mexican-American community in Texas. Am Anthropol 62:966-976

Romano O. 1969. The anthropology and sociology of the Mexican-American history. El Grito 2

Rubel AJ. 1990. Ethnomedicine. In Johnson TM, Sargent CF (eds). Medical Anthropology: Contemporary Theory and Methods. Praeger. New York. pp. 120-122

Rubel AJ, O'Neil CW. 1978. Difficulties of presenting complaints to physicians: Susto illness as an example. In Velimirovic B (ed). Modern Medicine and Medical Anthropology in the United States-Mexico Border Population. Washington, D.C.: Pan American Health Organization. Scientific Publication No. 359

Ruiz P, Langrod J. 1976. Psychiatry and folk healing: a dichotomy? Am J Psychiatry 133:95-97

Samora J. 1961. Conceptions of disease among Spanish Americans. Am Cath Soc Rev 22:314-323

Sanchez A. 1954. Cultural Differences and Medical Care: The Case of the Spanish-Speaking People of the Southwest. Russell Sage Foundation. New York

Sanchez A. 1971. The defined and the definers: A mental health issue. El Sol 4:10-32

Saunders L, Hewes GW. 1953. Folk medicine and medical practice. J Med Educ 28:43-46

Smithers WD. 1961. Nature's Pharmacy and the Curanderos. Sul Ross State College Bulletin. Alpine, Texas

Snow LF. 1974. Folk medical beliefs and their implications for care of patients. Ann Intern Med 81:82-96

Speilberg J. 1959. Social and Cultural Configurations and Medical Cure: A Study of Mexican-American's Response to Proposed Hospitalization for the Treatment of Tuberculosis. Masters Dissertation. University of Texas

Trotter RT II. 1978a. A case of lead poisoning from folk remedies in Mexican American communities. In Fiske S, Wulff R (eds). Anthropological Praxis. Westview Press. Boulder, Colorado

Trotter RT II. 1978b. Discovering New Models for Alcohol Counseling in Minority Groups. In Velimirovic B (ed). Modern Medicine and Medical Anthropology in the United States-Mexico Border Population. Scientific Publication No. 359. Pan American Health Organization. Washington, DC. pp. 164-171

Trotter RT II. 1986. Folk medicines and drug interactions. Migrant Health Newsline 3(171):3-5

Trotter RT II. 1986. Folk medicine in the Southwest: myths and medical facts. Postgrad Med 78(8):167-179

Trotter RT II. 1988. Caida de mollera: A newborn and early infancy health risk. Migrant Health Newsline

Trotter RT II. 1990. The cultural parameters of lead poisoning: a medical anthropologist's view of intervention in environmental lead exposure. Environ Health Perspect 89:79-84

Trotter RT II, Chavira JA. 1980. Curanderismo: an emic theoretical perspective of Mexican American folk medicine. Med Anthropol 4(4):423-487

Unknown. 1951. Rudo Ensayo. By an unknown Jesuit. Tucson: Arizona Silhouettes Publication. Original 1763 by Johann Nentuig

Uzzell D. 1974. Susto Revisited: illness as a strategic role. Am Ethnol 1(2):369-378

Wagner F. Remedios Caseros con Plantas Medicinales. D.F. Medicina, Mexico. Hermanos, S.A.

Weclew RV. 1975. The nature, prevalence and levels of awareness of "Curanderismo" and some of its implications for community mental health. Comm Ment Health J 11:145-154

CHAPTER 24

Southern African Healing Traditions and Professional Considerations

M A R I A N A   H E W S O N

We waited patiently for the healer to call us for the interview. The waiting room was small, containing only six chairs and a dresser. Prepared with the specified money and gift, we reviewed our questions, the way in which the interpretation would be handled, and how our notes would be taken. Eventually, the traditional healer appeared in full regalia: copious strands of white beads around her neck, wrists, and ankles; decorative strands of animal skins hanging from her waist; her legs clad in animal skins decorated with beads, shells, and beer bottle tops; and an impressive headdress (much like a bishop's miter) made of cowhide. She had several ceremonial tools, highly decorated with intricate beadwork: a fly whisk (made of a cow tail) to signify the healer's status, a long-handled spear for slaughtering animals, and a smoking pipe and drum that she used to contact ancestral spirits. Two younger apprentices in more modest dress stayed close at her side and ministered to her needs. To initiate my interview, I put the required fee (about $20) plus a gift on the floor of the waiting room. One of the apprentices burned a local dried plant, *bepo,* in an open dish, and the master healer ceremoniously smoked her long pipe to invoke the spirits to be present in our conversation. She tipped a little ash onto the money and

Continued

429

Continued

gifts to bless them, a necessary part of developing our relationship* (Hewson, 1998). ∾

In this chapter, I outline the professional components of traditional healing based on interviews with traditional healers (Hewson, 1998). The value of studying a phenomenon outside of one's own culture is to identify aspects of one's own culture that are not readily apparent to those who practice within that culture. By looking at the careers of non-Western but analogous healers, it is possible to identify similarities and differences in the way healers are professionalized and, indirectly, to learn important lessons concerning the professionalization of Western healers.

PROFESSIONALISM AND THE HEALING ARTS

Is traditional African healing a profession? In the Western view the medical profession consists of specialists who diagnose and prescribe in areas that draw on comprehensive knowledge and skills that transcend those available to nonspecialists (Goodlad, 1984). Education for the professions involves questions about legitimate knowledge, license to practice, arrangements for providing services, entry to education and training, the curriculum offered, standards of achievements, and assessment (Goodlad, 1984). Similarly, Cassidy describes professional considerations of a health care system in Chapter 3 of this volume. Following Cassidy's categories, we discuss (1) the explanatory model of illness that underlies traditional healing in southern Africa, (2) the educational process of healers, (3) the professional accreditation of the practitioners, (4) the professional organization of practitioners who monitor and maintain standards of care, and (5) the social mandate through which the community influences the provision of care. Finally, I highlight unique aspects of traditional healing that can transcend both the traditional and allopathic systems of healing.

*This interview was one of eight similar interviews with female traditional healers in Southern Africa.

THE EXPLANATORY MODEL UNDERLYING TRADITIONAL HEALING IN SOUTHERN AFRICA

Concepts of Health, Illness, and Healing

Traditional healing in southern Africa existed long before the arrival of modern medicine, and it remains an intact system of caregiving among many African people. This system of healing coexists in a modern society that subscribes to and practices allopathic medicine. Despite regional differences, there appears to be a common system aimed to relieve illness and disease (feelings of being out of sorts, or ill at ease socially and spiritually).

In the southern African view, illness is thought to be caused by psychological conflicts or disturbed social relationships with persons living or dead. The accompanying disequilibrium is expressed as physical or mental problems (Frank, 1973). Traditional healers believe that psycho-social-spiritual imbalances must be rectified before a patient can recover physically. Traditional healing thus focuses on psychological and spiritual suffering, as well as on physical suffering, and aims to correct the disequilibrium. Traditional healers view healing as the removal of impurities from the body or disequilibrium from the patient's mind, with the hope of reducing the anxieties it has produced. For example, a common concept of healing involves purification by draining the body of harmful substances with consequent wide use of purgatives and emetics. Healing also involves appeasing the patients' spirits (in particular, the recently departed members of the family), who might be angry with the patient for some reason. Warding off bad spirits, such as the *tokoloshe* (a mischievous or evil spirit responsible for life's misadventures and accidents), the curses from living people, or the ill will of angry ancestral spirits constitutes a version of preventive medicine. Furthermore, in several southern African groups, such as the Basotho of Lesotho, the state of disequilibrium manifests in the form of being "hot" (not feverish) (Hewson & Hamlyn, 1985), and treating people who are "hot" involves cooling with appropriate agents such as ash, water plants, or aquatic animals. These views are quite distinct from modern allopathic medical concepts of disease as the malfunctioning of physiological systems.

Traditional Healing Processes

Traditional healers hold an esteemed and powerful position in modern African societies, and their role is a combination of physician, counselor, psychotherapist, and priest. Traditional healers prevent and treat illnesses mainly with plant and some animal products in combination with divination. There are two kinds of traditional healers: those who are mainly herbalists and those who use divination. However, the distinction between the two is becoming increasingly blurred, and most traditional healers appear to practice both types of medicine. Sorcery (evil or malevolent doctoring) is practiced by some healers in southern Africa but is not considered further in this chapter.

Traditional healers appear to work most successfully with illnesses that have a high psychological or emotional content related to envy, frustration, or guilt (Frank, 1973), what in allopathic medicine might be called *somatic illnesses*. Today, they also appear to concentrate on illnesses for which allopathic medicine has little effective curative power, such as stroke, tuberculosis, cancer, and human immunodeficiency virus/acquired immunodeficiency syndrome HIV/AIDS. Traditional healers claim to be effective in helping to treat pregnancy, malaise, arthritis, and social problems, especially those involving interpersonal disputes. All the healers seemed to be able to distinguish between those illnesses that need to be helped by Western medicine (e.g., broken bones, hernias), and those that respond to traditional healing. The claims to heal illnesses such as stroke, cancer, and HIV/AIDS appear to relate to the psychosocial and emotional components of the illness rather than the pathological or pathophysiological conditions. For example, traditional healers make no claims to be able to deal directly with bacterial or viral impurities but rather with the patient's ability to cope with and eliminate them. This view of healing suggests that if one takes care of the psychodynamics of illness, the body will heal. This is in contrast to the modern view that if one takes care of the body, the mind will heal itself (Hewson, 1998).

As part of the diagnostic process, traditional healers "throw the bones." The "bones" consist of a set of 10 to 15 items, such as bones and shells and various collectibles (e.g., dice, coins, bullets, domino pieces). These are usually "thrown" (like dice) in the belief that clues to the problem can be read in the configuration of the items. The "bones" are made up of an idiosyncratic collection of items that have attributed

meanings, depending on the context and the meaning attributed by particular healers. Each item signifies an important aspect of a person's life (e.g., happiness, children, bad luck, ancestral spirits). The consistencies among these items is in the attributions of the items rather than in the items themselves. For example, a traditional healer from Mozambique had a red die signifying war (the country had experienced a civil war for many years), and a healer from South Africa had a bullet signifying death or misfortune (South Africa was, at that time, engulfed in violence).

Traditional healers use drumming and dance to augment the healing process through the spirits. To encourage their own dreams, they wash with herbal solutions, drink herbal potions, smoke a pipe, or use snuff (all of which appear to have psychotropic effects). They prepare and prescribe therapeutic herbal remedies for their patients. A traditional healer must know the symptoms of a disorder and the conditions of the patient's life before prescribing a treatment.

Traditional healers find out as much as they can about a patient to determine why the illness happened when it did. They ask questions such as the following: Does someone wish you ill? Do you want something you do not or cannot have? Do you have enemies? and Are your ancestors (the "recently departed") displeased with you for some reason? They inquire into every aspect of a patient's present and past activities, focusing on behaviors that would be most likely to provoke conflict with others in the community or with internal conflicts in personal values. This inquiry may not provide results, and the diagnostic process may take a long time. In this situation the healer may say, "The bones are not talking today," and request subsequent visits. When healers cannot find an answer to the patient's problems, they will refer the patient to another traditional healer or to a Western doctor. All healers are concerned with truth and trust in their relationship with a patient. If the healer discerns a lack of either, he or she will ask the patient to leave.

THE EDUCATIONAL PROCESS

Selection: The Call to Be a Healer

Traditional healers are "called" to become healers and need to be verified by the group's elders who check whether the call is real or not. First, the future healer experiences an unusual, mysterious illness that does not respond to usual herbal or allopathic treatment. Some examples recounted by my respondents included heart problems, lung problems, abdominal pain, swollen abdomen unrelated to pregnancy, amenorrhea, problems with feet, dizziness, headaches, mental problems (e.g., forgetfulness), pains all over the body, and "fevers that are not real fevers" (which may relate to the cultural metaphor of being "hot" (see also Hewson & Hamlyn, 1985).

The illness is often followed by dreams with significant, recognizable components. The future healer then asks his or her elders (e.g., parents, aunts, uncles, grandparents) about the dreams. If an elder recognizes the special components of the dream, he or she advises the future healer to consult a traditional healer. At the discretion of the traditional healer, the patient is then both treated and taken as an apprentice for several years. A traditional healer named Emily tells how she was called by her ancestral spirits to be a healer:

First I was sick for a whole year, like I didn't know where I was, like becoming mad, my mind wasn't working properly. I felt pains everywhere and I didn't know what to do. I was forgetful. I forgot what I did the day before, like washing dishes, and I felt like sitting alone and no one should come near me. I went to the doctors and they could not see what the problem was with me. Then I had a dream. In my sleep I saw three grand people, old people, sitting next to me. One was holding a bible. My father's mother was holding beads in a dish and some bones—little bones—with two hands. And my mother's father was holding a bible. They said to me I must wear a white dress. And I dreamed I was in this big hall and on the other side was a church. The people were dancing and preaching. And in the hall the *sangomas* and *nyangas* (widely used terms for traditional healers in southern Africa) were dancing and beating drums. And I said 'What kind of a dream is this?'

Then I told my aunty that I had this kind of funny dream. I described the old people and she said they really were my grand people who I had never seen before in life. And she called another woman [a healer], and I told her this same dream. Then she took me to the river and prayed and talked to my old people [ancestral spirits] who are called *amanyangas*. And then she prayed there for me and I took the water. She made beads for me and put them round my neck, and then I was alright. I never got sick again.

A second healer, Elizabeth, described her sickness (headaches and fevers that were not really fevers) followed by a dream in which her ancestor came to her and told her to go to the forest to find herbs. This she

did and encountered a man, sitting in the light, who instructed her. This dream was interpreted as being a call to be a healer. Yet another healer described her mysterious sickness and said that she went to consult a healer, who made a mixture of stringy roots mixed with a grated rhizomelike substance in water. Using a twig as a mixer, this solution created a profusion of bubbles. The future healer was asked to drink the bubbles by her trainer, which induced dreams that "helped me see what I should do to help people." She used the same techniques for inducing the spirits in her apprentices.

To refuse the calling by the ancestors is to invite worse sickness, madness, and possible death. One healer recounted the story of a woman who had denied the call and had become "mad." A man in Cape Town, a renowned drunkard, believed he was being called to be a healer, but the elders of his family disabused him of this idea, saying that his dreams and sickness were the consequence of alcohol.

Training

Training involves an apprenticeship, usually with a well-known master healer. If the master healer lives far away, the apprentices live in his or her master healer's compound (many small dwellings inhabited by extended family members) for the duration of the training. The art of the healer is thought to be transmitted through the ancestral spirits who speak to healers through dreams. Apprentices are encouraged to have dreams and to learn how to interpret them on behalf of their patients. Dreams can be induced by herbal potions, inhaled smoke, or snuff. As one traditional healer put it, "Through the dreams, your ancestors open your eyes to signs. I trust the dreams every time." Another said that anyone can learn about the practice of traditional healing, but "unless you have contact with the spirits through dreams, you cannot be a healer."

The master healer first demonstrates the use of herbs and animal parts and then teaches the apprentices how to administer them. Then, in a progressive weaning process, the master healer withdraws and expects the apprentices to perform independently. One healer described being taken into the bush by her teacher to find *muti* (medicinal substances, such as herbs, roots, and barks; and animal parts, such as hooves, bones, and horns) that are used for healing. She had to rise at 4:30 AM "because the spirits only come early in the morning." She had to prepare herself to get the *muti* by bringing on the ancestral spirits. This she did by taking a bath, drinking herbal concoctions, beating the drums, and dressing with a special wrap or *kapilano*.

The training process is strenuous and challenges the mental and physical strength of the apprentices. One healer said: "I went to the bush for many days with my teacher to seek *muti*, with only *putu* [corn meal porridge] and black tea. It was hard to live like that, but it is necessary for *nyangas* to suffer because this kind of work is *swarig* (Afrikaans word for heavy or burdensome)." Not every apprentice completes the training because it is so exacting.

Apprentices help their master healers with many patient consultations, seemingly acting as a team for the duration of the training program. One apprentice and master healer in a Lesotho mountain village entered a trancelike state in which both danced with extremely rapid movements to the accompaniment of drums and, in a trancelike state, called on the ancestors and revealed spiritual insights to the assembled small crowd (Hewson, 1993).

THE PROFESSIONAL ACCREDITATION OF THE PRACTITIONERS

Tests and Standards

Throughout training apprentices are tested on their ability to find things, to identify and administer herbs, and to contact the ancestors through dreams to discern people's physical, psychological, or spiritual problems. Some of the objects to be found become part of the "divining bones," and others are used as medicines. The things that needed to be found are often given to the apprentice by patients, friends, or family members in recognition of the demonstrated healing skills and power of the apprentice. The master healer may also help the apprentices find things they need. For example, one healer described how, on occasions, the very thing she had been instructed to find would be given to her by someone, apparently in a serendipitous manner (McCallum, 1992). Another described how she went to the beach with her teacher and collected the perfect shells for her set of "bones." Other objects must be gleaned from the countryside, found in the bush, or purchased from stores that specialize in the healers' equipment and accoutrements.

Several levels of tests must be passed by the apprentice healers. Tests of competence may involve oral examinations. For example, one healer described how her master healer asked all the apprentices in her cohort "to stand like a choir" and to answer numerous questions. Then each apprentice was asked to declare whether he or she was able to cure.

The final test often involves finding a hidden object. For her final test, one healer had to find an unknown object that had been hidden somewhere in the vicinity of a village (McCallum, 1992). Her success could be attributed to her powers of observation, for example, in noticing signs in the physical environment and getting clues from the people in the village, and it could involve the cooperation of the villagers—a subtle sign of their acceptance of her as a traditional healer. The final test also involves "finding" the animals that will be slaughtered as part of the graduation ceremony, such as a chicken, goat, or cow. The procurement of these animals may involve gifting the apprentice's family, friends, or satisfied patients and is an additional social accreditation that represents faith and trust in the apprentice as a healer.

An apprentice graduates when the master healer is satisfied that he or she has passed all the tests; that, through dreams, the ancestral spirits have confirmed the apprentice's readiness; and that the apprentice has paid the stipulated fees, including procuring the necessary animals for slaughter. The master healer consults his or her own ancestral spirits concerning the sufficiency of each apprentice's knowledge. When all of the criteria had been satisfied, the master healer gave each apprentice a gift, such as a set of bones or a braided bracelet. Thus both the teacher and apprentice, and indirectly, the community, assess the readiness for graduation. Patients also play a part in this judgment through their gifts.

More importantly, the ancestral spirits indicate, through dreams, when a trainee is ready. One healer explained that she knew that she was ready to graduate when she had a dream in which her ancestor (grandfather) "sent me to a *rondavel* (Afrikaans for a small round dwelling) that had a half door made of glass. There was a man standing behind the door who asked 'What do you want here? I don't know what you are doing here any more.'" Then she heard the words coming from behind her: "Go and help people." At this point she went through the final graduation ceremony, collected all her medicines and divining tools, and traveled back to her home, 300 miles away.

Graduation often involves a final test of slaughtering an animal with the ceremonial spears. The apprentice drinks the animal's blood and selects various body parts, such as pieces of hoof or bone, to become part of his or her healer's tools (bones) or as *muti*. For example, the skin of the slaughtered goat may be used as the mat for throwing bones, the animal's stomach may be used as a pouch for carrying other medicine, or a vertebrae may become part of the divining tools. The rest of the animal is then consumed by the group or village to celebrate the occasion.

PROFESSIONAL ORGANIZATION: MONITORING OF STANDARDS OF CARE

Continuing Education

Traditional healers engage in meetings with other healers. One group described meetings that occurred most weekends, in which they would assemble, fully dressed in their ceremonial costumes (clothing, wigs, necklaces, anklets), to discuss healing matters, to share their latest healing stories, and to compare notes. The group may collectively criticize certain healers for dangerous or unwise practices. The regular meetings also include singing, dancing, drumming, drinking herbal potions, and engaging the ancestral spirits. The meetings appear to be important social events in the lives of traditional healers.

The business of traditional healers includes their formal organization (South African healers are now organized and provide their healers with certificates), their practice in the context of new diseases, such as HIV/AIDS, and their relationship with Western medicine; the World Health Organization has recognized traditional healers in Mozambique and elsewhere, and increasingly traditional healers are being recognized and incorporated into the general medical system.

Ongoing Relationships with Teachers

Traditional healers typically maintain a lifelong relationship with their master healers who serve as mentors. These relationships appear to be deep and profound. One healer from Maputo in southern Mozambique returned approximately once a year to visit her teacher in northern Mozambique. These visits were casual in nature, and the master healer might teach "depending on his mood. If he is not happy he doesn't teach anything!" This particular healer had trained five of her own apprentices, and she used the same methods as those used by her own teacher. She liked to teach, but reflected that to be a teacher, "you have to be happy all the time," suggesting the essential relationship between teacher and learner involves enthusiasm and effort.

Mutual Caring

Mutual caring among healers becomes necessary under stressful or strained conditions, especially death. According to one healer, when a patient dies, the traditional healer becomes spiritually contaminated and loses his or her healing powers because the relationship with the patient has been broken and the healer, of necessity, grieves. In this situation the healer removes his or her necklaces, ceremonial clothes, and artifacts and does not practice as a healer. This afflicted healer must be treated by another healer in a purification ceremony that restores the healing powers.

THE SOCIAL MANDATE: COMMUNITY INFLUENCE ON THE PROVISION OF CARE

Community control is exerted through remuneration and accreditation systems. Traditional healers are paid according to the type of service they provide. For straightforward dispensing of *muti*, patients pay over-the-counter fees for the medicines they receive. For diagnosis of physical, psychological, social, or spiritual problems, the patient must first "open his or her pockets" and pay a flat fee at the beginning of the process. This amount is prorated on the approximate cost of one head of cattle and appears to be approximately one sixth of the total cost. When cured, the patients must pay an additional fee that appears to be independent of time spent or medicines dispensed but is measured in proportion to the patient's satisfaction with the care, the cure, or both. Thus a moderately satisfied patient might provide a modest offering, such as food bought from a store (sugar, flour, or vegetables) or picked from a vegetable garden, whereas a highly satisfied patient might offer a live animal, such as a chicken, goat, or cow, that would be ceremonially slaughtered at a later date.

For training services, an apprentice needs to pay a relatively large fee, equivalent to at least one head of cattle, and must also provide the animal(s) for the graduation ceremony. Apprentices are helped in paying the required fees by other people (patients, friends, or family members) who pay or provide necessary items in proportion to their belief in the healing powers of the apprentice. This linking of the payment, patient satisfaction, and the accreditation process provides a complex system of checks and balances in an otherwise unregulated training system.

The healers referred to their own satisfaction in terms of "happiness." For example, one healer said that "to heal someone is to give life to that person," and when the person is healed, "both the traditional healer and the patient become happy." This happiness is manifest at a celebration in which the food offered is consumed in thanksgiving for the healing

and for the continued goodwill of the spiritual beings whose power over the living is great.

UNIQUE ASPECTS OF TRADITIONAL HEALING

Differences between traditional and allopathic professionalism are summarized in Tables 24-1 and 24-2. Despite these differences, there are interesting phenomena that characterize traditional healing and the professionalization of the healers that are of importance to the fundamental, perhaps archetypic, contract between healer and patient.

The Spiritual Context of Healing

Spiritual powers are loosely defined within African cosmology as those spiritual powers that derive ultimately from God (within the African world view) and that are present in decreasing amounts through the various levels of spirits of the ancestors (the forefathers) and the recently departed, elders (old people),

TABLE 24-1

Steps to Becoming a Professional in Traditional Healing and in Western Medicine

Step	Traditional healing	Western medicine
Call to healing	Mysterious illness, significant dreams, interpreted and sanctioned by elders in community	Individual, personal "call" to become a clinician, family suggestion, augmented by academic counseling
Selection of trainees	Based on mysterious illness and recognizable evidence of healing capability and spiritual power	Based on standardized test scores, essay(s), and interviews with medical school personnel
Training	Rigorous, prolonged, relatively expensive; emphasis on subjective witness of healing powers by patients and/or trainers	Rigorous, prolonged, expensive; emphasis on objective measures of competence designed by professional Boards
Accreditation	Approval by master healer, community members, and guidance from ancestral spirits	Approval on basis of national test scores in certifying/licensing examinations
Continuing education	Regular and frequent meetings and celebrations with other healers, and regular ongoing communication with trainer	Regular and frequent conferences, with regulated continuing medical education (CME) accreditation
Professional relationships	Lifelong relationship with trainer and ongoing relationships with colleagues	Occasional mentors, ongoing relationships with professional colleagues, especially focused on research

TABLE 24-2

Characteristics of the Practice of Traditional Healing and Western Medicine

Characteristic	Traditional healing	Western medicine
Concepts of curing	Take care of the mind and the body will take care of itself.	Take care of the body and the mind will take care of itself.
Diagnosis	Use spiritual powers and psychological techniques to discern causes of spiritual, psychological, or social disequilibrium.	Use technological and scientific tools to directly or indirectly "see" the pathology/pathophysiology. Use clinical reasoning and evidence-based medicine.
Prevention	Very important to ward off negative spirits and harmful circumstances.	Becoming important to ward off potentially harmful agents and conditions.
Treatment	Resolve disequilibrium and return person to harmonious state.	Treat the biological causes of disease.
Relationship to patient	Subjective, interpersonal involvement, counselor, confessor.	Objective, scientific, rational, clinical relationship.
Relationship to community and individual patients	Paternalistic relationship based on healers' spiritual and social status and reputation.	Paternalistic relationship based on clinicians' accreditation level, social status, and reputation.
Professional satisfaction and rewards for healing	Directly linked with patient satisfaction and monetary payment or "in kind" gifts.	Indirectly linked with patient satisfaction, salary negotiated with health care organization.

people, animals, vegetation (e.g., trees), and the earth itself (Mbiti, 1969).

Traditional healing deals with spiritual powers that are manifest through an integrated conception of body and mind at all levels. For example, in the call to be a healer, the person experiences physical illness and has dreams that reveal a connection with ancestral spirits. In the training process the apprentice learns both the physical skills of an herbalist and the spiritual skills of interpreting problems through dreams that involve the ancestral spirits. When traditional healers graduate, the tests involve knowledge and skills in both herbal medicine and spiritual healing.

Truth and Trust in the Healer-Patient Relationship

The traditional system of healing in southern Africa is consistent with the worldview of the people indigenous to this region. This worldview constitutes a paradigm that emphasizes some ways of thinking (e.g.,

the body-mind connection) and deemphasizes others (e.g., the objective, rational scientific approach). To be effective, traditional healing requires that patients who seek healing within this paradigm must subscribe to it. Thus traditional healers are cautious in checking the adherence of patients to their traditional African way of thinking. In addition, there is the "dark side" to this practice: malevolent sorcery. For similar reasons that benevolent traditional medicine is effective, sorcery is powerful and greatly feared. Traditional healers need to discern the intentions of their patients, and they are alert to desires for dirty witch doctoring. If a patient is thought to be untruthful or distrustful, the healer will send him or her away. Western physicians currently pay little attention to their patient's health belief models or spiritual convictions. An increased focus on the commitment of their patients to the type of care physicians offer may pay dividends in increasing adherence and in improving mortality and morbidity. Moreover, the role of spirituality in healing is receiving increased attention throughout Western medicine (Suchman et al., 1993).

The Psychosocial Medical Model and Interpersonal Communications

Based on the central premises concerning the connection between body and mind and between the earthly and spiritual realms, traditional healing is a form of integrated bio-psycho-social healing in which the biomedical Western medical model is relatively weak. The healers pay close attention to the ways in which their patients describe their illnesses and to the contexts within which the illnesses occur. They listen to the attributions of the patient, or what Budd and Zimmerman (1986) describe as "the assumptions and principles that constitute the precepts by which the patient creates the reality in which he or she lives." They concentrate on looking for signs that indicate the reasons for the disequilibrium that causes sickness. The holistic approach allows traditional healers to integrate body-mind phenomena and to provide healing, despite being extremely limited in terms of modern medical science. As a result of historical influences, Western clinicians have largely dispensed with concern for the spiritual needs of their patients and focus only on the physical body, a split that handicaps the Western physician's ability and capacity to heal (Damasio, 1994; Fox, 1997). Without compromising the high standards of modern medicine, Western practitioners could augment and potentially improve their biomedical practice by reintroducing focus on the status of the patient's psychosocial and spiritual well-being.

Patients Contribute to the Accreditation of Professionals

In the training of traditional healers, patients have the opportunity to play a role in certifying the apprentice through the voluntary gifts they make. In Western medical training, there is little if any role for the patient in the forming of new professionals. A prevalent view assumes that patients are ignorant of what is best for themselves and are in no position to make judgments on the abilities of physicians. This paternalistic view is slowly changing as modern patients continue to gain unprecedented access to medical information, especially through the Internet. Public outrage against their physician's poor humanistic skills in the United States (indicated in part by

the number of lawsuits against physicians) raises the question of why patients have been so consistently overlooked and ignored in the healing process and in the training of physicians. The training of traditional healers suggests that patients can contribute the training and certification of individual healers through being asked to rate their satisfaction with care received.

The Establishment of Lifelong, Mentoring Relationship(s)

Traditional healers in southern Africa appear to engage in lengthy apprenticeships with one master healer. Although the length of training may last from one to many years, the relationship with the master healer does not end at graduation. Instead, these relationships are treasured and maintained for life, which suggests that trainees benefit from the deeper, more sustained relationships, similar to those in traditional apprenticeships. The cross-fertilization of styles and standards of practice takes place at regular meetings of traditional healers. These gatherings can be seen as analogs of Grand Rounds and national and regional conferences.

Apprenticeship Methods

The apprenticeships of traditional healers involved initially being shown how to do things (e.g., to recognize herbs, to interpret dreams) through role-modeling and coaching. As the apprentices become more competent, the master healer allows them more independence and takes on a role more akin to that of an evaluator, in which the apprentice is tested for knowledge and skills and for evidence of the power of healing. At the same time the teacher personally rewards the apprentice with small, highly desired gifts that are needed as part of the prescribed collection of accoutrements (e.g., the divining "bones" and various *medications*). In addition, some of the gifts from the master healer could be worn by the apprentice, a visible testament to the healer's skills. This apprenticeship style of teaching is effective in developing professional competence and supports several teaching approaches such as role-modeling (performing so that the learner can see what you do) and coaching (helping the learner by providing assistance as well as feedback) and are applicable to the way in which traditional healers are trained.

Hardship as a Necessary Part of Professional Training

The training of traditional healers is strenuous because the practice of medicine is hard. Healers are expected to lead a lifestyle characterized by a high level of personal and social responsibility, and their training is thus a test of physical and mental endurance. The requirement for this type of physical and mental testing is also present in the cultural initiation rites that take place at puberty for boys and girls in southern African cultures. Indeed, in Xhosa, the word for a healer-in-training is *mkweta,* which is the same word used for young boys and girls who undergo initiation. Western medical training is also exacting. In particular, the housestaff or resident training often involves hardships, such as frequent sleep deprivation and agonizingly long work hours, that make normal social interactions and even normal life difficult. A potential positive outcome of this feature of medical training for Western and traditional trainees is that enduring these hardships creates strong interpersonal bonds among the trainees, which may strengthen professional identities and commitment.

CONCLUSION

In this chapter, I have described the practice of traditional medicine in southern Africa and the training of these traditional healers. Despite the obvious and substantial differences between traditional African and Western healers, there are interesting similarities in the professionalization of the practitioners. These similarities may reduce the negative perceptions of traditional healers and offer possibilities for a synergism between the two traditions, with potential mutual benefits for both types of healers and for the training of these healers.

Acknowledgments

The author thanks Thomas Lang, The Cleveland Clinic, for his editorial help and useful suggestions concerning this topic.

References

Budd MA, Zimmerman ME. The potentiating clinician: combining scientific and linguistic competence. Advances 1986;3(3):40-55.

Damasio AR. Descartes' Error: Emotion, Reason and the Human Brain. New York: Avon Books, 1994.

Fox, E. Predominance of the curative model of medical care. JAMA 1997;278(9):761-763.

Frank JD. Persuasion and Healing: A Comparative Study of Psychotherapy. Baltimore: Johns Hopkins University Press, 1973, p. 46-77.

Goodlad S. (Ed.). Education for the Professions: Quis Custodiet . . . ? Guildford, United Kingdom: Society for Research in Higher Education & NFER-Nelson, 1984.

Hewson MG. Training in the traditional arts: some thoughts. Medical Encounter 1993;9(3):3-4.

Hewson MG. Traditional healers in southern Africa. Ann Intern Med 1998;128:1029-1034.

Hewson MG, Hamlyn D. Cultural metaphors: some implications for science education. Anthropology and Education Quarterly 1985;16:31-46.

Mbiti JS. African Religions and Philosophy (2nd ed.). London: Heinemann Educational Books Inc., 1969.

McCallum TG. White Woman Witchdoctor: Tales from the African Life of Rae Graham, as Told by Rae Graham. Miami: Fielden Books, 1992.

Suchman AL, Matthews DA, Branch WT. Making "connexions": Enhancing the therapeutic potential of patient-clinician relationship. Ann Intern Med 1993;118:973-977.

Suggested Readings

Cassel EJ. The Nature of Suffering and the Goals of Medicine. New York: Oxford University Press, 1991.

Collins A, Seely Brown J, Newman S. Cognitive apprenticeship: teaching the crafts of reading, writing and mathematics. In: Resnick LB. (Ed.) Knowing, Learning, and Instruction: Essays in Honor of Robert Glaser. Hillsdale, New Jersey: Lawrence Erlbaum Associates, Publishers, 1989.

Fadiman JA. Mountain witchcraft: Supernatural practices and practitioners among the Meru of Mount Kenya. African Studies Review 1977;20(1):87-101.

Ngubane H. Clinical practice and organization of indigenous healers in South Africa. In: S Feierman, JM Janzen (Eds.), The Social Basis of Health and Healing in Africa. Los Angeles, University of California Press, 1992.

Rantala E, Kodzwa GM, Viisainen K, Dlodlo R, Osaki S, Freling D. Baseline Study—Health Care: Manica Province Integrated Health Project (Vol 1). Report of the Ministry of Health, The Republic of Mozambique, December, 1992.

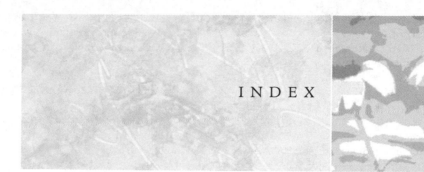

INDEX

Page numbers in italics indicate illustrations; *t* indicates tables.

Maharishi Ayurveda—cont'd
  future direction of, 377-378
  history of, 366-367
  pharmacology of, 373-374
  prevention, pathogenesis, and balance in, 370-372, *372t*
  theoretical basis (consciousness model) of, 367-369
  transcendental meditation in, 369-370
Maharishi Mahesh Yogi, 224, 366
Mal de ojo (evil eye), 411, 414, 424
Malaria, chloroquine-resistant, 76
Malas (waste products), in Ayurveda, 346-347
Manaka, Yoshio, 331
Manga Report, 48
Manipulation practices, 27, 100
  active vs. passive, 107
  basis concepts of, 101-107
  bilateral symmetry, 101
  compensation and decompensation, 106
  direct vs. indirect, 107
  fascia, 102-103
  gravity, 101
  osteopathic manipulative treatment (OMT), 109
  pain and guarding, muscle spasm and facilitation, 105-106
  postural maintenance and coordinated movement, 101-102
  range of motion and barrier concept, 106-107
  reflexes or autonomic nervous system, 103-105
  relative physical invasiveness of therapeutic techniques in, *28*
  segmentation/functional spinal unit, 103
Manipulative system, 29
Manka, Yoshio, 335
Mann, Felix, 331
Mantra-yoga, 363
Manual therapies, 100-125
  acupressure/jin shin do, 119-120
  Ayurvedic manipulation, 122-123
  balance, types of, 107
  bioenergetic explanations for, 13
  energy work, 123
  energy-based techniques, 125
  Feldenkrais (awareness through movement), 118-119
  neuromuscular therapy, 117
  qigong (China), 123
  reflexology, 120-121
  reiki, 123-124
  shiatsu (zen shiatsu), 120
  structural integration (rolfing), 119
  tenents of, 100
  therapeutic or healing touch, 124-125
  Trager method, 117-118
  Tui na, 121-122
Mao Tse-Tung, 14

Maslow, Abraham, 263
Mason, Arthur, 229
Massage, 13, 27, 73, 115-117
  with aromatherapy, 147, 149, 151-152
  confusion related to meaning of, 27
  effleurage, 116
  friction, 116-117
  mesmeric vital energy in origin of, 47-48
  other styles of, 116-117
  pétrissage, 116
  tapotement, 116
  Tui Na, 326-327
  vibration, 116
Mastalgia (cyclical/noncyclical), 140
Materia medica
  Chinese
    fundamental categories, 328-329
    research in, 336-337
  of homeopathy, 89-91
Materia Medica Pura (Hahnemann), 88, 93
Material level (nivel material)
  in curanderismo, 414-417
  natural illness and herbal cures in, 415-416
  ritual in, 415-417
  supernaturally caused illness and ritual cures in, 415-416
  types of healers in, 414
Materialism
  in biomedicine, 23-24, 38
  vs. nonmaterialism view of sickness, 33-34
  in physics, 367
Matter-energy duality, 4
Maury, Marguerite, 147-149
May, Rollo, 266
Mechanism, theory of, 174
Mechanistic view of healing, 202
Medical art therapy, 269
Medical botany, 130
Medical ecology, and adaptational model, 11-12
Medical Nemesis (Illich), 59
Medici, Catherine de, 148
Medicinal herb garden, 130
Medicine
  confusion related to meaning of, 27
  development of medical education, 58-60
  as human endeavor, 303-304
  new initiatives of, 59-60
  postmodern medicine, 57-70
Medicine for a small planet, 3
Medieval concept of vitalism, 44
Meditation, 27, 50-51, 73, 223-225
  eastern techniques and transcendental mediation, 224
  meditative exercises, 27
  in Mind Cure healing, 47